Bioethics, Justice, and Health Care

EDITED BY

Wanda Teays
Mount St. Mary's College

AND

Laura M. Purdy
University of Toronto

WADSWORTH
™
THOMSON LEARNING

Australia • Canada • Mexico • Singapore • Spain • United Kingdom • United States

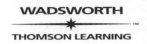

WADSWORTH

THOMSON LEARNING

Philosophy Editor: Peter Adams
Assistant Editor: Kara Kindstrom
Editorial Assistant: Mark Andrews
Marketing Manager: Dave Garrison
Print Buyer: Tandra Jorgensen
Permissions Editor: Joohee Lee

Production Service: Penmarin Books
Copy Editor: Kevin Gleason
Cover Designer: Liz Harasymczuk
Compositor: TBH Typecast, Inc.
Cover and text printer: Von Hoffmann Graphics

For permission to use material from this text, contact us:
Web: http://www.thomsonrights.com
Fax: 1-800-730-2215 **Phone:** 1-800-730-2214

Library of Congress Cataloging-in-Publication Data
Bioethics, justice, and health care / edited by Wanda Teays and Laura M. Purdy.
    p. cm.
Includes bibliographical references and index.
ISBN 0-534-50828-6
   1. Medical ethics.   2. Bioethics.   3. Medical ethics—Social apects.   4. Medical laws and legislation.
I. Teays, Wanda.   II. Purdy, Laura Martha.
R724.B4827 2000
174'.2—dc21   00-043471

Wadsworth/Thomson Learning
10 Davis Drive
Belmont, CA 94002-3098
USA

For information about our products, contact us:
Thomson Learning Academic Resource Center
1-800-423-0563
http://www.wadsworth.com

International Headquarters
Thomson Learning
International Division
290 Harbor Drive, 2nd Floor
Stamford, CT 06902-7477
USA

UK/Europe/Middle East/South Africa
Thomson Learning
Berkshire House
168-173 High Holborn
London WC1V 7AA
United Kingdom

Asia
Thomson Learning
60 Albert Street, #15-01
Albert Complex
Singapore 189969

Canada
Nelson Thomson Learning
1120 Birchmount Road
Toronto, Ontario M1K 5G4
Canada

To Silvio and John
With you dreams have become reality

Contents

Chapter 2
Rights and Obligations in Health Care   69

Chapter 3
Medical Experimentation:
Historical Considerations   163

Chapter 4
Contemporary Issues in Informed Consent and Experimentation   255

Chapter 5
Death and Dying   371

Chapter 6
Abortion and Reproductive Freedom   445

Chapter 7
Reproductive Technology and Surrogacy   533

Chapter 8
Genetics and Cloning   603

Introduction

To convince someone of the truth, it is not enough to state it,
but rather one must find the path from error to truth.
   —Ludwig Wittgenstein

Power at its best is love implementing the demands of justice.
Justice at its best is love correcting everything that stands against love.
   —Zora Neale Hurston

ETHICAL DECISION MAKING is a fact of our lives. At times we come face to face with ethical dilemmas involving good versus evil, loyalty versus betrayal, justice versus injustice, truth telling versus lying, and so on. Both as individuals and as a society, we have expectations about how we should treat one another and what we consider morally permissible behavior. This decision making goes beyond stating what we perceive to be truths: We must first find the path leading out of our errors, our misconceptions, our prejudices—not necessarily an easy task. As Wittgenstein said of his own quest for order in the world, "You are looking into fog and for that reason persuade yourself that the goal is already close. But the fog disperses and the goal is not yet in sight."

In this volume we look at the range of issues facing us in terms of health care resources, rights, responsibilities, and obligations. This inquiry leads us into areas of bioethics in which we have struggled to clarify problems, gain insight into important moral dilemmas, and arrive at solutions wherever possible. This calls us to reflect on our own set of values and what sort of society we want to live in. We need to develop an awareness, as the authors here demonstrate, that the decisions we make may have a significant impact in defining ourselves as moral agents and in giving shape to our collective ethical identity.

The task, therefore, is personal, since our choices may directly affect a single life. It is also global, since decisions made may serve as a precedent that others are expected to follow. Central to bioethics, therefore, is the examination of laws, policies, and guidelines shaping the ethical and legal framework of our lives and our institutions. And whether the focus on ideas, issues, and actions is narrow or broad, we cannot escape issues of justice and injustice.

Every day we see those who are marginalized or disenfranchised being denied access to medical resources. If we don't avert our eyes, we also see people shuffled off to clinics that are poorly equipped, understaffed, and overwhelmed by the needs of those too poor to afford even minimal health care for themselves and their families. We see a history of prejudice and discrimination woven into the very fabric of medical "care" giving. There are warning signs all around us that justice needs to be put right at the center of health care. As Zora Neale Hurston asserts, power at its best entails love serving the cause of justice. We do assume power, as the authors here show us, by looking at messy moral problems and finding paths to justice.

The journey starts with an overview of the moral terrain of bioethics, where we confront a myriad of issues that require reflection, clarification, and decision making. In fact, we are inundated with difficult moral questions regarding health, health care, and medical treatment. Does society have any duty to protect health? Should doctors assist patients who want to die? Should we be able to compel a woman to get a caesarian section against her will? Should the federal government fund abortions for poor women? Should the children of undocumented aliens be allowed access to health care? Should HMOs be prohibited from denying patients consultations with specialists? Is it justifiable to construct a health care system that denies care to those without insurance? These are just a few of the moral dilemmas facing us. Yet few of us have received any formal education in moral decision making. For that reason, it is important to become informed and develop our capacity for moral reasoning. We can then examine issues of morality, arrive at decisions that reflect our values, and think critically about those values.

OVERVIEW OF TOPICS

We want justice and fairness to be seen as at the heart of bioethics; otherwise, the "ethics" in bioethics lacks the integrity and power that it could have. We created this anthology to fulfill a vision: We wanted to compile a collection of readings that would address not only the issues already seen as pivotal to the field but also ones that go beyond the traditional. It is important not merely to listen to the voices of the greats, however insightful their thoughts may be. We need also to listen to those who have not always had a forum in which to speak. These voices and alternative perspectives deserve recognition.

We wanted to break down some of the complacency we see in the public and professional response to biomedical issues. Thus, we sought out readings that would make us more aware of the range of significant issues and of how important it is to seek solutions wherever possible. To achieve this goal, we include topics that tend to be relegated to the sidelines: justice and the health care system; the role of race, class, and gender in access to medical treatment; patient-provider relationships; bias in research; recent developments with respect to informed consent; changes brought about by advances in reproductive technology; and genetics and cloning.

Our authors in the eight chapters give us a solid overview of the issues, along with a greater appreciation for the ways they affect our lives. The articles collectively provide us with a framework for moral decision making. The variety of important viewpoints presented in the selections help us examine individual values, societal attitudes, and some of the preconceptions found in science, medicine, health care, and the law. They also help us reflect on the distribution of power and privilege, and what we must do to achieve a more just and compassionate system of health care.

We take it as a given that questions of justice are central to a wide range of issues in bioethics. We believe that both the issues and perspectives presented here help readers become aware of how social and political arrangements affect health, and how the practice of medicine and the health care system raise concerns about justice that are often ignored.

KEY FEATURES AND STRATEGIES OF THE BOOK

- An emphasis on justice and fairness to help us keep the goal of doing good work before us and to be aware of the potential impact of our decision making.

- The inclusion of voices not usually heard, giving a broader range of readings than is customarily seen in bioethics texts. They point to a range of systemic concerns, offer ideas for achieving more clarity, and identify what we need to do to arrive at solutions. They thus offer fresh insights into what are often deep-seated problems.

- A balance of the new and the old, groundbreaking pieces and classic articles, to provide a rich resource for readers and for instructors.

- Chapter introductions frame ways of examining the issues presented in the readings and suggest problem-solving techniques, to help clarify what's at stake, how the concerns have evolved over time, and how they are rooted in an ethical and historical context.

- Individual narratives among the readings that reflect the personal impact of health issues, medical decision making, and the ways illness and suffering touch our lives.

- Case study exercises present recent real-life moral dilemmas that can be used to provoke stimulating discussions, group projects, and individual assignments, or for an individual reader's own development. Some relate back to the issues raised in the chapter or the readings themselves, others present actual cases and ask readers to pull out the embedded concerns and formulate a response or set out recommendations.

- Chapters that are independent of one another. This independence offers instructors and readers the flexibility of using any one of the chapters as a jumping-off point to a study of bioethics, emphasizing areas and ordering topics as desired.

- Two chapters on the functioning of the health care system as a whole, with articles on the social construction of health and on rights and obligations.

- Two chapters on medical experimentation: one with a historical focus and one looking at contemporary issues of informed consent, medical experimentation, and property rights in the human body.

- Readings that focus on environmental and societal issues in which the chosen course of action (e.g., the human radiation studies) had devastating results or, in the case of some current controversies (e.g., xenotransplants), has the potential for global disaster.

- Medical codes and guidelines that reveal a set of values, beliefs, and expectations about medicine and health care.

- Thoughtful pieces for professional development. We also wanted the works included here to remind us of our own obligation, as ethicists, professors, and medical caregivers; for we too have a fiduciary duty to those who depend on us for guidance. We therefore need to be sensitive to the needs of others and aware of the potential repercussions of our own actions and policies.

- Inclusion of practical material, such as a Living Will form. This material is not only available for the reader's own personal use but also better enables us all to understand the clinical dimensions of bioethics.

- A Web site that complements the text by providing resources that don't go out of date. The site includes a range of material—an overview of moral theory, Supreme Court cases, legal opinions, public policy guidelines, articles, exercises, additional reference material, and so on.

- Also on the Web site is a list of *InfoTrac College Edition* articles that supplement each chapter, providing a range of additional readings. Thus, our text is an ongoing project that is both a text and an on-line resource.

ORGANIZATION OF THE TEXT

We wanted this volume to present issues and perspectives that range across the spectrum of bioethics, with enough diversity to function both as a primary text and an excellent supplementary text. This diversity also enables instructors to construct quite different courses using our text.

Chapter 1 looks at the health care system as a totality, emphasizing societal assumptions and attitudes that help define the way we conceptualize health care in this country. The impact of culture on medicine, issues around managed care, institutional racism, and gender disparities in the health care system are addressed.

Chapter 2 takes on the issue of rights and obligations, starting with the question of whether society should take steps to protect the health of every individual. It looks at some of the causes of ill health and how the health care system has negatively affected different groups in our society. It focuses particularly on how factors such as race, class, gender, and disability affect health. Two articles examine violence: one on the medicalization of violence against women and the other on health care issues arising from gun-related violence.

Chapter 3 sets out medical codes and guidelines, philosophical considerations regarding medical experimentation, and a look at some of the more infamous cases in history, such as the Nazi experiments, the Tuskegee syphilis study, the use of slaves in nineteenth-century experiments, and the Willowbrook experiment on retarded children.

Chapter 4 focuses on informed consent, examining decision making in such cases as breast implants, performance-enhancing drugs, and use of third world subjects. We then turn to property issues around the body, such as organ sales and transplants, before looking at such societal and environmental issues as the human radiation studies and the use of animals in experimental research.

Chapter 5 goes into death and dying, ethical guidelines, and legal conundrums (and related concerns, such as some disability rights advocates' opposition to physician-assisted suicide), and ends with personal narratives. It includes a detailed examination of physician-assisted suicide and issues regarding autonomy and freedom in controlling when and how we will die.

Chapter 6 looks at reproductive ethics, focusing on contraception, abortion, and maternal-fetal conflicts. In addition to core issues, there are related ones regarding access to abortion, professional obligations, minors' right to abortion, and abortion clinic violence. In the second section authors examine the history of how the courts have addressed maternal-fetal conflicts and compulsory medical treatment for pregnant women, such as forced caesarians, and the question of what sorts of moral standards should be applied to pregnant women.

Chapter 7 examines recent issues in reproductive technology, such as those arising from in vitro fertilization, multiple births, and surrogacy. Authors here consider the ethics of contraceptive technologies, reproductive freedom, potential harm to children conceived through surrogacy arrangements, and contracts used in reproductive technology and surrogacy arrangements.

Our last chapter, Chapter 8, presents articles on genetics and cloning. Authors in the first section examine genetic testing and counseling, eugenics concerns, somatic and germ-line therapy, and genetics and reproduction. Authors in the second section present a variety of perspectives on cloning: arguments for and against the banning of cloning, the applicability of the U.S. Constitution to the cloning debate, and ethical and religious issues raised by cloning. The chapter ends with an article on biotechnology and society.

VOICES NOT USUALLY HEARD

One of our goals was to create a textbook that would balance the traditional approaches and classical readings with new ways of seeing issues and voices not often heard in bioethics. Each chapter is shaped by this goal in the selection of topics, material, narratives, and case study exercises and in the organization of material. The result is a combination of in-depth journal articles offering carefully reasoned and thoughtful analyses of issues and short pieces — focused discussions on an issue or individual narratives. This combination provides a nice balance of the abstract and the concrete; for example, works that are more theoretical and those that bring in actual cases and applications.

NEW VOICES IN JUSTICE AND HEALTH CARE AND RIGHTS AND OBLIGATIONS

In the areas of both justice and health care and rights and obligations, we bring in voices speaking about the following:

- Institutionalized racism in health care and bias in health providers

- Ethical issues with managed care

- Gender disparities in medical treatment and research

- Public health, justice, and access to health care

- Wealth and poverty and health care

- Violence against women and gun-related violence

Prejudice and injustice have deep roots. In health care, these roots are often overlooked or trivialized, and have been hard to eradicate. It is time to bring them out into the light and look at them in a systematic way. That the examination may be messy or painful cannot be allowed to stop us.

NEW VOICES IN MEDICAL EXPERIMENTATION AND INFORMED CONSENT

In the areas of medical experimentation and informed consent, we wanted to include, along with pivotal articles in the field, readings that raise new issues for our consideration, such as:

- The harvesting and selling of sperm, eggs, and body tissue

- The commercialization of the body

- The ethics of performance-enhancing drugs

- The marketing of breast implants

- The ethics of using animal organ transplants in humans

- Human radiation studies and the treatment of Gulf War vets

- The use of animals as research subjects

Some of these concerns, such as injustices suffered by vulnerable populations and oppressed groups, are not new to bioethics. What *is* new, however, is our growing realization that these matters warrant close attention, and that not only Nazis but also well-meaning individuals can violate human rights.

NEW VOICES IN REPRODUCTIVE ETHICS AND REPRODUCTIVE TECHNOLOGY

In the area of reproductive ethics, we consider contraception, abortion, maternal-fetal conflicts, reproductive technology, and surrogacy. This is an area in which many already hold strong positions. Even so, we include related issues that are rarely examined:

- Abortion clinic violence

- Abortion, forced labor, and war

- Historical issues around racism and reproductivity

- Minors' rights to abortion

- Substance abuse and pregnancy

- Ethical issues around the various "parents" in surrogate arrangements

- Fertility drugs and multiple births

All raise concerns not easily answered by the traditional approaches to the area, and yet the issues have considerable impact, as seen with minors' rights to abortion and late-term abortion. Moreover, even though abortion is legal in this country, the decreasing number of abortion providers raises serious problems. Terrorist threats and acts of violence against doctors and clinic workers aiding abortions also raise concerns. Our discussions of reproductive technology cover such topics as in vitro fertilization, reproductive freedom, and biological surrogacy versus gestational surrogacy (in which the birth mother is not genetically related to the child she bears). How we respond to these concerns in terms of societal attitudes, laws, and policies has the potential to completely reshape our society and our notions of what constitutes a mother, father, and a family.

NEW VOICES IN GENETICS

In addition to mainstream concerns in genetics, we also look at others that have not been given much attention. These include:

- Genetic testing and germ-line therapy

- Genetic engineering
- Sex selection
- Cloning

Each of these is highly controversial. And since scientists have made ground-breaking advances with the human genome project, and some researchers are even patenting genes and entire organisms, genetics is an important new area of bioethics. For instance, genetic testing may make it possible to predict some aspects of our own futures and intervene to address medical conditions before they have surfaced as medical *problems*. This power could be a dream for some, a nightmare for others. Also genetic testing brings genetic knowledge, resulting in a need for genetic counselors and spiritual advisors. Other aspects of genetics are genetic engineering or manipulation, sex selection, privacy rights, and the distribution and sale of genetic information. Knowing more about this area helps us sort out fears and fantasies, and provides us with the conceptual and ethical tools for further examination of the topic. In addition, getting a sense of the ethical issues surrounding cloning provides us with the intellectual tools for grasping the advances in technology that lie ahead.

Preface

WHAT JOY TO complete this volume. This book has been a labor of love, both a source of satisfaction at compiling a work representing our conviction of the need to hear new voices, and a source of frustration as the need to squeeze it all into a reasonable-sized volume periodically reasserted itself. We have sought to provide mainstream and alternative perspectives on the recognized areas of the field, as well as to include areas that are less often recognized but merit attention. For this reason, we have included voices and bioethics issues often omitted in traditional texts.

This variety of perspectives includes those of the individual, society, medical professionals, researchers, and institutions and professional organizations like the American Medical Association and the American Nurses Association. The reader thus gets a broader view of the territory and an understanding of how very significant are each of these perspectives in our lives.

Our choice of readings also emphasizes questions of justice. There are serious issues still to be addressed in this respect, such as racism, sexism, and unequal access of the affluent and the poor to health care. Selections throughout the book raise issues of justice and keep us aware of how much more work lies ahead to rectify current patterns. We are pleased to have included a range of readings that examine the role of ethnicity, gender, sexual orientation, and disability in health care and hope to include more in future editions.

Narratives are valuable in helping readers gain a more imaginative perspective on health care issues: They can provide a direct and in-depth look at the personal and experiential side of medicine. These insightful and reflective pieces, presenting a variety of frames of reference—those of patients, doctors, family members, and so on—play the important role of allowing us to understand bioethics issues and concerns more concretely than abstract analyses alone can do, and thus to see that these issues here directly impact our lives.

Supplementing this text as a resource is our Web page: an on-going source of relevant links, on-line reference material, and bioethics organizations. As we find more material in any and all areas, we can add links, articles, and case studies that expand on each of our chapter topics. The Web page is also a useful source for instructors, having additional exercises, suggested syllabi, tests, writing assignments, and so on. With your participation, we can also put in place a network of those of us who teach bioethics—we can share insights on teaching, discuss pedagogical concerns, and become an on-line bioethics community. We also hope that readers will use the site to suggest issues and writings to us for possible inclusion. The *InfoTrac College Edition* articles should also prove very useful to both students and instructors.

And so we are delighted to bring this new book to life. Doing so has been a shared effort. Wanda approached Wadsworth with the initial idea and has acted as our liaison with our editor, Peter Adams, and the production staff, and is thankful that Laura agreed to be her partner on this journey. We are both pleased with the result. Wanda's areas of expertise in bioethics are medical experimentation, informed consent, reproductive technology, surrogacy, and cloning. Laura's areas of expertise are the concept and value of health, access to health care, reproductive ethics (contraception, abortion, maternal-fetal conflicts), and genetics. Our division of labor went as follows: We selected and edited the readings as a joint effort, and each edited the other's introductions to produce a common voice. Wanda developed case study exercises to provide practical application.

We are very pleased with the range of excellent articles we present in this anthology and are grateful to their authors that such high-quality work is being done in the field. We thank them all. Our gratitude also goes to colleagues, friends, readers, and family members who made suggestions. Particular thanks go to our reviewers: Robert Baker, Union College (NY); Deborah Blake, Regis University (CO); Kathleen Marie Dixon, Bowling Green State University; and William E. Stempsey, College of the Holy Cross.

Special thanks are due Willow Nardoni-Teays, who contributed her expertise in navigating the library resources at the University of Michigan and in helping with the bibliography and permissions. We also thank Jennifer Purvis at the University of Toronto for helping tabulate publishers' addresses. And for helping with the production stage, thanks go to copy editor Kevin Gleason, and to Hal Lockwood and Connie Hathaway of Penmarin Books.

We are especially grateful to our editor, Peter Adams for his vision, guidance, and support. For just being there, Wanda's thanks go to Silvio, Willow, and Carla, and Laura's go to John. Your love sustains us.

Chapter 1

Social Construction of Health

IN THE LAST 25 YEARS, bioethics has become one of the most significant areas in philosophy in terms of its social impact. From modest beginnings in the 1970s, bioethics has grown into a huge practical and scholarly enterprise in the 1990s. There are now specialists in ethics working in medical centers doing "real-life" bioethics. There are university-affiliated centers for research. There are graduate programs in bioethics, and a range of other channels through which philosophers, ethicists, legal scholars, clergy, and public-policy analysts work in medical ethics.

To understand why there has been such enormous growth in this field, we could point to innovative medical treatments and technologies, skyrocketing costs in health care, and shifts in demographics. However, the most fundamental reason for the rise of bioethics is that it is about health. It is about our bodies, about procreation and birth, about suffering and well-being, about who controls decisions about medical treatment. In short, bioethics is about life and about death.

These dimensions of life and death are so crucial to us because in some sense we are our bodies, and what happens to them—how we are born, how we feel while we are alive, and how we die, affects everything we do. For instance, ill health, broadly construed, generally causes pain and can limit our activities. Pain is unpleasant and can make our lives miserable; disability may make it difficult or impossible to do things we want to do. Health can be seen as a basic good: It is something we desire for its own sake, as well as something that helps us attain many other goals.

This centrality of health has important consequences. First, we need to consider what we mean by "health," for, as the readings show, its definition can affect us in surprising ways. A sufficiently expansive conception of health can, when joined with other beliefs, put us in for extreme therapies, cause us to be shunned as "sickies," or make us into second class citizens. It can also determine whether we are regarded as persons in need of treatment or as criminals. We saw this, for example, when, with a stroke of the pen, the Supreme Court changed heroin addiction from an illness to criminality. Not only did this decision reshape the way drug use was understood in this country, but it set new boundaries around who was eligible or ineligible for state benefits.

Our ignorance about particular health conditions factors into this equation as well. For instance, until fairly recently epileptics were routinely put in mental hospitals and treated as if they were mentally retarded. Furthermore, our conception of health gives rise to numerous justice issues. Among them are the distribution of care, and social arrangements that impinge on health. For instance, if we consider health benefits and treatment an option available only for people under a certain age, then we consign the elderly to a veritable no-man's-land. Or if, instead, we consider health benefits and treatment an option only for U.S. citizens, then we consign illegal aliens and other noncitizens to a world without prenatal care or anything beyond emergency health care (and sometimes not even that). Where we draw the lines around who qualifies for health services has significant consequences in terms of justice or injustice.

We first need to come to some understanding of what "health" entails. The World Health Organization (WHO) asserts its definition of health as no less than "a state of complete physical, mental and social well-being, and not merely the absence of disease or infirmity." WHO further asserts that governments are responsible for providing "adequate health and social measures." If we consider access to health care a fundamental right, then we are forced to re-examine public-policy guidelines.

The WHO definition of health has provoked substantial debate. Central to critics' worries are the moral, political, and social implications inherent in such sweeping demands. Simply eradicating physical disease and infirmity would be a tall order. If we took the definition to its logical conclusion, it would require developing cures not now known to us, ensuring an equitable distribution of care, and, more generally, remedying the broader social conditions that contribute to diseases that require medical attention. Although embracing an ideal of positive physical well-being is, in some ways, an attractive proposition, it also has drawbacks. To the extent that it encourages people to take up good health habits, it is obviously desirable. But it may also encourage them to engage in worrisome forms of perfectionism—whether it be excessive exercise programs or risky surgery for conditions that can be adequately controlled by less invasive means. There are also resource allocation decisions that cannot be derived from the definition itself.

In addition, the WHO definition provides neither discussion of the nature of mental or social well-being nor any guidelines about how to achieve them. If the definition helps us to see the connections among the physical, mental, and social components of our lives, that is all to the good. However, if this definition encourages us to redefine psychological and social issues as medical ones, that could be dangerous: Physicians are relatively untrained in these areas, and many issues involve unresolved value questions. People's whole lives come into question. As readings in this section show, we need to carefully examine our notions of health and sickness and what well-being requires. As we will see in this text, our assumptions and concepts regarding health and health care can result in disparities regarding access to resources, options, and information and can affect our values, such as trust, dignity, and integrity, that are of fundamental importance to health care. Moreover, those values do not exist in a vacuum, for they have very real consequences in terms of behavior (e.g., in relationships between patients and health caregivers) and in systemic concerns (e.g., in creating a just health care system).

Conceptions about individuals' "proper" station in life also influence views about health and disease. Gender, race, class, and, to some extent, age result in patients' being offered inferior medical care. The history of oppression and prejudice in the medical profession in particular and society in general led to what now seem to be astounding conclusions about the health of members of these groups.

For example, one of the catalysts of the Tuskegee syphilis study was the prevailing medical view that blacks were physiologically different from whites, and were uniquely more vulnerable than whites to sexual diseases such as syphilis. Today, these assumptions are generally more muted and covert, yet, as we shall see, they still affect health in significant ways. For instance, prisoners found guilty of a felony are generally unable to qualify for an organ transplant, even when they will die without it. The assumption is that such persons do not warrant access to such a precious, limited resource.

We see what happens when issues come up against common stereotypes and societal norms. A case in point is homosexuality. Although it has often been viewed as a sin, medical models turned such alleged sins into diseases. On the one hand, this prevents "sinners" from being punished as criminals. On the other, this medicalization "creates" disease, generating extreme "cures." Although not comparable in scope to the damaging effects of female genital mutilation, social history shows the struggles to think critically about sexuality. Only in 1973 did the American Psychiatric Association cease categorizing homosexuality as a medical problem. Yet many people still see it as a disease that ought to be eradicated. Those who judge homosexuality to be a disease consequently recommend genetic engineering, "healthier" families, or behavior modification as remedies.

Another illustration of the ways in which societal stereotypes affect medicine is found in the creation and development of breast implants. A product that has no clear health benefits other than those that may follow from pleasure with one's own appearance, was developed and introduced on the market with little research. What research was done tended to be short range and mostly done on beagles, not humans. With over one million American women effectively acting as research subjects, concerns about risks vs. benefits have tended to be viewed more as a litigious matter than a medical one.

As well, there are issues regarding social worth that creep into medical decision making. For instance, those in prison and in the military have had diminished rights to individual autonomy compared to the typical citizen. To some degree, they have been seen as either less deserving of health care services (e.g., prisoners' lack of access to organ donations) or viewed as more expendable (e.g., use of members of the military as atomic guinea pigs).

Making distinctions among individuals on the basis of apparent group membership is still no simple matter, however. Cultural presuppositions affect our conceptions about health and disease in yet more fundamental ways. For example, in the United States we tend to be highly individualistic, activist in the face of perceived problems, and trusting of technological solutions. We also tend to see deep divisions between mind and body, and between different body parts and systems.

These approaches have led to unique understandings of disease and well-being, and ones that are in contrast to those of other cultures. For example, the French put a great deal more emphasis on the state of the organism at risk, whereas we have tended to concentrate wholly on the threat from outside it; more recently the focus has shifted to narrow genetic explanations. Similarly, Chinese medicine (especially herbal medicine) employs a much less invasive approach to medicine than Western approaches.

Furthermore, religion, culture, and ethnicity can even shape attitudes about treatment options and what extraordinary measures are morally acceptable. For instance, look at how religious beliefs shaped attitudes to medical treatment. Jehovah's Witnesses routinely refuse blood transfusions, even in the face of life-threatening medical conditions. Buddhists tend to oppose surgery, particularly when alternatives are available. Christian Scientists regularly recommend prayer over medical treatment, sometimes even denying medical treatment to minors despite the threat of legal action. Moreover, articulated position papers on medical issues have been set out by such diverse groups as the Catholic Bishops, the American Jewish Congress, the Unitarian-Universalist Association, and Islamic groups.

Such diverse outlooks can make a huge difference in both how we conceive of health and how disease is treated. Indeed, a major issue we face as a society is how to balance respect for diverse religious or cultural beliefs and attitudes that are in conflict with mainline views about protecting patient health, especially in minors. Becoming aware of such differences is essential for thinking critically and constructively about these matters.

This chapter is structured so as to illuminate three approaches to the social construction of health. First we look at the conceptual issues; i.e., how health has been understood in terms of how it has been defined and how it functions in practice. In this way we can see what factors shaped our understanding of health. In the second section, we examine a number of systemic concerns, such as the growth of health maintenance organizations (HMOs), the role of bias and prejudice in the health care system, and the degree to which such fundamental notions as autonomy are socially constructed. In the last section, we see how people have come face to face with the health care system. Here we look at the interpersonal relationships and the ways in which individuals have been transformed by their experiences.

THE READINGS

The readings in the first section of the chapter look at the concept of health. Readings include:

1. The WHO definition of health argues for a broad notion of the concept.

2. Daniel Callahan raises serious objections to this broad WHO definition.

3. James Goodwin shows how assumptions we take for granted—but that are not necessarily shared by other cultures—shape mainstream American medicine.

4. Dan E. Beauchamp argues that individual-based "market justice" undermines society's ability to address social and political sources of poor health and disability.

5. Edmund D. Pellegrino argues for the centrality of trust in professional ethics.

6. Finally, going from a specific case, Joseph Carrese, Kate Brown, and Andrew Jameton comment on the role of culture in healing and the moral issues that arise around professional duties.

In the second section we look at a range of issues that challenge us to continue to examine and work for a more just health care system.

1. Suzanne Gordon and Timothy McCall examine some of the problems with the managed care system and proposals for ways to make HMOs more human-centered.

2. Erica Goode points out the discrepancy between the quality of health care and general health between those who are wealthy and those who are not and notes a variety of problems that warrant our attention.

3. An editorial from *The Lancet* brings to our attention the extent to which racism infects the health care system and why it is so crucial that we address it.

4. The American Medical Association's Council on Ethical and Judicial Affairs reports on its examination of gender disparities in medicine, focusing on clinical decision making and revealing some disturbing sexist trends in clinical studies.

5. Virginia Warren argues for a new conception of autonomy, one that replaces "power-over" with a shared sense of power, thereby empowering the patient to become a more active participant in health care decision making.

6. Lisa I. Iezzoni comments on what it is like for a disabled person to try to communicate with those in the medical profession. In addition to detailing some of the problems she has experienced, she sets out a series of suggestions to improve the doctor-disabled patient relationship.

In the third section, three narratives offer different perspectives on the personal impact of health care.

1. N. Ann Davis describes what it was like to get cataracts on her eyes, causing severe problems with her vision, and how this experience affected her view of her health and her life.

2. David S. Shimm writes about treating a patient who is a chronically ill smoker.

3. Nancy V. Raine gives us a personal look at the effects of violence against women by describing how her own life has been permanently marked by her rape years ago.

Concept of Health

Preamble to the Constitution of the World Health Organization

THE STATES PARTIES to this Constitution[1] declare, in conformity with the Charter of the United Nations, that the following principles are basic to the happiness, harmonious relations and security of all peoples:

Health is a state of complete physical, mental and social well-being and not merely the absence of disease or infirmity.

The enjoyment of the highest attainable standard of health is one of the fundamental rights of every human being without distinction of race, religion, political belief, economic or social condition.

The health of all peoples is fundamental to the attainment of peace and security and is dependent upon the fullest co-operation of individuals and States.

The achievement of any State in the promotion and protection of health is of value to all.

Unequal development in different countries in the promotion of health and control of disease, especially communicable disease, is a common danger.

Healthy development of the child is of basic importance; the ability to live harmoniously in a changing total environment is essential to such development.

The extension to all peoples of the benefits of medical, psychological and related knowledge is essential to the fullest attainment of health.

Informed opinion and active cooperation on the part of the public are of the utmost importance in the improvement of the health of the people.

Governments have a responsibility for the health of their peoples which can be fulfilled only by the provision of adequate health and social measures.

NOTES

1. The Constitution was adopted by the International Health Conference held in New York from 19 June to 22 July 1946, and signed on 22 July 1946 by the representatives of 61 States (*Off. Rec. Wld Hlth Org.* 2, 100). Amendments adopted by the Twentieth World Health Assembly (resolution WHA20.36) came into force on 21 May 1975 and are incorporated in the present text.

Reprinted from World Health Organization: Basic Documents, *26th ed. (Geneva: World Health Organization, 1976), p. 1.*

The WHO Definition of Health

DANIEL CALLAHAN

. . . IT MAY JUST BE that the WHO definition has more than a grain of truth in it, of a kind which is as profoundly frustrating as it is enticingly attractive. At the very least it is a definition which implies that there is some intrinsic relationship between the good of the body and the good of the self. The attractiveness of this relationship is obvious: it thwarts any movement toward a dualism of self and body, a dualism which in any event immediately breaks down when one drops a brick on one's toe; and it impels the analyst to work toward a conception of health which in the end is resistant to clear and distinct categories, closer to the felt experience. All that, naturally, is very frustrating. It seems simply impossible to devise a concept of health which is rich enough to be nutritious and yet not so rich as to be indigestible.

One common objection to the WHO definition is, in effect, an assault upon any and all attempts to specify the meaning of very general concepts. Who can possibly define words as vague as "health," a venture as foolish as trying to define "peace," "justice," "happiness," and other systematically ambiguous notions? To this objection the "pragmatic" clinicians (as they often call themselves) add that, anyway, it is utterly unnecessary to know what "health" means in order to

DANIEL CALLAHAN is director of international programs for the Hastings Center. He is an honorary professor at the Charles University School of Medicine, Prague, the Czech Republic. He won the 1996 Freedom and Scientific Responsibility Award of the American Association for the Advancement of Science.

treat a patient running a high temperature. Not only that, it is also a harmful distraction to clutter medical judgment with philosophical puzzles.

Unfortunately for this line of argument, it is impossible to talk or think at all without employing general concepts; without them, cognition and language are impossible. More damagingly, it is rarely difficult to discover, with a bit of probing, that even the most "pragmatic" judgment (whatever *that* is) presupposes some general values and orientations, all of which can be translated into definitions of terms as general as "health" and "happiness." A failure to discern the operative underlying values, the conceptions of reality upon which they are based, and the definitions they entail, sets the stage for unexamined conduct and, beyond that, positive harm both to patients and to medicine in general. . . .

[T]he most specific complaint about the WHO definition is that its very generality, and particularly its association of health and general well-being as a positive ideal, has given rise to a variety of evils. Among them are the cultural tendency to define all social problems, from war to crime in the streets, as "health" problems; the blurring of lines of responsibility between and among the professions, and between the medical profession and the political order; the implicit denial of human freedom which results when failures to achieve social well-being are defined as forms of "sickness," somehow to be treated by medical means; and the general debasement of language which ensues upon the casual habit of labeling everyone from Adolf Hitler to student radicals to the brat next door

Hastings Center Studies *1, no. 3 (1973): 77–78. Reprinted by permission of Daniel Callahan and The Hastings Center. Copyright The Hastings Center* as "sick." In short, the problem with the WHO definition is not that it represents an attempt to propose a general definition, but that it is simply a bad one.

That is a valid line of objection, provided one can spell out in some detail just how the definition can or does entail some harmful consequences. Two lines of attack are possible against putatively hazardous social definitions of significant general concepts. One is by pointing out that the definition does not encompass all that a concept has commonly been taken to mean, either historically or at present, that it is a partial definition only. The task then is to come up with a fuller definition, one less subject to misuse. But there is still another way of objecting to socially significant definitions, and that is by pointing out some baneful effects of definitions generally accepted as adequate. Many of the objections to the WHO definition fall in the latter category, building upon the important insight that definitions of crucially important terms with a wide public use have ethical, social, and political implications; defining general terms is not an abstract exercise but a way of shaping the world metaphysically and structuring the world politically.

Wittgenstein's aphorism, "Don't look for the meaning, look for the use," is pertinent here. The ethical problem in defining the concept of "health" is to determine what the implications are of the various uses to which a concept of "health" can be put. We might well agree that there are some uses of "health" which will produce socially harmful results. To carry Wittgenstein a step further, "Don't look for the uses, look for the abuses." We might, then, examine some of the real or possible abuses to which the WHO definition leads, recognizing all the while that what we may term an "abuse" will itself rest upon some perceived *positive* good or value. . . .

HEALTH AND HAPPINESS

Let us examine some of the principal objections to the WHO definition in more detail. One of

them is that, by including the notion of "social well-being" under its rubric, it turns the enduring problem of human happiness into one more medical problem, to be dealt with by scientific means. That is surely an objectionable feature, if only because there exists no evidence whatever that medicine has anything more than a partial grasp of the sources of human misery. Despite Dr. Chisholm's optimism, medicine has not even found ways of dealing with more than a fraction of the whole range of physical diseases; campaigns, after all, are still being mounted against cancer and heart disease. Nor is there any special reason to think that future forays against those and other common diseases will bear rapid fruits. People will continue to die of disease for a long time to come, probably forever.

But perhaps, then, in the psychological and psychiatric sciences some progress has been made against what Dr. Chisholm called the "psychological ills," which lead to wars, hostility, and aggression? To be sure, there are many interesting psychological theories to be found about these "ills," and a few techniques which can, with some individuals, reduce or eliminate antisocial behavior. But so far as I can see, despite the mental health movement and the rise of the psychological sciences, war and human hostility are as much with us as ever. Quite apart from philosophical objections to the WHO definition, there was no empirical basis for the unbounded optimism which lay behind it at the time of its inception, and little has happened since to lend its limitless aspiration any firm support.

Common sense alone makes evident the fact that the absence of "disease or infirmity" by no means guarantees "social well-being." In one sense, those who drafted the WHO definition seem well aware of that. Isn't the whole point of their definition to show the inadequacy of negative definitions? But in another sense, it may be doubted that they really did grasp that point. For the third principle enunciated in the WHO Constitution says that "the health of all peoples is fundamental to the attainment of peace and security. . . ." Why is it fundamental, at least to peace? The worst wars of the 20th century have been waged by countries with very high standards of health, by nations with superior life-expectancies for individuals and with comparatively low infant mortality rates. The greatest present threats to world peace come in great part (though not entirely) from developed countries, those which have combatted disease and illness most effectively. There seems to be no historical correlation whatever between health and peace, and that is true even if one includes "mental health."

How are human beings to achieve happiness? That is the final and fundamental question. Obviously illness, whether mental or physical, makes happiness less possible in most cases. But that is only because they are only one symptom of a more basic restriction, that of human finitude, which sees infinite human desires constantly thwarted by the limitations of reality. "Complete" well-being might, conceivably, be attainable, but under one condition only: that people ceased expecting much from life. That does not seem about to happen. On the contrary, medical and psychological progress have been more than outstripped by rising demands and expectations. What is so odd about that, if it is indeed true that human desires are infinite? Whatever the answer to the question of human happiness, there is no particular reason to believe that medicine can do anything more than make a modest, finite contribution.

Another objection to the WHO definition is that, by implication, it makes the medical profession the gate-keeper for happiness and social well-being. Or if not exactly the gate-keeper (since political and economic support will be needed from sources other than medical), then the final magic-healer of human misery. Pushed far enough, the whole idea is absurd, and it is not necessary to believe that the organizers of the WHO would, if pressed, have been willing to go quite that far. But even if one pushes the pretension a little way, considerable fantasy results. The

mental health movement is the best example, casting the psychological professional in the role of high priest.

At its humble best, that movement can do considerable good; people do suffer from psychological disabilities and there are some effective ways of helping them. But it would be sheer folly to believe that all, or even the most important, social evils stem from bad mental health: political injustice, economic scarcity, food shortages, unfavorable physical environments, have a far greater historical claim as sources of a failure to achieve "social well-being." To retort that all or most of these troubles can, nonetheless, be seen finally as symptoms of bad mental health is, at best, self-serving and, at worst, just plain foolish.

A significant part of the objection that the WHO definition places, at least by implication, too much power and authority in the hands of the medical profession need not be based on a fear of that power as such. There is no reason to think that the world would be any worse off if health professionals made all decisions than if any other group did, and no reason to think it would be any better off. That is not a very important point. More significant is that cultural development which, in its skepticism about "traditional" ways of solving social problems, would seek a technological and specifically a medical solution for human ills of all kinds. There is at least a hint in early WHO discussions that, since politicians and diplomats have failed in maintaining world peace, a more expert group should take over, armed with the scientific skills necessary to set things right; it is science which is best able to vanquish that old Enlightenment bogeyman, "superstition." More concretely, such an ideology has the practical effect of blurring the lines of appropriate authority and responsibility. If all problems — political, economic and social — reduce to matters of "health," then there cease to be any ways to determine who should be responsible for what.

THE TYRANNY OF HEALTH

The problem of responsibility has at least two faces. One is that of a tendency to turn all problems of "social well-being" over to the medical professional, most pronounced in the instance of the incarceration of a large group of criminals in mental institutions rather than prisons. The abuses, both medical and legal, of that practice are, fortunately, now beginning to receive the attention they deserve, even if little corrective action has yet been taken. (Counterbalancing that development, however, are others, where some are seeking more "effective" ways of bringing science to bear on criminal behavior.)

The other face of the problem of responsibility is that of the way in which those who are sick, or purportedly sick, are to be evaluated in terms of their freedom and responsibility. Siegler and Osmond [*Hastings Center Studies*, vol. 1, no. 3, 1973, pp. 41–58] discuss the "sick role," a leading feature of which is the ascription of blamelessness, of non-responsibility, to those who contract illness. There is no reason to object to this kind of ascription in many instances — one can hardly blame someone for contracting kidney disease — but, obviously enough, matters get out of hand when all physical, mental, and communal disorders are put under the heading of "sickness," and all sufferers (all of us, in the end) placed in the blameless "sick role." Not only are the concepts of "sickness" and "illness" drained of all content, it also becomes impossible to ascribe any freedom or responsibility to those caught up in the throes of sickness. The whole world is sick, and no one is responsible any longer for anything. That is determinism gone mad, a rather odd outcome of a development which began with attempts to bring unbenighted "reason" and free self-determination to bear for the release of the helpless captives of superstition and ignorance.

The final and most telling objection to the WHO definition has less to do with the definition itself than with one of its natural historical consequences. Thomas Szasz has been the most eloquent (and most singleminded) critic of that sleight-of-hand which has seen the concept of health moved from the medical to the moral arena. What can no longer be done in the name of "morality" can now be done in the name of "health": human beings labeled, incarcerated, and dismissed for their failure to toe the line of "normalcy" and "sanity."

At first glance, this analysis of the present situation might seem to be totally at odds with the tendency to put everyone in the blame-free "sick role." Actually, there is a fine, probably indistinguishable, line separating these two positions. For as soon as one treats all human disorders — war, crime, social unrest — as forms of illness, then one turns health into a normative concept, that which human beings must and ought to have if they are to live in peace with themselves and others. Health is no longer an optional matter, but the golden key to the relief of human misery. We *must* be well or we will all perish. "Health" can and must be imposed; there can be no room for the luxury of freedom when so much is at stake. Of course the matter is rarely put so bluntly, but it is to Szasz's great credit that he has discerned what actually happens when "health" is allowed to gain the cultural clout which morality once had. (That he carries the whole business too far in his embracing of the most extreme moral individualism is another story, which cannot be dealt with here.) Something is seriously amiss when the "right" to have healthy children is turned into a further right for children not to be born defective, and from there into an obligation not to bring unhealthy children into the world as a way of respecting the right of those children to health! Nor is everything altogether lucid when abortion decisions are made a matter of "medical judgment" (see *Roe* vs. *Wade*); when decisions to provide psychoactive drugs for the relief of the ordinary stress of living are defined as no less "medical judgment"; when patients are not allowed to die with dignity because of medical indications that they can, come what may, be kept alive; when prisoners, without their consent, are subjected to aversive conditioning to improve their mental health. . . .

MODEST CONCLUSIONS

Two conclusions may be drawn. The first is that some minimal level of health is necessary if there is to be any possibility of human happiness. Only in exceptional circumstances can the good of self be long maintained in the absence of the good of the body. The second conclusion, however, is that one can be healthy without being in a state of "complete physical, mental, and social well-being." That conclusion can be justified in two ways: (a) because some degree of disease and infirmity is perfectly compatible with mental and social well-being; and (b) because it is doubtful that there ever was, or ever could be, more than a transient state of "complete physical, mental, and social well-being," for individuals or societies; that's just not the way life is or could be. Its attractiveness as an ideal is vitiated by its practical impossibility of realization. Worse than that, it positively misleads, for health becomes a goal of such all-consuming importance that it simply begs to be thwarted in its realization. The de-

mands which the word "complete" entail set the stage for the worst false consciousness of all: the demand that life deliver perfection. Practically speaking, this demand has led, in the field of health, to a constant escalation of expectation and requirement, never ending, never satisfied.

What, then, would be a good definition of "health"? I was afraid someone was going to ask me that question. I suggest we settle on the following: "Health is a state of physical well-being." That state need not be "complete," but it must be at least adequate, i.e., without significant impairment of function. It also need not encompass "mental" well-being; one can be healthy yet anxious, well yet depressed. And it surely ought not to encompass "social well-being," except insofar as that well-being will be impaired by the presence of large-scale, serious physical infirmities. Of course my definition is vague, but it would take some very fancy semantic footwork for it to be socially misused; that brat next door could not be called "sick" except when he is running a fever. This definition would not, though, preclude all social use of the language of "pathology" for other than physical disease. The image of a physically well body is a powerful one and, used carefully, it can be suggestive of the kind of wholeness and adequacy of function one might hope to see in other areas of life.

Culture and Medicine: The Influence of Puritanism on American Medical Practice

JAMES S. GOODWIN

> Research must be held accountable for the choice of its rationality; its basis—which we know is not the established objectivity of science—must be questioned.—Michel Foucault [1]

INTRODUCTION

We are in a period of rapid transition in medicine, not just in issues of financing but also in methods of assessing the effectiveness of what we do. However, this critical examination of effectiveness takes place within a cultural context. If we do not recognize that context, we are at risk for selectivity in our evaluations. A failure to appreciate the cultural context may result in uncritical acceptance of much in American medical practice which, while it may accurately reflect our cultural values, does not improve the health of the populace.

Medicine is taught and described and contemplated within the scientific model. The language and attire of medicine is that of science, with "P" values and white lab coats. Thus, there is some resistance to the idea that medical practice is an expression of cultural values. In the Western world the body of scientific information is virtually the same in all countries. American scientists studying leukotriene biosynthesis or DNA repair are studying the same processes as their Italian, German, Swedish, or French colleagues. They attend the same international conferences, publish in the same journals, and talk the same language (English). An American scientist has little trouble adjusting to working in a western European laboratory, and vice versa. But at the level of the *practice* of medicine there is an entirely different story. Here each country is unique, reflecting strong cultural and historical influences. A few examples will illustrate this point.

In the late 1970s, I came upon a list of the 10 most widely prescribed medications in the United States and several Western European countries. It was remarkable how little overlap there was, not just by specific drug but by indication for their use. In the United States, three of the top 10 were sedative hypnotics, and the rest were antibiotics, NSAIDS, and antihypertensives. In France, liver preparations topped the list. In the United States, a patient with malaise is depressed or nervous or has a virus; in France, the cause is a weak liver, and many popular and seemingly efficacious medications address that need. In Italy, five of the most popular medications were hormonal preparations. In Germany,

JAMES S. GOODWIN is a medical doctor at the University of Texas Medical Branch. The author thanks Marilyn Brodwick; Thomas Cole; Clifford Goodwin; Jean Goodwin; Patricia Jakobi; Jeanne St. Pierre; and William Winslade for their helpful comments.

Perspectives in Biology and Medicine *38, 4 (Summer 1995)* © *1995 by The University of Chicago.*
All rights reserved.

a large number of medicines are given not orally but by rectal suppository.

Another example is spinal manipulation. In this country people who manipulate spines are considered quacks by many in the medical establishment [2], though the Federal Trade Commission has recently enjoined us from continuing to state so publicly [3]. In northern European countries, such as Belgium, the Netherlands, and the Scandinavian countries, spinal manipulation has been recognized and utilized as an efficacious treatment throughout the present century, and is an important component of the therapeutic armamentarium of physiatrists and rheumatologists [4, 5].

A related example is spa therapy [6]. The benefits of spa therapy have been recognized in many European countries for centuries, and the national health insurance plans in Germany, Switzerland, France, and other countries cover the cost of extended spa therapy for a variety of medical conditions from arthritis to angina. In the United States, spas died out with the introduction of effective antituberculous chemotherapy.

If therapies differ greatly among Western countries, so do diseases. Low blood pressure is a popular diagnosis in Germany and other continental European countries; there are careful studies on its causes, consequences, and effects of treatment [7]. It does not exist in the United States and Britain except as a disreputable diagnosis [8]. On the other hand, the U.S. preoccupation with pills and programs to lower blood cholesterol is not matched in most Western European countries.

The point in listing these differences is not to make value judgments, nor to come to a conclusion as to which treatments or diseases are truly valid. Rather, the fact that major differences exist in medical practice should remind us that medical practitioners are products of their culture. A similar but much broader point was made by Foucault, who argued that the current orientation of all of Western medicine is a product of the cultural values of late eighteenth-century Europe [9].

If one accepts the above arguments, it would seem useful to describe the cultural influences that shape American medicine. Currently, there is considerable concern both within and without the medical community about standardizing care, improving quality, and controlling costs. Such efforts would benefit from a clearer understanding of all the influences on American medicine—why we do what we do. The discussion that follows will focus on one such influence, Puritan ideals adhered to by the early colonists and transmitted to later generations and to immigrants from diverse cultural backgrounds.

AMERICAN PURITANISM

If medicine is culturally determined, what is American culture? We Americans proudly see ourselves as a polyglot product of all the world's cultures; but who got here first? Who established the dominant culture that the other immigrant groups more or less accepted as the "real" American culture, the culture into which to be assimilated? The answer is the Puritans. The Puritans dominated early America: 85 percent of the churches in the original thirteen colonies were Puritan in spirit [10]; major institutions of higher learning, such as Harvard and Yale, were founded and run by the Puritan ministry; and Puritanism was responsible for the foundation of the public school system in America [11]. Puritan values form the bedrock of our culture. These were more lately leavened with the value systems of other religions and other ethnic groups, but no one can ignore the fundamental importance of Puritanism in American culture.

This makes us very different from most European countries, which, with the exception of German-speaking areas of Switzerland, Flemish Belgium, and parts of the Netherlands, do not manifest major Puritan influences.

How should one describe the nature of that Puritan influence? What are Puritan values? In my brief summary I hope to avoid a caricature; nor is it my intention to demean these values. The *Encyclopedia Britannica* describes Puritanism as "noted for a spirit of moral and religious earnestness that determined their whole way of life" [10]. The Puritan idea was one of emulation. The saints' lives could be achieved by all of us: "Saints' lives are valuable not for themselves but because they make the true norms of identity accessible to all good men" [12, p. 15]. This contrasted with the traditional church practice of venerating the saints. Early Puritans defined theology as the doctrine of living well [13]. A fundamental tenet of Puritanism is that the individual has a covenant with God. Individual or group success bespeaks God's favor and indicates that the individual has kept the covenant. Conversely, individual or group failure was usually seen as a manifestation of God's displeasure for failure to keep the covenant. Worthiness and righteousness were important concepts.

Another tenet of Puritanism is the responsibility of each individual member of the community for the behavior of the other members of the community. If you lead a virtuous life, but your neighbors are sinners, you share in the responsibility. An important liturgy for Puritans was from the Gospel of Matthew 18:15–17, an admonition to confront fellow believers with their faults, and, if they are unresponsive, to reject them. Someone else's incorrect behavior is offensive to the entire community.

One aspect of Puritanism is difficult to describe without risking the charge of bias: it is not much of an oversimplification to characterize the Puritan way of life as pleasure-averse. Life was serious, earnest, and somewhat grim. Pleasure, particularly external manifestations of pleasure, was suspect. At this point, the reader might note that many values related to Puritanism are shared to a greater or lesser extent by the other major Christian denominations as well as by Islam and Judaism. However, compared to other Christian denominations, Puritanism was more insistent on incorporating these values into enforceable community standards.

PURITANISM IN AMERICAN MEDICINE

The argument that American medicine incorporates Puritan values can be viewed as almost trivial. There are many jokes about how doctors proscribe all that is pleasurable in life. The Puritan metaphor became more concrete when the man who was arguably the most effective surgeon general in modern times had an appearance reminiscent of Captain Ahab. But the trivial aspects of this analysis should not obscure the important Puritan influences on American medicine. A major influence of Puritanism is an earnest preparation for a future bliss at the expense of current earthly pleasures. Nowhere in American public health literature is there the concept of pleasure, of contentment, of happiness. Only very recently have these ideas been mentioned anywhere in American medicine, and only under the well-circumscribed and sanitized rubric of "quality of life." What is more natural, more basic than the question "Are you enjoying life?" Is this not as fundamental an issue as any other in public health?

I will focus on four areas where American medical practice clearly differs from that in some other Western countries and seems to reflect or has been presumably influenced by Puritan values. These four areas are alcohol use, pain control, pregnancy, and preventive medicine.

Alcohol Use

The 1990 *Dietary Guidelines for Americans* contains the following statement: "Drinking [alcoholic beverages] has no net health benefit, is linked with many health problems, is the cause of many accidents, and can lead to addiction. Their consumption is not recommended" [14].

The repeat of Prohibition in America was not accompanied by any lessening of the dread with which most physicians regard alcohol. Like many Puritan values, our view of alcohol is conflicted. Most American physicians consume it, as do most Americans. But our message is still one reminiscent of prohibition: "If you *must* drink, do so only in moderation." Medical organizations supported the successful efforts to require health warnings on all advertising of and containers for alcoholic beverages.

This attitude flies in the face of compelling epidemiologic evidence that moderate alcohol consumption is beneficial. Cardiac and all-cause mortality is significantly and substantially lower in moderate (one to three drinks/day) drinkers compared to abstainers [15]. The efforts of the public health community to either ignore or explain away these results [16, 17] involve reasoning so convoluted that it would be rejected as absurd if found in another setting. The effect of alcohol on mortality is by no means trivial. Certainly no such decline in all-cause death rate has ever been demonstrated from, for example, programs to lower cholesterol [18, 19]. If one were to chance on these data afresh, devoid of American cultural values, one might conclude that the prescription of regular alcohol might have a substantial beneficial effect on the public health. One third of Americans abstain from alcohol [20], and a disproportionately high percentage of these have heart disease; so the potential benefit to the population is very large. Yet there have been no controlled trials of alcohol administration. Might it not be reasonable to assess the effects of daily alcohol in non-drinkers with cardiovascular disease? Abstention from alcohol is associated with an increase in risk of cardiac death and a higher overall mortality rate. This association may or may not be causal. If it is causal, then an alcohol intervention program could save many lives each year. Of course, there may be toxicities of such therapy, such as an increase in accidental deaths and deaths from liver disease,

particularly if some individuals given alcohol became heavy drinkers. In this regard alcohol does not differ from any other therapeutic intervention. The only way to assess risks and benefits is in a controlled trial. The repugnance of such a suggestion stems from cultural values, not scientific ones.

Alleviation of Pain

In the 1970s, my colleagues and I documented the widespread fallacy among health professionals that a positive response to placebo medication was evidence that a patient's complaint of pain was not "real" [21, 22]. More recently, the Agency for Health Care Policy and Research has issued guidelines to physicians and nurses in an attempt to overcome the underutilization of narcotic analgesics in hospitalized patients [23]. The attitude of American medicine towards pain control is clearly conflicted. Pain is seen as good, useful, even noble: "no pain, no gain." But the well-documented undertreatment of pain by American health professionals is not, in my opinion, secondary to a belief in its benefits. Rather, the primary problem is that medications for pain are pleasurable. Many people given morphine enjoy the experience. This makes pain control a tricky and somewhat dirty business. It is generally recognized that the fear of producing addicts is exaggerated [21]. At one time, even high-dose salicylates were discouraged in patients with rheumatoid arthritis out of the fear that patients would become addicted to them [25]. The continued undertreatment of pain and the underutilization of patient-controlled narcotic delivery systems cannot be fully understood unless one addresses the powerful cultural forces in American medicine that discourage use of narcotics. No program to promote the humane treatment of people in pain can hope to succeed if it addresses only the scientific issues such as pharmacokinetics and ignores the value our culture places on asceticism and the wariness with which we view unbridled, unearned, and undeserved pleasure.

Pregnancy and Childbirth

Puritanism viewed pregnancy with discomfort; while it was not strictly sinful, it was clearly not a socially accepted state. Modern American medicine has transformed the near-sin into a near-disease. The efforts of modern medicine to re-define pregnancy as a medical illness have been so successful that it is probably difficult for most American physicians to see this as a cultural rather than a scientific issue. Until recently, any weight gain in pregnancy was rigorously con-trolled. Fetuses are scanned and monitored. Am-niocentesis is routinely performed, initially in women over age 40, then over age 35, and more recently in those aged 30 or above. One in four babies are delivered by major surgery; prior to the routine Caesarian section, we routinely used forceps. Until recently all babies were delivered in an operating room atmosphere, with gowns, masks, and sterile fields.

One might imagine that strong evolutionary forces have acted to optimize the process of childbirth over the past hundreds of thousands of years. And yet, over the space of a century, Amer-ican medicine has managed to redefine preg-nancy and childbirth from a natural process to a pathologic one. Pregnancy has become a very se-rious business. Any alcohol consumption is for-bidden, and the pregnant woman who smokes becomes a social pariah. In order to appreciate the cultural bases for these attitudes, it would be useful to review the scientific data on the effects of alcohol or tobacco use during pregnancy. There are no data—absolutely no data—suggest-ing that a drink of wine or beer or whiskey daily in pregnancy is harmful to the fetus. And the lack of evidence is not from want of trying [26, 27]. Nevertheless, the American Medical Association has strongly stated that pregnant women should consume no alcohol. Such a prohibition is not found in Western European countries.

The issue of pregnant women smoking is more complex, because cigarette smoking is clearly a major threat to the health of the smoker. However, our severe reaction to pregnant women smoking seems disproportionate to the threat. It is not an overstatement to say that the picture of an eight months pregnant woman puffing on a cigarette would make many physi-cians physically uncomfortable and perhaps angry. I doubt if an obviously pregnant woman could smoke in public without being accused of harming her baby. What is the harm to the fetus? The babies, on average, are a little smaller; the placentas are a little bigger—an effect, in short, similar to residence at high altitude [28]. For ex-ample, in a recent study the average birth weight of babies of smokers was 3043 grams, versus 3141 grams for babies from nonsmoking woman [29]. This hardly seems a major health threat to the fetus, not comparable to the impact of smoking on the pregnant woman herself.

Any member of society has the right to tell a pregnant woman how to act. This attitude is fa-cilitated by the fact that pregnant individuals are women, and women are given no leeway in Puri-tan society. I would argue that the righteousness with which educated society upbraids the preg-nant smoker is a manifestation of cultural values, our Puritan tenet to confront and correct the bad behavior of others.

Preventive Medicine

It is not difficult to recognize the strong Puritan influence in the American preventive medicine movement. Preventive medicine practice in this country involves a series of prohibitions— against smoking, against eating certain foods— combined with recommendations for difficult activities such as regular aerobic exercise and weight loss. There is no doubt that many of these activities improve the health of the public, but what is of interest is the selectivity of the concerns of preventive medicine. For example, poor availability of social support has been shown to be associated with increased morbidity and mortality, even after controlling for income, comorbidity, and other factors [30–33]. Evidence that such an association is causal is provided by intervention studies [34–37], as well as by animal experiments [38]. Based on these findings, House has estimated that the magnitude of the effect of availability of good social support is equal (and opposite) to the effect of cigarette smoking on the health of an individual [39]. Simply being married confers substantial protection from deaths from cancer and other diseases [40]. Why are there no public health recommendations about getting married or about ways to avoid social isolation? We might be as successful in increasing social support as our current programs are in lowering cholesterol.

At this point I can hear the reader objecting that I am making a large leap of faith in assuming that encouraging social support would improve public health. One might say that the causal relationship between adequate social support and good health is not definitively established, that no one has demonstrated in a prospective trial a decrease in all-cause mortality from providing social support. That is a correct objection. It would also be a correct objection to our current national effort to lower blood cholesterol. I am not arguing that one program is good and another one bad, only that the selectivity in our public health emphasis reflects our cultural values. Why are we so obsessed with weight loss, when the available evidence suggests that chubby people live longer than lean ones [41]? Yes, maybe there are explanations, confounding factors which when fully accounted for would show it really *is* better to be skinny. but why do we only search for those factors, and believe in them even when we cannot quite prove they are there, when the issue involves self-denial and not when it involves pleasure?

Certainly, there are European cultures that do not see asceticism as a worthy public health goal. Even our emphasis on enforcing personal safety is not shared in European countries. I do not recall seeing a bicycle helmet during a week of cycling in Belgium. Indeed, a common sight was of one or two toddlers balanced precariously on the handlebars of a parent's bicycle on a family outing. There is similar lack of concern, relative to the United States, for speed limits or for safety in amusement park rides. All this is somewhat counterintuitive; the United States is a country steeped in individualism, while European countries have many state controls on individuals that would be unacceptable here—national identity cards, strict libel laws, etc. The point is, in some European countries unsafe behavior by an individual is not an affront to the entire society, as it is in a Puritan culture.

CONCLUSION

Nobel Laureate Jacques Monod once described the reaction of the scientific community to his ideas as comprising two stages: the first was, the proffered concept was absurd; the second was, it was obvious. I fear a similar response to my thesis that much of what we do in American medicine is culturally determined, and that a dominant cultural influence is that of Puritanism. On the other hand, this plea for some perspective in the examination of American medical practice is not occurring in a vacuum. Several recent analyses and commentaries have challenged the American medical love affair with technology [42–44] and our overestimation of the benefits of health screening examinations [45].

Cross-cultural studies have taught us much about disease. For example, Japanese men in Japan have an incidence of prostate cancer one-tenth that of American Caucasian men, while the rate for men of Japanese ancestry in America is approximately one-half that of American Caucasian men [46]. This simple fact is all one needs to conclude that prostate cancer is largely environmentally determined [47]. We can achieve similar benefits applying cross-cultural methods to the study of medical practice. It is no fault to be a product of one's culture. The fault lies in resisting self-examination, in cloaking ourselves with the certainty, or pseudo-certainty, of science [48].

Why do we do circumcisions? Why do we do Caesarian sections? Why do we give chemotherapy to cancer patients where no one has been able to demonstrate benefit? Why do we combine a moralistic approach to some safety issues with a tolerance for violence and death by guns and automobiles? Why do we perform screening proctoscopies, sigmoidoscopies, colonoscopies? Why do we need to visualize every ulcer, every clogged coronary? It is not because such procedures have been shown to improve the public health. There are of course many answers, many factors that affect what we do, including economic forces, our understanding of disease mechanisms, and the intrinsic attractiveness of some medical technologies. And surely there are many uniquely American cultural traits other than Puritanism, the understanding of which will give us insight into our practices. To this great national debate on the future of the American health care system we should add a deep appreciation for the influences our cultural value systems exert on the practice of medicine.

REFERENCES

1. Foucault, M. *La recherche scientifique et la psychologie.* In *Michel Foucault,* edited by D. Eriban, and translated by B. Wing. Cambridge: Harvard Univ. Press, 1991, p. 43.

2. Bollantine, H. Will the delivery of health care be improved by the use of chiropractic services? *N. Engl. J. Med.* 286:237–242, 1972.

3. Getzendanner, S. Wilk vs. American Medical Association: Permanent injunction order against AMA. U.S. Dist. Court, North Dist Il, East Div, No 76 C, 3777. Reprinted in *JAMA* 259:81–82, 1988.

4. Koes, B. W.; Assendelft, W. J.; VanderHeigden, G. J.; et al. Spinal manipulation and mobilization for back and neck pain: A blinded review. *BMJ* 303:1298–1303, 1991.

5. Stevens, A. Manual medicine: A description of some strategies. *Acta Belgica Medica Physica* 11:151–163, 1988.

6. Porter, R., ed. The medical history of waters and spas. *Medical History* 10(Suppl.):1–44, 1990.

7. Pilgrim, J. A.; Mansfield, S.; and Marmot, M. Low blood pressure, low mood? *BMJ* 304:75–78, 1992.

8. Meador, C. K. The art and science of non disease. *N. Engl. J. Med.* 272: 92–94, 1965.

9. Foucault, M. *The Birth of the Clinic: An Archeology of Medical Perception,* translated by S. Smith. New York: Pantheon, 1973.

10. Spalding, J. C. Puritanism. In *Encyclopaedia Britannica,* 15th ed. 15:304–308, 1981.

11. Meyer, A. E. History of education: British America. In *Encyclopaedia Britannica,* 15th ed. 6:357–358, 1981.

12. Bercovitch, S. The Puritan origins of the American self. New Haven: Yale Univ. Press, 1975.

13. Emerson, E. Puritanism in America 1620–1750. Boston: Twayne Pub., 1977.

14. Peele, S. The conflict between public health goals and the temperance mentality. *Am. J. Public Health* 83:805–810, 1993.

15. Stampfer, M. J.; Rimm, E. B.; and Walsh, D. C. Commentary: Alcohol, the heart, and public policy. *Am. J. Public Health* 83:801–804, 1993.

16. Shaper, A. G. Editorial: Alcohol, the heart, and health. *Am. J. Public Health* 83:799–801, 1993.

17. Blackburn, H.; Waganaar, A.; and Jacobs, D. R. Alcohol: Good for your health? *Epidemiology* 2: 230–231, 1991.

18. Muldoon, M. F.; Manuck, S. B.; and Mathews, K. A. Lower cholesterol concentrations and mortality: A quantitative overview of primary prevention trials. *BMJ* 301:309–314, 1990.

19. Canadian Task Force on the Periodic Health Examination. Periodic health examination, 1993 update: Lowering the blood total cholesterol level to prevent coronary heart disease. *Can. Med. Assoc. J.* 148:521–538, 1993.

20. The Gallup Poll News Service. Princeton, NJ: Gallup, 7 Feb. 1992.

21. Goodwin, J. S.; Goodwin, J. M.; and Vogel, A. Knowledge and use of placebos by house officers and nurses. *Ann. Intern. Med.* 91:106–110, 1979.

22. Goodwin, J. M., and Goodwin, J. S. Le placebo: Histoire d'un concept. *Cahiers Médicaux* 7:1325–1327, 1982.

23. Laery, W. E. U.S. urges doctors to fight surgical pain (and myths). *New York Times* (6 March 1992): A1.

24. Von Roenn, J. H.; Cleeland, C. S.; Gonin, R.; et al. Physician attitudes and practice in cancer pain management. *Ann. Intern. Med.* 119:121–126, 1992.

25. Goodwin, J. S., and Goodwin, J. M. Failure to recognize efficacious therapies: A history of salicylate

use for rheumatoid arthritis. *Perspect. Biol. Med.* 25:78–92, 1981.

26. Zuckerman, B. S., and Hingson, R. Alcohol consumption in pregnancy: A critical review. *Dev. Med. Child. Neurol.* 28:649–661, 1986.

27. Larroque, B.; Kaminsky, M.; Lelong, N.; et al. Effects on birth weight of alcohol and caffeine consumption during pregnancy. *Am. J. Epidemiol.* 137: 941–950, 1993.

28. McClung, J. *Effects of High Altitude on Human Birth.* Cambridge: Harvard Univ. Press, 1969.

29. Qing, C.; Windsor, R. A.; Perkins, L.; et al. The impact of an infant birth weight and gestational age of cotinine-validated smoking reduction during pregnancy. *JAMA* 269:1519–1524, 1993.

30. Berkman, L. F., and Syme, S. L. Social networks, host resistance, and mortality: A nine year follow-up study of Alameda County residents. *Am J. Epidemiol.* 109:186–204, 1979.

31. House, J. S.; Robbins, C.; and Metzner, H. L. The association of social relationships and activities with mortality: Prospective evidence from the Tecumseh community health study. *Am. J. Epidemiol.* 116:123–140, 1982.

32. Schoenbach, V. J.; Kaplan, B. H.; Fredman, L.; et al. Social ties and mortality in Evans County, Georgia. *Am. J. Epidemiol.* 123:577–591, 1986.

33. Blazer, D. G. Social support and mortality in an elderly community population. *Am. J. Epidemiol.* 115:680–696, 1982.

34. Gruen, W. Effect of brief psychotherapy during the hospitalization period on the recovery process in heart attacks. *J. Consult. Clin. Psychol.* 43:223–232, 1975.

35. Raphael, B. Preventive intervention with the recently bereaved. *Arch. Gen. Psychiatry* 34:1450–1454, 1977.

36. Sosa, R.; Kennell, J.; Klaus, M.; et al. The effect of a supportive companion on perinatal problems, length of labor, and mother-infant interaction. *N. Engl. J. Med.* 303:597–600, 1980.

37. Spiegel, D.; Bloom, J. R.; Kraemer, H.; and Gottheil, E. Effect of psychosocial treatment on survival of patients with metastatic breast cancer. *Lancet* 2:888–891, 1989.

38. Cassel, J. The contribution of the social environment to host resistance. *Am. J. Epidemiol.* 104:107–123, 1976.

39. House, J. S.; Landis, K. R.; and Umberson, D. Social relationships and health. *Science* 241:540–546, 1988.

40. Goodwin, J. S.; Hunt, W. C.; Key, C. R.; and Samet, J. M. The effect of marital status on stage, treatment, and survival of cancer patients. *JAMA* 258:3125–3130, 1987.

41. Harris, T.; Cook, E. F.; Garrison, R.; et al. Body mass index and mortality among nonsmoking older persons. *JAMA* 259:1520–1524, 1988.

42. Grimes, D. A. Technology follies: The uncritical acceptance of medical innovation. *JAMA* 269:3030–3033, 1993.

43. Diamond, G. A., and Denton, T. A. Alternative perspectives on the biased foundations of medical technology assessment. *Ann. Intern. Med.* 118:455–464, 1993.

44. Black, W. C., and Welch, H. G. Advances in diagnostic imaging and overestimations of disease prevalence and the benefits of therapy. *N. Engl. J. Med.* 328:1237–1243, 1993.

45. Lee, J. M. Screening and informed consent. *N. Engl. J. Med.* 328:438–440, 1993.

46. Holnszel, W., and Kurihoro, M. Studies of Japanese migrants. *J. Nat. Cancer Inst.* 40:43–68, 1968.

47. Meikle, A. W. and Smith, J. A. Epidemiology of prostate cancer. *Urol. Clinics N. America* 17:709–718, 1990.

48. Goodwin, J. S., and Goodwin, J. M. The tomato effect: Rejection of highly efficacious therapies. *JAMA* 251:2387–2390, 1984.

Public Health as Social Justice

DAN E. BEAUCHAMP

ANTHONY DOWNS has observed that our most intractable public problems have two significant characteristics. First, they occur to a relative minority of our population (even though that minority may number millions of people). Second, they result in significant part from arrangements that are providing substantial benefits or advantages to a majority or to a powerful minority of citizens. Thus solving or minimizing these problems requires painful losses, the restructuring of society and the acceptance of new burdens by the most powerful and the most numerous on behalf of the least powerful or the least numerous. As Downs notes, this bleak reality has resulted in recent years in cycles of public attention to such problems as poverty, racial discrimination, poor housing, unemployment or the abandonment of the aged; however, this attention and interest rapidly wane when it becomes clear that solving these problems requires painful costs that the dominant interests in society are unwilling to pay. Our public ethics do not seem to fit our public problems.

It is not sufficiently appreciated that these same bleak realities plague attempts to protect the public's health. Automobile-related injury and death; tobacco, alcohol and other drug damage; the perils of the workplace; environmental pollution; the inequitable and ineffective distribution of medical care services; the hazards of biomedicine—all of these threats inflict death and disability on a minority of our society at any

DAN E. BEAUCHAMP, professor emeritus, dept. of health policy, management and behavior in the school of public health at the State University of New York (SUNY), Albany.

given time. Further, minimizing or even significantly reducing the death and disability from these perils entails that the majority or powerful minorities accept new burdens or relinquish existing privileges that they presently enjoy. Typically, these new burdens or restrictions involve more stringent controls over these and other hazards of the world.

This somber reality suggests that our fundamental attention in public health policy and prevention should not be directed toward a search for new technology, but rather toward breaking existing ethical and political barriers to minimizing death and disability. Thus is not to say that technology will never again help avoid painful social and political adjustments. Nonetheless, only the technological Pollyannas will ignore the mounting evidence that the critical barriers to protecting the public against death and disability are not the barriers to technological progress— indeed the evidence is that it is often technology itself that is our own worst enemy. The critical barrier to dramatic reductions in death and disability is a social ethic that unfairly protects the most numerous or the most powerful from the burdens of prevention.

This is the issue of justice. In the broadest sense, justice means that each person in society ought to receive his due and that the burdens and benefits of society should be fairly and equitably distributed. But what criteria should be followed in allocating burdens and benefits: Merit, equality or need? What end or goal in life should receive our highest priority: Life, liberty or the pursuit of happiness? The answer to these questions can be found in our prevailing theories or models of justice. These models of justice, roughly speaking, form the foundation of our politics and public policy in general, and our health policy (including our prevention policy) specifically. Here I am speaking of politics not as partisan politics but rather the more ancient and venerable meaning of the political as the search for the common good and the just society.

These models of justice furnish a symbolic framework or blueprint with which to think about and react to the problems of the public, providing the basic rules to classify and categorize problems of society as to whether they necessitate public and collective protection, or whether individual responsibility should prevail. These models function as a sort of map or guide to the common world of members of society, making visible some conditions in society as public issues and concerns, and hiding, obscuring or concealing other conditions that might otherwise emerge as public issues or problems were a different map or model of justice in hand.

In the case of health, these models of justice form the basis for thinking about and reacting to the problems of disability and premature death, in society. Thus, if public health policy requires that the majority or a powerful minority accept their fair share of the burdens of protecting a relative minority threatened with death or disability, we need to ask if our prevailing model of justice contemplates and legitimates such sacrifices.

MARKET-JUSTICE

The dominant model of justice in the American experience has been market-justice. Under the norms of market-justice people are entitled only to those valued ends such as status, income, happiness, etc., that they have acquired by fair rules of entitlement, e.g., by their own individual efforts, actions or abilities. Market-justice emphasizes individual responsibility, minimal collective action and freedom from collective obligations except to respect other persons' fundamental rights.

While we have as a society compromised pure market-justice in many ways to protect the public's health, we are far from recognizing the principle that death and disability are collective problems and that all persons are entitled to health protection. Society does not recognize a general obligation to protect the individual against disease and injury. While society does prohibit individuals from causing direct harm to others, and has in many instances regulated clear public health hazards, the norm of market-justice is still dominant and the primary duty to avert disease and injury still rests with the individual. The individual is ultimately alone in his or her struggle against death.

Barriers to Protection

This individual isolation creates a powerful barrier to the goal of protecting all human life by magnifying the power of death, granting to death an almost supernatural reality. Death has throughout history presented a basic problem to humankind, but even in an advanced society with enormous biomedical technology, the individualism of market-justice tends to retain and exaggerate pessimistic and fatalistic attitudes toward death and injury. This fatalism leads to a sense of powerlessness, to the acceptance of risk as an essential element of life, to resignation in the face of calamity, and to a weakening of collective impulses to confront the problems of premature death and disability.

Perhaps the most direct way in which market-justice undermines our resolve to preserve and protect human life lies in the primary freedom this ethic extends to all individuals and groups to act with minimal obligations to protect the common good. Despite the fact that this rule of self-interest predictably fails to protect adequately the safety of our workplaces, our modes of transportation, the physical environment, the commodities we consume, or the equitable and effective distribution of medical care, these failures have resulted so far in only half-hearted attempts at regulation and control. This response is explained in large part by the powerful sway market-justice holds over our imagination, granting fundamental freedom to all individuals to be left alone—even if the "individuals" in question are giant producer groups with enormous capacities to create great public harm through sheer inadvertence. Efforts for truly effective controls over these perils must constantly struggle against a prevailing ethical paradigm that defines as threats to fundamental freedoms attempts to assure that all groups—even powerful producer groups—accept their fair share of the burdens of prevention.

Market-justice is also the source of another major barrier to public health measures to minimize death and disability—the category of voluntary behavior. Market-justice forces a basic distinction between the harm caused by a factory polluting the atmosphere and the harm caused by the cigarette or alcohol industries, because in the latter case those that are harmed are perceived as engaged in "voluntary" behavior. It is the radical individualism inherent in the market model that encourages attention to the individual's behavior and inattention to the social preconditions of that behavior. In the case of smoking, these preconditions include a powerful cigarette industry and accompanying social and cultural forces encouraging the practice of smoking. These social forces include norms sanctioning smoking as well as all forms of media, advertising, literature, movies, folklore, etc. Since the smoker is free in some ultimate sense to not smoke, the norms of market-justice force the conclusion that the individual voluntarily "chooses" to smoke; and we are prevented from taking strong collective action against the powerful structures encouraging this so-called voluntary behavior. . . .

The prestige of medical care encouraged by market-justice prevents large-scale research to determine whether, in fact, our medical care technology actually brings about the result desired— a significant reduction in the damage and losses

suffered from disease and injury. The model conceals questions about our pervasive use of drugs, our intense specialization, and our seemingly boundless commitment to biomedical technology. Instead, the market model of justice encourages us to see problems as due primarily to the failure of individual doctors and the quality of their care, rather than to recognize the possibility of failure from the structure of medical care itself. Consequently, we seek to remedy problems by trying to change individual doctors through appeals to their ethical sensibilities, or by reshaping their education, or by creating new financial incentives. . . .

Public Health Measures

I have saved for last an important class of health policies—public health measures to protect the environment, the workplace, or the commodities we purchase and consume. Are these not signs that the American society is willing to accept collective action in the face of clear public health hazards?

I do not wish to minimize the importance of these advances to protect the public in many domains. But these separate reforms, taken alone, should be cautiously received. This is because each reform effort is perceived as an isolated exception to the norm of market-justice; the norm itself still stands. Consequently, the predictable career of such measures is to see enthusiasm for enforcement peak and wane. These public health measures are clear signs of hope. But as long as these actions are seen as merely minor exceptions to the rule of individual responsibility, the goals of public health will remain beyond our reach. What is required is for the public to see that protecting the public's health takes us beyond the norms of market-justice categorically, and necessitates a completely new health ethic.

I return to my original point: Market-justice is the primary roadblock to dramatic reductions in preventable injury and death. More than this, market-justice is a pervasive ideology protecting the most powerful or the most numerous from the burdens of collective action. If this be true, the central goal of public health should be ethical in nature: The challenging of market-justice as fatally deficient in protecting the health of the public. Further, public health should advocate a "counter-ethic" for protecting the public's health, one articulated in a different tradition of justice and one designed to give the highest priority to minimizing death and disability and to the protection of all human life against the hazards of this world. . . .

Ideally . . . the public health ethic is not simply an alternative to the market ethic for health — it is a fundamental critique of that ethic as it unjustly protects powerful interests from the burdens of prevention and as that ethic serves to legitimate a mindless and extravagant faith in the efficacy of medical care. In other words, the public health ethic is a *counter-ethic* to market-justice and the ethics of individualism as these are applied to the health problems of the public.

This view of public health is admittedly not widely accepted. Indeed, in recent times the mission of public health has been viewed by many as limited to that minority of health problems that cannot be solved by the market provision of medical care services and that necessitate organized community action. It is interesting to speculate why many in the public health profession have come to accept this narrow view of public health — a view that is obviously influenced and shaped by the market model as it attempts to limit the burdens placed on powerful groups.

Nonetheless, the broader view of public health set out here is logically and ethically justified if one accepts the vision of public health as being the protection of all human life. The central task of public health, then, is to complete its unfinished revolution: The elaboration of a health ethic adequate to protect and preserve all human life. This new ethic has several key implications which are referred to here as "principles": 1) Controlling the hazards of this world, 2) to prevent death and disability, 3) through organized collective action, 4) shared equally by all except where unequal burdens result in increased protection of everyone's health and especially potential victims of death and disability. . . .

I do not see these goals of public health as hopelessly unrealistic nor destructive of fundamental liberties. Public health may be an "alien ethic in a strange land." Yet, if anything, the public health ethic is more faithful to the traditions of Judeao-Christian ethics than is market-justice.

The image of public health that I have drawn here does raise legitimate questions about what it is to be a professional, and legitimate questions about reasonable limits to restrictions on human liberty. These questions must be addressed more thoroughly than I have done here. Nonetheless, we must never pass over the chaos of preventable disease and disability in our society by simply celebrating the benefits of our prosperity and abundance, or our technological advances. What are these benefits worth if they have been purchased at the price of human lives?

Trust and Distrust in Professional Ethics

EDMUND D. PELLEGRINO

Ademantus. "I wonder men dare trust themselves with men."

— *Timon of Athens*, 1.2.43

INTRODUCTION

Trust is ineradicable in human relationships.
Without it, we could not live in society or attain
even the rudiments of a fulfilling life. Without
trust, we could not anticipate the future and we
would therefore be paralyzed into inaction. Yet
to trust and entrust is to become vulnerable and
dependent on the good will and motivations of
those we trust. Trust, ineradicable as it is, is also
always problematic.

To be sure, there have always been professionals who violated trust but they were the moral
renegades and pariahs. Not until recently has the
central place of trust in professional ethics been
seriously doubted or attacked, not only as an illusion, but even as a radical impossibility.[1] Indeed,
what amounts to an ethics of distrust has been
gathering force. It would place higher restraints
on professionals or eliminate the need for trust
entirely. To this end, alternatives to trust in the
ethics of the professions are proposed—reducing
professional relationships to contracts or appointing ombudsmen or other intermediaries to
monitor the advice and actions of professionals.

EDMUND D. PELLEGRINO is a John Carroll professor of
medicine and medical ethics at Georgetown University.
He was also awarded Georgetown's 1998 Laetare Medal.

To advance the ethics of trust against the
ethics of distrust we shall first examine the phenomenon of trust, both in general and in the
professional context. Then we shall examine the
rise of the ethics of distrust and its inherent falla-
cies, and finally, the inescapable obligations that
the ineradicability of trust imposes on professionals and on patients as well.

Bernard Barber, a sociologist, identifies trust
with the expectation that social actors will observe three conditions: (1) they will act within a
persistent moral order, (2) they will perform
their technical roles competently, and (3) roles
that require a special concern for others, such as
the fiduciary role, will be faithfully fulfilled.[2] So
far as professions go, Barber sees three distinctive characteristics that have a special bearing on
trust: (a) their possession of powerful knowledge, (b) the autonomy necessary to their practice, and (c) their fiduciary obligation to individuals and society.[3] Barber's analysis is largely
descriptive, and it treats the moral foundations
of trust only indirectly. . . .

While trust aims to reduce complexity, it also
unavoidably involves contingency. Some attempt to avoid contingency by distrust—by
withdrawing confidence in the expectation that
the person trusted will not abuse that confidence. But, at the same time, distrust reduces the
range of possible human relationships and thus
the fulfillment one can attain in life. Obviously,
all but the most reclusive humans can, or would
want to, rule their lives by trust rather than distrust.

From Edmund D. Pellegrino, Robert M. Veatch, and John P. Langan, S.J., Editors, Ethics, Trust,
and the Professions: Philosophical and Cultural Aspects. *(1991). Permission granted by Georgetown
University Press.*

Luhmann seeks a possible way out of the risks inherent in trust by transferring trust from person-to-person relationships to "system trust." Confidence is placed in institutional and social structures to reduce complexity by the restraints they impose on individuals who function within them. This seems a highly problematic solution, given that the relationships between individuals and institutions are neither less notably complex nor more notably reliable than person-to-person relationships.

Annette Baier has undertaken the ambitious task of a formal inquiry into the nature of trust, a subject that has been neglected in philosophical discourse.

Baier defines trust as "reliance on others' competence and willingness to look after, rather than harm, the things one cares about which are entrusted to their care."[4] She defines different kinds of trust relationships; the differences between promise, contracts, and trust, and the conditions that make trust "morally decent." She emphasizes the vulnerability involved in trusting another person, the indispensability and dangers of discretionary power given the one trusted, and the necessity of confidence that the trusting person's vulnerability will not be exploited, even if the one trusted has motives for doing so. Baier's inquiry illustrates the complexity of trust and the need for a better understanding of the philosophical foundations for morally valid trust relationships. . . .

Most construals of trust involve several elements, the strength and combinations of which vary with the nature of the relationship between the person trusted and the person trusting. One element is confidence that expectations of fidelity to what is entrusted will be fulfilled. Second, is the sense that the person trusted has explicitly or implicitly made a promise to act well with respect to the interests of the person trusted. Third, is the belief that discretionary latitude of certain proportions is necessary if trust is to be fulfilled, and that the one trusted will use it well, neither assuming too much nor too little. Fourth, is the congruence of understanding on these first three

elements between the one trusting and the one trusted. Finally, underlying all of these aspects is an act of faith in the benevolence and good character of the one trusted. Each of these five elements takes on a special meaning in the special context of relationships with professionals.

Trust in Relationships with Professionals

Like other human relationships, our relationships with professionals ineradicably involve trust. Here, trust has special moral dimensions which are the foundation for professional ethics, what Barber has called "fiduciary relationships."[5] Trust in the helping professions—medicine, law, ministry, and teaching—has many features in common. Each relationship deserves examination in its own right, but only one will be examined here. The medical relationship will serve to illustrate the way trust shapes the ethical relationships between patients and physicians, and by analogy the relationships between lawyers and clients, ministers and parishioners, and teachers and students.

People seek out physicians when some adverse sign or symptom threatens their conception of their health sufficiently to impel them to seek expert advice. As soon as persons decide they need help, they become "patients"—they "bear" a burden of anxiety, pain, or suffering. To seek professional help is to trust that physicians possess the capacity to help and heal. From the very first moment, the patient makes an act of trust: first, in the existence and utility of medical knowledge itself, and then in its possession by the one who is being consulted. Trust at this initial level is more like what Baier calls "reliance," the kind of trust we place in airline pilots, firemen, or policemen—a trust inspired less by the person than the common recognition of a defined social role.[6] It is an expression of general confidence somewhat akin to Luhmann's "system trust."

If we take medical relationships as our paradigm case, we recognize a certain amount of trust in the system of education, credentialing, and the processes of licensure. But the intimacy, specificity, and personal nature of relationships with physicians compel us to be more concerned with personal qualities—with personality, but most of all with character.[7] Except in emergencies, at the earliest stages of a medical relationship, we are freer than we are in the choice of our pilot. We can consult other physicians, former patients, and credentials, as well as do research on the advice we receive. Here, the system can serve to establish or reinforce trust.

But before we engage this presumably competent physician, we are interested in much more. We expect to open the most private domains of our bodies, minds, social and family relationships to her probing gaze. Our vices, foibles, and weaknesses will be exposed to a stranger. Even our living and dying will engage her attention and invite her counsel. This is not at all like our trust in the pilot. The "system" cannot provide the reassurances we may want. Ultimately, we must place our trust in the person of the physician. We want someone who knows about us and treats us nonjudgmentally and is still concerned with our welfare. We will want someone who will use the discretionary latitude our care requires with circumspection—neither intruding nor presuming too much nor undertaking too little. We must be able to trust her to do what she is trusted to do, i.e., to serve the healing purposes for which we have given our trust in the first place.

We must trust also that our vulnerability will not be exploited for power, profit, prestige, or pleasure. The physician or lawyer's superior knowledge and skill foreordains inequality in the relationship. Even if we are physicians or lawyers ourselves, our capacity for objectivity is compromised when we are ill or named in a lawsuit. We know we can be deceived or led to the choice the lawyer or physician wants by the way he or she selects the facts about what can be done to help us. We can, to be sure, elicit other opinions, read for ourselves about our illnesses, or speak to other patients. But, ultimately, we must decide not only what we should do, but who will do it.

What we want and what the doctor prescribes may be in conflict. We have to choose between our own judgment and that of someone we trust to have knowledge and a commitment to our well-being.

No professional can function properly without discretionary latitude. The more discretionary latitude we permit our professionals, the more vulnerable we become. Yet to limit that latitude is to limit the capacity for good as much as it may limit the capacity for harm. When all is said and done, we cannot anticipate every contingency even in a disease we understand well. Chronically ill patients often understand their illnesses better than physicians. Yet they can also be distressingly misinformed. At some point even our intimate knowledge of our needs must be translated into action. That action will be taken by another person, the physician, or lawyer, or minister on whom we are forced to depend if our goals are to be realized.

We can consult different authorities about our medical, legal, or spiritual problems. We may evaluate their logic, the evidence they adduce, or their compatibility with our personal values. Yet when there are differences among experts we must choose among them. And when we do, we really are choosing the professional we think we can trust to carry out our wishes and respect our values in carrying them out. Even then, every iota of our evaluation of our own situation may not be perfectly congruent with that of our physician, lawyer or minister. . . .

Let us suppose that a physician has been chosen because his opinion and recommendation after our investigations seem more credible than his colleague's. We still have the question of skill in carrying out the recommendations. How does one check on skill? Some patients seek out a surgeon's morbidity and mortality statistics or the opinions of her peers. Here we must trust the surgeon's honesty in reporting or the objectivity of her peers. We would find out that all surgeons have a certain irreducible mortality and morbidity. We must trust that the one we have chosen will have the skill requisite for a beneficial outcome.

Even the most distrustful and skeptical patient must at some point confront the fact that the physician is the final pathway through which all things medical must funnel. It is the physician who writes the orders, performs the procedure, and interprets the recommendations of other health professionals. The physician is a de facto "gatekeeper" who we trust to be the patient's advocate, and not simply an instrument of social, institutional, or fiscal policies.[8] Depending on his character and fidelity of trust, he may treat the patient as a statistical entity or he may be the patient's last protection against the "system." These contingencies are all exacerbated by the fact that trust in professional relationships is forced; it is trust generated by our need for help. When we need a doctor, lawyer, or minister, we have no choice but to trust someone, though we might prefer to trust none.

Living wills are a good example of attempts to supplant trust by contractual agreement. They seek to make the wishes of patients explicit to family and physician, particularly regarding terminal care. Morally and legally they have the same force as a competent patient's decision. They can settle or avoid disputes about what is in the patient's best interests. They also forewarn the physician, who may choose not to enter the relationship if he or she disagrees with the patient's values.

But living wills cannot specify every detail and every contingency. They are open to interpretation, particularly the physician's or family's understanding of what the patient meant by "ordinary" or "extraordinary" measures or doing "everything possible."

If living wills are written too tightly, they limit the physician's discretionary latitude in ways the patient might not really want. If written too broadly, they leave too much room for dispute and presumption. Living wills must be implemented through human agency. Those who write them must trust that those who eventually carry out their wishes act out of good will. In short, living wills cannot supplant trust because their execution depends on it.

Replacing trust relationships by contracts for care is equally dependent upon trust. Contracts can diminish the risk of frustration of the patient's will, but again they are based on trust that the things agreed to will, in fact, be performed. Contracts cannot envision all contingencies. They must allow discretionary latitude to the professional or they are self-defeating.

Moreover, the whole concept of a contract between someone who is ill, in need of justice, or worried about salvation, and the professional who can help meet those needs, is illusory. Contracts are negotiated between equals or near equals. This is simply not the case in relationships with doctors, lawyers, or ministers. Contractors must also trust that there is understanding of mutual interest beyond the phraseology of the contract. The same words only too often carry different meanings. The frequency with which breach of contract is alleged is ample testimony that there is implicit trust even in the most explicitly worded agreement.

It is clear from the empirical and from the conceptual points of view that trust cannot be eliminated from human relationships, least of all relationships with professionals. Given this fact, an ethic based on mistrust and suspicion must, by the nature of human relationships, ultimately fail. To be sure, living wills, contracts if one wants them, durable powers of attorney, or appointment of a patient advocate or health care manager can diminish some of the vulnerability of trust relationships. In the end, however, all of these arrangements displace trust from the physician or professional and locate it elsewhere—but trust remains. . . .

THE ETHOS AND ETHICS OF DISTRUST

The Milieu of Medical Practice

Distrust of professionals, especially doctors, is not a new phenomenon. Venal, greedy, incompetent, dishonest, and insensitive professionals have never been a rarity. They have been the satirists' favorites for a long time.[9] Their acid comments had their origins in real experiences of the sick. In part, they arose from the gross misbehavior of professionals themselves and in part from the hostility of the sick to fate which forces them to seek out physicians and then to pay for something they do not want in the first place. Because of our resentment at our loss of freedom, and at the powerlessness that serious illness imposes on all of us, the physician, good or bad, has always been a lightning rod for the frustrations of the sick.

In the last two or three decades, these perennial sources of distrust have been reinforced and expanded by a wide variety of events within and outside medicine—the malpractice crisis; the commercialization of medical care by advertising and entrepreneurism; the excessive income and free-spending life-style of some physicians; the bottom-line, marketplace, "pay-before-we-treat" policies of hospitals and some doctors; the depersonalization of large group prepayment practices; physicians' growing preferences for nine-to-five jobs and time off; the retreat from general to specialty practice; the early retirements—the list is long and growing daily.

As a result, patients, as the opinion polls show, increasingly think doctors are less available and less interested in them and more interested in money than they used to be. In self-defense, patients feel they must take charge of their own care, do their own research about their symptoms and their doctors, and even order their own tests to become as informed as the doctor to be sure of getting good care. The doctor is, in this view, merely one resource among many.

The eroding effect of these attitudes on the trust relationship is clear. Wariness replaces trust. Physicians and patients approach each other as potential enemies rather than friends. Patients perceive doctors as less interested in them than in their money, more interested in time off than service, and more the exploiters than stewards of medical knowledge. For many, the whole enterprise of medicine has increasingly called forth the principle of "caveat emptor" rather than the principles of fidelity to trust, beneficence, and effacement of self-interest.

These erosive tendencies within medicine have been reinforced by powerful forces within the social fabric of our times. Participatory democracy, better public education, the attention of the media, a mistrust of authority and experts in general—all have weakened the trust relationship. On the positive side, they encourage greater independence in patient decisions and thus help to neutralize the traditional paternalism of the professions. This is a salubrious move to more adult, open, and honest relationships. Indeed, now the problem is often the absolutization of autonomy which must be tempered by the interests of third parties, and the moral right of physicians to refuse to do what they consider to be unethical. The line between healthy protection of patients' autonomy and dangerous depreciation of medical expertise is becoming more difficult to define.

The Ethos and Ethics of Distrust

An ethos of distrust asserts the radical impossibility of trust to professional relationships. Using medicine as an example, the ethics of distrust asserts that physicians cannot know all of a patient's values, that medicine deals only with a subset of things important to human fulfillment, and that physicians by the very nature of their profession necessarily place medical values over all other values. Moreover, since physicians are human they have personal values which they cannot suppress. Physicians, therefore, select and weigh the facts to be presented on the basis of their own rather than the patient's perceptions of what is good. Even so-called medical facts are tinged with value desiderata to such a degree that there are no value-free facts. Finally, we cannot trust in some standard of virtues inherent in professional practices which will protect the patient against the doctor's value system. The virtues of a profession are not intrinsic to that profession but derivative from a wide variety of ethical and philosophical systems. There is nothing in the nature of medicine, law, or ministry per se that entails honesty, compassion, fidelity to trust, or suppression of self-interest; the so-called internal morality of the professions is a fiction. On this view, an ethos of distrust assumes the formal character of an ethics of distrust.

An ethics of distrust entails that professionals and those who seek their help assume primarily a self-protective stance. Patients must seek strict contractual relationships with their doctors. Specific instructions as to care must be spelled out by patients and must be observed to the letter by physicians. In addition, for further protection, some insist on the interjection of a presumably objective third party who will be the patient's advocate in place of the physician and who will monitor the physician's compliance with the terms of the contract.

The ethos and ethics of distrust confers a legalistic quality on relationships with professionals— one which leads to ethical minimalism. Professionals will tend to limit themselves to the precise letter of agreement. They will feel free of the expectation that they are advocates, counsellors, and protectors of the patient's welfare. The professional's necessity to efface self-interest will be blunted since legalistic and contractual relationships call upon the participants to protect their own self-interest, not that of the other party—except to the extent the contract requires. The impetus to do the "extra" that requires some compromise of self-interest is blunted if not destroyed entirely. These attitudes are already evident in professional relationships. They will be legitimated and reinforced by an ethos based in mistrust. . . .

THE ETHICS OF TRUST RESTRUCTURED

Trust in professionals can no longer be absolute or open ended, much as physicians and even some patients might wish it to be. Public education about medicine and medical ethics, the prominence of patient autonomy as a central principle of professional ethics, the potential conflict between the physician's and patient's best interests—all necessitate a more restricted and realistic view. Nevertheless, the ineradicability of trust mandates that it remain a central element in any coherent ethic of the professions.

Since trust is a permanent feature of human relating, fidelity to trust is an indispensable virtue of the good professional—lawyer, doctor, minister, or teacher. Without this virtue, the relationship with a professional cannot attain its end. It becomes a lie and a means of exploitation of vulnerability rather than a means of helping and healing. If there is any meaning to professional ethics, it must revolve around the obligation of fidelity to trust.

In an ethic of trust the physician is impelled to develop a relationship with the patient from the very outset which includes developing familiarity with who, and what, the patient is and how he or she wants to meet the serious challenges of illness, disability, and death. It is essential that the physician help the patient to anticipate certain critical decisions such as withholding or withdrawing life-sustaining treatments, cardiopulmonary resuscitation, request for assisted death, abortion, and the like. The physician must prepare for these eventualities before they become urgent or the patient loses competence. Patients should be able to rely on the physician for the proper timing, sensitivity, and degree of detail appropriate in each case. These cannot be written into a contract. They must be entrusted to the physician or some physician substitute.

In an ethics of trust, the physician is obliged to present clinical data as free as possible of personal or professional bias. Fidelity to trust precludes manipulation, coercion, or deception in obtaining consent. It requires assisting patients to perform the calculus of effectiveness, benefit, and burden as carefully as the situation permits. What is known must be distinguished from what is uncertain, or simply, unknown. The indispensability of keeping information up to date is obvious. Consultation with or reference to those with more experience or skill or with closer congruence with the patient's values is required. When patient and physician values are sharply at variance, the physician should decline to enter the relationship or withdraw from it graciously, with candor, and without recrimination.

A realistic ethic of trust does not absolutize the professional's fiduciary role. Nor does it ignore the realities that may compromise trust— for example, the potential intrusion of the physician's personal and professional values, the complexity of the notion of the patient's best interests, the difficulty of disassociating fact and value.

Nor does an ethic of trust ignore the sad facts of incompetence, quackery, fraud, inadequate self-regulation, and peer review of the addicted and alcoholic professional. To recognize the ineradicability of trust is not therefore to argue against regulation of the professional by licensure, educational and certification procedures, quality controls, periodic relicensure, and liability laws. Professionals are ordinary humans called by the nature of the activities in which they engage to extraordinary degrees of obligation and trust. Living wills, durable power of attorney, and inquiries into competence are all legitimate measures those who seek professional help are entitled to invoke. A certain degree of distrust based on experience of the caprices of human behavior is unavoidable.

But these reasonable constraints on trust do not justify an ethic of distrust which takes fidelity to trust relationships to be invalid and impossible. That trust may be violated in varying degrees does not entail the inevitability of its violation. Moreover, even if all the current measures which

place restraint on trust were implemented, an ineffaceable residuum of trust would remain. It is with the acknowledgement of this residuum, its enhancement and strengthening, that an ethic of trust is most concerned. A restructured ethic of trust therefore recognizes simultaneously the origins of distrust and the ineradicability of trust.

On balance, an ethic of trust is more realistic, conceptually sounder, and phenomenologically more consistent than an ethic of distrust. To highlight trust in professional relationships, to make it explicit and more precise, is to provide the very protection an ethic of distrust seeks but cannot reach. Older notions of absolute trust are inadequate and were always so. What is needed is a redefinition of trust relationships consistent with the contemporary context of autonomy, participatory democracy, and the moral pluralism of the interacting parties in professional relationships. . . .

NOTES

1. R. M. Veatch, "Is Trust of Professionals a Coherent Concept?"

2. Bernard Barber, *The Logic of Limits of Trust* (New Brunswick, NJ: Rutgers University Press, 1983), 9.

3. Ibid., 135.

4. Annette Baier, "Trust and Anti-Trust," *Ethics* 96 (January 1986): 259.

5. Barber, 14–16.

6. Baier, 245.

7. E. D. Pellegrino, "Character, Virtue and Self-Interest in the Ethics of the Professions," *The Journal of Contemporary Health Law and Policy* 4 (Spring 1989): 53–73.

8. E. D. Pellegrino, "Rationing Health Care: The Ethics of Medical Gate-keeping," *The Journal of Contemporary Health Law and Policy* 2 (1986): 23–45.

9. Mary B. Mahowald, "The Physician," in R. W. Clarke and R. O. Lawry, eds., *The Power of the Professions* (Lanham, Md.: University Press of America, 1988), 119–31.

Culture, Healing, and Professional Obligations

JOSEPH CARRESE, KATE BROWN, ANDREW JAMETON

DR. LEIGH MUSED silently over a cup of coffee after a busy day at the Oakside Community Clinic. "So how far am I supposed to go with cultural sensitivity, anyway?" she asked herself. This question arose from the lingering doubt she felt about how she had responded earlier that day to a patient's mother, Ms. Ying Saeto.

Ms. Saeto had brought her youngest child, Marie, into the clinic for her four-month immunizations. Marie is a lively, healthy baby who is growing normally, in the 65th percentile for her age. Dr. Leigh usually enjoys Ms. Saeto's visits and has learned much about the Iu Mien culture of Ms. Saeto's native Laos from their conversations. Ms. Saeto's excellent English and her willingness to share information about Mien cultural heritage have allowed Dr. Leigh to understand better the many Mien living in the vicinity, who use the clinic for (at least some of) their health care needs.

Ms. Saeto was born in Laos, but at the end of the Vietnam War she fled with her family and neighbors and was finally resettled in the U.S. with her grandparents when she was fourteen. Her first year in America was hard for Ms. Saeto. When she became more comfortable with her new environment, she went through what she now calls a "rebellious stage." She refused to speak Mien except with her grandparents, who never learned English. A part-time job provided money and independence, enabling her to feel less like an outcast in school. But Ms. Saeto did not have many years in this new life as an American high school student. She became pregnant before graduating and she left school. The father of her baby drifted away, leaving her without support except for her grandparents and the Iu Mien community. She was welcomed home.

Ms. Saeto has since married a Mien man. They live with his mother and their three babies and her first child. She says, "Now I am a Mien woman." She finds great value in the sense of belonging. She is proud of her growing knowledge of Mien traditions and beliefs and eagerly informs Dr. Leigh about Mien spirits, ceremonies, and cures during her visits to the clinic.

Today Ms. Saeto had not hesitated to explain the meaning of the burns on her baby's stomach. "Burns?!" Dr. Leigh asked incredulously as she looked at the five red and blistered quarter-inch round markings on the child's abdomen. Ms. Saeto explained that she had used a traditional Mien cure for pain because she suspected that Marie had a case of "Gusia mun toe." This is a rare folk illness among Mien babies characterized by restlessness, unremitting crying, agitation, constipation, and loss of appetite. A particular characteristic of the syndrome is that a baby will keep "throwing her head back" when held.

The cure she used involves burning a "string" of the inner pulp found in a special reed. The pulp is dipped lightly in pork fat and then lit. The flame is then passed quickly over the skin

From the Hastings Center Report (July–Aug. 1993): 15–17. Reprinted by permission of Joseph Carrese, Kate Brown, Andrew Jameton, and The Hastings Center. Copyright The Hastings Center.

above the pain site, raising a blister that pops— "like popcorn," she said—indicating that the illness is not related to spiritual causes. If no blisters arise, then it is possible that a shaman will be needed to conduct a spirit ritual for a cure.

Depending on the severity of illness, 3, 5, 7, or even 11 burns might be made. Before the flame is extinguished, it is used to burn a spot on a wall of the room (or a block of wood) systematically, transferring the pain. "The wall doesn't feel, so let the wall suffer instead of this person," the person performing the cure says. "Wall, let the pain go on in you forever, let the pain off this person." The burns are then covered with Tiger Balm, a mentholated cream.

Ms. Saeto explained that the original pain will usually subside within a half-hour and any pain from the burning will be gone within the hour. In her experience infection is rare, and the burns heal in a week or so. Sometimes scars remain afterward, but these are not thought to be disfiguring; they are simply recognized as the result of this treatment.

Ms. Saeto explained that this method of cure was dangerous for children. Dr. Leigh readily concurred, but soon discovered that their ideas about the dangerousness of burning children did not match at all. Ms. Saeto explained that this cure must be done by someone skilled in burning, like her mother-in-law, because if a burn is placed too near to the line between the baby's mouth and her bellybutton, the baby could become mute or even retarded. In Marie's case the cure had been successful, according to Ms. Saeto. The child had stopped crying immediately, calmed down, and regained her appetite uneventfully. Upon examination, Dr. Leigh found no reason to suspect otherwise.

Dr. Leigh had gone ahead with Marie's immunizations, noting to herself that the procedure considerably disturbed the baby's contentment, and wondering—not for the first time— about the pain she routinely inflicted upon children in the course of her practice. She had not mentioned her misgivings about Ms. Saeto's

practice of burning her baby. But now, at the end of the day, Dr. Leigh wondered if she should have said something. After all, didn't she think it was cruel to burn babies? Didn't she *know* it was dangerous, and not for the reasons that Ms. Saeto had stated?

COMMENTARY BY JOSEPH CARRESE

Doing the right thing in clinical medicine, always a challenge, is even more complicated when providers and patients are from different cultures. Our ability to consider this case in an informed and thoughtful manner may be hindered by our lack of knowledge of Mien culture generally and Ying Saeto's local world particularly. Mutual unfamiliarity, of course, is paradigmatic of cross-cultural encounters. Nonetheless, we can raise several points to consider when addressing moral conflicts in cross-cultural settings.

One is that the meaning we assign to various ideas and concepts is culturally based. For example, in the Hippocratic tradition physicians are admonished to benefit patients, or at least do no harm. This seemingly straightforward maxim is rendered ambiguous in the cross-cultural setting precisely because abstract concepts like benefit and harm take on meaning only in the context of culture, and in the give and take of peoples' everyday lives, relationships, and experiences. What a Mien person considers beneficial or harmful may differ profoundly from Western biomedical notions of benefit and harm.

Not only may people from different cultures attach different meanings to similar concepts and principles, but additionally unfamiliar—even unimaginable—concepts and principles may be a central feature of the moral landscape. For exam-

JOSEPH CARRESE, M.D. is an assistant professor of medicine, Johns Hopkins Bayview Medical Center.

ple, an important concept in traditional Navajo culture is *hózhǫ́*, which is approximated in meaning by combining the Western notions of beauty, harmony, order, good, and happiness. There is no equivalent concept in Anglo-American culture. Conversely, in traditional Navajo culture there is nothing comparable to the Western concept of risk, an idea that fundamentally shapes and permeates Western medicine. The broader point here is that Western biomedicine too is a cultural system, reflecting a particular set of concepts and principles and a unique way of construing the world. Confronting that which appears strange and different invites refection on that which is familiar; both exist and can only be appreciated in context.

The fact that the patient in this case is a child complicates matters further. Some providers may be comfortable with the idea of respecting cultural differences when the patient is a competent adult, but with children they may be unwilling to tolerate decisions that result in what they perceive to be compromised care or harm, even when these decisions make sense in the context of a particular culture. There is certainly precedent for this distinction in American law, most notably in cases involving Jehovah's Witnesses and Christian Scientists. Yet one might ponder in what sense we truly respect another culture if we interfere with its transfer to the next generation.

Mapping unfamiliar moral landscapes and interpreting foreign moral vocabularies may benefit from an ethnographic approach. Ethnography positions itself at the interface of different traditions and different systems of meaning, and may be useful for: (1) identifying the culturally relevant values, principles, and concepts of a particular group; (2) discerning the meaning(s) the cultural group assigns to those principles and concepts; (3) gaining insight into the culturally appropriate way of doing things; and (4) beginning to understand the social, political, and historical forces that constitute the larger context in which individual cross-cultural relationships are embedded. This information is crucial to determining what the ethical course of action is when providers and patients do not share a common cultural background.

An ethnographic approach to ethics in the cross-cultural setting need not result in a strict ethical relativism. One can be respectful of cultural differences *and* recognize that there are atrocities and violations of fundamental human rights which agents from diverse perspectives would judge as morally unacceptable. Here the perceived degree of harm is critical: if great enough it may outweigh our duty to respect cultural differences.

In deciding "how far to go with cultural sensitivity," ethical limits should be set only after a careful, thoughtful, and imaginative effort to understand and interpret, in context, that which appears strange and problematic. This decision should be accompanied by a sincere and critical reflection on one's own position and its historical and cultural underpinnings. Attention should also be given to who is at the table and which perspectives are represented when decisions are made about the fundamental rights and principles to be respected.

Finally, Western physicians caring for non-Western patients should acknowledge that in the cross-cultural setting they are representatives of a dominant culture and thus may have the power to impose and enforce their views in ways their patients do not. Health care providers must therefore be sensitive to inequities of power and manage them responsibly.

In the case presented, the physician's first response to Ms. Saeto should not be to educate her, thereby disabusing her of her "folk beliefs." Rather, the physician's effort should be directed primarily to understanding Ms. Saeto in the context of her world, and to explaining the physician's perspective to her. Interpretation in both directions is required.

A cross-cultural ethical conflict, like ethical dilemmas in other settings, may not have a single, ethically correct resolution, but many possible resolutions, each with ethical costs and advantages. However, which resolutions are ultimately considered will depend on which voices are included in the moral dialogue — and in the cross-cultural setting more than one voice must be heard.

COMMENTARY BY KATE BROWN AND ANDREW JAMETON

This case illustrates a number of complex issues clinicians face when patients' culturally appropriate treatments are at odds with the clinician's methods of therapy. Our general view in such cases is that there are good reasons for respecting culturally differing practices, particularly when they fit into a larger rationale of explanations for health and illness, good and evil. Ms. Saeto's belief, as recounted here, appears to be well grounded in her culture; it is practiced widely; the reasons for it are widely understood among the Iu Mien; the procedure, from a Mien point of view, works; Ms. Saeto's application of the procedure, as recounted here, appears in accordance with Mien customs and not merely a personal and culturally unaccepted practice. This rules out concerns that her actions stemmed from ill-will, insanity, irrationality, and the like.

One reason for respecting cultural diversity rests on the observation that community membership, participation, and shared symbolism are important sources of human happiness and health, apart from any validity of the symbols with reference to science or to reality. In this case, Ms. Saeto clearly derives a sense of identity and security from her status within the Mien community. Given Ms. Saeto's history and social circumstances, it might be destructive for Dr.

KATE BROWN is an associate professor, Center for Health Policy and Ethics, Creighton University, Omaha, Neb.; Andrew Jameton is associate professor and head of the section on humanities and law, Department of Preventive and Societal Medicine, University of Nebraska Medical Center.

Leigh to undermine Ms. Saeto's affiliation with this cultural group.

A second justification for respect in such cases is that they offer opportunity to extend human knowledge by finding wisdom in dissimilar cultural practices, especially ones as ancient as the Chinese tradition, thought to be the source of the Mien practice of moxibustion. Many traditional therapies have provided theoretical clues and practical remedies for the treatment of disease. These traditional sources create a presumption of seriousness and warrant investigating possible applications to contemporary settings.

Furthermore, openness to other paradigms can stimulate clinicians like Dr. Leigh to examine critically the cultural norms of their own practices. Dental and injection pain and vaccination scars are seen as easily justified from a Western medical perspective. And she can reflect ironically on more questionable practices, such as the widespread use of painful and highly technological procedures, many of questionable benefit, against a background of dismal public health figures as compared with other industrialized nations. An unreflective challenge to moxibustion could rightly be seen as ethnocentric or even racist against the background of Dr. Leigh's professional culture.

On the other hand, as also voiced by Dr. Leigh, it may be impossible and inappropriate to suspend clinical training and judgment in favor of "cultural sensitivity," even when based on the good reasons we have mentioned. The need for membership in community has also been used to justify much cruelty in the past — were someone to argue that we should tolerate the torture and murder of children simply because it has a cultural foundation, we would disagree. Health practitioners should not abstain from involvement in conflict with their own or other cultures where they are concerned about basic offenses against humanity and human health. We note that respect for autonomy fares no better against cruelty and evil than does respect for culture.

Dr. Leigh has several choices about how to respond. The worst of these would be simply to tolerate the practice as a primitive cultural artifact and to take no further interest in it. We would particularly oppose a referral of child abuse to the police or Child Protective Services. In general, we think there is scope for interpreting the law in cases where there are cultural disagreements over the nature of harm. It is unlikely that harm is intended in the application of a traditional remedy—the obverse is more likely true. In this case, the mother's actions do not constitute intentional abuse; the child's welfare is a priority for her. Neither could her actions be read as neglect since she is obviously attentive and seeking care for her child.

Rather than trying to prohibit this practice directly, which might alienate Ms. Saeto, a clinician could discuss the risk of and protection against secondary infection and suggest safer pain remedies. Dr. Leigh should be more worried about being able to monitor the baby's symptoms of illness than the Mien therapy (the "head thrown back" symptom reported with the folk illness could become worrisome with a high fever). Part of her commitment to patients is to teach what, from a medical point of view, may damage health. Maximally, Dr. Leigh could try to learn more about the rationale for and techniques of moxibustion herself. If after her inquiry she is still concerned about the procedure, she should consider sharing her concerns with the local Mien community, not Ms. Saeto alone.

The Health Care System

Healing in a Hurry:
Hospitals in the Managed-Care Age

SUZANNE GORDON, TIMOTHY MCCALL

SINCE THE TRANSITION to managed care, hospital stays for everything from bypass surgery to hip replacements to mastectomies for breast cancer have shortened dramatically. Such reductions are a central cost-cutting strategy of insurance companies and of employers, who are the major purchasers of health insurance. As a result, nurses and doctors are under increasing pressure —with financial incentives frequently dangling before them—to discharge patients more quickly. The driving force behind recent reductions in hospital stays—leading to the infamous "drive-through delivery"—has been financial.

Patients are ejected from the hospital when they are on ventilators or unable to walk; when they have fevers, urinary catheters, draining wounds or conditions that could destabilize within minutes. They have been assured professional nurses and home health aides will care for them at home. At the same time, however, HMOs have initiated draconian cuts in home care and Congress has followed suit. Home-care agencies are responding to the financial crunch by closing their doors, limiting services or simply refusing to care for patients who are more expensive because they are sicker, frailer or have more complex problems. . . .

This situation is a predictable consequence of allowing decisions about hospital admissions to be based largely on cost. To be sure, hospitalization is one of the most expensive components of healthcare. . . . To make the reductions, HMOs use a three-pronged strategy. First, many routinely deny coverage for some elective procedures—such as cataract surgery and bone-marrow transplants for advanced breast cancer—that traditional insurance would have paid for. A *Journal of the American Medical Association* study of California hospitals found that in hospitals in markets with the highest penetration of HMOs, the number of operations dropped 14.8 percent between 1983 and 1993. Second, HMOs shift many other procedures to outpatient settings. The *JAMA* study noted that in high-HMO mar-

Reprinted with permission from the March 1, 1999, issue of The Nation, *pp. 199–201.*

kets the number of inpatient procedures was almost halved, while outpatient surgeries almost doubled. Third, HMOs discharge patients sooner. In the same study the total number of hospital days in high-HMO markets plummeted from 4.9 million to 2.8 million in the ten-year period.

Because childbirth is the number-one cause of hospitalization, managed-care plans saw that if they could cut mothers' time in the hospital they could save billions of dollars. In 1970 women having normal vaginal deliveries stayed an average of four days; those undergoing caesarean sections stayed eight days. By 1994 most HMOs were limiting stays for C-sections to two or three days and for vaginal deliveries to one day. Some California plans, like Kaiser Permanente's, were encouraging new mothers to leave the hospital after only eight hours.

For traditional heart bypass surgery, hospital stays of two or more weeks were common as recently as a few years ago. Now four days is considered the goal. Women having mastectomies have gone from more than a week in the hospital to receiving the procedure on an outpatient basis in some recent cases. According to oncologist Glenn Bubley of Boston's Beth Israel Deaconess Medical Center, patients undergoing radical prostate surgery used to stay in the hospital between seven and nine days. Now they are out in two or three days—and must go home before their urinary catheters have been removed.

The logic seems to be that if cutting a little time was good, then cutting more is better. "There is a 'can we get away with it' attitude among insurers," Bubley says. Indeed, researchers in a number of studies have concluded that cuts in lengths of stay are safe. Typically, however, these studies have excluded more seriously ill patients. Also, most of the studies didn't include a control group. And most included so few patients that they would have lacked sufficient statistical power to detect important differences in quality even if control groups had been used.

. . . A 1991 JAMA study compared the effects of various lengths of stay for six common medical and surgical conditions. No significant differences were found in deaths, likelihood of readmission or patient satisfaction. But given today's standards the study was way off the mark: In the case of bypass surgery, in the hospital with the shortest length of stay, patients stayed 8.9 days on average. In 1999, that would be considered the height of luxury.

Moreover, the things that matter most to patients and their families don't show up on the radar screens of most researchers. Take pain control. Dr. Kathleen Foley, attending neurologist at Memorial Sloan-Kettering Cancer Center, explains, "Today's shortened average length of stay has altered the kind of pain management that doctors can use because they are trying to get patients out of the hospital so quickly." And according to Colleen Dunwoody, clinical coordinator for pain management at the University of Pittsburgh Medical Center, "Patients are leaving the hospital with more pain because they are leaving earlier." Ironically, failing to control pain adequately could ultimately increase costs.

. . . According to a 1994 study, HMOs cover about half as many home visits per hospital discharge as traditional Medicare. Cutting hospital stays and home-care services reduces some governmental and corporate costs for healthcare—at least in the short term—but the effect on overall costs to society remains unclear. "When insurers and the government consider the safety of shortening length of stay, patients' and families' comfort and convenience do not figure into calculations at all," Dr. Bubley explains. "It's simply not in insurers' interest to know about the myriad problems patients have at home." It's also not in insurers' and employers' interest to calculate the financial costs to family members who must take time off work to care for a sick relative. . . .

In a 1997 study sponsored by the American Hospital Association, patients reported "a feeling of being abandoned when they are released from the hospital—like 'jumping off into nowhere,' as one patient described it." Thirty percent were not told what danger signals to watch for after discharge, and 28.7 percent said they had problems with continuity and transition. In February 1998 the medical journal *Lancet* published an article that found an eightfold increase in deaths in the United States due to outpatient medication errors. In other words, when patients act as their own nurse or doctor, they often make mistakes and may die as a result. And when family members are required to fill in for professional nurses there are similar hazards.

But even excluding the added costs to patients and their families, there is evidence that cutting length of hospital stays hasn't saved the country much money. According to Princeton economist Uwe Reinhardt, from 1980 to 1993 real per capita spending on hospital inpatient care rose by nearly 53 percent even though inpatient days plummeted by 36 percent. Hospitals have traditionally negotiated their services at a flat daily rate—say, $1,000 a day. In the hospital, however, the earliest days of care tend to be much more costly. That's because a patient who has just undergone a surgical procedure or who has an acute illness will need more tests, more medication and more intensive nursing care. As the patient recuperates, his or her needs decrease. The actual cost of a day later in the hospitalization might be only $150. Professor Alan Sager of the Boston University School of Public Health concludes that it may cost as little as $30 to $60 to care for a mother and her newborn in the hospital after the first day. This figure may seem startlingly low, but if little nursing and physician time is needed, few tests are done and the bed would otherwise lie empty, the costs are negligible. Yet whether care costs $30 or $300, that day will still be billed at $1,000.

. . . George LeMaitre, [a] Massachusetts surgeon, describes how he was effectively fired by one of the largest HMOs in his area after refusing to discharge a patient recovering from a major operation for colon-cancer surgery after what was in his judgment too little time in the hospital. LeMaitre says, "Were I a younger surgeon, just getting started, I might choose to wimp out, beg the forgiveness of the HMO and promise to make amends in the future."

When one looks at healthcare costs in other nations, it's clear that hospitalization is not the most important factor. In Germany hospitalization averages seven days longer, while that country spends 10.5 percent of its GDP on healthcare compared to our 13.6 percent. England and Canada also have much lower overall healthcare costs than the United States but more generous lengths of stay.

Clearly, the problem will not go away until medical decisions are based on the patient's health. Some type of comprehensive universal health program could achieve this, in addition to saving money and solving the problems facing the 43 million uninsured Americans. Our highly fragmented approach to healthcare allows hundreds of insurance companies to take anywhere from 16 to 40 percent of premium dollars off the top for profit, administration and multimillion-dollar CEO salaries. Each insurer has its own rules, its own forms to be filled out and its own bevy of "utilization reviewers" to determine which patients can have tests, see specialists and stay in the hospital.

The reality is that Congress is unlikely to enact anything more than piecemeal reform unless it is forced by overwhelming public opinion to do otherwise. Only a mass movement to change our healthcare system has the potential to force the politicians' hands. The hundreds of small and medium-sized groups working more or less independently to reform healthcare must come together. . . . But the focus must be on the needs of patients—every one of us.

For Good Health,
It Helps to Be Rich and Important

ERICA GOODE

DOCTORS USUALLY EVALUATE patients' vulnerability to serious disease by inquiring about risk factors like cigarette smoking, obesity, hypertension and high cholesterol. But they might be better off asking how much money those patients make, how many years they spent in school and where they stand relative to others in their offices and communities.

Scientists have known for decades that poverty translates into higher rates of illness and mortality. But an explosion of research is demonstrating that social class — as measured not just by income but also by education and other markers of relative status — is one of the most powerful predictors of health, more powerful than genetics, exposure to carcinogens, even smoking. What matters is not simply whether a person is rich or poor, college educated or not. Rather, risk for a wide variety of illnesses, including cardiovascular disease, diabetes, arthritis, infant mortality, many infectious diseases and some types of cancer, varies with *relative* wealth or poverty: the higher the rung on the socioeconomic ladder, the lower the risk. And this relationship holds even at the upper reaches of society, where it might seem that an abundance of resources would even things out.

Social class is an uncomfortable subject for many Americans. "I think there has been a resistance to thinking about social stratification in our society," said Dr. Nancy Adler, professor of medical psychology at the University of California at San Francisco and director of the John T. and Catherine D. MacArthur Foundation Research Network on Socioeconomic Status and Health. Instead, researchers traditionally have focused on health differences between rich and poor, or blacks and whites (unaware, in many cases, that race often served as a proxy for socioeconomic status, since blacks are disproportionately represented in lower income brackets). But the notion that a mid-level executive with a three-bedroom, split-level in Scarsdale might somehow be more vulnerable to illness than his boss in the five-bedroom colonial a few blocks away seems to have finally captured scientists' attention.

In the past five years, 193 papers addressing aspects of socioeconomic status and health have appeared in scientific journals — twice the number in the previous five-year period. The National Institutes of Health last year declared research on disparities in health related to social class or minority status one of its highest priorities, said Dr. Norman Anderson, associate director of the N.I.H. And a recent conference in Bethesda, Md., on the topic, sponsored by the New York Academy of Sciences and the MacArthur Foundation network, drew more than 250 participants from a wide variety of disciplines.

EXECUTIVE PRIVILEGE INCLUDES LONGEVITY

A study following 18,133 male civil servants over 25 years shows that the grade of employment was a strong predictor of mortality, especially before retirement. What first compelled researchers' interest was a now-classic study, begun in the late 1960's, of men in the British civil service. The Whitehall study, directed by Dr. Michael Marmot, director of the International Center for Health and Society at University College London, tracked mortality rates over 10 years for 17,530 male civil service employees. When the data were analyzed, the researchers were astonished to discover that mortality rates varied continuously and precisely with the men's civil service grade: the higher the classification, the lower the rates of death, regardless of cause.

This finding was as perplexing as it was intriguing. The men all had jobs, and equal access to health care under Britain's national health system. But mortality rates for men in the lowest civil service classification, the researchers found, were three times higher than those for men in the highest grade. And a 25-year follow-up of the Whitehall subjects, some results of which were published in 1996, found the social class gradient persisted well past retirement, even among men into their late 80's. Subsequent studies demonstrated a similar relationship between socioeconomic status and mortality in the United States and Canada. What could account for such startling findings? One plausible explanation was that lower-ranked men might engage in more risky behaviors, like smoking. But the same health disparity from pay grade to pay grade that was evident in smokers held for nonsmokers, too. And all coronary risk factors combined, the researchers found, accounted for only a third of the differences between grades.

Stress, or other aspects of psychological life that can have an impact on a person's vulnerability to disease, the Whitehall group reasoned, might also play a role in the results. Prolonged exposure to stress, researchers have found, can lead to abnormalities in immune function and glucose metabolism, and destroy brain cells involved in memory. And studies show that the

lower one's social status, the more stressed people feel, and the more stressful events they encounter in their lives. Dr. Sheldon Cohen, professor of psychology at Carnegie Mellon University in Pittsburgh, has demonstrated a link between social status and vulnerability to infectious disease in male macaque monkeys. In a study carried out in conjunction with primate researchers at Wake Forest University School of Medicine, Dr. Cohen found that males at the lower end of the dominance hierarchy were more susceptible to a cold virus than dominant males.

Dr. Cohen and his colleagues at Carnegie Mellon then replicated those findings in humans. Subjects in the study were asked to rate their relative standing in their community on a social status ladder, then were exposed to a mild respiratory virus. People who ranked themselves low on the ladder were more likely to become infected with the virus than those who ranked themselves higher up on the ladder. In another study, the researchers found that people who had been unemployed for one month or more under highly stressful conditions were 3.8 times more susceptible to a virus than people who were not experiencing a significant stressful situation.

At least in primates, the interaction of stress with social class and illness, however, depends both on the nature of the stress and the context in which it occurs, as demonstrated in a series of studies by Dr. Jay R. Kaplan, a professor of pathology and anthropology at Wake Forest. In a crowded situation where resources are scarce, for example, male monkeys at the lowest end of the dominance hierarchy, who must scramble hardest to survive, are likely to feel the most stress. And in studies of primates in the wild, researchers find that subordinate animals show higher levels of stress hormones.

But when Dr. Kaplan and his colleagues fed male monkeys a "luxury" diet, high in fat and cholesterol, and moved them each month for two years into a new group of strange males, it was the dominant animals, forced to reassert their position continually, who suffered the most stress. Under such conditions, Dr. Kaplan finds, dominant males show a hypervigilant response, and have higher rates of coronary artery disease than subordinates. For humans and primates, a sense of control over life events is intimately related to stress. And control seems to have been one factor at work in the Whitehall study.

In 1985, Dr. Marmot and his colleagues launched Whitehall II, a second large-scale study, which included civil servants of both sexes and which collected more detailed information on the participants. As part of the study, employees were asked to rate the amount of control they felt over their jobs. Managers also rated the amount of control employees had. Job control, the researchers found, varied inversely with employment grade: the higher the grade, the more control. And the less control employees had, as defined either by their own or managers' ratings, the higher the employees' risk of developing coronary disease. Job control, in fact, accounted for about half the gradient in deaths from pay grade to pay grade.

To some extent, people's ability to withstand stress, and the ways in which they interpret and respond to life events, are shaped by early life, the product of what one social scientist, Dr. Clyde Hertzman of the University of British Columbia, calls "the long arm of childhood." Genetics play a role, as does nutrition. (In the Whitehall study, height—which varies with social class—was used as a rough indicator of childhood influences on development, and accounted for a small portion of the association between mortality and employment grade.) And scientists have found that early life experiences—abuse and neglect, for example—can alter brain development and influence responses to stressful events.

Any discussion of socioeconomic status in the United States of necessity involves a discussion of race, since the two are entwined in complex, sometimes inextricable, ways. Proportionally, far more African-Americans live in poverty than whites: 28.4 percent of blacks fell below the poverty line in 1996, compared with 11.2 percent of whites, according to Government data. Death rates for African-Americans from all causes are 1.6 times higher than for white Americans, Dr. David R. Williams of the University of Michigan's Institute for Social Research, said at the Bethesda conference.

Life expectancy for blacks and whites also varies. At age 45, a white man can expect to live five years longer than an African-American man, and white women can expect to live 3.7 years longer than their black counterparts. If socioeconomic status is taken into account, health differences between blacks and whites decrease substantially: Black men in the highest income brackets, for example, have a life expectancy 7.4 years longer than black men in the lowest brackets, Dr. Williams said. White men at top income levels live 6.6 years longer than their lowest-income counterparts. But race and to some extent sex still have an impact on health that is independent of social class. The gap in infant mortality rates between blacks and whites, for example, actually increases with higher social status. And being black or female discounts some of the advantages afforded by education: white men accrue health advantages with every additional year of schooling they receive. But black men and women, though they also show gains, show them only through high school, according to an analysis of Federal data by Dr. Adler and Dr. Burton Singer of Princeton University's Office of Population Research. White women, the researchers found, continue to gain in health status through college, but unlike white men, do not receive the gains in health bestowed by postgraduate education.

Social exclusion, residential segregation and other expressions of institutional racism magnify the impact of socioeconomic status. Several studies, for example, have shown higher adult and infant mortality rates for people living in segregated areas. For both blacks and whites, living in a neighborhood where social bonds have eroded may have negative effects on health. Dr. Robert Putnam of Harvard University coined the term "social capital" to describe the elements that contribute to social cohesion.

Dr. Ichiro Kawachi, director of the Harvard Center for Society and Health, has explored one aspect of social capital—interpersonal trust—and its relationship to national and community rates of illness and death.

Dr. Kawachi and his colleagues correlated mortality rates in states with the percentage of state residents who agreed with the statement, "Most people would try to take advantage of you if they got the chance." Death rates, Dr. Kawachi reported at the Bethesda conference, were strongly linked to level of social trust, with the most mistrustful ratings clustering in southern and northeastern states. Another study, of Chicago neighborhoods, yielded similar findings: neighborhoods in which more residents

agreed with the statement "Neighbors can be trusted" had lower mortality rates.

Why are neighborhoods or states with higher levels of trust healthier? Dr. Kawachi suggests that in neighborhoods where social trust is high, negative health behaviors—smoking and alcohol consumption, for example—might be discouraged through community pressure. Residents in high trust neighborhoods may also share more resources, be more willing to help one another out and offer one another more emotional support. "It is speculation," Dr. Kawachi said, "but probably these little things add up to quite important health differences."

Even so, the relationship between social class and health is unlikely to be entirely explained by social capital, or by any other single dimension of life experience. Said Dr. Adler, "There isn't going to be a single explanation or an easy solution, but we've started mapping out some of the places where we can intervene."

Institutionalised Racism in Health Care (Editorial)

"Institutionalised racism" consists of the collective failure of an organisation to provide an appropriate and professional service to people because of their colour, culture or ethnic origin. It can be seen or detected in processes, attitudes and behaviour which amount to discrimination through unwitting prejudice, ignorance, thoughtlessness, and racist stereotyping which

disadvantage minority ethnic people—The Stephen Lawrence Inquiry, London: Stationery Office, 1999

HEALTH CARE is a largely humanitarian effort. So any suggestion of racial bias is extremely worrying. Sadly, medicine has a history of racism. Hippocrates thought Asiatics were fee-

The Lancet, *March 6, 1999. Copyright 1999 by The Lancet Ltd. Reprinted with permission.*

ble, Down associated trisomy 21 with a perceived inferior Mongoloid race, and in the infamous Tuskegee study, black men were denied an available cure for syphilis.

It can be difficult to distinguish racism from differences between ethnic groups in socioeconomic, educational, cultural, and genetic factors. Do ethnic minorities receive less than their fair share of health services because they do not present to doctors as often as the majority do? Or, having presented, do such minorities get treated unfairly because of their race? Poorer socioeconomic status and lower educational attainment may well lead to less access to and treatment from health services. Even so, institutionalised racism in society as a whole and, therefore, in employment, education, and welfare systems is potentially contributing to unfairness.

In 1990, the Council on Ethical and Judicial Affairs of the American Medical Association concluded that blacks were less likely than whites to receive certain treatments. The Council called for greater access to health care for African-Americans and for greater awareness among doctors of differences in treatment between blacks and whites. The New England Journal of Medicine, in its Feb 25 issue this year, reports a survey of doctors presented with videotapes of actors as patients with chest pain. The "patients" were white or black, male or female. Blacks, and women, were significantly less likely to be offered cardiac catheterisation than whites and men. The participating doctors may have been overtly prejudiced or acting subconsciously, but this finding was independent of other explanatory factors and is as close to a definition of institutionalised racism as doctors and health-care providers may dare to get.

The life expectancy of African-Americans, at 70.2 years, is shorter than that of white Americans, at 76.8 years. The Committee on Cancer Research among Minorities and the Medically Underserved, a committee of the US Institute of Medicine, recently called for increased funding to research why some ethnic groups are more likely to die from cancer. The Committee also recalculated the amount the US National Cancer Institute says it spends on research and training in minority programmes. The NCI puts the 1997 figure at US$ 124 million. But the Committee says this sum includes studies that enrol participants from ethnic minorities, and recalculates the figure at US$ 24 million, to reflect the projects focused on minority health. Is this difference in financial perception an example of institutionalised racism, albeit subconscious?

The spectre of institutionalised racism, raised by the Lawrence inquiry, looms over all organisations, which now need to scrutinise themselves carefully for overt and covert racial biases.

Gender Disparities in Clinical Decision Making

COUNCIL ON ETHICAL AND JUDICIAL AFFAIRS, AMERICAN MEDICAL ASSOCIATION

RECENT EVIDENCE has raised concerns that women are disadvantaged because of inadequate attention to the research, diagnosis, and treatment of women's health care problems. In 1985, the US Public Health Service's Task Force on Women's Health Issues reported that the lack of research data on women limited understanding of women's health needs.[1]

One concern is that medical treatments for women are based on a male model, regardless of the fact that women may react differently to treatments than men or that some diseases manifest themselves differently in women than in men. The results of medical research on men are generalized to women without sufficient evidence of applicability to women.[2-4] For example, the original research on the prophylactic value of aspirin for coronary artery disease was derived almost exclusively from research on men, yet recommendations based on this research have been directed to the general populace.[4]

Some researchers attribute the lack of research on women to women's reproductive cycles. Women's menstrual cycles may constitute a separate variable affecting test results.[5] Also, researchers are reluctant to perform studies on women of childbearing age, because experimental treatments or procedures may affect their reproductive capabilities. However, the task force pointed out that it is precisely because medications and other therapeutic interventions have a differential effect on women according to their menstrual cycle that women should not be excluded from research.[6] Research on the use of antidepressant agents was initially conducted entirely on men, despite apparently higher rates of clinical depression in women.[6,7] Evidence is emerging that the effects of some antidepressants vary over the course of a woman's cycle, and as a result, a constant dosage of an antidepressant may be too high at some points in a woman's cycle, yet too low at others.[2,3]

In response to the task force, the National Institutes of Health promised to implement a policy ensuring that women would be included in study populations unless it would be scientifically inappropriate to do so.[4] However, in June 1990, the General Accounting Office reported that the National Institutes of Health had made little progress in implementing the policy and that many problems remained.[4]

In addition to these general concerns raised by the task force about women's health, recent studies have examined whether a patient's gender inappropriately affects the access to and use of medical care. Three important areas in which evidence of gender disparities exists are (1) access to kidney transplantation, (2) diagnosis and treatment of cardiac disease, and (3) diagnosis of lung cancer. Other studies have also revealed gender-based differences in patterns of health care use. Although biological factors account for some differences between the sexes in the provision of medical care, these studies indicate that nonbiological or nonclinical factors may affect clinical decision making. There are not enough data to identify the exact nature of nonbiological or nonclinical factors. Nevertheless, the existence

Journal of the American Medical Association 266 (1990): 559–562. Reprinted with permission. Copyrighted 1991, American Medical Association of these factors is a cause for concern that the medical community needs to address.

EVIDENCE OF DISPARITIES

Gender Differences in Health Care Use

Some evidence indicates that, compared with men, women receive more health care services overall. In general, women have more physician visits per year and receive more services per visit.[8] Several studies have examined the issue of differences in health care use between men and women.[8-14] The results of these studies vary and some are contradictory. One of the most extensive studies on gender differences in the use of health care services found that when medical care differs for men and women (in approximately 30% to 40% of cases), the usual result is more care for women than for men. Women seem to receive more care even when both men and women report the same type of illness or complaint about their health.[8] Women undergo more examinations, laboratory tests, and blood pressure checks and receive more drug prescriptions and return appointments than men. However, the reasons for this are not clear.

Studies that have examined gender as a factor for receiving several major diagnostic or therapeutic interventions, however, suggest that women have less access than men to these interventions.

Disparities in Providing Major Diagnostic and Therapeutic Interventions

Kidney Dialysis and Transplantation

Gender has been found to correlate with the likelihood that a patient with kidney disease will receive dialysis or a kidney transplant. . . .

Disparities based on gender are more pronounced for the likelihood of receiving a kidney transplant. An analysis of patient dialysis data from 1981 through 1985 indicated that women undergoing renal dialysis were approximately 30% less likely to receive a cadaver kidney transplant than men.[16] Another study, done during the period 1979 through 1985, showed that a female dialysis patient had only three-quarters the chance of a male patient to receive a renal transplant.[17] Controlling for age did not significantly reduce gender as a factor in the likelihood of receiving a transplant. Men were more likely to receive a transplant in every age category. The discrepancy between sexes was most pronounced in the group 46 to 60 years old, with women having only half the chance of receiving a transplant as men the same age.[18]

Diagnosis of Lung Cancer

Recent autopsy studies have revealed that in as many as a quarter of patients with lung cancer, a diagnosis is not made while they are alive.[18-20] A comparison between the population in which lung cancer is diagnosed and the population in which it is not diagnosed shows that a detection bias favors the ordering of diagnostic testing for lung cancer in patients who are smokers, have a recent or chronic cough, or are male.[20]

One study compared the rates of lung cancer detected at autopsy with the way cytologic studies of sputum were ordered in a hospital setting to detect lung cancer. Men and women have relatively equal rates of previously undiagnosed lung cancer detected during autopsy. In addition, other studies have shown that women and men with similar smoking practices are at essentially equivalent risk for lung cancer.[21] However, men were twice as likely to have cytologic studies of sputum ordered as women. Once smoking status and other medical considerations were taken into account, men still had 1.6 times the chance of having a cytologic test done.[20]

Catheterization for Coronary Bypass Surgery

Men seem to have cardiac catheterizations ordered at a rate disproportionately higher than women, regardless of each gender's likelihood of having coronary artery disease. A study done in

1987 showed that in a group of 390 patients, of those with abnormal exercise radionuclide scans, 40% of the male patients were referred for cardiac catheterization, while only 4% of the female patients were referred for further testing.[22] The study showed that once researchers controlled for the variables of abnormal test results, age, types of angina, presence of symptoms, and confirmed previous myocardial infarction, men were still 6.5 times more likely to be referred for catheterization than women, although men have only three times the likelihood of having coronary heart disease than women. . . .

POSSIBLE EXPLANATIONS

Biological Differences between the Sexes

Differences in biological needs between male and female patients probably account for a large part of the differences in the use of health care services. The kind and number[23] of illnesses that are reported differ somewhat for women and men. Possibly, women get more care because they have more illnesses or because the types of illnesses they have require more overall care. Some figures show that the generally lower socioeconomic status of women may be associated with poorer health. Also, women tend to live longer than men and individuals of older ages may have more morbidities.[8] However, real differences in morbidity and mortality between the sexes would not explain the fact that women seem to receive more care than men for the same type of complaint or illness.[8]

Real biological differences also cannot account for the gender disparities in rates of cardiac catheterization, kidney transplantation, or lung cancer diagnoses. For instance, the discrepancy in dialysis rates might be explained by the existence of coexisting diseases in women that lessen the potential effectiveness of dialysis. However, the Health Care Financing Administration reports that female patients receiving dialysis have a slightly better survival pattern than male patients.[24]

Also, biological differences between the sexes, such as the level of cytotoxic antibodies, number of complications after transplantation, or differences in the type of renal disease between men and women did not explain the disparity in the likelihood of receiving a kidney transplant.[17] It is unlikely that the difference reflects either patient or physician preference; successful transplantation is generally considered superior to lifetime dialysis by both patients and physicians.[16,17]

The difference in sputum cytologic findings between male and female patients may reflect the historical association between male sex and cigarette smoking. Traditionally, more men than women have been smokers.[21] In fact, past demographic data showed that men were more likely to have lung cancer than women. Physicians, in turn, may view smoking and being male as independent risk factors for lung cancer and therefore tend to suspect cancer more readily in patients who either smoked or were men even though gender is not an independent risk factor. . . .[21]

Other evidence also suggests that women may be disadvantaged by inadequate attention to the manifestations of cardiovascular disease in women. There is some evidence that cardiovascular disease is not diagnosed or treated early enough in women. Studies show that women have a higher operative mortality rate for coronary bypass surgery[25,26] and a higher mortality rate at the time of an initial myocardial infarction.[27–29] The higher mortality rates reflect the fact that cardiovascular disease is further advanced in women than men at both the time of surgery and the time of an initial attack.[27]

Societal Attitudes May Affect Decision Making in the Health Care Context

Data that suggest that a patient's gender plays an inappropriate role in medical decision making raise the question of possible gender bias in clinical decision making. Gender bias may not necessarily manifest itself as overt discrimination based on sex. Rather, social attitudes, including stereotypes, prejudices and other evaluations based on gender roles may play themselves out in a variety of subtle ways.

For instance, some evidence suggests that physicians are more likely to attribute women's health complaints to emotional rather than physical causes.[30–32] Women's concerns about their health and their greater use of health care services have been perceived to be due to "overanxiousness" about their health.[32] However, characterizing women's use patterns as a result of emotional excess or overuse risks providing inadequate care for women. For example, in the study of catheterization rates, attributing a disproportionate percentage of women's abnormal nuclear scan results to psychiatric or noncardiac causes for their symptoms may have compromised their care. . . .[22]

Societal value judgments placed on gender or gender roles may also put women at a disadvantage in the context of receiving certain major diagnostic and therapeutic interventions, such as kidney transplantation and cardiac catheterization. A general perception that men's social role obligations or of their contributions to society are greater than women's may fuel these disparities.[9] For instance, altering one's work schedule to accommodate health concerns may be viewed as more difficult for men than women. Overall, men's financial contribution to the family may be considered more critical than women's. A kidney transplant is much less cumbersome than dialysis. Coronary bypass surgery, for which catheterization is a prerequisite, is a more efficient and immediate solution to the problem of coronary artery disease than continuous' antianginal drug therapy. However, judgments based on evaluations of social worth or preconceptions about the probable roles of men and women are clearly inexcusable in the context of medical decision making.

Role of the Medical Profession in Examining Gender Disparities and Eliminating Biases

Available data do not conclusively demonstrate a connection between gender bias and gender disparities in the provision of health care. Designing a study that can control for the myriad social, economic, and cultural factors that might influence decision making in a clinical context has proved extraordinarily difficult.

Historically, societal perceptions regarding women's health status have often disadvantaged women. Throughout the mid-19th and well into the 20th century, women's perceived disposition toward both physical and mental illness was used as a rationale for keeping them from worldly spheres such as politics, science, medicine, and law. For women, behavior that violated expected gender-role norms was frequently attributed to various physical or mental illnesses[33,34] and in turn often was treated in a variety of ways, including gynecological surgeries, such as hysterectomies and, occasionally, clitoridectomies.[35] Society and medicine have addressed and are working to remedy sex stereotypes and biases. Yet, many social and cultural attitudes that endorse sex-stereotyped roles for men and women remain in our society.

The medical community cannot tolerate any discrepancy in the provision of care that is not based on appropriate biological or medical indications. The US Public Health Service's Task Force on Women's Health Issues concluded that "[b]ecause health care is a legitimate concern of all people, the health professions are obligated to seek ways of ensuring that clinical decisions are based on science that adequately pertains to all people."[6] Insufficient research on women is not only discriminatory but may be dangerous; medical care or drug treatments that prove effective in men may not always be safely generalizable to women.[4] The influence that social attitudes and perceptions have had on health care in the past suggest that some biases could remain and affect modern medical care. Such attitudes and perceptions may disadvantage both women and men by reinforcing gender-based stereotypes or inhibiting access to care. Current evidence of possible discrepancies indicates a need for further scrutiny.

SUMMARY OF RECOMMENDATIONS

Physicians should examine their practices and attitudes for the influence of social or cultural biases that could affect medical care. Physicians must ensure that gender is not used inappropriately as a consideration in clinical decision making. Assessments of need based on presumptions about the relative worth of certain social roles must be avoided. Procedures and techniques that preclude or minimize the possibility of gender bias should be developed and implemented. A gender-neutral determination for kidney transplant eligibility should be used.

More medical research on women's health and women's health problems should be pursued. Results of medical testing done solely on men should not be generalized to women without evidence that results can be applied safely and effectively to both sexes. Research on health problems that affect both sexes should include male and female subjects. Sound medical and scientific reasons should be required for excluding women from medical tests and studies, such as that the proposed research does not or would not affect the health of women. An obvious example would be research on prostatic cancer. Also, further research into the possible causes of gender disparities should be conducted. The extent to which physician-patient interactions may be influenced by cultural and social conceptions of gender should be ascertained.

Finally, awareness of and responsiveness to socio-cultural factors that could lead to gender disparities may be enhanced by increasing the number of female physicians in leadership roles and other positions of authority in teaching, research, and the practice of medicine.

REFERENCES

1. US Public Health Service. *Women's Health: Report of the Public Health Service Task Force on Women's Health Issues.* Washington, DC: US Dept of Health and Human Services; 1985;2.

2. Cotton P. Is there still too much extrapolation from data on middle-aged white men? *JAMA.* 1990;263:1049–1050.

3. Cotton P. Examples abound of gaps in medical knowledge because of groups excluded from scientific study. *JAMA.* 1990;263:1051–1052.

4. *Hearings Before the House Energy and Commerce Subcommittee on Health and the Environment,* 101st Congr, 1st Sess (1990) (testimony of Mark V. Nadel, associate director, US General Accounting Office).

5. Hamilton J, Parry B. Sex-related differences in clinical drug response: implications for women's health. *J Am Med Wom Assoc.* 1983;38:126–132.

6. Hamilton JA. Guidelines for avoiding methodological and policy-making biases in gender-related health research in Public Health Service. *Women's Health: Report of the Public Health Service Task Force on Women's Health Issues.* Washington, DC: US Department of Health and Human Services; 1985;2.

7. Raskin A. Age-sex differences in response to antidepressant drugs. *J Nerv Ment Dis.* 1974;159:120–130.

8. Verbrugge LM, Steiner RP. Physician treatment of men and women patients: sex bias or appropriate care? *Med Care.* 1981;19:609–632.

9. Marcus AC, Suman TE. Sex differences in reports of illness and disability: A preliminary test of the 'fixed role' hypothesis. *J Health Soc Behav.* 1981;22:174–182.

10. Gove WR, Hughes M. Possible causes of the apparent sex differences in physical health: an empirical investigation. *Am Sociol Rev.* 1979;44:126–146.

11. Cleary PD, Mechanic D, Greenley JR. Sex differences in medical care utilization: an empirical investigation. *J Health Soc Behav.* 1982;23:106–119.

12. Hibbard JH, Pope CR. Another look at sex differences in the use of medical care: illness orientation and the type of morbidities for which services are used. *Women Health.* 1986;11:21–36.

13. Armitage KJ, Schneiderman LF, Bass RA. Response of physicians to medical complaints in men and women. *JAMA.* 1979;241:2186.

14. Natanson CA. Illness and the feminine role: a theoretical review. *Soc Sci Med.* 1975;9:57–63.

15. Kjellstrand CM, Logan GM. Racial, sexual and age inequalities in chronic dialysis. *Nephron.* 1987;45:257–263.

16. Held PJ, Pauly MV, Bovbjerg RR, et al. Access to kidney transplantation. *Arch Intern Med.* 1988;148:2594–2600.

17. Kjellstrand CM. Age, sex, and race inequality in renal transplantation. *Arch Intern Med.* 1988;148: 1305–1309.

18. McFarlane MJ, Feinstein AR, Wells CK. The 'epidemiologic necropsy': unexpected detections, demographic selections, and the changing rates of lung cancer. *JAMA.* 1987;258:331–338.

19. McFarlane MJ, Feinstein AR, Wells CK. Necropsy evidence of detection bias in the diagnosis of lung cancer. *Arch Intern Med.* 1986;146:1695–1698.

20. Wells CK, Feinstein AR. Detection bias in the diagnostic pursuit of lung cancer. *Am J Epidemiol.* 1988;128:1016–1026.

21. Schoenberg JB, Wilcox HB, Mason TJ, et al. Variation in smoking-related lung cancer risk among New Jersey women. *Am J Epidemiol.* 1989;130:688–695.

22. Tobin JN, Wassertheil-Smoller S, Wexler JP, et al. Sex bias in considering coronary bypass surgery. *Ann Intern Med.* 1987;107:19–25.

23. Verbrugge LM. Sex differentials in health. *Prevention.* 1982;97:417–437.

24. Eggers PW, Connerton R, McMullan M. The Medicare experience with end-stage renal disease: trends in incidence, prevalence, and survival. *Health Care Fin Rev.* 1984;5:69–88.

25. Khan SS, Nessim S, Gray R, Czer LS, Chaux A, Matloff J. Increased mortality of women in coronary artery bypass surgery: Evidence for referral bias. *Ann Intern Med.* 1990;112:561–567.

26. Wenger NK. Gender, coronary artery disease, and coronary bypass surgery. *Ann Intern Med.* 1990;112:557–558.

27. Wenger NK. Coronary disease in women. *Ann Rev Med.* 1985;36:285–294.

28. Fiebach NH, Viscoli CM, Horwitz RI. Differences between women and men in survival after myocardial infarction. *JAMA.* 1990;263:1092–1096.

29. Dittrich H, Gilpin E, Nicod P, Cali G, Henning H, Ross J. Acute myocardial infarction in women: influence of gender on mortality and prognosis variables. *Am J Cardiol.* 1988;62:1–7.

30. Bernstein B, Kane R. Physicians' attitudes toward female patients. *Med Care.* 1981;19:600–608.

31. Colameco S, Becker L, Simpson M. Sex bias in the assessment of patient complaints. *J Fam Pract.* 1983;16:1117–1121.

32. Savage WD, Tate P. Medical students' attitudes towards women: a sex-linked variable? *Med Educ.* 1983;17:159–164.

33. Waisberg J, Page P. Gender role nonconformity and perception of mental illness. *Women Health.* 1988;14:3–16.

34. Broverman IK, Broverman DM, Clarkson FE, et al. Sex-role stereotypes and clinical judgments of mental health. *J Consult Clin Psychol.* 1970;34:1–7.

35. Barker-Benfield B. 'The spermatic economy.' In: Gordon M, ed. *The American Family in Sociohistorical Perspective.* New York. NY: St Martin's Press; 1973.

From Autonomy to Empowerment: Health Care Ethics from a Feminist Perspective

VIRGINIA L. WARREN

THIS ESSAY CONCERNS power. Health care ethics should place more emphasis on physicians'

VIRGINIA WARREN is a Philosophy professor at Chapman University.

power and authority over others, and on the social structure of hospitals and medical schools. See Paul Starr (1982) for an astute sociological account of how American medicine came to be structured as it is. Brody (1992, ixx, 12) describes

Unpublished paper. Printed by permission of Virginia L. Warren

how power came to be omitted from contemporary health care ethics. Health care ethics should do more to challenge the power of institutions: hospitals, HMOs and other insurers, pharmaceutical companies, medical and nursing schools, and government. Asserting patients' autonomy against what physicians deem best is insufficient to confront the issue of power in health care, especially with health insurance policies becoming increasingly restrictive. My thesis is that replacing the standard concept of autonomy in health care ethics with the politically charged concept of empowerment used by feminists and others engaged in liberation struggles would be a good first step toward better health care. We need to recognize existing power relationships in health care, to identify the interests protected by existing health care institutions, and, where necessary, to change those institutions. An apolitical ethics, such as we have now in health care ethics, is only seemingly apolitical. It is Stealth politics; it flies beneath the radar.

Autonomy is on a short list of moral principles (along with beneficence, non-maleficence, justice, and utility) that has become firmly established in Anglo-American health care ethics since the late 1960's. See Brody (1992, 36–41, 48–49) for an overview of how health care ethics developed in the past thirty years. Autonomy has had a host of meanings in Western moral and political philosophy (Dworkin, 1988, 3–6; Hill, 1991, 25 and 44). However, within health care ethics, one conception of autonomy has reigned. On this standard view, being autonomous involves making uncoerced decisions according to values of one's own choosing; one is autonomous if one has thought through a decision oneself without undue outside interference, and without an inner, psychological compulsion.

Autonomy is a political metaphor applied to one's relations with others, and to the self. Autonomy has been used to limit the physician's "power-over" the patient. To be autonomous is also to have "power-over" oneself. Many feminist authors contrast "power-over" with an alternative form of power. For example, French (1985, 505–512) calls this alternative "power-to"; Daly (1986, 199) calls it the "power of presence"; Christ (1986, 213) refers to the female power symbolized by the Goddess; Collins (1991), Sherwin (1992, 84–95) and Mahowald (1993) speak of empowerment. Mahowald (1993, 255–271) makes astute observations about the effects of power. However, she does not clearly identify a sense of empowerment distinct from having "power-over" others. I have chosen to call this alternative "empowerment" in order to highlight the connection to politics, and the way that the personal and the political intertwine.

I see four problems with the standard autonomy model. First, because the autonomy-paternalism debate focuses narrowly on who has final control, the aspects of the physician-patient relationship which do not concern control are often overlooked or distorted. It is not surprising that, as part of the autonomy-paternalism debate, the non-control aspects of the physician-patient relationship are de-emphasized, for the goal of medicine is often thought primarily to be curing disease rather than caring for patients (Warren, 1991; Mahowald, 1993, 269). I once heard a physician comment: "If I give patients the chance to autonomously choose their treatment, there's nothing left for me to do. I'm abandoning the patient." Brody (1992, 49–52) makes a similar comment.

Second, emphasizing patient autonomy vs. physician paternalism has overshadowed other power relationships. In my view, one of the most explosive moral issues in health care is the nurse-physician relationship. It concerns not only money, but status, identity, and power. It is a "housekeeping issue" (Warren, 1989, 78–80), [involving] moral issues which are on-going (rather than resolved once and for all) and seemingly trivial (when compared with "crisis issues," such as withdrawal of life support. Addressing this relationship may require unraveling the fabric of daily hospital life: the hierarchical social structure of hospitals. Third, autonomy has been used to examine one-to-one relationships rather than institutions. The power of hospitals, HMO's and other insurers, drug companies, and government tends to be hidden. Informed consent focuses on which alternative is chosen from among those available, not on why some choices are available and not others. If the only power at issue is "power-over" one other person, then patients and the public generally are less likely to think in terms of a different kind of power: empowerment.

The basic features of becoming empowered are these: 1) it is an on-going process involving, 2) developing and exercising a capacity for shaping one's life, 3) a feeling of energy and wholeness, 4) an integration of different aspects of the self, and, 5) being social in one or more of the following senses (a) being supported by others while (b) developing community and (c) attending to the social and political context, including how power affects relationships.

First, becoming empowered is an on-going process central to becoming a moral person. Second, like autonomy, becoming empowered involves developing and exercising a capacity for shaping one's life. Even if one's outward actions are severely restricted, one may resist by fashioning a new self-definition. Nedelsky (1989) and Collins (1991, ch. 5). Because one's story may be interwoven with the story of a group, Collins, who is writing about African American women, sees self-definition as both an individual and a group project. Third, to be empowered one must feel empowered, [. . .] to feel energized by one's capacity to make things happen. Nedelsky (1989, 24–25) wants to include feeling in her Reconceived autonomy: Fourth, becoming empowered involves a process of self-integration. Regarding self-acceptance, note: (a) that acceptance of a tendency or feature of self does not mean that one must like it, develop it, or allow it free rein; (b) that the process of self-integration is not always additive, since self-integration requires periods of self-disintegration (I thank Linda LeMoncheck for this insight); and (c)

that, like self-definition, self-acceptance can be at once personal and political. Fifth, while the standard view of autonomy is individualistic, empowerment is paradigmatically social in one or more senses. Becoming empowered is typically (a) accomplished with the support of others. Becoming empowered also typically involves (b) aiming at developing bonds of community. Lastly, becoming empowered typically (c) focuses on the social and political context, including how power affects relationships. Sources of power, especially institutional power, are identified and, where necessary, challenged. By contrast, standard autonomy remains at the level of individualistic psychology.

To develop a health care system in which people are empowered, we need an ethics of empowerment. In this last section, I will discuss (A) knowledge and (B) power—the two main features of a health care ethics based on empowerment—and then consider (C) some objections to replacing autonomy with empowerment in health care ethics. The first advantage of the empowerment model is that the public would know much more. Truly educating patients about health care would go far beyond the explanations of alternative treatments central to informed consent.

On the empowerment model, one would also know how to choose a physician and how to evaluate his/her performance, including being able easily to find out whether he or she has a track record of being sued for malpractice. A "Consumer Reports" (1996, 62) article says: "it's not all that easy to tell good doctors from bad. Sources like these [cited] can help, but the information you might want is scattered and incomplete. The more negative the information, the harder—and more expensive—it is to find. Currently it is one-sided: physicians can check to see if a prospective patient has a record of suing physicians for malpractice, but patients cannot easily get malpractice information about physicians. And physician peer review is not working well. General information about how health care operates overall—e.g., how health care professionals are selected, trained, and compensated; how hospitals are organized; how physicians get information about drugs; how, in practice, health care policies and laws may be influenced by the public; how other countries structure their health care, with what results; how to get information from sources other than physicians. On the current autonomy model, the public knows much too little, much too late. What is hidden tends to protect powerful interests.

A second advantage over autonomy is that the empowerment model focuses on who controls knowledge. As Brody (1992, 121) notes: "Authors as far removed in time as Plato and Oliver Wendell Holmes used precisely the same analogy to describe the physician's skill: truth and falsehood should be doled out to patients with the same care, precision, and foresight called for by the administration of medications." While the current autonomy model has increased the amount prescribed, knowledge is still a controlled substance. By contrast, on an empowerment model of health care, the public would take more initiative in educating itself. Gaining knowledge can empower in two ways: through the acquisition of knowledge, and through the process of gaining knowledge in partnership with others. Through this process one may develop assertive skills, and develop bonds of community. As the public develops more sources of health care information, we grow less dependent on our own physicians for information. As AIDS activists know, gaining knowledge can empower.

Empowerment asks bigger questions of the whole health delivery system than does standard autonomy. The empowerment model makes it easier to consider the broader social, historical, and political context, and to search out underlying values and interests (e.g., profit, status, power). It encourages us to challenge the system: to influence which treatment options and research data are available, and to shape policies and institutions. Thus, empowerment calls for changes that are more radical, political, and cre-

ative than does standard autonomy. First, the specific options offered to patients should be examined. There should be more public debate about what standard care should be. Second, empowerment may require changing institutions. Third, the education of health care professionals should be reassessed in order to empower future patients and health care professionals alike. Fourth, we should find ways for health insurance plans to empower clients. Instead of battling gatekeepers and cost-cutting administrators, the public needs more input in shaping policy—making health care not only cost-effective, but responsive and humane. Fifth, we should "decompartmentalize" our thinking, blurring the line between medical and non-medical concerns.

I will end by considering four objections. First, by refocusing health care ethics on empowerment, which is explicitly political, makes the definition of health care too broad. [However, a] middle ground exists, and we should debate where the boundary around health care should be drawn. Second, it may be objected that redesigning health care to empower people is an expensive luxury in an era of scaled-back health coverage and choice. My first reply is that a valuable thing is worth some expense. I have never heard the complaint that autonomy is too expensive. My second reply is that, while some attempts to empower may prove too expensive, others may be cheaper in the long run (Okazawa-Rey, 1994, 231). A third objection also concerns priorities: the struggle for the more radical demands of empowerment should wait until standard patient autonomy has been consistently achieved. While the principle of autonomy is widely accepted, many would reject empowerment as too radical. My reply is, first, to concede that, for some purposes and for some audiences, arguing for standard autonomy may be the more effective strategy for change; sometimes, it is the best we can do. Second, however, we must recognize that, even were physician paternalism to vanish tomorrow, patient autonomy would not thereby prevail. The gains desired by those who want a robust patient autonomy will be best achieved by using empowerment to challenge the status quo. For example, while autonomy focuses on patients knowing the risks and benefits of taking a particular drug, empowerment asks, in addition, whether the experimental subjects were both females and males, and how much of what physicians know about this drug was supplied by the company producing it. Then we can work to change what is known, and how this information is disseminated.

REFERENCES

Anzaldua, Gloria. 1987. *Borderlands: La frontera; the new mestiza.* San Francisco: Aunt Lute Books.

Brody, Howard. 1992. *The Healer's Power.* New Haven: Yale University Press.

Christ, Carol P. 1986. Why women need the Goddess: Phenomenological, psychological, and political reflections. In *Women and values: Readings in recent feminist philosophy.* Marilyn Pearsall, ed. Belmont, CA: Wadsworth.

Collins, Patricia Hill. 1991. *Black feminist thought: Knowledge, consciousness, and the politics of empowerment.* New York: Routledge.

Consumer Reports 1996. Your health: Checking up on your doctor; what can you find out? Nov., 1996, pp. 62–63.

Daly, Mary. 1986. The qualitative leap beyond patriarchal religion. In *Women and values: Readings in recent feminist philosophy,* Marilyn Pearsall, ed. Belmont, CA: Wadsworth

Dworkin, Gerald. 1988. *The Theory and Practice of Autonomy.* Cambridge: Cambridge University Press.

French, Marilyn. 1985. *Beyond power: On women, men, and morals.* New York: Ballantine Books.

Hill, Jr., Thomas E. *Autonomy and Self-respect.* Cambridge: Cambridge University Press.

Mahowald, Mary. 1993. *Women and children in health care: An unequal majority.* New York: Oxford University Press.

Nedelsky, Jennifer. 1989. Reconceiving autonomy. *Yale Journal of Law and Feminism.* 1 (1): 7–35.

Okazawa-Rey, Margo. 1994. Grandparents who care: An empowerment model of health care. In *"It just ain't fair": The ethics of health care for African Americans,* Annette Dula and Sara Goering, eds. Westport, Conn.: Praeger.

Sgarro, Amy Arner. 1993. *A surgeon and her community.* Vassar Quarterly. Spring, 1993: 10–13.

Sherwin, Susan. 1992. *No longer patient: Feminist ethics and health care.* Philadelphia: Temple University Press.

Starr, Paul. 1982. *The social transformation of American medicine.* New York: Basic Books.

Warren, Virginia L. 1989. Feminist directions in medical ethics. *Hypatia: A Journal of Feminist Philosophy,* 4 (2): 73–87.

Warren, Virginia L. 1991. The "medicine is war" metaphor. *HEC Forum: An Interdisciplinary Journal on Hospitals' Ethical and Legal Issues,* 3 (1): 39–50.

What Should I Say?
Communication around Disability

LISA I. IEZZONI, M.D., M.SC.

EVERY SO OFTEN, we all experience moments that crystallize an essential truth about our lives. Last spring, I had one in the cramped interstices of a federal office building in Washington, D.C. Before a meeting, I hurried to a back office to use the telephone, but a man was already there. We recognized each other instantly. "It's been 20 years," I said. "You taught that great course on patients' experiences of illness. It helped me decide to go to medical school." "I remember you well." He paused, eyeing me with momentarily unguarded sadness. "I heard about your troubles." My mind raced. What troubles? "Oh, you mean my multiple sclerosis [MS]? I don't think of that as a trouble. I'm doing fine!"

Why had I not immediately understood what he meant by "your troubles"? I felt that he was saddened to see me in my wheelchair; when he knew me 20 years ago, I ran everywhere. Although this encounter held many layers of meaning for me, one aspect is shared by all persons with visible disabilities: the implicit embargo on spoken words and the volumes of unspoken thoughts permeating our relationships with others, even our passing greetings. Communicating around disability is hard on both sides. People often don't know what to say or where to look. Silence frequently subsumes a complex tangle

LISA I. IEZZONI, M.D., M.Sc., Beth Israel Deaconess Medical Center, Boston, MA.

of fears, discomforts, and uncertainties. Other times, similarly complicated feelings prompt spoken words of many stripes: generous, tentative, hurtful, intrusive. As Sally Ann Jones,[1] a woman with MS, said to me: "Some people see you're in a wheelchair, and immediately they raise their voice as if you are deaf. I mean, you're some kind of handicapped. They're not quite sure what to do. People aren't comfortable with handicapped people."

For those of us with disabilities, silence is often the default position. We ourselves are uncomfortable talking about our disability, concerned about breaching that invisible barrier circumscribing socially acceptable discourse. We think, generally erroneously, that silence protects our precious privacy. But silence carries consequences. Silence reinforces the stigmatization of disability, the sense of shame and guilt, and the idea that disability is something to hide.

Persons in wheelchairs live below the eye level of most standing adults. Nonetheless, something other than this physical fact must make us sometimes invisible. Positioned strategically in full view of others, we often remain unnoticed. People don't want to see you; they're not going to see you.

Although seen, sometimes we are not heard. For example, returning to Boston after a business trip, a colleague pushed my airport-issue wheelchair to the gate. The agent processed our tickets and addressed my colleague. "Here's a

From Iezzoni, L. What Should I Say? Communication Around Disability. *Ann Intern. Med. 1998;
129:661–665. Permission granted by The American College of Physicians.*

sticker to put on her coat," the agent said, gesturing toward me with a round, red-and-white-striped sticker. "Why?" I asked. "It will alert the flight attendants that she needs help," the agent replied to my colleague. "Thanks. If I need help, I'll ask for it." "But the sticker indicates she needs assistance." My bemused colleague remained silent. "When I need help, I'll ask for it." "So she won't wear the sticker?" "No, I won't." "Why won't she?" "Because I can ask for help." "Why won't she wear it?" This was going nowhere. I looked at my colleague, imploring her to stop this silliness. "Because it's demeaning," she said and rolled me away.

Admittedly, many people with disabilities hesitate to ask for help. We are often proudly self-sufficient, and requesting assistance is hard. Sometimes we are stopped by implicitly being on the lower rung of that inevitable hierarchy of human relationships. In these instances, the right thing would be for the other person to ask us what we need, as suggested by these two examples.

During a third-year clerkship in medical school, my MS flared up. I could no longer use the stairs when rounds with the attending physician traveled among beds scattered across several floors. As the team entered the stairwell, I went to the elevators, hoping to arrive at the next floor in time to see the team down the hallway en route to the next room. I was still in my "tough it out, don't talk about it" mode, but it nonetheless hurt that neither the attending nor the residents seemed to notice my visible difficulty in walking and left me behind. I was also timid. At that point, my attendings seemed to hold my destiny in their hands. I did not speak up until the attending paused during the closing of a fairly brutal exit interview at the end of his month. "Didn't you notice I was having trouble walking?" I ventured. "I did," he responded. "But because I understood you wanted to be treated just like other students, I didn't ask."

Persons with physical disabilities are frequently grabbed or touched by persons unknown and unasked. In general, this seems to be motivated by genuine efforts to help. Sometimes it preserves our physical safety, as it did when I was lifted off a busy Washington, D.C., street by several strangers after my wheelchair tipped over in a pothole. Nonetheless, unrequested physical contact can be unnerving and physically uncomfortable. Similarly, conversations can cross acceptable boundaries even if others are trying to be kind.

Nowadays, attitudes about so-called "entitlement" can filter down into individual encounters. The major contact that many physicians have with disability is filing forms for patients anxious to obtain dispensation from the government or employers. Physicians tell me that this often makes them suspicious of patients' motivations. Certainly, some patients do manipulate the system. However, suspicions are readily communicated nonverbally, especially to persons sensitized by embarrassment about their impairments. Judgmental disbelief is hurtful. Proving that what we experience is real can become a daunting task. As Mabel Bickford, an obese woman with bad knees who uses a wheelchair, said tearfully about talking to her physicians: "A lot of times I don't say anything, because if things get too out of control with my doctor, then emotionally I'm drained for the rest of the day. They just think that you don't want to walk. You just want to be in the wheelchair; it's comfortable. Well, you try it! I'm sure this plastic cuts my legs."

A common thread of failed communication is that persons with disabilities are somehow invalidated. In the most egregious instances, the invalidation is explicit, as suggested by two examples from medical school. One day, I encountered an attending physician, Dr. Winston, in a hospital lobby. "Hi, Lisa," he greeted me in a friendly way. "It's so good to see you." "Hello, Dr. Winston," I smiled. "You always seem so cheerful when I see you," he said, pausing thoughtfully. "That must be one of the benefits of the inappropriate euphoria of MS. The inconvenience of MS is compensated by you always feeling happy. That must be why you are so generally pleasant."

On my first day in the operating room during my surgical rotation, the attending surgeon let me hold a finger retractor during a delicate procedure. After the concentrated silence broke and closing began, the surgeon turned to me. "What's the worst part of your disease?" he inquired. Embarrassed by the assembled team of residents and nurses, I replied, "It's hard to talk about." "Do you want my opinion?" he asked. The scrub nurse rolled her eyes at me empathetically. "You will make a terrible doctor," he continued. "You lack the most important quality in a good doctor: accessibility. You should limit yourself to pathology, radiology, or maybe anesthesiology." He turned to the anesthesiologist. "What do you think?" They planned my career.

Finally, in the "politically correct" 1990s, disability has joined those topics in which language matters. Some disability advocates emphasize words, preferring, for example, "person who uses a wheelchair" to "wheelchair-bound patient." Although these preferences have solid rationales (for example, focusing on persons, not assistive devices), heightened semantic sensitivities undoubtedly chill some efforts at conversation with people who have disabilities. Our conversational partners are afraid of offending.

The 1990 signing of the Americans with Disabilities Act brought the possibility that speech could convey discriminatory attitudes and presage actions that are now illegal. In retrospect, some positions expressed to me and actions taken during my 4 years in medical school (1980 to 1984) would probably be illegal under the Americans with Disabilities Act, which requires reasonable accommodations for persons with disabilities. For example, late in my third year, I began thinking about applying for an internal medicine residency. At a student dinner, I sat next to a leader at an affiliated teaching hospital, and I boldly asked his advice. I could not stay up all night, but few other accommodations seemed necessary. "What would your hospital think of my situation?" I asked. "Frankly," he replied in a conversational tone, "there are too many doctors in the country right now for us to worry about training handicapped physicians. If that means certain people get left by the wayside, that's too bad." There was silence around the table. During the next months, I received little support from my medical school, and after a wrenching internal debate (which was joined by my caring and realistic husband), I decided to go straight into research.

Communication is a two-way street. Both partners control—albeit sometimes unequally—conversational directions and outcomes. Therefore, my suggestions address persons on both sides of the issue.

For persons with disabilities: We should realize that many people have difficulty talking to us because of deeply embedded, complex emotions. Although overly simplistic, one explanation is certainly fear. Disability defines the one historically disadvantaged group that everyone can join in a flash. Perhaps the most obvious stigmata of disability is loss of control; this prospect terrifies Americans, who are used to being in charge. One way to forestall this horrific possibility is to invalidate those who personify it.

Persons with disabilities constantly teach others about what our lives are like and, thus, what theirs may become. However, although it is desirable to aim for patience in frustrating situations, total equanimity is unrealistic. Sometimes people seem oblivious to the effect of their words or actions; saying something tart and corrective may vent our irritation and improve the situation (for example, motivate someone blocking our way to move). We must contend with being dismissed: "She's just upset because she's handicapped." Nonetheless, sometimes we should lighten up. Especially in casual contacts, one cannot alter firmly rooted attitudes.

Communication with physicians deserves special mention. Persons with disabilities, especially those progressively impaired by chronic illness, must talk directly to their physicians about their functional needs. For these patients, the discussion of acute concerns often consumes clinical encounters, and functional issues remain unaddressed. Certainly, many physicians skillfully evaluate functional impairments and intercede to improve lives (for example, by prescribing physical therapy, assistive devices, or home modifications). Others, however, do not. Part of the problem is medical education. Many physicians know little about assessing and addressing functional problems. Until recently, most medical students were trained exclusively in inpatient settings, where acute illnesses or acute exacerbations of chronic disease are the focus. Nevertheless, another explanation is that physicians are people, too. Physicians also experience fears, discomforts, and uncertainties about confronting disability that they cannot cure. In many instances, we must educate them.

For persons without disabilities: My first advice is to offer us choices and options. "Do you want help?" "How can we make things better for you?" Listen, and then respect our answers, even if they are a repeated, "No, thank you." My second suggestion is for you to ask yourself: "Why does talking to this person make me uncomfortable?" The reasons will probably be obvious; potential solutions will readily follow. For example, many people tell me that they fear saying "the wrong thing." Acknowledge this fear openly: "Look, forgive me if I say something stupid." Remember that those of us with disabilities are

awkward with words, too. Third, avoid doing what I did here—framing the argument as "us against them." I used this rhetorical device to explicate my arguments. Nonetheless, the well-worn phrase "we are all human," although trite, is true. The most visible feature that distinguishes you from me, perhaps, is my wheelchair. Each of us, however, carries private histories that differentiate us from all others; for some of us, only this one distinguishing feature is visible. Communication among people is always challenging for innumerable reasons. Identifying the role that disability plays is the first step in removing it from that complex mix of impediments.

Finally, if words and actions are obviously caring and respectful, communication will almost always be positive. For example, near the end of my first year of medical school, I was hospitalized briefly when I became completely unable to walk. Although I had tried to keep my situation secret, a classmate whom I barely knew came to my bedside one night. "Gosh," he said reverentially, "I hear you have a really serious disease." He paused again, obviously lost for words, but then he rallied. "I brought you a cheesecake," he said. He handed me a big box and retreated hastily. When spoken with warmth, even awkward words are wonderful.

NOTE

1. All proper names in this paper are pseudonyms.

The Experiential Dimension

Second Sight

N. ANN DAVIS

AS A CHILD, I was quite analytical in my efforts to understand physical impairments and disabilities, particularly those that were a part of my everyday life. My paternal grandfather wore thick glasses, with strangely-shaped lenses; when I put them on, the room curved in bizarre ways. Things came into hyper-focus, and they seemed impossibly small and distant. It was an alien, rather lunar view of the world that was revealed to me through my grandfather's glasses; what, I wondered, did the world look like to him without them? . . . [M]y understanding of disability and correction was essentially mechanical, and compensatory. . . . I thought the remedy lay in effecting balance, a thing that could be achieved by the implementation of equal and opposite force.

Recollection of my childhood attempts at understanding impairment came back to me years later with the sudden revelation of my own. Early in my 40s, I learned that I had cataracts in

both eyes, ones that would probably be operable at some point, but were not so at the time. I learned, too, that in the interim my vision would be only partly correctable, and that things would probably get a lot worse before they could get better. But the world without my glasses was not the obverse of the world I had seen through my glasses; the simple translation scheme I had used as a child was clearly inadequate. The world I saw without my glasses was simply a different world; in some profound sense, it was not the world at all.

Nor could I really remember my pre-cataract world, or chart the history of its disappearance. I had known for some time that I was not seeing as well as I used to see, but I had not drawn the obvious conclusion. For two years, I had been embroiled in the struggles of a failing marriage and its aftermath: a bitter, exhausting, and financially ruinous divorce. The process took a heavy toll upon me, both physically and psychically. . . .

I knew that I was not seeing well; my eyes burned when I read for any length of time, and I was prone to headaches. But I attributed these things to stress and fatigue; when the legal wars

N. ANN DAVIS is an Associate Professor of Moral Theory and Applied Ethics at Pomona College. She is also the Associate Editor of the University of Chicago's *Ethics* journal.

A slightly different form of this essay appeared under the title "Cataracts" in the literary journal of the University of Colorado Health Sciences Center, Fetishes, *3 (1997), 9–10. Reprinted with permission from the author.*

were over, and I could sleep again, I thought the problems would abate. I postponed medical check-ups and my vision exam, both to save money and conserve energy, and to allow my body time to regain its former balance.

I continued to have problems reading and driving at night, but the edifice of evasion and denial that I had crafted during the separation remained firmly in place. I thus let nearly a year pass after the divorce before I went to have my eyes checked. One day, as I was walking to my office and looking up at the trees just coming into leaf, I stopped in disbelief. Though I could tell by the size and general shape of the green blur before me that the leaves were coming out, I could not actually see individual leaves. And I could not really discern where one tree ended and another began, not because I was walking in a grove layered thick with different sorts of trees, but because something had happened to my depth perception.

In my work, I had always made a point of attending carefully to nuance and detail. Now there I was, no longer living in a physical world rich with subtlety and depth, but stumbling through one that was flat and impressionistic. Nor was it just my perception of the world that was awry; somehow my sense of my own presence in the world had become blurred as well.

I cannot say whether the divorce, or its physical aftermath, is what changed me, or my body. Nor can I separate the physical consequences of stress and suffering from the more basic facts of aging. No one really knows why I happened to develop cataracts so young, and thus no one can reassure me that their emergence bore no relation to the events in my life. I see my physical affliction as inextricably bound up with the misfortune of a bad marriage, and the misery of divorce. My vision failed, perhaps, because my experience of the public world came, in salient respects, to mirror my private life.

And I know that my childhood attempts to construct my grandfather's . . . were kind, yet off the mark. Even when we love them, we cannot see the world as others do, through their eyes, or understand what it is like to walk in their shoes, with their feet. With the added dimension of disability must come the acknowledgment of a larger private space around the individual, and the recognition of greater, possibly even unbridgeable, distance. . . .

Even portions of my own experiences have been lost to me: in some respects, the world before disability is essentially unrecoverable to the person who experiences disability. As I have learned, we do not easily acknowledge that things have changed, that details have blurred or faded. We may choose to live in darkness and denial for a long time before we will admit the light has dimmed. And even then, the suspicion—the certainty—is that the world itself remains the same, but that we have somehow lost it. It is as if we were sifting sand through a sieve: when the very texture of things blurs and coarsens, we doubt our ability to recall the finer objects that now lie buried. . . .

We cannot bridge the gaps that lie between our own experience and others' simply by coming to understand that there are gaps there, or even why they are there: we must learn somehow to feel our way across them. Whatever we are taught about the causes of disability, and in whatever detail we try to reconstruct the perceptions and sorrows of people who have experienced it, we cannot really understand what it is like for them to see or stumble as they do, and we cannot really imagine ourselves seeing or walking or feeling as they do.

In the end, all we can know by understanding is that they cannot see detail or dimension, or cannot walk without pain; that their world is shaped by such things, and they wish that it were otherwise. For such affliction, it is not simply the pursuit of understanding, but the cultivation of simple kindness that may be the better remedy.

Chained Smoker

DAVID S. SHIMM, M.D.

THE MAN SAT in the examination chair as the physician talked to him. He could feel the sunlight coming through the window, warming his face. . . . Although in his fifties, he looked like an old man. His face was tanned and wrinkled, and his cheeks and lips were sunken because he had no teeth to fill them out. His gaunt temples emphasized his dark, sunken eyes. He had a full head of oily, unkempt black hair that was peppered with gray. On his hands and forearms were several crude tattoos in faded ballpoint pen. One spelled his ex-wife's name, and another represented the torso of a nude, headless woman. Various cellmates had etched these tattoos as they passed monotonous hours in the county jail for petty offenses: fighting, public drunkenness, driving under the influence of alcohol. The index and middle fingers of both his hands were stained brown, one of the stigmata of his years of smoking. His hands were calloused, and there were deep cracks in his skin around his knuckles. His left ring finger was missing above the first joint. His life had been rough, and his body bore the scars of the abuse that had been done to him by others and by himself.

He had gone to the physician because of pain in his tongue and an ache in his ear when he swallowed. Although he initially brushed it off, the pain became so bad when he swallowed that he had stopped eating; he had already lost 15 pounds. He had seen this physician for the first time 2 days earlier. The physician spent an eternity asking questions and examining him. After

DAVID S. SHIMM, M.D., University of Arizona, Tucson, AZ.

he finished, he told the man that he probably had a malignant tumor in his tongue, but he needed to do a biopsy to be sure.

. . . Although the biopsy itself did not hurt, the feeling of tissue being torn from his tongue without pain was almost worse than the pain of the injection. After that, he was aware of the metallic taste of blood and, later, a dull ache as the anesthetic wore off.

"The results of your biopsy are back," said the physician. . . . "I'm sorry, it doesn't look good. You have a malignant tumor in your tongue." . . . "There are two ways of treating this. The first way is to operate. We would have to take out most of your tongue, part of your jaw, and the lymph glands in your neck. It's a fairly big operation, and you'd probably be in the hospital for a couple of weeks, maybe even a month if you had problems healing. The other way would be to treat you with chemotherapy and radiation. With those, you'd probably have some nausea, you'd have a bad sore throat, and afterwards your mouth would be permanently dry. With either treatment, you've got about a 50–50 chance." "No good choices, I guess. What if I do nothing?"

The physician paused before responding. "Well, the tumor would continue to grow." "And how would it kill me?" "Well, in this location, it would either grow big enough to choke off your airway or keep you from swallowing, or it would eat into a blood vessel and you'd bleed to death. Not very gentle ways to go. I really wouldn't recommend doing nothing. There's still a reasonable chance of curing this tumor." The two stared

Annals of Internal Medicine 129 (1998): 331–332. Reprinted by permission of the American College of Physicians.

at one another for a moment before the physician continued. "Another thing . . . it's really important for you to quit smoking. I know it's hard, but if you do, you'll tolerate the treatment better, and you'll be less likely to get another kind of cancer later."

The man sat staring at the wall, focusing on one of the spots of drywall showing through. He felt numb, just as he did whenever his foot fell asleep, a numbness that took his strength away. But this time it wasn't his foot: It was his mind and his soul that were numb. . . . "How much time do I have to decide?" "You really need to make a decision in the next few days," answered the physician. "Time isn't on your side, but this is an important decision, and you need to feel comfortable with your choice. Let's make an appointment for you to come in and talk right after lunch, the day after tomorrow."

The man nodded and sat in the chair for a few more moments. . . . He swallowed, and there was the pain again, stabbing into his ear. He reached into his shirt pocket and took out his pack of cigarettes. Holding the pack between thumb and forefinger, he examined it. He closed his hand around the pack to crush it but then stopped. He removed a cigarette, put it in his mouth, and pulled a nearly empty book of matches from between the cardboard and the cellophane. Striking a match, he lit the cigarette, took it from his mouth, and held it to the stoma he had breathed through since he had lost his larynx to cancer. He inhaled deeply.

Returns of the Day

NANCY V. RAINE

ON AN AUTUMN AFTERNOON in Boston seven years ago, when the cherry tree in my garden was the color of orange marmalade and the sky was a flawless blue, a man slipped through the back door of my ground-floor apartment while I was taking out the trash.

I don't know how long he skulked in my home, or in what shadows. Long enough for me to lock the back door, turn my back, walk over to the sink and begin to wash the pan I'd cooked oatmeal in that morning. I was scrubbing it

NANCY V. RAINE is the author of *After Silence: Rape and My Journey Back*. New York: Crown, 1998.

when he grabbed me from behind. "I'm going to kill you," he said. He dragged me into my bedroom and, using duct tape, blindfolded and bound me. He then beat me and raped me. I never saw him. Only his enormous feet.

The anniversary of my rape is the brooding axis of my year, more significant than my birthday. After all, I don't remember my own birth struggle. But I remember even second of those three hours. Like the majority of rapists, he was never caught, tried or imprisoned. Like all survivors, I am growing accustomed to living with an anniversary that can be marked only by silence, a silence that tastes a lot like shame.

New York Times Magazine, *October 2, 1994, p. 34. Reprinted by permission of Nancy V. Raine.*

Every year I feel the anniversary coming even before my conscious mind recognizes it. When the air crisps and the leaves begin to turn, I get this thing about taking out the trash. About oatmeal. The eyes in the back of my head, the ones that are never shut, begin to burn like the autumn colors, filling me with emotions I still can't encompass.

I know how to mark my birthday, my wedding anniversary, even the anniversary of my brother's death. But the day I was raped? How should I observe the passing of another year? After all, I did take the trash out yesterday, and just this morning—*the* morning—I ate oatmeal standing at my kitchen window while contemplating the wild plum trees in my California garden that were turning the color of . . . orange marmalade.

Of course, anniversaries are celebrations. Celebrate is what I do on my birthday, with friends and family who make a fuss that I outwardly protest and secretly relish. Celebrate is what I do on my wedding anniversary, when my husband and I slip out of the humdrum and go off and do something silly that makes us appreciate our routine again. And on the anniversary of my kid brother's death, I call my mother and we retell the story of how he carried his pet alligator to the zoo when it outgrew the bathtub—in a paper bag on a Washington bus. I am never alone when I celebrate these anniversaries, because someone else remembers them, too.

Is it possible to celebrate this anniversary alone, as alone as I was that afternoon? Celebrate in silence my slow coming to terms with the fact that I can never again be that woman who locked her door and felt safe. My husband, my mother, my friends still suffer their own brand of helplessness when they try to imagine the content of my memory. My father, who spent his life in law enforcement, leaves the room if the subject of rape in general, or my rape in particular, creeps into the conversation. Why remind them? And dare they remind me, when they secretly hope I might be "over it" at last?

Silently every year on this date I remember with particular lucidity what it was like to be only mindless instinct, a collection of synapses and fibers, muscle and bone, organized around a single desire: to live another second. This reduction to such bare necessities of body was an alchemy that spun not gold but something dark and polar, a terrible knowledge that to this day sits in the center of my heart like glacial ice. Why remind people who love me it is still there?

On this anniversary, more or less safe in the cradle of the day's routine, I began to think back. To the first anniversary, when I realized that I had to stop talking about what happened to me because the people who loved me could not bear to hear it. The second, when I pretended to myself I was "over it." The third, when I realized I wasn't. The fourth, when I was in treatment for post-traumatic stress syndrome. The fifth, when I was convinced my treatment wasn't helping and secretly wondered if I had the guts to kill myself. The sixth, during a lunch date, when I told a woman I barely knew that our meeting was occurring on the anniversary of my rape. I spoke matter-of-factly, afraid she might gather up her black briefcase and suddenly remember a dentist's appointment. "My 10th was in June," she replied.

As the seventh anniversary hour, 3:30 P.M., approached, I made a cup of tea. I remembered a story I'd heard 25 years earlier from my friend George. In those days, work crews marked construction sites by putting out smudge pots with open flames. George's 4-year-old daughter got too close to one and her pants caught fire like the Straw Man's stuffing. The scars running the length and breadth of Sarah's legs looked like pieces of a jigsaw puzzle. In the third grade she was asked, "If you could have one wish, what would it be?" Sarah wrote: "I want everyone to have legs like mine."

Yes, I thought.

When George first told this story I knew it contained a profound truth, but not what that truth was, nor that I would need it someday. Today, I understand that the self consumes misfortune like a sacred potion until the glass is empty. And this bitter elixir changes who we are.

Sarah could not imagine herself without her scars. But she *could* imagine those scars not setting her apart. She could imagine not being alone. She was not wishing her misfortune on others, but wishing they could share it with her.

I finished my tea and realized I was too anxious to take my daily walk The odds of being raped don't go down because you've been raped once. A little past 3:30, the doorbell rang. I crept to the peep hole and looked out. It was only the local florist, a woman. The bouquet she presented was huge — yellow roses, pale orange lilies and blue irises. It was from my goddaughter, a university student, who was viciously attacked and sexually molested two years ago by a pack of American college boys in a bar in Mexico. The note read: "You are not alone. Love K."

No. I am not alone. There are millions of us celebrating our silent anniversaries, I thought.

Someday we will all march to the Capitol carrying flowers, and we will leave them on the steps. We will celebrate our anniversaries. We will give our names. The month, the day, the year, the hour. We will stop being silent. We will stop being alone. It doesn't have to be in autumn. I'm not picky.

Case Study Exercises

1. What do you believe are the most pressing health care issues we face? What do you think our priorities should be as a society, and what should we do in order to achieve justice in health care?

2. What should we do about the concerns raised by the following information about poverty and health?

   The U.S. Conference of Mayors reports that requests for emergency food increased an average of 14% during the period 1997–1998. One out of five requests for food assistance went unmet. The American Journal of Public Health in 1998 reported that 10 million Americans — including more than four million children — do not have enough to eat; a majority are members of families with at least one member working. All members of Congress enjoy publicly financed health care, but they refuse to extend these same benefits to their constituents. And the private sector is walking away: in 1985 nearly two-thirds of all businesses with 100 or more employees paid the full cost of health care coverage. Today fewer than one-third still do. (See "Wealth and Health," in *Rachel's Environment and Health Weekly*, no. 654, June 10, 1999)

3. What is the best way to regulate health insurance companies? Include your ideas for regulating health insurance to prevent abuses like this case:

   National Medical Care struck deals worth hundreds of thousands of dollars a year with kidney specialists and other doctors who determined both where dialysis patients went for care and how hospital contracts to treat the sickest patients were awarded. For example, National Medical paid the insurance on the Rolls Royce owned by Dr. Arnold Roland, the supervisor of a kidney dialysis clinic. Deals like these helped National Medical become the country's largest provider in the competitive (kidney) dialysis business. This is true, even as it has been accused by patients' groups and government investigators of using procedures and equipment that, they contend, bolster profits while placing the health of patients at risk. (See Kurt Eichenwalk, "Doctors' Highest-Paid Skill: Steering in Kidney Patients," *New York Times*, 5 December 1995.)

4. In April 1996 the AMA recommended that investors dump tobacco stocks — the most sweeping call yet by a major public health group for divestiture of tobacco stocks. They suggested all investors sell their shares in 13 tobacco companies and 1,474 mutual funds

holding tobacco securities. One AMA official, Dr. Randolph Smoak, Jr., said, "All people interested in the health and welfare of our children should review their investments and divest of tobacco" and that tobacco is "a ruinous and enslaving product that has brought misery, disease, anguish and death." Scott D. Ballin of the American Heart Assn. responded, "It's the appropriate thing to do, and long overdue. . . . We should not be supporting companies that continue to sell disease and death in this country and overseas." (See Hiltzik and Jackson, "AMA Calls on Investors to Dump Tobacco Stocks," *Los Angeles Times,* 24 April 1996.)

   a. What could be said in support of the AMA recommendation?
   b. What could be said in support of the tobacco industry?
   c. To what extent should we consider such lifestyle choices as smoking in ethical decision making around health care resources?

5. Studies by researchers from the Harvard school of Public Health report that reducing economic inequality could reduce mortality rates.
   a. Given that income inequality increases death rates at all ages, from infants to the elderly, what should be done?
   b. Set out three or four recommendations that might be offered by a group representing the rights of poor patients.
   c. Set out three or four recommendations that might be offered by a group representing the rights of doctors and other health care givers.
   d. Set out three or four recommendations that might be offered by a group representing the interests of the more affluent members of society.
   e. If you were hired to negotiate a plan drawing from the various recommendations set out in b–d, what would you propose?

6. How can we keep "mad cow disease" (also known as Creutzfeldt-Jakob disease) away from American and Canadian blood supplies? Mad cow disease (so named in Britain because it was found in cows) kills brain cells and leaves the brain full of holes, like a sponge. Thirty-four humans in Britain have come down with the disease, presumably from eating contaminated meat. One issue before the Food and Drug Administration (FDA) is whether people who have traveled to or lived in Britain since 1980 be prohibited from donating blood and organs. Although the risk of transmission of the disease through blood appears to be very low, scientists fear that failing to take steps now may lead to later epidemics (much as the failure to take AIDS more seriously early on contributed to its spread). Set out your recommendations.

7. Should a surgeon be able to patent surgical techniques? Discuss the concerns raised by the following case and then set out your recommendations for resolving the dilemma:

Dr. Jack Singer, a Vermont ophthalmic surgeon who removes cataracts about 250 times a year specializes in an incision that removes the need for an incision. Dr. Samuel Pallin, an Arizona ophthalmic surgeon, claims to own the procedure for stitchless cataract surgery. He has a patent to support his claim that Dr. Singer and others who use the technique patented by Dr. Pallin should pay him royalties. Patents for techniques used to be very rare, but are now issued several times a week. However, the AMA says it knows of no doctor who has paid another one royalties. Dr. John Glasson, Chair of the AMA Council on Judicial and Ethical Affairs raised questions, saying, "How can anyone claim to own the way one turns one's knife when performing surgery?" Some claim that, no more can a painter own the way she holds her brush or a golfer own the way he handles a club, should it be possible for a surgeon to own a technique. The AMA council fears that patents will restrict access to treatment, obstruct peer review of new therapies, add to the cost of health care, and be impossible to enforce. However, within the field of medicine patents are common and for decades medical techniques have been patented as the directions for using a device that was patented at the same time. Given this, Dr. Pallin asks, "How can the AMA rationally take the position that a pure method patent is unethical, while a combined method and device patent is not?" He also notes that the Hippocratic oath says nothing about intellectual property. (See Sabra Chartrand, "Why Is This Surgeon Suing?," *New York Times,* 8 June 1995.)

8. On February 1st, 1996, it was reported that the length of time a patient survives from AIDS is directly proportional to a doctor's experience in treating the disease. (See Lawrence K. Altman, "AIDS Survival Linked to Doctors' Experience," *New York Times,* 1 Feb 96). University of Washington researchers found that median survival of patients after AIDS was diagnosed was 26 months when treated by the most experienced AIDS doctors and only 14 months for those treated by the least experienced doctors. In light of this study and the fact that doctors need to treat patients to gain experience, what would you recommend be done to give recognition to the study?

9. In *Arato v. Avedon,* a 1993 California Supreme Court case, the question is raised regarding the doctor's duty to disclose to the patient the known statistical odds of the patient's life expectancy:

The case centers on the failure of Arato's doctors to inform him that he had a very high probability of a short life expectancy. The case was not about the medical treatment that was given; it was about the boundaries around the duty to inform the patient about his condition. Arato had been informed about his medical condition (which involved a non-functioning kidney and a pancreatic tumor) and the facts and risks of the radiation and chemotherapy that was part of his treatment. He was told the cancer might recur and, if so, it would be incurable. He was also told that the recommended experimental treatment might have no benefit. However, he was not told that he had a 50-50 chance of being dead within a year, even though he had filled out a questionnaire that doctors gave him and marked "yes" when asked whether he wanted to be told the truth even if his condition were serious. (See Marjorie M. Shultz, "Restoring Informed Consent," *Los Angeles Daily* [Law] *Journal,* 8 September 1993.)

a. In light of this request and the fact that Arato had personal, medical, and professional decisions to make, do you think the California Supreme Court should rule in favor of requiring the doctors to disclose such statistical odds?

b. Should such disclosure be left to the doctor's discretion, given that such odds are never a guarantee of certainty and may cause a patient to become listless or depressed?

c. What do you think the policy should be on disclosing such prognoses to patients?

10. Do patients with tuberculosis (TB), a contagious and debilitating disease, have the right to refuse medication, although others are put at risk? For example, a California woman, Hongkham Souvannarath, was jailed for refusing to take her tuberculosis medication. As David Hadden, a Fresno County California health officer, said, "How do you protect the public? You can't put a sign around her neck telling everyone to steer clear of this woman because if she sneezes she could be spewing out a deadly disease." Jailing TB patients who refuse to take medication is not unheard of; in the mid-1990s officials hunted down and incarcerated such individuals in a special unit of the Fresno county jail. In Souvannarath's case, it seems that she was the victim of "an inadvertent but illegal detention." (See Mark Arax, "Woman Jailed 10 Months for Refusing TB Medicine," *Los Angeles Times,* 31 May 1999.)

The issue centers on patient rights vs. the society's right to be protected. Where should we draw the line? Share your thoughts.

11. Given the problems with access to health care, should groups form their own HMOs? In an article in *Health Line* (9 July 1998), "New Mexico: Tribal Groups May Start Own HMO," it was reported that tribes are negotiating with the state of New Mexico about setting up their own managed care health organization in conjunction with the state's Medicaid SALUD! Program.
    a. What do you recommend we do to reach groups that have traditionally had limited, if any, health care coverage?
    b. Is it better to address the issue state by state or attempt some kind of nationalized or socialized medicine?

12. How should we address racism in health care services and distribution? What are some methods the different organizations (such as the AMA, the Canadian Medical Association, the American Nurses Association, American Physical Therapy Association) might adopt to effect some changes in this regard?

13. To what degree do you think violence (domestic violence, rape, incest, gang violence, shootings in schools, and so on) should be treated as a *medical* problem and not just a social issue? Set out your thoughts on this and any recommendations you might have.

14. A Maryland man, Kevin Knussman, was awarded $375,000 for being denied extended leave to care for his newborn child on account of his gender. In the first sex discrimination case under the Federal Family and Medical Leave Act, a jury recognized that fathers also have rights to parental leave. He testified that a personnel manager told him, "unless your wife is in a coma or dead, you can't be the primary care provider." (See Tama Lewin, "Father Awarded $375,000 in a Parental Leave Case," *New York Times,* 3 February 1999.) Discuss how our attitudes about men, women, and family relationships affect how we view health care.

15. Looking over the readings in this chapter, what are your impressions about our collective view of health and the sorts of systemic problems we face in addressing health care and the relationships between patients and health care givers?

16. In 1999 the American Philosophical Association asked its members to vote on a public statement opposing the death penalty. Should professional organizations in medicine, such as the AMA and ANA, take public stands on bioethical issues? This dilemma gets raised by cases like the following: Biostatistician Dr. Peter S. Gartside conducted a study of workers at an atomic weapons factory in Fernald, Ohio. He found they died at significantly younger ages (the median life expectancy of the workers was 58 years) and suffered higher rates of cancer than the average American. When a study such as this comes out, do you think groups like the AMA or the ANA have an ethical obligation to issue a response and give their recommendations? How politically active should medical professionals be when they become aware of injustices?

17. In an article on the mind's effect on a person's health, Erica Goode reports on a study publicized in the *Journal of the American Medical Association* showing that writing about traumatic experiences measurably improves the health of patients with chronic asthma or rheumatoid arthritis. Other scientists found that veterans with post-traumatic stress disorder were more likely to suffer several health problems like heart disease and respiratory diseases than were veterans without post-traumatic stress. (See Erica Goode, "Your Mind May Ease What's Ailing You," *New York Times,* 18 April 1999.) Goode wonders why, if scientists are discovering such evidence of reciprocity between mind and body, doctors remain distrustful of treatments, such as kinds of alternative medicine, that use psychological means to achieve physical results. And we might also ask, to what degree should evidence of a mind-body connection affect our view of health care?

InfoTrac College Edition

1. Sev S. Fluss, "Ethics in Health: Some Current Perspectives"
2. Kevin P. Glynn, "Can We Still Earn a Living Caring for Sick People?"
3. John M. Luddin, "Can the Patient Be the Focus of Managed Care?"
4. Elizabeth Brown, "Who Should Be Responsible? [For the Payment of Investigational Therapy]"
5. Donna Vavala, "The New Academic Health Center Hybrids: Part Business, Part Academic"
6. Eugene Feingold, "Public Health versus Civil Liberties"
7. U.S. Dept. of Health and Human Resources Report, "Eliminating Racial and Ethnic Disparities in Health: Response to the Presidential Initiatives on Race"
8. Ren-Zong Qiu, "Bioethics in an Asian Context"
9. John Hornberger, Haruka Itakura, and Sandra R. Wilson, "Bridging Language and Cultural Barriers between Physicians and Patients"
10. Jay Noren, David Kindig, and Audrey Sprenger, "Challenges to Native American Health Care"
11. Trude Bennett, "Racial and Ethnic Classification: Two Steps Forward and One Step Back?"
12. Ralph W. Hingson, "College-Age Drinking Problems"
13. Liana B. Winett, "Constructing Violence as a Public Health Problem"

Web Connections

For links to Social Constructions of Health Care Web sites, articles, cases, and more exercises go to our Justice page at philosophy.wadsworth.com /teays.purdy/justice.

Chapter 2

Rights and Obligations in Health Care

CONSIDERATIONS ABOUT THE NATURE and concept of health lead us quite naturally to examining the value of health. Health surely is among the most basic and important of goods. It influences both how we feel at any given moment and what we are capable of doing. It is also morally significant: Our state of health is crucially important to our well-being, and yet health is not just a given. We can assume neither continued good health nor a life free of suffering. Furthermore, health concerns are rarely solitary, in the sense that others are involved and may be directly affected by decisions about medical treatment and access to care. Thus it follows that health status is something to which the concept of justice is relevant.

In general, justice dictates that people have equal shares of health, other things being equal. Unfortunately, this isn't the case. Whatever forces are at work in the universe have yet to address inequities in the distribution of physical well-being. Consequently, applying considerations of justice to health requires understanding the factors that affect health, rendering it better or worse. We tend to focus on health care as the primary determinant of health, and consequently much of our concern about justice has been channeled into discussions about the distribution of health care. Although this is an important topic, we need to think more broadly about the causes of ill health and disability. Only then can we consistently practice prevention rather than focusing on patching people up, as does much of contemporary medical science.

The power to cure, although extensive, has inherent limitations. And even if we found cures for all known diseases, others — as we have seen with AIDS — can appear. Even if we could anticipate new diseases, we cannot prevent suffering and death. For this reason, there will never be a "magic bullet" in health care. There will always be threats to our health and the reality that death is inevitable for each of us. This fact is both obvious and hard to face; this may be one reason people spend, on average, 70% of their health care dollars in the last six months of life.

How we live, how we deal with medical problems, and how we die are deeply woven into the social fabric. Because of this, in our society we emphasize patient autonomy and self-determination. However, as Virginia Warren discussed in Chapter 1, those very concepts warrant examination, in light of questions regarding power and empowerment and the consequences for decision making in health care.

One way these issues have been framed is by focusing on the question whether we have a right to health. Oddly enough, there is little debate about this topic, although people do comment that there is no way to guarantee health to people. Nevertheless, the question is a good jumping-off point for deeper inquiry: What, if anything, does society owe us in the way of health protection? To what extent must society keep track of the health consequences of various policies? Where policies endanger health, how should conflicts be resolved? Last, but not least, do we have equal claims to protection, and what does such equality imply? If we don't have equal claims, why not? In short, what are the justice dimensions of health care? As we draw the boundaries of medical ethics, we have a moral obligation to pay attention to underlying issues of justice.

Let us therefore begin with what we can rightfully assume about justice and health care. In democratic societies, it seems reasonable to start with the assumption that the health of each individual is to be considered equally important. Exceptions to this rule should be restricted to those who freely and voluntarily undertake greater risks, and to those who must, in times of emergency, act to protect society as a whole. The risks undertaken by such individuals must surely be kept to a minimum, and be compensated. Judging how to balance the costs of risk minimization and compensation where they come into conflict with other values is a matter to be democratically decided.

This line of argumentation requires of us a very fundamental discussion about social and political arrangements. Why? Because there is coming to be more and more evidence that factors like the degree of overall inequality a society tolerates are relevant to health. And that relation should not be too surprising: health is greatly affected by a huge array of factors. A good diet, plenty of exercise, good preventive care, toxin-free environments, occupational safety, and protection from crime are among the factors that enhance health; their opposites put health at risk.

Good health education is clearly crucial, for it helps people make healthy choices. But many people cannot make those choices because they lack access to the material resources to secure these goods for themselves. In our society, members of disadvantaged groups are much less likely to enjoy these basic protections. Their rates of illness and death reflect their powerlessness: They cannot buy their way out of dangerous situations, and they often get substandard health care.

These facts press us to probe our values, since safety often comes into conflict with such values as a business-friendly environment, convenience, or a powerful military establishment. A business-friendly environment means less regulation of businesses. For example, look at the 1990 decision in the case of *John Moore v. Regents of University of California*. A patient whose unique properties in his blood cured his leukemia was considered to have no property rights in the commercialization of a potentially enormously profitable cell line that was created on the basis of Moore's blood and tissues. In effect, the court gave a green light to biotechnology firms, even though it was a setback for patient rights.

However encouraging the environment may be, businesses can be dangerous for those who work in them, dangerous for the consumers of their products, or dangerous for society at large. For example, in the case of Film Recovery Systems, Inc., a worker died from exposure to cyanide used in stripping the silver off x-ray film. An investigation of the death revealed conditions so appalling that the district attorney of Illinois prosecuted the president, vice-president, plant manager, and plant foreman on murder charges.

There are many other examples of workers suffering death or serious bodily harm. For instance, just look at pesticide accidents affecting farm workers, exposure of Navajo miners to uranium, construction workers' exposure to asbestos, nuclear workers' exposure to low-level radiation, or exposure to second-hand smoke by those working in smoke-ridden environments with poor ventilation. Consider, too, the many examples of workplace accidents that are also environmental disasters on a global scale, such as the Bhopal gas leak, the Chernobyl nuclear accident, and the Exxon Valdez oil spill.

The workplace is not the only concern. Consumers cannot assume that the commodities they buy are safe. For example, we saw numerous cases of Ford Pintos bursting into flames in rear-end collisions because of the lack of an $11 part that would have acted as a buffer between the gas tank and the rear of the car. Look too at tobacco: Smokers are sold a nicotine delivery system in the form of cigarettes and face all the risks that follow. And there is the example of women who have breast implants and who now face an uncertain health future because of possible links between breast implants and autoimmune diseases and other health problems.

We also tolerate many health threats, such as high speed limits, in the name of convenience. For that matter, public transportation is much safer than our current transportation system emphasizing individually owned cars: Most of the 40,000–50,000 deaths a year in the U.S. alone could be avoided. Likewise, there was the exposure of men and women to safety hazards like radiation, Agent Orange, and the biowarfare-chemical vaccines now thought to be the cause of the Gulf Vet Syndrome.

In short, a thoroughgoing and informed concern for health puts into question many ways of doing things that we take for granted. Improving health clearly requires much heightened awareness of the health consequences of basic social arrangements. Thus it is necessary to look more systematically at such arrangements, perhaps by means of independent review committees whose sole charge is to raise ethical and social concerns. Reason requires that we be aware of the trade-offs we are making and that we be prepared to change social arrangements resulting in health costs that are too high or unfairly distributed.

It is also important to consider how to pursue justice with respect to health in more traditional ways. Health care may not be the primary determinant of health. Nevertheless, it can help prevent disease or disability, sometimes it can cure, and it can often alleviate pain and suffering. It is therefore an important component in health, and justice seems to require that it be equally available to all. In the United States and Canada, physicians are usually the first, and most significant, contact patients have with the health care establishment. Because of this, a number of concerns arise regarding justice and patient care. For instance, we need to ask whether physicians are morally required to care for patients unable to pay for care, and, if not, whether health care is merely a commodity like any other.

The answers to these questions are intimately related to our conception of medicine as a profession. For instance, what role should profit play in the enterprise? And, more generally, do members of the profession have special duties in virtue of their education and society's trust in them? If so, what duties? We might wonder, for example, whether physicians should be prohibited from doing research on a patient because of the potential conflicts of interest involved. The AMA code, however, is silent on this issue.

Likewise, should physicians be held to the Hippocratic oath that they should provide care even if they are not compensated? In the past, most people sought care and paid the bill when they could. More recently, as medicine has become more dependent upon technology, and thus more expensive, many people bought insurance to cover their bills. Unfortunately, medical insurance itself has become too expensive for many people. Consequently, the reality now is that some people have private medical insurance, some have group medical insurance, some have Medicare (or similar basic-needs government insurance), and some have no medical insurance whatsoever.

In 1996, some 41 million people in the U.S. had no insurance at all, and many others were poorly covered. As costs rise and fewer social resources are allocated toward providing care, there are fewer and fewer sources of free or inexpensive care. Many people have enrolled in so-called health maintenance organizations (HMOs). Many of these are for-profit businesses, providing all care for a single, monthly fee, with perhaps some small co-payments for additional services. Their emphasis on prevention and careful control over access to high-tech and high-cost medical treatment holds costs down. However, questions have arisen about their ability to provide high-quality care to those who do get sick.

The fundamental moral problem here is whether justice requires equal access to appropriate care, without either age restrictions or the application of explicit or implicit social worth criteria. Explicit criteria have been used to deny care to prisoners, undocumented aliens, or substance abusers. More implicitly, such factors as gender, race, or sexual orientation have affected both the quantity and quality of care available to members of certain groups.

Many people believe that society has no duty to provide care for those who cannot pay, or who are deemed insufficiently worthy. For example, in California there have been attempts to restrict medical care so that undocumented aliens or others of questionable legal status cannot obtain prenatal care. Similarly, although prisoners have access to medical care, they cannot ordinarily receive organ transplants.

Many others believe that health is a fundamental human good and that both justice and care for others put health care in a special category, like basic education. Taking this right seriously motivates the drive for universal access to quality care. A central challenge for any civilized society, according to this view, is finding ways to achieve that goal. No society can be considered just that disregards it.

THE READINGS

The readings in this chapter are divided into two parts; the first focuses on the right to health and the second looks at the right to care. The right to health considers the broader social context within which health evolves, such as inequalities based on race, gender, or class that, for example, discourage healthy lifestyle choices or increase exposure to environmental toxins. The right to health care considers the more traditional bioethics questions about the delivery of care.

The first section contains the following readings.

1. In the first reading Suzanne Gordon argues that patients are getting worse care because HMOs emphasize profit.

2. Annette Dula argues that bioethics has largely ignored the needs and interests of those, like African Americans, who are for the most part excluded from positions of power and influence.

3. Gregory Pappas elaborates on the relationships among race, socioeconomic status, and health.

4. The AMA Council on Scientific Affairs provides additional food for thought on this topic, with specific reference to the health of Hispanics.

5. Nancy Krieger and Mary Bassett investigate arguments used to explain the differential between the health of black and white Americans.

6. Carol Jonann Bess examines gender (and to a lesser degree, age) bias in health care, focusing on the disparity she sees in all levels of health care related to coronary heart disease, with examples of the extent of the problem.

In the second section we examine the right to care and the issue of professional obligations and access to health care.

1. Tom H. Christoffel makes the argument that health care is a human right, thus deserving of a set of protections (and a constitutional provision) not currently recognized. He uses as a case in point the dire health needs seen in Garfield Park, a ghetto on the west side of Chicago.

2. Harry Schwartz, assessing the question of professional duties, denies that individual physicians have any special obligation toward indigent patients.

3. In a contrasting article, Steven H. Miles looks at the treatment of indigent patients in terms of their medical care, arguing for a more compassionate system.

4. Addressing the ways in which people have access to health care, the American College of Physicians sets out a proposal that can help clarify for us what sorts of things we might do to change the status quo.

5. The American Nurses Association has also addressed some of the deep-seated prejudices played out in health care, and offers specific suggestions for addressing racism and discrimination.

6. Sidney D. Watson tackles the issue of minority access to health care and asserts that this is a right that has not been given its due, and that, consequently, health care reform is in order.

7. Abby L. Wilkerson examines the intersection of violence and health care. She argues that the mainstream medical paradigm is questionable, showing how it harms women in the way it conceptualizes rape and setting out some recommendations.

8. In the last article of the chapter, Leigh Turner looks at the silence of bioethicists on gun-related violence and argues that the issue warrants our attention, especially in light of the extent of the problem.

The Right to Health

Is There a Nurse in the House?

SUZANNE GORDON

LATE LAST OCTOBER [1994], an advertisement appeared in several national and California newspapers. Alongside pictures of nurses standing at the bedside of acutely ill patients was the following statement: "Hospitals and HMOs are cutting care to make record profits. Patients are paying the price. Just ask any registered nurse who provides direct care."

The ad launched a California Nurses Association (C.N.A.) campaign called "Patient Watch." It is an attempt to reach out to patients and families and elicit Congressional action to address what nurses — and increasingly many physicians — feel is a trend that is literally endangering the lives of thousands of patients: Responding to market pressures, hospitals are "restructuring" or downsizing. By pitting hospitals against one another in the bidding for managed-care contracts, the new lords of the health care market — insurers and H.M.O.s — are winning drastic discounts, often below the hospitals' actual costs. To make up their losses, hospitals are cutting their nursing

SUZANNE GORDON is an adjunct professor at the McGill University School of Nursing.

staffs, which represent about 28 percent of hospital labor costs.

Competition, says John O'Brien, C.E.O. of the Cambridge Hospital and chairman-elect of the Massachusetts Hospital Association, is forcing hospitals to "squeeze down on our costs at every possible level." O'Brien is a longtime supporter of single-payer health care and a vocal critic of competition. "Nursing has been hard hit. Nursing is the backbone of the hospital. But the pressures we're putting on our nurses are inordinate. I'm doing it, like everyone else is. It certainly can't continue."

According to a 1994 study done in conjunction with the American Hospital Association's *Hospitals and Health Networks* magazine, nearly three-fourths of American hospitals of every kind — private nonprofits, for-profit hospital chains, public hospitals, small community and large teaching hospitals — are engaged in or developing plans for "restructuring." In 1994 the American Nurses Association conducted a survey of nursing layoffs. Preliminary findings of the yet-unpublished study report on data provided by 1,835 nurses from all fifty states. Seventy percent

Permission from the February 12, 1995, issue of The Nation, *pp. 199–201.*

of the respondents said their employers were cutting back on staffing by leaving vacated positions unfilled, 66 percent said hospitals had laid off nurses or were planning to do so, and 45 percent said that the use of unlicensed assistive personnel (U.A.P.s) was increasing. Three-quarters of the nurses in hospitals with reduced nursing staff said patient care had eroded and more than two-thirds said patient safety was compromised.

These nurses are being replaced with lower-wage and less-skilled employees, like nursing assistants and technicians who may have no health care background and yet are asked to make complex nursing decisions. Aides are not required to meet any educational or licensing requirements. Nurses who remain at the bedside must now care for more patients and supervise these techs as well. Moreover, they are legally responsible for any mistakes the U. A.P.s make.

In Massachusetts and California, which have the highest penetration of managed care in the country, this trend is increasingly common. In 1993, Boston's prestigious nonprofit Brigham and Women's Hospital laid off more than forty registered nurses. The hospital wiped out its entire continuing care department, laying off seven clinical nurse specialists, one nurse practitioner and one staff educator. They were replaced by less expensive social workers who had no formal medical education. Brigham and Women's nurses are now required to work mandatory overtime and have had to give up the kinds of flexible scheduling arrangements that had been marked improvements in their working conditions and job satisfaction.

When Brigham and Women's announced its historic merger with Massachusetts General Hospital in December 1993, the heads of those two institutions—each of whom earned close to a million dollars that year—announced even further staff cuts. They trumpeted that they were going to cut 20 percent of their budgets, which could entail the loss of at least 4,000 hospital jobs. At Massachusetts General, nurses' anecdotal reports suggest that vacated positions aren't being filled and that many units are understaffed. Massachusetts General and Brigham and Women's are hardly struggling hospitals. These nonprofit hospitals have constructed palatial new facilities, added redundant and unnecessary services, hired outside consultants, and spent enormous sums buying up primary physician practices, as well as on advertising and marketing.

In California, R.N.-to-patient ratios have declined precipitately. Even in critical-care units— developed specifically to provide intensive nursing care—staffing has suffered, nurses say, as hospitals try to game the system to slash costs. Some hospitals, nurses report, have renamed units to disguise the intensity of patient needs. In others, patients may be transferred out of critical-care units prematurely just to reduce the number of R.N.s employed in those units.

Deborah Bayer, a staff nurse in the critical-care unit at Children's Hospital in Oakland, said that in 1993 the hospital replaced 20 percent of its medical surgical R.N.s with aides on a one-to-one ratio. (The hospital recorded a $6.2 million profit and has finished construction of a large ambulatory care center.) These aides were given eleven days of training before replacing R.N.s with years of schooling and bedside experience. On medical surgical floors, says Bayer, administrators insist that because nurses now have "helpers," they can carry a caseload of five or six patients, sometimes even six or seven patients, rather than three or four.

Even the nonprofit H.M.O. Kaiser Permanente is now developing a radical redesign of its health care delivery system, referred to as the Gateways Operational Planning Project. Literature on the project presents a design that faithfully mirrors industrial mass-production techniques. The process of patient care is broken down into its constituent parts. Each moment of the patient's day is plotted in advance and each fragment of care is assigned to a different assembly-line worker. Nurses are replaced by "multi-skilled caregivers," most of whom will be lower-paid aides. Streamlined to move along a well-oiled factory conveyor belt, patients will have less and less contact with skilled nurses. Those nurses who remain in the hospital will function not as repositories of intimate knowledge about and connection with the patient but as detached managers who supervise less educated and less experienced members of the "care team."

Periodic attempts to de-skill nurses have long concerned members of that profession. But today, this trend is particularly dangerous. Patricia Benner, professor of physiological nursing at the University of California at San Francisco School of Nursing, says "there is no one in a hospital today who is not in that hospital because they are very sick. We rarely put patients in hospitals just for observation. We rarely admit them prior to surgery and we discharge them faster after their surgeries. This means that the acuity level of patients is far higher than it used to be and that most of these patients have conditions where there is very little room for error. They need instantaneous interventions and great skill."

Administrators claim that their new policies are intended to help patients by liberating nurses from unnecessary tasks so they can spend more time doing "real nursing"—redefined as managing the patient from afar. Less costly aides, not expensive nurses, should be the ones taking temperatures, giving bedpans and feeding patients, insist administrators and insurers. Again, most nurses argue vehemently against this corporate redefinition of their profession. "Administrators tell us that you don't really need nurses to change a baby's diaper or feed a baby. Aides can do that, and we can stand back and assess the patient, devise a plan of care and supervise the aide who carries it out," says Bayer. But how, she asks, can you evaluate patients if you no longer have the relationship with them over time that is the hallmark of nursing?

When she's feeding a baby, Bayer explains, she's engaged in a whole series of complex cognitive activities. "I'm learning if the baby has energy to suck. I'm determining what her color is while she's sucking. When I'm changing a baby I'm diagnosing that baby's condition. Does he cry out in pain when I touch him? What does his skin look like? Babies can't verbally tell you how they feel. How you learn is through interactions around their bodily care."

In the Orwellian doublespeak of corporate-driven health care reform this denial of critical care is recast as "patient-driven" or "patient-centered care." The results, however, are often far from "patient-centered." According to the C.N.A., a labor and delivery nurse at a Berkeley hospital related the following incident: "On a very busy night when we were already understaffed, a patient whom we didn't know showed up and said she was in labor. The ward clerk directed her to a room and notified the charge nurse of her arrival. The patient used the bell twice to complain that she was in pain and needed a nurse, but the ward clerk could not find anyone free who could see her. When the patient had been there about twenty to thirty minutes, her husband came out to say that she had to push. Our ward clerk called two of us and said it was an emergency, so we left our patients and ran to the new patient's room. When we arrived, she had delivered a very small baby into the toilet, head first. The baby was too small to survive and died of prematurity."

Similar stories are now surfacing in hospitals, and are reminiscent of the horrors of the nursing crisis of the mid-1980s, when a critical shortage of nurses resulted in significant problems with patient care. Take the case of a 72-year-old man who was diagnosed with lung cancer. The man was well-insured, and his family included several health care professionals who should have been able to get him the very best treatment. He was admitted to a large teaching hospital to have a lung removed. The operation went extremely well, and the surgeons announced that he was making a remarkable recovery. When he left the recovery unit for a general medical surgical floor, his physicians believed he could be discharged a day early. Unfortunately, the hospital had targeted the medical surgical floor for drastic cuts in its nursing staff. The patient developed pneumonia, which went undetected and untreated until it was too late. He died three days later.

Stunned at the outcome, one of his family members, who is a nurse, said, "At the end, he was surrounded by all this incredible high-tech medical equipment. But the tragic thing was that all he needed was the most rudimentary piece of medical equipment—a stethoscope—and a nurse who had the time and experience to check on him, listen to his chest and hear the unmistakable wheezing of pneumonia. If he had gotten that kind of routine attention, he would probably be alive today."

Research studies documenting what happens when nursing care is eliminated are beginning to appear. Boston College nursing professor Judith Shindul-Rothschild studied nurses' working conditions and patient care in a geographical cross section of Massachusetts hospitals in 1989 and 1994. The 1994 study reported that the numbers of R.N.s decreased and unlicensed personnel increased. In the same study, 43 percent of nurses polled reported recent increases in unsafe staffing levels, and nurses reported fifteen patient deaths because of inadequate staffing. One of these occurred in a sub-acute unit; because of understaffing, no one responded when an alarm light sounded on a patient's respirator, signaling that the patient was going into respiratory arrest. The patient died. In another incident, a patient who had been disconnected from a respirator died because not enough nurses were on duty. Six patients committed suicide while unattended.

A clear sign of the seriousness of the problems in hospitals is that a number of physicians are speaking out to defend nursing. Traditionally, physicians have downplayed nurses' importance. But Dr. John Merritt O'Donnell, chairman of the Department of Surgical Intensive Care at The Lahey Clinic outside Boston, points out that in medical and surgical intensive-care units, nurses constantly re-evaluate patients and "rec-

ognize the most subtle changes in vital signs, mental status and sophisticated monitors that may herald a catastrophic event. Their role has become even more crucial recently because the dramatic reduction in residency training programs has depleted the number of interns and residents previously providing twenty-four-hour-a-day in-hospital coverage. Physicians now, more than ever, rely on nursing assessments and recommendations when making diagnostic and therapeutic decisions. There are certainly deserving targets for cuts—physician spending, pharmaceuticals, hospital middle management and insurance. But don't cut nursing care."

Not only does competition eliminate expert nurses at the bedside, it also deprives patients of nursing care through the dramatic acceleration of the trend toward early hospital discharge that began with the introduction of controls on Medicare payments in the mid-1980s. The United States now has the shortest length of hospital stay of any industrialized country—a development that has done nothing to curtail soaring health care costs. Patients in this country stay in hospitals 20 to 40 percent fewer days than in countries with single-payer systems. Managed care groups have embraced early discharge with religious fervor: They discharge patients from the hospital much more quickly than traditional fee-for-service plans.

"You would not believe what people are going home with today," Dr. Ruth McCorkle, American Cancer Society Professor of Nursing at the University of Pennsylvania School of Nursing and a researcher on the home care needs of cancer patients, exclaims with undisguised outrage. "We're doing mastectomies on an outpatient basis. Mastectomies!" She pauses, almost with disbelief. "Women are going home with complex dressing changes, with drains from their wounds, with injections they have to give themselves. Men are going home after prostate surgery with inadequate education about the consequences of their surgery. And I haven't even gotten to the emotional needs of these patients, who are faced with life-threatening illnesses and whose bodies may have been dramatically altered.

"In our ongoing study of testing nursing interventions in elderly postsurgical cancer patients, a fifth of our sample has deep-vein thrombosis [blood clots in the leg]. Out of that group, four have been re-admitted with pulmonary emboli [clots that travel from the leg to the pulmonary arteries, where they can cause instant death]. This means we're getting them out of the hospital so fast that we're forgetting the fundamentals about the dangers of blood clots after surgery and the need for nurses to initiate walking with supervision after surgery."

"Taking care of patients today is an exercise in frustration," says Martha Griffin, almost in despair. A nurse for twenty-four years who works as a cardiac thoracic critical-care nurse at Brigham and Women's Hospital, Griffin reports that over the past year and a half, some patients having open-heart surgery are now being discharged after four to five days, rather than six to ten. "Patients used to leave the hospital because they were ready to leave. Now the goal is to get them out, to move patients along the continuum, whether they are ready to go or not. We used to send people home with things that a patient or family member could take care of. Today we're sending people home who need complicated wound care. They have stitches in their chest and leg where they were cut open or drains were put in. They have staples in their chest. They have wounds with a high risk for infection. They go home with physical therapy referrals because they can't get out of bed alone. They have com-

plicated drug regimens. What we are doing is turning the home into a hospital."

Hospital administrators and insurance executives rationalize away their responsibilities to patients and families. After a *Boston Globe* editorial criticized Harvard Community Health Plan's newly mandated labor and delivery policy— which forces women to leave the hospital twenty-four hours after a normal vaginal delivery — several of its medical directors responded in a letter to the editor: "The *Globe* may believe there is no substitute for an extra day free of worries about preparing meals, housekeeping or child care, but that is not what medical coverage is supposed to provide, especially in this era of grave concern about the rising costs of health care."

The directors of one of the most prominent H.M.O.s in the nation are explicitly segregating treatment from the process of recovery and coping. "It is as though they are saying that their only job is to extract the baby from the womb, and then their responsibility to the patient is over," commented Joan Lynaugh, associate dean and director of graduate studies at the University of Pennsylvania School of Nursing. "Our health care system has never done very well with the concept of convalescence," Lynaugh continued, "but when people who run a community health care plan explicitly argue that we shouldn't plan for the fact that people who are ill are tired and weak and can't get out of bed and need help with activities of daily living—when they say that it is not our job to care for the sick—then we have to ask, What is their job, what are they taking our money to do?"

Bioethics: The Need for a Dialogue with African Americans

ANNETTE DULA

INTRODUCTION

OVER THE LAST TWENTY YEARS, the field of bioethics has assumed major importance, as advances in medical technology and rising costs of health care have forced society to come to terms with difficult ethical choices surrounding life and death, allocation of resources, and doctor-patient relationships. Today, we find university departments and academic programs, hospital ethics committees, bioethics think tanks, and presidential task forces devoted to medical ethics policy and decision making. Furthermore, numerous conferences, journals, and books disseminate information and knowledge generated by the new profession.

Yet, the mainstream literature emerging from this influential new field rarely includes discussions of race, class, and gender. Influential ethics centers, such as the Hastings Center in Briarcliff Manor, New York, do address cultural issues but primarily from an international perspective. One reason for the dearth of critical discussion of cultural and social issues here in the United States may be the demographic makeup of bioethicists. Although feminist bioethicists are beginning to have a louder voice, the field is dominated by

ANNETTE DULA is a research associate at the University of Colorado.

white, male, middle-class professionals and academics. These men decide what is important, they frame questions, and they make policy recommendations. The voices of those outside of the power circle—racial minorities, the poor, and women—have been excluded from ongoing debates on ethics and health care policy. At best, such exclusion from decision making results in paternalistic decisions made for the "good" of the powerless. At worst, it victimizes the powerless. As Renee Fox points out in her discussion of the sociology of bioethics, "relatively little attention has been paid [by bioethicists] to the fact that a disproportionately high number of the extremely premature, very low birthweight infants, many with severe congenital abnormalities, [who are] cared for in NICU [neonatal intensive care units], are babies born to poor, disadvantaged mothers, many of whom are single nonwhite teenagers" (Fox 1989, p. 231).

I intend to show that the articulation and development of professional bioethics perspectives by minority academics are necessary to expand the narrow margins of debate. Without representation by every sector of society, the powerful and powerless alike, the discipline of bioethics is missing the opportunity to be enriched by the inclusion of a broader range of perspectives. Although I use African-American perspectives as an example, these points apply to other racial and ethnic groups—Hispanics, Native Americans, and Asians—who have suffered similar health care experiences.

In the first section of this chapter, I suggest that an African-American perspective on bioethics has two bases: (1) our health and medical experiences and (2) our tradition of black activist philosophy. In the second section, through examples, I show that an unequal power relationship has led to unethical medical behavior toward blacks, especially regarding reproductive issues. In the third section, I argue that developing a professional perspective not only gives voice to the concerns of those not in the power circle, but also enriches the entire field of bioethics.

MEDICAL AND HEALTH EXPERIENCES

The health of a people and the quality of health care they receive reflect their status in society. It should come as little surprise, then, that the health experiences of African Americans differ vastly from those of white people. These differences are well documented. Compared to whites, more than twice as many black babies are born with low birthweight and over twice as many die before their first birthday (CDC 1993a). Fifty percent more blacks than whites are likely to regard themselves as being in fair or poor health (Blendon et al. 1989). Blacks are included in fewer trials of new drugs—an inequity of particular importance for AIDS patients, who are disproportionately black and Hispanic (El-Sadr and Capps 1992). The mortality rate for heart disease in black males is twice that for white males; research has shown that blacks tend to receive less aggressive treatment for this condition (Wenneker and Epstein 1989). More blacks die from cancer, which, unlike the situation in whites, is likely to be systemic by the time it is detected (Rene 1987). African Americans live five fewer years than do whites (Department of

Health and Human Services 1985). Indeed, if blacks had the same death rate as whites, 59,000 black deaths a year would not occur (Miller 1987). Colin McCord and Harold P. Freeman, who reported that black men in Harlem are less likely to reach the age of 65 than are men in Bangladesh, conclude that the mortality rates of inner cities with largely black populations "justify special consideration analogous to that given to natural-disaster areas" (McCord and Freeman 1990, p. 173).

These health disparities are the result of at least three forces: institutional racism, economic inequality, and attitudinal barriers to access (Jones and Rice 1987). Institutional racism has roots in the historically unequal power relations between blacks and the medical profession, and between blacks and the larger society. It has worked effectively to keep blacks out of the profession, even though a large percentage of those who manage to enter medicine return to practice in minority communities—where the need for medical professionals is greatest. Today, institutional racism in health care is manifested in the way African Americans and poor people are treated. They experience long waits, are unable to shop for services, and often receive poor quality and discontinuous health care. Moreover, many government programs do not target African Americans as a group. As a result, benefits to racially defined populations are diffused. There is hope: Healthy People 2000 complemented by the Clinton health care proposal can go a long way to reducing these problems.

Black philosopher W.E.B. Du Bois summed up the economic plight of African Americans: "To be poor is hard, but to be a poor race in a land of dollars is the very bottom of hardships" (Du Bois 1961, p. 20). Poor people are more likely to have poor health, and a disproportionate number of poor people are black. African Americans tend to have lower paying jobs and fewer income-producing sources such as investments. Indeed, whites on average accumulate eleven times more wealth than do blacks (Jaynes and Williams 1989). Less money also leads to substandard housing—housing that may contain unacceptable levels of lead paint, asbestos insulation, or other environmental hazards. Thus, both inadequate employment and subpar housing available to poor African Americans present health problems that wealthier people are able to avoid. In addition, going to the doctor may entail finding and paying for a babysitter and transportation, and taking time off from work at the risk of being fired, all of which the poor cannot afford.

Attitudinal barriers—perceived racism, different cultural perspectives on health and sickness, and beliefs about the health care system—are a third force that brings unequal health care. Seeking medical help may not have the same priority for poor people as it has for middle-class people. One study in the *Journal of the American Medical Association* revealed that, compared to whites, blacks are less likely to be satisfied with how their physicians treat them, more dissatisfied with their hospital care, and more likely to believe that their hospital stay was too short (Blendon et al. 1989). In addition, many blacks, like people of other racial and ethnic groups, use home remedies and adhere to traditional theories of illness and healing that lie outside of the mainstream medical model (Watson 1984). Institutional racism, economic inequality, and attitudinal barriers, then, contribute to inadequate access to health care for poor and minority peoples. These factors must be seen as bioethical concerns. Bioethics cannot be exclusively medical or even ethical. Rather, it must also deal with beliefs, values, cultural traditions, and the economic, political, and social order. A number of medical sociologists have severely criticized bioethicists for ignoring cultural and societal particularities that limit access to health care (Fabrega 1990; Fox 1989; Keyserlingk 1990; Marshall 1992).

This inattention to cultural and societal aspects of health care may be attributed in part to

the mainstream Western philosophy on which the field of bioethics is built. For example, renowned academic bioethicists such as Robert Veatch, Tom Beauchamp, and Alasdair MacIntyre rely on the philosophical works of Rawls, Kant, and Aristotle (Beauchamp and Childress 1989; MacIntyre 1981; Veatch 1981). In addition, until recently the mainstream Western philosophic method has been presented primarily as a thinking enterprise, rarely advocating change or societal transformation. Thus, for the most part, Western philosophers have either gingerly approached or neglected altogether to comment on such social injustices as slavery, poverty, racism, sexism, and classism. As pointed out in *Black Issues in Higher Education,* until recently mainstream philosophy was seen as above questions of history and culture (Brodie 1990).

BLACK ACTIVIST PHILOSOPHY

The second basis for an African-American perspective on bioethics is black activist philosophy. Black philosophy differs from mainstream philosophy in its emphasis on action and social justice (Boxill 1992). African-American philosophers view the world through a cultural and societal context of being an unequal partner. Many black philosophers believe that academic philosophy devoid of societal context is a luxury that black scholars can ill afford. Moreover, African-American philosophers have purposely elected to use philosophy as a tool not only for naming, defining, and analyzing social situations, but also for recommending, advocating, and sometimes harassing for political and social empowerment—a stance contrary to mainstream philosophic methods (Harris 1983). Even though all bioethicists would do well to examine the thinking of such philosophers as Alain Locke, Lucius Outlaw, Anita Allen, Leonard Harris, W.E.B. Du Bois, Bernard Boxill, Angela Davis, Cornel West, William Banner, and Jorge Garcia, references to the work of these African Americans are rarely seen in the bioethics literature.

Although the professionalization of bioethics has frequently bypassed African-American voices, there are a few notable exceptions. Mark Siegler, director of the Center for Clinical Medical Ethics at the University of Chicago, included three African-American fellows in the 1990–91 medical ethics training program; Edmund Pellegrino of the Kennedy Institute for Advanced Ethics co-sponsored three national conferences on African-American perspectives on bioethics; and Howard Brody at Michigan State University is attempting to diversify his medical ethics program. In addition, a number of current publications offer important information for bioethicists. For example, the National Research Council's *A Common Destiny: Blacks and American Society* (Jaynes and Williams 1989) provides a comprehensive analysis of the status of black Americans, including discussions on health, education, employment, and economic factors, as does the National Urban League's annual *The State of Black America;* Marlene Gerber Fried's *From Abortion to Reproductive Freedom* (Fried 1990) presents many ideas of women of color concerning abortion; and several journals (e.g., *Ethnicity and Disease,* published by the Loyola University School of Medicine, and *The Journal of Health Care for the Poor and Underserved*) call particular attention to the health experiences of poor and underserved people. Finally, literature and narrative as forms of presenting African-American perspectives on bioethics are now being explored (Dula 1994; Secundy 1992).

Clearly, bioethics and African-American philosophy overlap. Both are concerned with distributive justice and fairness, with autonomy and paternalism in unequal relationships, and with both individual and societal ills. African-American philosophy, therefore, may have much to offer bioethics in general and African-American bioethics in particular.

MAINSTREAM ISSUES RELEVANT TO AFRICAN AMERICANS

A shocking history of medical abuse against unprotected people is also grounds for African-American perspectives in bioethics. In particular, reproductive rights issues—questions of family planning, sterilization, and genetic screening—are of special interest to black women.

A critical examination of the U.S. birth control movement reveals fundamental differences in perspectives, experiences, and interests between the white women who founded the movement and African-American women who were affected by it. Within each of three phases, the goals of the movement implicitly or explicitly served to exploit and subordinate African-American as well as poor white women (Gordon 1990).

The middle of the nineteenth century marked the beginning of the first phase of the birth control movement, characterized by the rallying cry "Voluntary Motherhood!" Advocates of voluntary motherhood asserted that women ought to say "no" to their husbands' sexual demands as a means of limiting the number of their children. The irony, of course, was that, while early white feminists were refusing their husbands' sexual demands, most black women did not have the same right to say "no" to these and other white women's husbands. Indeed, African-American women were exploited as breeding wenches in order to produce stocks of enslaved people for plantation owners. August Meier and Elliott Rudwick comment on slave-rearing as a major source of profit for nearly all slaveholding farmers and planters: "Though most Southern whites were scarcely likely to admit it, the rearing of slaves for profit was a common practice. [A] slave woman's proved or anticipated fecundity was an important factor in determining her market value; fertile females were often referred to as 'good breeders'" (Meier and Rudwick 1970, p. 56).

The second phase of the birth control movement gave rise to the actual phrase "birth control," coined by Margaret Sanger in 1915 (Gorton 1990). Initially, this stage of the movement led to the recognition that reproductive rights and political rights were intertwined; birth control would give white women the freedom to pursue new opportunities made possible by the vote (Davis 1981). This freedom allowed white women to go to work while black women cared for their children and did their housework.

This second stage coincided with the eugenics movement, which advocated improvement of the human race through selective breeding. When the white birth rate began to decline, eugenists chastised middle-class white women for contributing to the suicide of the white race: "Continued limitation of offspring in the white race simply invites the black, brown, and yellow races to finish work already begun by birth control, and reduce the whites to a subject race preserved merely for the sake of its skill" (Popenoe 1926, p. 144).

Eugenists proposed a twofold approach for curbing "race suicide": imposing moral obligations on middle-class white women to have large families and on poor immigrant women and black women to restrict the size of theirs. For the second group, geneticists advocated birth control. The women's movement adopted the ideals of the eugenists regarding poor, immigrant, and minority women, and it even surpassed the rhetoric of the eugenists. Margaret Sanger described the relationship between the two groups: "The eugenists wanted to shift the birth-control emphasis from less children for the poor to more children for the rich. We went back of that [sic] and sought first to stop the multiplication of the unfit" (Sanger 1938). Thus, while black women have historically practiced birth control (Collins 1990; Rodrique 1990), they learned to distrust the birth control movement as espoused by white feminists—a distrust that continues to the present day (Collins 1990).

The third stage of the birth control movement began in 1942 with the establishment of the Planned Parenthood Federation of America. Although Planned Parenthood made valuable contributions to the independence, self-esteem, and aspirations of many women, it accepted existing power relations, continuing the eugenic tradition by defining undesirable "stock" by class or income level (Gorton 1990). Many blacks were suspicious of Planned Parenthood; men, particularly, viewed its policies as designed to weaken the black community politically or to wipe it out genetically (Littlewood 1977). From the beginning of this century, both public and private institutions attempted to control the breeding of those deemed "undesirable." The first sterilization law was passed in Indiana in 1907, setting the stage for not only eugenic, but also punitive sterilization of criminals, the feebleminded, rapists, robbers, chicken thieves, drunkards, and drug addicts. By 1931 thirty states had passed sterilization laws, allowing more than 12,145 sterilizations. By the end of 1958, the sterilization total had risen to 60,926. In the 1950s several states attempted to extend sterilization laws to include compulsory sterilization of mothers of "illegitimate" children (Morrison 1965). As of 1991, sterilization laws were still in force in twenty-two states (Reilly 1991). They are seldom enforced, and where they have been, their eugenic significance has been negligible (Collins 1990).

Numerous federal and state measures perpetuated a focus on poor women and women of color. Throughout the United States in the 1960s, the federal government began subsidizing family planning clinics designed to reduce the number of people on welfare by checking the transmission of poverty from generation to generation. The number of family planning clinics in a given geographical area was proportional to the number of black and Hispanic residents (Mass 1976). In Puerto Rico, a massive federal birth control campaign introduced in 1937 was so successful that by the 1950s, the demand for sterilization exceeded facilities (Presser 1973), and by 1965 one-third of the women in Puerto Rico had been sterilized (Gould 1984).

In 1972 Los Angeles County Hospital, a hospital catering to large numbers of women of color, reported a sevenfold rise in hysterectomies (Mass 1976). Between 1973 and 1976, almost 3,500 Native American women were sterilized at one Indian Health Service hospital in Oklahoma (Fried 1990). In 1973 two black sisters from Montgomery, Alabama, 12-year-old Mary Alice Relf and 14-year-old Minnie Lee Relf, were reported to have been surgically sterilized without their parents' consent (Aptheker 1974).[1] An investigation revealed that in the same town, eleven other young girls of about the same age as the Relf sisters had also been sterilized; ten of them were black. During the early 1970s in Aiken, South Carolina, of thirty-four Medicaid-funded deliveries, eighteen included sterilizations, and all eighteen involved young black women (Aptheker 1974). In 1972 Carl Schultz, director of the Department of Health, Education, and Welfare's Population Affairs Office, acknowledged that the government had funded between 100,000 and 200,000 sterilizations (Payne 1974). These policies aroused black suspicions that family planning efforts were inspired by racist and eugenist motives.

The first phase of the birth control movement, then, completely ignored black women's sexual subjugation to white masters. In the second phase, the movement adopted the racist policies of the eugenics movement. The third stage saw a number of government-supported coercive measures to contain the population of poor people and people of color. While blacks perceive birth control per se as beneficial, blacks have historically objected to birth control as a method of dealing with poverty. Rather, most blacks believe that poverty can be remedied only by creating meaningful jobs, raising the minimum wage so that a worker can support a family, providing health care to working and nonworking people through their jobs or through universal coverage, instituting a high-quality day care system for low- or no-income people, and improving educational opportunities (Edelman 1987).

INFORMED CONSENT

Informed consent is one of the key ethical issues in bioethics. In an unequal patient-provider relationship, informed consent may not be possible. The weaker partner may consent because he or she is powerless, poor, or does not understand the implications of consent. And when members of subordinate groups are not awarded full respect as persons, those in positions of power then consider it unnecessary to obtain consent. The infamous Tuskegee experiment is a classic example. Starting in 1932, over 400 poor and uneducated syphilitic black men in Alabama were unwitting subjects in a Public Health Service experiment, condoned by the surgeon general, to study the course of untreated syphilis. Physicians told the men that they were going to receive special treatment, concealing the fact that the medical procedures were diagnostic rather than therapeutic. Although the effects of untreated syphilis were already known by 1936, the experiment continued for forty years. In 1969 a committee appointed by the Public Health Service to review the Tuskegee study decided to continue it. The Tuskegee experiment did not come to widespread public attention until 1972, when the *Washington Star* documented this breach of medical ethics. As a result, the experiment was halted (Jones 1980). Unfortunately, however, the legacy of the experiment lingers on, as several chapters in this volume illustrate.

It may be tempting to assume that such medical abuses are part of the distant past. However, there is evidence that violations of informed consent persist. Of 52,000 Maryland women screened annually for sickle cell anemia between 1978 and 1980, 25 percent were screened without their consent, thus denying these women the benefit of prescreening education or followup counseling, or the opportunity to decline screening (Farfel and Holtzman 1984). A national survey conducted in 1986 found that 81 percent of women subjected to court-ordered obstetrical interventions (Caesarean section, hospital detention, or intrauterine transfusion) were black, Hispanic, or Asian; nearly half were unmarried; one-fourth did not speak English; and none were private patients (Kolder et al. 1987). When in 1981, a Texas legislator asked his constituency whether they favored sterilization of women on welfare, a majority of the respondents said that welfare benefits should be tied to sterilizations (Reilly 1991).

HOW A PROFESSIONAL PERSPECTIVE MAKES A DIFFERENCE

Thus far, I have shown some grounds for African-American perspectives on bioethics, based on black activist philosophy and the unequal health status of African Americans. I have also argued that a history of medical abuse and neglect toward people in an unequal power relationship commands our attention to African-American perspectives on bioethics issues. In this final section, I will argue that a professional perspective can voice the concerns of those not in the power circle. Two examples—black psychology and the white women's movement—illustrate that professional perspectives can make a difference in changing society's perceptions and, ultimately, policies regarding a particular population.

Black Psychology

Until recently, mainstream psychology judged blacks as genetically and mentally inferior, incapable of abstract reasoning, culturally deprived, passive, ugly, lazy, childishly happy, dishonest, and emotionally immature or disturbed. Mainstream psychology owned these definitions and viewed African Americans through a deficit-deficiency model—a model it had constructed to explain African-American behavior (Billingsley 1968; Dodson 1988; Edelman 1987; Jones 1980; Moynihan 1965). When blacks entered the profession of psychology, they challenged that deficit model by presenting an African-American perspective that addressed the dominant group's assessments and changed, to a certain extent, the way society views blacks. Real consequences of black psychologists' efforts to encourage self-definition, consciousness, and self-worth have been felt across many areas: professional training, intelligence and ability testing, criminal justice, and family counseling. Black psychologists have presented their findings before professional conferences, legislative hearings, and policy-making task forces. For example, black psychologists are responsible for the ban in California on using standardized intelligence tests as a criterion for placing black and other minority students in classes for the mentally retarded. The Association of Black Psychologists publishes the *Journal of Black Psychology,* and black psychologists contribute to a variety of other professional journals (White 1984). As a result of these and other efforts, most respected psychologists no longer advocate the deficit-deficiency model.

The Women's Movement

The women's movement is another example of a subordinated group defining its own perspectives. The perspectives of white women have historically been defined largely by white men; white women's voices, like black voices, have traditionally been ignored or trivialized. A mere twenty years ago, the question, "Should there be a woman's perspective on health?" was emotionally debated. Although the question is still asked, a respected discipline of women's studies has emerged, with several journals devoted to women's health. Women in increasing numbers have been drawn to the field of applied ethics, specifically to bioethics (Griffiths and Whitford 1988; Holmes 1989), and they debate issues such as maternal and child health, rights of women versus rights of the fetus, unnecessary hysterectomies and Caesareans, the doctor-patient relationship, and the absence of women in clinical trials of new drugs. Unfortunately, however, the mainstream women's movement is largely the domain of white women. This, of course, does not mean that black women have not been activists for women's rights; on the contrary, African-American women historically have been deeply involved in fighting both racism and sexism, believing that the two are inseparable. Many black women distrust the movement, criticizing it as racist and self-serving, concerned only with white middle-class women's issues (Collins 1990; Davis 1990; Giddings 1984). Black feminists working within the abortion rights movement and with the National Black Women's Health Project, an Atlanta-based self-help and health advocacy organization, are raising their voices to identify issues relevant to African-American women and men in general, and reproductive and health issues in particular (Fried 1990). Like black psychologists, these black feminists are articulating a perspective that is effectively promoting pluralism.

CONCLUSION

The disturbing health inequities between blacks and whites—differences in infant mortality, average life span, chronic illnesses, and aggressiveness of treatment—suggest that minority access to health care should be recognized and accepted as a *bona fide* concern of bioethics. Opening the debate can only enrich this new field, thereby avoiding the moral difficulties of exclusion. Surely the serious and underaddressed health concerns of a large and increasing segment of our society are an ethical issue that is at least as important as such esoteric, high-visibility issues as the morality of gestational surrogacy. The front page of the August 5, 1991, *New York Times* headlined an article, "When Grandmother Is Mother, Until Birth." Although interesting and worthy of ethical comment, such sensational headlines undermine the moral seriousness of a situation in which over 37 million poor people do not have access to health care.

There is a basis for developing African-American perspectives on bioethics, and I have presented examples of medical abuse and neglect that suggest particular issues for consideration. Valuable as our advocacy has been, our perspectives have not gained full prominence in bioethics debates. Thus, it is necessary to form a community of scholars to conduct research on the contributions as well as the limitations of perspectives of African-Americans and other poor and underserved peoples in this important field.

NOTE

1. More recently, Reilly has reported that, while the literature states that two sisters were sterilized, in fact only one of them, Minnie Relf, was. See P. R. Reilly, *The Surgical Solution* (Baltimore: Johns Hopkins University Press, 1991), p. 151.

REFERENCES

Aptheker, H. "Sterilization, Experimentation and Imperialism." *Political Affairs* 53 (1974):37–48.

Beauchamp, T. F., and J. F. Childress. *Principles of Biomedical Ethics.* 3rd ed. New York: Oxford University Press, 1989.

Billingsley, A. *Black Families in White America.* Englewood Cliffs, N. J.: Prentice-Hall, 1968.

Blendon, R. J., L. H. Aiken, H. E. Freeman, and C. Corey. "Access to Medical Care for Black and White Americans: A Matter of Continuing Concern." *Journal of the American Medical Association* 261, no. 2 (1989): 278–281.

Boxill, B. R. *Blacks and Social Justice.* Revised ed., Totowa, N.J.: Rowman and Littlefield Publishers, 1992.

Brodie, J. M. "In Locke's Footsteps: Black Philosophers Search for Wisdom and Validation." *Black Issues in Higher Education,* 1990, 1, 23–27.

Centers for Disease Control (CDC). "Prevention and Control of Tuberculosis in the U.S. Communities with At-Risk Minority Populations: Recommendations for the Elimination of Tuberculosis." *Morbidity & Mortality Weekly Report* 41 (No. RR-5) (1992e):1–11.

Collins, P. H. *Black Feminist Thought: Knowledge, Consciousness, and the Politics of Empowerment.* Boston: Unwyn Hyman, 1990.

Davis, A. *Women, Race & Class.* New York: Vintage Books, 1981.

——. "Racism, Birth Control and Reproductive Rights." In *From Abortion to Reproductive Freedom: Transforming a Movement,* ed. M. G. Fried, 15–26. Boston: South End Press, 1990.

Department of Health and Human Services. *Report of the Secretary's Task Force on Black and Minority Health.* 1985.

Dodson, J. "Conceptualizations of Black Families." In *Black Families, Second Edition,* ed. H. P. McAdoo, 77–90. Newbury Park, Calif.: Sage Publications, 1988.

DuBois, W. E. B. *The Souls of Black Folk: Essays and Sketches.* Greenwich, Conn.: Fawcett Publications, 1961.

Dula, A. "Miz Mildred's Story: The PSDA." *Clinical Geriatrics.* Forthcoming (1994).

Edelman, M. W. *Families in Peril: An Agenda for Social Change.* Cambridge, Mass.: Harvard University Press, 1987.

El-Sadr, W., and L. Capps. "The Challenge of Minority Recruitment in Clinical Trials for AIDS." *Journal of the American Medical Association* 267, no. 7 (1992):954–957.

Fabrega, H. "An Ethnomedical Perspective of Medical Ethics." *Journal of Medicine and Philosophy* 15 (1990): 593–625.

Farfel, M. R., and N. A. Holtzman "Education, Consent, and Counseling in Sickle Cell Screening Programs: Report of a Survey." *American Journal of Public Health* 74 (1984):373–375.

Fox, R. *The Sociology of Medicine.* Englewood Cliffs, N.J.: Prentice-Hall, 1989.

Fried, M. G., ed. *From Abortion to Reproductive Freedom.* Boston: South End Press, 1990.

Giddings, P. *When and Where I Enter: The Impact of Black Women on Race and Sex in America.* Toronto: Bantam Books, 1984.

Gordon, L. *Woman's Body, Woman's Rights: Birth Control in America.* Revised ed., New York: Penguin Books, 1990.

Gould, K. H. "Black Women in Double Jeopardy: A Perspective on Birth Control." *Health and Social Work* (1984):96–105.

Griffiths, M., and M. Whitford, ed. *Feminist Perspectives in Philosophy.* Bloomington: Indiana University Press, 1988.

Harris, L., ed. *Philosophy Born of Struggle.* Dubuque, Iowa: Kendall Hunt Publishing Co., 1983.

Holmes, H. B. "Can Clinical Research Be Both Ethical and Scientific?" *Hypatia* 4, no. 2 (1989):156–168.

Jaynes, G. D., and R. M. Williams, Jr., eds. *A Common Destiny: Blacks and American Society.* Washington, D.C.: National Academy Press, 1989.

Jones, R. *Black Psychology.* New York: Harper & Row, 1980.

Jones, W., and M. F. Rice. "Black Health Care." In *Health Care Issues in Black America: Policies, Problems, and Prospects,* ed. W. Jones and M. F. Rice, 3–20. Westport, Conn.: Greenwood Press, 1987.

Keyserlingk, E. "Ethical Guidelines and Codes: Can They Be Universally Applicable in a Multi-Cultural Society?" *In Ethics in Medicine: Individual Integrity Versus Demands of Society,* ed. P. Allebeck and B. Jansson, 137–150. New York: Raven Press, 1990.

Kolder, V., J. Gallagher, and M. T. Parsons. "Court-ordered Obstetrical Interventions." *New England Journal of Medicine* 316 (1987):1192–1196.

Littlewood, T. B. *The Politics of Population Control.* Notre Dame, Ind.: University of Notre Dame Press, 1977.

Marshall, P. "Anthropology and Bioethics." *Medical Anthropology Quarterly* 6, no. 1 (1992):49–73.

Mass, B. *Population Target: The Political Economy of Population Control in Latin America.* Toronto: Women's Press, 1976.

McCord, C., and H. P. Freeman. "Excess Mortality in Harlem." *New England Journal of Medicine* 322, no. 3 (1990):173–177.

Meier, A., and E. Rudwick. *From Plantation to Ghetto.* New York: Hill & Wang, 1970.

Miller, S. M. "Race in the Health of America." *The Milbank Quarterly* 65, suppl. 2 (1987):500–531.

Morrison, J. L. "Illegitimacy, Sterilization, and Racism: A North Carolina Case History." *Social Science Review* 39 (1965):1–10.

Moynihan, D. *The Negro Family: The Case for National Action.* U.S. Department of Labor, Office of Policy Planning and Research, 1965.

Payne, L. "Forced Sterilization for the Poor." *San Francisco Chronicle,* February 26, 1974.

Popenoe, P. *The Conservation of Family.* Baltimore: Williams & Wilkins Co., 1926.

Presser, H. B. *Sterilization and Fertility: Decline in Puerto Rico.* Berkeley, Calif.: Institute of International Studies, 1973.

Reilly, P. R. *The Surgical Solution.* Baltimore: Johns Hopkins University Press, 1991.

Rodrique, J. M. "The Black Community and the Birth Control Movement." In *Unequal Sisters: A Multi-Cultural Reader in U. S. Women's History,* ed. E. C. Du Bois and V. L. Ruiz, 333–344. New York: Routledge, 1990.

Sanger, M. Autobiography. New York: W. W. Norton, 1938.

Secundy, M. G., with L. L. Nixon, ed. Trials, *Tribulations, and Celebrations: African American Perspectives on Health, Illness, Aging and Loss.* Yarmouth, Me.: Intercultural Press, 1992.

Veatch, R. M. *A Theory of Medical Ethics.* New York: Basic Books, 1981.

Watson, W. H., ed. *Black Folk Medicine: The Therapeutic Significance of Faith and Trust.* New Brunswick, N.J.: Transaction Books, 1984.

Wennecker, M. B., and A. M. Epstein. "Racial Inequalities in the Use of Procedures for Patients with Ischemic Heart Disease in Massachusetts." *Journal of American Medical Association* 261 (1989): 253–257.

White, J. L. *The Psychology of Blacks: An Afro-American Perspective.* Englewood Cliffs, N.J.: Prentice-Hall, 1984.

Elucidating the Relationships between Race, Socioeconomic Status, and Health

GREGORY PAPPAS

THE PUBLIC HEALTH FIELD is committed to decreasing social disparities in health.[1] Growing differences in death rates among racial and socioeconomic groups have heightened our concern about the disadvantages that have consequences for the public's health.[2-4] In this issue of the journal, the articles on social disadvantage in health contribute to our knowledge of health disparities and give direction to programs that may help close the gaps.

GREGORY PAPPAS is an associate professor of philosophy at Texas A&M University.

One of the most disturbing trends of the last decade is the increasing difference in life expectancy between Blacks and Whites. Kochanek et al. have investigated the causes of death associated with this inequality;[5] they have found that heart disease is the No. 1 cause of death fueling the disparity. The relative widening of the racial gap must first be distinguished from the absolute decline in life expectancy for Blacks. The causes of death among Black men that contributed most to the tragic decrease in life expectancy between 1984 and 1989 were human immunodeficiency virus (HIV) infection and homicide.

American Journal of Public Health, *Vol. 84 (6), June 1994, pp. 892–893. Copyright 1994. Reprinted with permission of the American Public Health Association.*

Among Black women, the leading contributors were HIV infection and cancer. However, although the number of deaths due to heart disease has been declining for both Blacks and Whites, the decline among Whites is so much more rapid than that among Blacks that heart disease is the chief contributor to the widening racial gap in life expectancy.

Such disparities in health status between Blacks and Whites are best understood in terms of the groups' underlying living circumstances.[6] Race is often used as a proxy for social class; we know that the poorer education, lower income, and lower occupational standing of Blacks have important effects on the survival of both adults and children.[7-9] In a study of a national sample of deaths, Rogers demonstrated that the racial differences in death rates were eliminated after an adjustment for income, marital status, and household size.[10] When these socioeconomic factors are controlled in cause-specific mortality, Blacks are at lower risk than Whites for death from respiratory disease, accidents, and suicide; they are equally at risk for cancer and circulatory diseases; and Blacks are at higher risk for infectious diseases, homicide, and diabetes.

The complex ways in which social and economic class and race create disadvantages and produce disparities in health must be more fully investigated. The recent pace of social and economic change has increased the intensity and range of the debate on class.[11] Income, education, occupation, and place of residence (geo-codes) are the usual indicators for measuring its health effects.[12]

However, "class" is a word with many meanings and one whose use has been contentious for a long time. "Socioeconomic status" is the preferred term in public health, perhaps because it seems to avoid the complexities of class analysis. Occupation has consequences on a person's health through work conditions or through the prestige associated with the job (as mediated by a reaction to the job's stress). Yet the grade of a person's occupation is in part determined by that person's education, and the prestige of an occupation is largely determined by the position's usual income. Income and education both have direct causal links to health (e.g., as manifested in the ability to afford healthy environments and in knowledge of healthy behavior patterns). In the sociological literature, income, education, and occupation have been shown to relate differently to the strata of our society, but in public health these distinctions have been generally overlooked. Despite these intricacies of social-class theories and the difficulty in measuring social factors' true impact on individuals, we can ill afford to ignore stratification in our society because it structures much of our everyday life and has profound effects on our health.

If social positions have an effect on individual health, movement between such positions may also hold some significance. In this issue, Waitzman and Smith examine the relationship, in men, between occupational class mobility and blood pressure in data from the National Health Examination Follow-up Survey, a national longitudinal cohort study followed over a decade.[13] Declining occupational status and low occupational status were associated with increased incidence of hypertension for both Blacks and Whites. For each kind of occupational status, work-associated stress and failed expectations for job improvement may be the source of the increased incidence of hypertension. Remaining in or moving into low-status jobs are patterns of disadvantage that traditionally relate to poor health. This pathway is but one of the many ways in which social class is thought to affect health.

Earlier historical explanations of the relationship between social stratification and health—explanations such as poor housing, poor nutrition, and inadequate medical care—must still be considered alongside newly emerging reasons. Evidence for the importance of individual health risk behavior has long been conclusive, but the importance of the social distribution of that behavior has come to be appreciated more recently.[14] Individual behaviors cannot be isolated from the social patterns in which they are embedded. Variations in stress at work and home and in smoking, alcohol use, activity levels, and other health-related behaviors have striking patterns, and these patterns depend on the society's social and economic arrangements. The changing social distribution of risk behavior may be one of the important factors that underlie and explain growing disparities in health among people with lower income and education. Thus, higher levels of health risk attach to certain populations' tobacco and alcohol use, activity levels, and obesity.

In order to gain an even more sophisticated understanding of the social distribution of health risk, ethnic and cultural patterns of health beliefs must also be considered. This important area has yet to be fully investigated. Using telephone survey data from San Francisco, Pérez-Stable et al. demonstrate differences between Latinos and non-Latino Whites in behavioral risk factors.[15] With age, sex, education, and employment adjusted, Latinos were less likely to drink any alcohol or to smoke and were more likely to be sedentary. Latino women were less likely to have ever had a Pap test or clinical breast examination than non-Latino White women. The authors emphasize that appropriate health-promotion campaigns require an appreciation of the audience's ethnicity.

The articles in this issue begin to map out the complex mechanism through which social disadvantage works. Yet if public health research is to help turn the tide of increasing disparities in health status, it must do more than simply demonstrate them. Explaining racial health differences by controlling for some measure of social class — and thus closing the gap statistically — is only a first step.

It will be important to apply our understanding of the dynamics of race and class as we try to improve access to health care, change behaviors through health promotion, and reform the health system. However, attempts to change behavior are bound to have only limited success because health risk behaviors are embedded in economic and social arrangements that reinforce those behaviors. Ultimately, closing the gaps between racial/ethnic and class groups will require altering the socioeconomic conditions of the disadvantaged in the United States.

REFERENCES

1. Lee PR. Speech delivered before Carter Center forum on reinventing public health; February 21–22, 1994; Atlanta, Ga.

2. National Center for Health Statistics. Advance report of final mortality statistics, 1989. *Month Vital Stat Rep.* 1990;40(8) (suppl 2).

3. Pappas G, Queen S, Hadden W, Fisher G. The increasing disparity in mortality between socioeconomic groups in the United States, 1960 and 1986. *N Engl J Med* 1993; 329:103–109.

4. Feldman JJ, Makuc DM, Kleinman JC, Corponi-Huntley J. National trends in educational differentials in mortality. *Am J Epidemiol.* 1989;129: 919–933.

5. Kochanek KD, Maurer JD, Rosenberg HM. Why did Black life expectancy decline from 1984 through 1989 in the United States? *Am J Public Health.* 1994;84:938–944.

6. Navarro V. Race or class versus race and class: mortality differentials in the United States. *Lancet,* 1990;336:1238–1240.

7. Otten MW Jr, Teutsch SM, Williamson DF, Marks JS. The effect of known risk factors on the excess mortality of black adults in the United States. *JAMA.* 1990; 263:845–850.

8. Haan MN, Kaplan GA. The contribution of socioeconomic position to minority health. In: *Report of the Secretary's Task Force on Black and Minority Health. Vol. 2. Crosscutting Issues in Minority Health.* Washington, DC: US Dept of Health and Human Services; 1985;69–103.

9. Kleinman JC. The slowdown in the infant mortality decline. *Paediatr Perinat Epidemiol.* 1990;4: 373–381.

10. Rogers RG. Living and dying in the U.S.A.: sociodemographic determinants of death among blacks and whites. *Demography.* 1992;29:287–303.

11. Crompton R. *Class and Stratification: An Introduction to Current Debates.* Cambridge, England: Policy Press; 1993.

12. Susser MW, Watson W, Hopper K. *Sociology in Medicine*. 3rd ed. New York, NY: Oxford University Press; 1985.

13. Waitzman NJ, Smith KR. The effects of occupational class transitions on hypertension: racial disparities among working-age men. *Am J Public Health*. 1994;84:945–950.

14. Williams DR. Socioeconomic differentials in health: a review and redirection. *Soc Psychol Q*. 1990;53:81–99.

15. Pérez-Stable EJ, Marín G, Marín BV. Behavioral risk factors: a comparison of Latinos and Non-Latino Whites in San Francisco. *Am J Public Health*. 1994;84:971–976.

Hispanic Health in the United States

COUNCIL ON SCIENTIFIC AFFAIRS

POVERTY, LACK OF EDUCATION, and access barriers to health care predispose many American minorities to disproportionate mortality and morbidity. Hispanics are the fastest growing minority in the United States. Since 1980, the Hispanic population has increased 34%, while the non-Hispanic population has increased only 7%. In March 1988, there were 19.4 million Hispanics in the United States.[1,2] By 2000, Hispanics will number an estimated 31 million, the largest minority group in the United States.[3]

Certain factors contributing to morbidity and mortality features are endemic among Hispanics, particularly when examined by subgroup. In addition, cultural norms, poor knowledge of English, and socioeconomic status affect Hispanics' use of health care. Compared with non-Hispanics, Hispanic families are more than 2½ times as likely to live below the poverty level.[1] Poverty and lack of health insurance contribute to the Hispanic health care challenge of today. This report examines these concerns and suggests ways for the American Medical Association to educate physicians about the health needs of this growing population.

BACKGROUND

Demographics

The Hispanic population has diverse national origins and cultures. The literature divides Hispanics into five subgroups: Mexican American, Puerto Rican, Cuban American, Central or South American, and "other" Hispanics.

Persons of Hispanic descent may have recently moved to the United States or their families may have lived here for centuries. Hispanics may be bilingual, speak only English, speak only Spanish, or speak a little of both. When Spanish is spoken, Hispanics often use different idioms among subgroups, which makes communication confusing among the different groups. In addition, cultural values, education, and family income vary by subgroup. Most of the literature focuses on Mexican Americans, Puerto Ricans, and Cubans. Scant data exist on Central or South Americans and other Hispanic subgroups.

Of the 19.4 million Hispanics in the United States, 62.3% are of Mexican origin, 12.7% are Puerto Rican, 5.3% are Cuban, 11.5% are Central or South American, and 8.1% are of other Hispanic origin. Subgroups tend to concentrate in different geographic areas, with Mexicans in California and Texas, Puerto Ricans in New York, and Cubans in Florida. Chicago has the most diverse cultural groupings, with proportions similar to the national divisions.[1,2] The Table further breaks down the Hispanic population by state.[4]

High birthrates and immigration account for the rapid Hispanic population growth in the United States. Compared with the fertility rate of the general population (65 of 1000 births), Hispanics have a higher fertility rate (97 of 1000 births), give birth to children at younger ages, and have more children.[3] Since the median age of Hispanics is 25 years and males and females are proportionally distributed, the high birthrate is expected to continue.

As of 1988, about half of all Hispanics completed 12 years of schooling. However, more than twice as many non-Hispanics as Hispanics finished 4 or more years of college. Less education predisposes Hispanics to high unemployment rates and poverty. Lack of education may also limit Hispanic understanding and use of the US health system.

Employment rates differ slightly between Hispanics and non-Hispanics, but proportionally many more Hispanics (8.5%) are unemployed compared with non-Hispanics (5.8%). For Hispanics, the 1988 mean income was $25 736, in contrast to $37 388 for non-Hispanics. Compared with non-Hispanics, Hispanics are more than 2½ times as likely to live below the poverty level. Of the subgroups, Cuban Americans have the highest incomes, while Puerto Ricans have the lowest. Nearly 40% of Puerto Ricans live below the poverty level, in contrast to about 14% of Cubans.[1]

Despite their lower incomes, Hispanics spend proportionally more of their disposable income on health care. Yet as a group, Hispanics are more likely than the general population to be uninsured. Cuban Americans, with the most education and highest incomes, are the most likely to have private health insurance (74%). Puerto Ricans, with the lowest incomes and highest unemployment rates, are most likely to have Medicaid coverage (32%). Although more Mexican Americans than Puerto Ricans are employed, they are the most likely to be uninsured (30%).[5,6] Mexican Americans who work tend to have jobs with no insurance benefits and/or they cannot afford insurance premiums for their large families.[4]

Use of Health Care

Use of health care by Hispanics is affected by perceived health care needs, insurance status, income, culture, language, and other factors that are beyond the scope of this report. Based on data from the National Health Interview Survey, Mexican Americans, who have the least insurance, visit physicians least often. Puerto Ricans have the highest physician visit rates, suggesting that persons on Medicaid have greater access to care than other poor, uninsured groups and that they tend to have more severe illnesses than those who are employed and insured.[6,7]

Preliminary data from the Hispanic Health and Nutrition Examination Survey (HHANES) of the National Center for Health Statistics, conducted in 1982 to 1984, confirm these trends. Compared with whites, about half as many Hispanics have a regular source of health care.[8] Thirty-nine percent of Puerto Ricans had a physical examination within a year, compared with 34% for Cubans and 25% for Mexican Americans.[3] Excluding Cubans, only about 60% of Hispanics initiate prenatal care in the first trimester, compared with 80% of whites. Hispanics are three times as likely as non-Hispanics to receive no prenatal care. Among the subgroups, Puerto Ricans received prenatal care later and less often.[3] Variation in Medicaid coverage may exist because of concentrations of Hispanics of different national subgroups in states with high Medicaid eligibility requirements.

Compared with whites, twice as many Hispanics report using the emergency department as a source of primary care. Digestive disorders and physical impairment constitute the most frequent presenting problems vs other potentially more serious conditions, such as circulatory and respiratory difficulties.[9] In addition, Hispanics are more apt to enter hospitals via emergency departments. Compared with whites, Hispanics have longer and more expensive hospital stays.[10]

Health care use is also governed by access to comprehensive and preventive health care. Overall, Hispanics are less likely to have private insurance than either whites or blacks.[11] Working Hispanics are more likely to be underemployed, employed part-time, or have jobs with no insurance benefits. Jobs that do offer insurance may impose high copayments for employees, which Hispanics often cannot afford to pay because of their large families. This lack of insurance restricts Hispanic access to adequate health care.[11,12] As an urban and poor minority, Hispanics receive the most health care from large, public hospitals that have rotating staffs, particularly for patients on Medicaid or other public funding.[13] In such settings, patients rarely experience continuity of health care. Hispanics who have no insurance or have public funding find themselves seeking care from institutions that focus on tertiary rather than primary care.

Low incomes and lack of health insurance restrict Hispanic access to primary health care more than any other variables.[11] Expanding Medicaid coverage to include everyone below the federal poverty level and mandating that employers offer health insurance for reasonable premiums would help Hispanics who have little or no insurance coverage.

In addition, Hispanics face cultural and language barriers. Although Hispanics constitute 7.9% of the US population, less than 5% of all US physicians and students in medical schools are Hispanic.[14] Differences in culture and language from that of most health care workers contribute to a lack of use of preventive care by Hispanics. For example, Hispanic patients who speak English are more likely to have a regular source of medical care compared with those who speak only Spanish.[15] Because Hispanics, blacks, and other minorities are underrepresented in medical schools, the American Medical Association has encouraged the recruitment and retention of these students.[16,17]

Furthermore, patients who are poor and do not speak English well or at all and who feel estranged from the complicated US health care system encounter complex obstacles to accessing preventive care. Acculturation, or the adaptation of persons from one culture to another, influences Hispanic use of health care. A recent study of Mexican Americans showed that less acculturated persons had significantly lower likelihoods of outpatient care for physical or emotional problems. Even when controlling for need, the less acculturated patients with Medicaid used inpatient services four times less than the more acculturated patients with Medicaid.[18] Other research supports the hypothesis that Hispanics need services but are reluctant to use them because of barriers related to culture and language. When researchers manipulated variables by minimizing cultural and language obstacles, Hispanic use of the health services at that facility increased.[19]

At times, Hispanic patients may be more likely to perceive their illnesses according to folk practices. Folk-defined illnesses or culture-bound syndromes have intrigued researchers over the years, and as a result they may be more of an artifact in the literature than a prevalent cultural influence. Hispanic patients may describe their illnesses according to their cultural understanding. For example, patients may complain of a fright sickness known as *susto* or a fighting attack called *ataque.* Often these complaints have biologic bases that need careful and sensitive medical exploration to accurately diagnose and treat the illness.[20-22]

Controversy exists among Hispanic health experts concerning the frequency with which folk healers, or *curanderos,* are used. Anderson et al.[23] note that while up to 20% of Hispanics may regularly use home remedies, the use of folk healers may be infrequent. Pedro Poma, MD, believes this practice varies considerably among the cultural subgroups and that the practice is fairly widespread in some subsets (oral communication, April 1990).

When communicating with a Hispanic patient, health care providers are often, either directly or indirectly, communicating with the patient's family. Most Hispanic families emphasize interdependence, affiliation, and cooperation. Important decisions are made by entire families, not individuals.[3] Thus, Hispanic patients may discuss the physician's diagnosis and treatment recommendations with their families before deciding to follow them.

HISPANIC HEALTH STATUS

Mortality

Accurate estimates of Hispanic death rates are impossible to determine because, until 1988, the national model death certificates did not contain Hispanic identifiers.[3] Although some states incorporated Hispanic origin on their death certificates, such reporting is not uniform and lacks precision. For example, funeral directors completing death certificates may indicate ethnic origin by observation rather than by inquiry with family.[24] The standardized collection of consistent vital statistics on Hispanics by designated state agencies would provide more accurate data.

Nevertheless, researchers have attempted to study Hispanic mortality rates by examining surnames on death certificates and by reviewing 1979 to 1981 mortality data tapes from the National Center for Health Statistics, which classified deaths by age, sex, cause of death, and place of birth.[3,25,26] Overall, Hispanics die of the major national killers: heart disease, cancer, and stroke.[3] Compared with the general population, Hispanics suffer from excess incidence of cancer of the stomach, esophagus, pancreas, and cervix.[27] Death due to stomach cancer is twice as high for Hispanics as for whites.[3,27,28] Hispanic women suffer from cervical cancer twice as often as white women,[3,27,29] but their 5-year survival rates slightly exceed those of whites.[30]

Alcoholism and cirrhosis are prevalent among Hispanics, particularly Mexican Americans and Puerto Ricans.[3,31,32] Mexican-born men have a 40% higher risk of death due to cirrhosis than white men. A review of autopsies from the University of Southern California Medical Center between 1918 and 1970 revealed that 52% of all deaths of Mexican-American men aged 30 to 60 years were due to alcoholism, compared with 24% for white men.[31] In addition to alcoholism, Hispanics share a disproportionate number of deaths due to narcotic addictions.[3]

Violent deaths account for high mortality rates among male adolescents and young adults of Mexican-American, Puerto Rican, and Cuban origin.[25,26] All three Hispanic male subgroups exceed white male deaths due to homicide. Puerto Rican males have higher death rates due to homicide than black males. Cuban and Puerto Rican males surpass white males for suicides. Accidents occur most frequently among Mexican-American males and least often among Cubans.[25]

Morbidity

Of the three major subgroups, Puerto Ricans report the worst health status. In 1979 to 1980, more Puerto Ricans reported chronic health problems as a limitation of their major activities than blacks, Mexican Americans, and Cubans. At the same time, compared with whites and other Hispanic subgroups, Puerto Ricans had the highest incidence of acute medical conditions.[6,20]

Compared with whites, Hispanics have three times the risk of diabetes.[12,33] Obesity and diet are largely correlated with diabetes in Hispanics. The HHANES study revealed that 26.1% of Puerto Ricans, 23.9% of Mexican Americans, and 15.8% of Cubans aged 45 to 74 years have diabetes.[31] In addition, approximately 30% of males and 39% of females of Mexican-American descent are overweight, as are 29% of males and 34% of females of Cuban descent and 25% of males and 37% of females of Puerto Rican backgrounds.[34] Mexican-American women suffer from gallstones twice as frequently as white women. In addition, Mexican Americans have a higher incidence of gallbladder cancer than whites.[12,35]

Not only do more Mexican Americans have diabetes than whites, but their disease is also of greater metabolic severity and places them at higher risk for complications. For example, Mexican Americans suffer a higher prevalence of diabetic retinopathy. In addition, the incidence of diabetes-related end-stage renal disease has been reported to be six times that of whites.[35] Given the Mexican-American propensity for obesity and diabetes, it is not surprising that this group also tends to have higher levels of cholesterol and triglycerides than whites.[36,37] Despite these potential risks, the incidence of cardiovascular mortality is not greater for Mexican Americans than whites.[3,35,37]

In general, Hispanics who are poor exhibit a higher risk for unrecognized and untreated hypertension.[3,37-39] Also, hypertension is more prevalent among Hispanics than whites.[3,12,37] Data from the HHANES study indicated that almost half of the Puerto Ricans surveyed with hypertension did not know they had it.[40] Cigarette smoking among Hispanics contributes to their risk for cardiovascular disease. According to data from the HHANES study, 43.6% of adult

Mexican-American men smoked compared with 41.8% of Cuban men, and 41.3% of Puerto Rican men.[41] A San Francisco (Calif) study revealed that men who are less acculturated have higher smoking rates and women who are more acculturated smoke more than their less culturally adapted counterparts.[42] Researchers link smoking with the nearly doubling of lung cancer rates among Hispanic men and women from 1970 to 1980.[31]

In addition to an increased risk for lung cancer, the incidence for tuberculosis is 4.3 times greater for Hispanics than whites.[43] From 1980 to 1987, New York City experienced a marked increase in tuberculosis cases, especially among 30- to 39-year-old Hispanics. Researchers suggest this increase relates to latent tuberculosis infection, which is activated by the human immunodeficiency virus (HIV) among Hispanics in that city.[43]

Although Hispanics constitute only 7.9% of the US population, they account for 14% of reported acquired immunodeficiency syndrome (AIDS) cases, nearly 21% of AIDS cases among women, and 22% of all pediatric AIDS cases.[3,44] Hispanics are at greater risk for HIV infection, not because of their race and culture, but because of underlying factors such as living in high-prevalence areas and exposure to intravenous drug use.[44] Most of the Hispanic AIDS cases in the Northeast are among intravenous drug users. Heterosexual transmission of HIV from intravenous drug users to their sexual partners is more prevalent among Hispanics because of cultural restrictions against the use of condoms[45] (Navarro M. AIDS and Hispanic people: a threat ignored. *The New York Times.* December 29, 1989:1, 4). The 1987–1988 National Center for Health Statistics Survey indicates that Hispanics know less about HIV and AIDS than non-Hispanics.[46] An Oregon survey of Hispanic outpatients revealed that only 50% thought condoms could help prevent transmission of HIV.[47] Because certain groups are at greater risk for HIV infection through drug use and because cultural differences may affect the understanding of HIV transmission, the American Medical Association suggests that AIDS prevention education programs be tailored to subgroups (such as Mexican Americans and Puerto Ricans) considering their cultural and language differences.[48]

Perhaps related to cultural restrictions on the use of condoms and the cultural importance of motherhood and child rearing, Mexican-American females tend to have high rates of teenaged pregnancies and high-parity births. According to 1983 and 1984 data from 23 states, 31% of Mexican-American females and 30% of Puerto Rican females aged 15 to 19 years have given birth.[3] Despite the young ages at the time of pregnancy and the lack of prenatal care, Hispanic females, especially Mexican Americans, have lower rates of premature deliveries and low birth weight.[3,49,50] Among the subgroups, Puerto Ricans have the highest birthrates for unmarried young women and the highest infant mortality attributed to low birth weight. Puerto Rican poverty and its effect on access to health care contribute to this group's lack of prenatal care and concomitant infant mortality.[12,51] As Hispanic women become more acculturated, the risk of giving birth to low birth weight babies increases.[50] In addition, increased acculturation is associated with decreased breast-feeding of infants. These trends, combined with the fact that Hispanics are three times more likely than non-Hispanics to receive *no* prenatal care, contribute to the morbidity of urban, poor Hispanic mothers and infants.[3]

SUMMARY

Hispanics are the fastest growing minority in the United States. As a heterogeneous group, Hispanics are multicultural and can be monolingual or bilingual. They are divided into five subgroups: Mexican American, Puerto Rican, Cuban, Central and South American, and other Hispanics. Poverty, little education, lack of insur-

ance, and high unemployment rates pose barriers to health care for Hispanics.

Poverty and lack of health insurance are the greatest impediments to health care for Hispanics. Use of health care services by Hispanics is affected by perceived health needs, socioeconomic status, insurance, language, and culture. Many Hispanics who work cannot afford insurance premiums. Those without insurance who report health needs avoid the health system until they are ill. The literature suggests that as Hispanics adjust to the US health system, both culturally and linguistically, they will use health services more often and more beneficially.

The literature also suggests that as Hispanics become more acculturated, their health status worsens. Hispanics increase their use of tobacco and consume a less healthy diet as they adapt to the US culture. As Hispanics live longer in the United States, their morbidity and mortality rates for certain diseases increase. Hispanics suffer a disproportionate share of AIDS cases, and males are more likely to die of violence. Diabetes, hypertension, tuberculosis, certain cancers, and alcoholism rates are higher for Hispanics than for whites.

By working with Hispanic health organizations on health promotion and disease prevention through community advertisement and education and by increased recruitment and retention of Hispanic medical students, the medical system can help Hispanics become more involved with their own health care. In addition, Spanish-language preventive health literature can help the less acculturated understand and use the health system appropriately. Finally, medical research geared toward decreasing the disproportionate rates of mortality and morbidity among Hispanics will contribute to the greater well-being of all Hispanics and to the knowledge and skill of all health providers.

REFERENCES

1. US Bureau of the Census. *The Hispanic Population in the United States: March, 1988.* Washington, DC:

US Dept of Commerce; 1988. Current Population Reports series P-20, No. 438.

2. Arnold CB. From the editor's desk. *Stat Bull.* 1988;69:1.

3. *Delivering Preventive Health Care to Hispanics: A Manual for Providers.* Washington, DC: The National Coalition of Hispanic Health and Human Services Organizations; 1988.

4. US Bureau of the Census. Washington, DC: US Dept of Commerce; 1989. Current Population Report series P-20, No. 444.

5. Lipton B, Katz M. Understanding the Hispanic market. *Med Market Media.* 1989;24:9, 10, 12, 18.

6. Trevino FM, Moss AJ. Health insurance coverage and physician visits among Hispanic and non-Hispanic people. In: *Health — United States, 1983.* Washington, DC: Public Health Service; 1983:45–48. US Dept of Health and Human Services publication PHS 84-1232.

7. Trevino FM, Moss AJ. *Health Indicators for Hispanic, Black, and White Americans.* Washington, DC: Public Health Service; 1984. US Dept of Health and Human Services publication PHS 84-1576. National Center for Health Survey series 10, No. 148.

8. The Robert Wood Johnson Foundation. Access to health care in the United States: results of a 1986 survey. *Spec Rep.* 1987;2:3–11.

9. White-Means SI, Thornton MC, Yeo JS. Sociodemographic and health factors influencing black and Hispanic use of the hospital emergency room. *J Natl Med Assoc.* 1989;81:72–80.

10. Munoz E. Care for the Hispanic poor: a growing segment of American society. *JAMA.* 1988;260:2711–2712.

11. Andersen RM, Giachello AL, Aday LU. Access of Hispanics to health care and cuts in services: a state-of-the-art overview. *Public Health Rep.* 1986;101:238–252.

12. Secretary's Task Force on Black and Minority Health. *Hispanic Health Issues, VIII.* Washington, DC: US Dept of Health and Human Services; 1986.

13. Secretary's Task Force on Black and Minority Health. *Crosscutting Issues in Minority Health, II.* Washington, DC: US Dept of Health and Human Services; 1985.

14. Poma PA. The Hispanic health challenge. *J Natl Med Assoc.* 1988;80:1275–1277.

15. Hu DJ, Covell, RM. Health care usage by Hispanic outpatients as function of primary language. *West J Med.* 1986;144:490–493.

16. Jonas HS, Etzel SI, Barzanski B. Undergraduate medical education. *JAMA.* 1989;262:1011–1019.

17. American Medical Association Board of Trustees. *Minority Students and Faculty in US Medical Schools.* Chicago, Ill.: American Medical Association 1989:41. Report F, A-89.

18. Wells KB, Golding JM, Hough RL, et al. Acculturation and the probability of use of health services by Mexican Americans. *Health Serv Res.* 1989;24:237–257.

19. Trevino FM, Bruhn JG, Bunce H. Utilization of community mental health services in a Texas-Mexico border city. *Soc Sci Med.* 1979;13A:331–334.

20. *Crosscultural Medicine: Clinical and Cultural Dimensions in Health Care Delivery to Hispanic Patients.* Chicago, Ill: Crosscultural Pathways and the Hispanic Health Alliance; 1990.

21. Trotter RT. Folk medicine in the Southwest: myths and medical facts. *Folk Med.* 1985;78:167–179.

22. DeLaCancela V, Guarnaccia PJ, Carrillo E. Psychosocial distress among Latinos: a critical analysis of *ataques de nervios. Humanity Soc.* 1986;10:431–447.

23. Anderson RM, Lewis SZ, Giachello AL, Chiu G. Access to medical care among the Hispanic population of the southwestern United States. *J Health Soc Behav.* 1981;22:78–79.

24. Trevino FM. Vital and health statistics for the US Hispanic population. *Am J Public Health.* 1982;72:979–981.

25. Rosenwaike I. Mortality differentials among persons born in Cuba, Mexico, and Puerto Rico residing in the United States, 1979–1981. *Am J Public Health.* 1987;77:603–606.

26. Shai D, Rosenwaike I. Violent deaths among Mexican-, Puerto Rican- and Cuban-born migrants in the United States. *Soc Sci Med.* 1988;26:269–276.

27. Secretary's Task Force on Black and Minority Health. *Cancer, III.* Washington, DC: US Dept of Health and Human Services; 1986.

28. Public Health Service. *Cancer and Minorities: Closing the Gap.* Washington, DC: Dept of Health and Human Services; 1987.

29. DeLaRosa M. Health care needs of Hispanic Americans and the responsiveness of the health care system. *Health Soc Work.* 1989;14:104–113.

30. Freeman HP. Cancer in the socioeconomically disadvantaged. *CA.* 1989;39:266–287.

31. Hispanic health risks. Maxwell B, Jacobson M. In: *Marketing Disease to Hispanics.* Washington, DC: Center for Science in the Public Interest; 1989:7–26.

32. Schinke SP, Moncher MS, Palleja J, et al. Hispanic youth, substance abuse, and stress: implications for prevention research. *Int J Addict.* 1988;23:809–826.

33. Public Health Service. *Diabetes and Minorities: Closing the Gap.* Washington, DC: Dept of Health and Human Services; 1987.

34. Centers for Disease Control. Prevalence of overweight for Hispanics — United States, 1982–1984. *MMWR.* 1989;38:838–843.

35. Diehl AK, Stern MP. Special health problems of Mexican-Americans: obesity, gallbladder disease, diabetes mellitus, and cardiovascular disease. *Adv Intern Med.* 1989;34:73–96.

36. Vega WA, Sallis JF, Patterson TL, et al. Predictors of dietary change in Mexican-American families participating in a health behavior change program. *Am J Prev Med.* 1988;4:194–199.

37. Secretary's Task Force on Black and Minority Health. *Cardiovascular and Cerebrovascular Disease, IV.* Washington, DC: US Dept of Health and Human Services; 1986.

38. Barrios E, Iler E, Mulloy L, et al. Hypertension in the Hispanic and black population in New York City. *J Natl Med Assoc.* 1987;79:749–752.

39. Kumanyika S, Savage DD, Ramirez AG, et al. Beliefs about high blood pressure prevention in a survey of blacks and Hispanics. *Am J Prev Med.* 1989;5:21–26.

40. Munoz E, Lecca PJ, Goldstein JD. *A Profile of Puerto Rican Health in the United States: Data From the Hispanic Health and Nutrition Examination Survey, 1982–1984.* New York, NY: Long Island Jewish Medical Center; 1988.

41. Escobedo LG, Remington PL. Birth cohort analysis of prevalence of cigarette smoking among Hispanics in the United States. *JAMA.* 1989;261:66–69.

42. Marin G, Perez-Stable EJ, Marin BV. Cigarette smoking among San Francisco Hispanics: the role of acculturation and gender. *Am. J Public Health.* 1989;79:196–198.

43. Rieder HL, Cauthen GM, Kelly GD, et al. Tuberculosis in the United States. *JAMA.* 1989;262:385–389.

44. Centers for Disease Control. Acquired immunodeficiency syndrome (AIDS) among blacks and Hispanics—United States. *MMWR.* 1986;35:655–666.

45. Schilling RF, Schinke SP, Nichols SE, et al. Developing strategies for AIDS prevention research with black and Hispanic drug users. *Public Health Rep.* 1989;104:2–11.

46. National Center for Health Statistics. AIDS knowledge and attitudes in the black and Hispanic populations. *Public Health Rep.* 1989;104:403–404.

47. Hu DJ, Keller R, Fleming D. Communicating AIDS information to Hispanics: the importance of language and media preference. *Am J Prev Med.* 1989;5:196–200.

48. American Medical Association Council on Scientific Affairs. *Reducing Transmission of Human Immunodeficiency Virus (HIV) Among and Through Intravenous Drug Abusers.* Chicago, Ill: American Medical Association; 1988. Report C, A-88.

49. Poma PA. Pregnancy in Hispanic women. *J Natl Med Assoc.* 1987;79:929–935.

50. Scribner R, Dwyer JH. Acculturation and low birthweight among Latinos in the Hispanic HANES. *Am J Public Health.* 1989;79:1263–1267.

51. Secretary's Task Force on Black and Minority Health. *Infant Mortality and Low Birthweight, VI.* Washington, DC: US Dept of Health and Human Services; 1986.

The Health of Black Folk:
Disease, Class, and Ideology in Science

NANCY KRIEGER and MARY BASSETT

SINCE THE FIRST crude tabulations of vital statistics in colonial America, one stark fact has stood out: black Americans are sicker and die younger than whites. As the epidemic infectious diseases of the nineteenth century were vanquished, the black burden of ill health shifted to the modern killers: heart disease, stroke, and cancer. Today black men under age 45 are ten times more likely to die from the effects of high blood pressure than white men. Black women suffer twice as many heart attacks as white women. A variety of common cancers are more frequent among blacks—and of cancer victims, blacks succumb sooner after diagnosis than whites. Black infant mortality is twice that of whites. All told, if the mortality rates for blacks and other minorities today were the same in the United States as for whites, more than 60,000 deaths in minority communities could be avoided each year.

What is it about being black that causes such miserable odds? . . .

THE GENETIC MODEL

Despite overwhelming evidence to the contrary, the theory that "race" is primarily a bio-

NANCY KRIEGER is an associate professor of health and social behavior at Harvard University.

MARY BASSETT is a faculty member in medicine and epidemiology, specializing in women's health issues, in the division of epidemiology at the Joseph L. Mailman School of Public Health, Columbia University.

logical category and that black-white differences in health are genetically determined continues to exert profound influence on both medical thinking and popular ideology. For example, an editorial on racial differences in birth weight (an important determinant of infant mortality) in the January 1986 *Journal of the American Medical Association* concluded: "Finally, what are the biologic or genetic differences among racial or ethnic groups? Should we shrink from the possibility of a biologic/genetic influence?" Similarly, a 1983 handbook prepared by the International Epidemiologic Association defined "race" as "persons who are relatively homogeneous with respect to biological inheritance." Public health texts continue to enshrine "race" in the demographic triad of "age, race, and sex," implying that "race" is as biologically fundamental a predictor of health as aging or sex, while the medical literature remains replete with studies that examine racial differences in health without regard to class.

The genetic model rests on three basic assumptions, all of which are flawed: that "race" is a valid biological category; that the genes which determine "race" are linked to the genes which affect health; and that the health of any community is mainly the consequence of the genetic constitution of the individuals of which it is composed. In contrast, we will argue that the health of the black community is not simply the sum of the health of individuals who are "genetically black" but instead chiefly reflects the social

Monthly Review, 38 (July–Aug 1986: 74–86 (12). Copyright 1986. Reprinted by permission of Monthly Review Foundation.

forces which create racially oppressed communities in the first place.

It is of course true that skin color, hair texture, and other visible features used to identify "race" are genetically encoded—there is a biologic aspect to "race." The importance of these particular physical traits in the spectrum of human variation, however, has been determined historically and politically. People also differ in terms of stature and eye color, but these attributes are rarely accorded significance. Categories based primarily on skin color correlate with health because race is a powerful determinant of the location and life-destinies of individuals within the class structure of U.S. society. Ever since plantation owners realized that differences in skin color could serve as a readily identifiable and permanent marker for socially determined divisions of labor (black runaway slaves were easier to identify than escaped white indentured servants and convicts, the initial workforce of colonial America), race and class have been inextricably intertwined. "Race" is not a natural descriptive category, but a social category born of the antagonistic relation of white supremacy and black oppression. The basis of the relative health advantage of whites is not to be found in their genes but in the relative material advantage whites enjoy as a consequence of political prerogative and state power. As Richard Lewontin has pointed out, "If, after a great cataclysm, only Africans were left alive, the human species would have retained 93 percent of its total genetic variation, although the species as a whole would be darker skinned." The fact that we all know which race we belong to says more about our society than about our biology.

Nevertheless, the paradigm of a genetic basis for black ill health remains strong. In its defense, researchers repeatedly trot out the few diseases for which a clear-cut link of race is established: sickle cell anemia, G&PD deficiency, and lactose intolerance. These diseases, however, have a tiny impact on the health of the black population as a whole—if anything, even less than those few diseases linked to "whiteness," such as some forms of skin cancer. Richard Cooper has shown that of the tens of thousands of excess black deaths in 1977, only 277 (0.3 percent) could be attributed to diseases such as sickle cell anemia. Such uncommon genetic maladies have become important strictly because of their metaphoric value: they are used to support genetic explanations of racial differences in the "big diseases" of the twentieth century—heart disease, stroke, and cancer. Yet no current evidence exists to justify such an extrapolation.

Determined nonetheless to demonstrate the genetic basis of racial health differences, investigators today—like their peers in the past—use the latest techniques. Where once physicians compared cranial capacity to explain black-white inequalities, now they scrutinize surface markers of cells. The case of hypertension is particularly illustrative. High blood pressure is an important cause of strokes and heart attacks, contributing to about 30 percent of all deaths in the United States. At present, the black rate of hypertension in the United States is about twice that of whites. Of over five hundred recent medical journal articles on the topic, fewer than a dozen studies explored social factors. The rest instead unsuccessfully sought biochemical-genetic explanations— and of these, virtually none even attempted to "define" genetically who was "white" and who was "black" despite the alleged genetic nature of their enquiry. As a consequence of the wrong questions being asked, the causes of hypertension remain unknown. Nonetheless, numerous clues point to social factors. Hypertension does not exist in several undisrupted hunter-gatherer tribes of different "races" but rapidly emerges in these tribes after contact with industrial society: in the United States, lower social class begets higher blood pressure.

Turning to cancer, the authors of a recent major government report surmised that blacks have poorer survival rates than whites because they do not "exhibit the same immunologic reactions to cancerous processes." It is noteworthy, however, that the comparably poor survival rates of British breast cancer patients have never elicited such speculation. In our own work on breast cancer in Washington state, we found that the striking "racial" difference in survival evaporated when we took class into account: working-class women, whether black or white, die sooner than women of higher social class standing.

To account for the persistence of the genetic model, we must look to its political significance rather than its scientific content. First used to buttress biblical arguments for slavery in a period when science was beginning to replace religion as sanction for the status quo, the genetic model of racial differences in health emerged toward the end of the eighteenth century, long before any precise theory of heredity existed. In well-respected medical journals, doctors debated whether blacks and whites were even the same species (let alone race), and proclaimed that blacks were intrinsically suited to slavery, thrived in hot climates, succumbed less to the epidemic fevers which ravaged the South, and suffered extraordinary rates of insanity if allowed to live free. After the Civil War effectively settled the argument about whether blacks belonged to the human species, physicians and scientists began elaborating hereditarian theories to explain the disparate health profiles not only of blacks and whites, but of the different white "races"—as defined by national origin and immigrant status. Virtually every scourge, from TB to rickets, was postulated to be inherited. Rheumatic fever, now known to be due to strep bacteria combined with the poverty which permits its expression in immunocompromised malnourished people, was long believed to be linked with the red hair and pale complexions of its Irish working-class victims. Overall, genetic explanations of differences in disease rates have politically served to justify existing class relations and excuse socially created afflictions as a result of immutable biology.

Nowadays the genetic model—newly dressed in the language of molecular genetics—continues to divert attention from the class origin of disease. Genetic explanations absolve the state of

responsibility for the health profile of black America by declaring racial disparities (regrettably) inevitable and normal. Intervention efforts based on this model founder for obvious reasons: short of recombinant DNA therapies, genetic screening and selective reproduction stand as supposed tools to reduce the racial gap in health.

Unfortunately, the genetic model wields influence even within the progressive health movement, as illustrated by the surge of interest in sickle cell anemia in the early 1970s. For decades after its initial description in 1925, sickle cell anemia was relegated to clinical obscurity. It occurs as often in blacks as does cystic fibrosis in whites. By linking genetic uniqueness to racial pride, such groups as the Black Panther Party championed sickle cell anemia as the number one health issue among blacks, despite the fact that other health problems—such as infant mortality—took a much greater toll. Because the sickle cell gene provides some protection against malaria, sickle cell seemed to link blacks to their African past, now three centuries removed. It raised the issue of racist neglect of black health in a setting where the victims were truly blameless: the fault lay in their genes. From the point of view of the federal government, sickle cell anemia was a uniquely black disease which did not raise the troubling issues of the ongoing oppression of the black population. In a period of political turmoil, what more could the government ask for? Small wonder that President Nixon jumped on the bandwagon and called for a national crusade.

THE ENVIRONMENTAL MODEL

The genetic model's long history and foundations in the joint race and class divisions of our society assure its continued prominence in discussions on the racial gap in health. To rebut this model, many liberals and progressives have relied upon environmental models of disease causation—only to encounter the Right on this turf as well.

Whereas the rise of slavery called forth genetic models of diseases, environmental models were born of the antagonistic social relations of industrial capitalism. In the appalling filth of nineteenth-century cities, periodic epidemics of yellow fever and cholera would attack the entire populace. A sanitary reform movement arose, advocating cleaner cities (with sewer systems and pure water) to protect the well-being of the wealthy as well as the poor, and also to engender a healthier, more productive workforce.

In the United States, most of the reformers were highly moralistic and staunchly procapitalist, seeing poverty and squalor as consequences of individual intemperance and ignorance rather than as necessary correlates of capital accumulation. In Europe, where the working-class movement was stronger, a class-conscious wing of the sanitary reform movement emerged. Radicals such as Frederick Engels and Rudolph Virchow (later the founder of modern pathology) argued that poverty and ill health could only be eliminated by resolving the antagonistic class relations of capitalism.

The early sanitary reform movement in the United States rarely addressed the question of racial differences in health per se. In fact, environmental models to explain black-white disparities emerged only during the mid-twentieth century, a consequence of the urban migration of blacks from the rural South to the industrial North and the rise of the civil-rights movement.

Today's liberal version of the environmental model blames poverty for black ill health. The noxious features of the "poverty environment" are catalogued and decried—lead paint from tenement walls, toxins from work, even social features like discrimination. But as in most liberal analyses, the unifying cause of this litany of woes remains unstated. We are left with an apparently unconnected laundry list of problems and no explanation of why blacks as a group encounter similar sickening conditions.

The liberal view fetishizes the environment: individuals are harmed by inanimate objects, physical forces, or unfortunate social conditions (like poverty)—by *things* rather than by people. That these objects or social circumstances are the *creations* of society is hidden by the veil of "natural science." Consequently, the "environment" is viewed as a natural and neutral category, defined as all that is external to individuals. What is not seen is the ways in which the underlying structure of racial oppression and class exploitation—which are relationships among people, not between people and things—shape the "environments" of the groups created by these relations.

The debilitating disease pellagra serves as a concrete example. Once a major health problem of poor southern farm and mill laborers in the United States, pellagra was believed to be a genetic disease. By the early 1920s, however, Joseph Goldberger had proved that the disease stemmed from a dietary deficiency in niacin and had also demonstrated that pellagra's familial nature existed because of the inheritance of nutritional options, not genes. Beyond this, Goldberger argued that pellagra, in essence, was a *social* disease caused by the single cash-crop economy of the South: reliance on cotton ensured seasonal starvation as food ran out between harvests, as well as periodic epidemics when the cotton market collapsed. Southern workers contracted pellagra because they had limited diets—and they had limited diets *because* they were southern workers. Yet governmental response was simply to supplement food with niacin: according to this view, vitamin deficiency—not socially determined malnutrition—was the chief cause of pellagra.

The liberal version of the environmental model also fails to see the causes of disease and the environment in which they exist as a historical product, a nature filtered through, even constructed by, society. What organisms and chemicals people are exposed to is determined by both the social relations and types of production which characterize their society. The same virus may cause pneumonia in blacks and whites alike, just as lead may cause the same physiologic damage—but *why* the death rate for flu and pneumonia and *why* blood lead levels are consistently higher in black as compared to white communities is not addressed. While the liberal conception of the environment can generate an exhaustive list of its components, it cannot comprehend the all-important assemblage of features of black life. What explains why a greater proportion of black mothers are single, young, malnourished, high-school dropouts, and so on?

Here the Right is ready with a "life-style" response as a unifying theme: blacks, not racism, are the source of their own health woes. Currently, the Reagan administration is the chief promoter of this view—as made evident by the 1985 publication of the Report of the Secretary's Task Force on Black and Minority Health. Just one weapon among many in the government's vicious ideological war to justify its savage gutting of health and social service programs, the report shifts responsibility for the burden of disease to the minority communities themselves. Promoting "health education" as a panacea, the government hopes to counsel minorities to eat better, exercise more, smoke and drink less, be less violent, seek health care earlier for symptoms, and in general be better health-care consumers. This "life-style" version of the environmental model accordingly is fully compatible with the genetic model (i.e., genetic disadvantage can be exaggerated by life-style choices) and echoes its ideological messages that individual shortcomings are at the root of ill health.

In focusing on individual health habits, the task force report ironically echoes the language of many "health radicals," ranging from iconoclasts such as Ivan Illich to counterculture advocates of individually oriented self-help strategies. United in practice, if not in spirit, these apparently disparate camps all take a "holistic" view, arguing that disease comes not just from germs or chemicals but from life-style choices about food, exercise, smoking, and stress. Their conflation of life-style choices and life circumstance can

reach absurd proportions. Editorializing on the task force report, the *New York Times* agreed that: "Disparities may be due to cultural or lifestyle differences. For example, a higher proportion of blacks and hispanics live in cities, with greater exposure to hazards like pollution, poor housing, and crime." But what kind of "life-style" causes pollution, and who chooses to live in high-crime neighborhoods? Both the conservative and alternative "life-style" versions of the environmental model deliberately ignore free choice and locate minority communities in the most hazardous regions of cities. What qualitatively constrains the option of blacks to "live right" is the reality of being black and poor in the United States.

But liberals have had little response when the Right points out that even the most oppressed and impoverished people make choices affecting their health: it may be hard to eat right if the neighborhood grocer doesn't sell fresh vegetables, but teenage girls do not have to become pregnant. For liberals, it has been easier to portray blacks as passive, blameless victims and in this way avoid the highly charged issue of health behaviors altogether. The end result is usually just proposals for more health services for blacks, Band-Aids for the gaping wounds of oppression. Yet while adequate health services certainly are needed, they can do little to stem the social forces which cause disease.

Too often the Left has been content merely to trail behind the liberals in campaigns for health services, or to call only for social control of environmental and occupational exposures. The Right, however, has shifted the terrain of battle to the issue of individual behavior, and we must respond. It is for the Left to point out that society does not consist of abstract individuals, but rather of people whose life options are shaped by their intrinsic membership in groups defined by the social relations of their society. Race and class broadly determine not only the conditions under which blacks and whites live, but also the ways in which they can respond to these conditions and the political power they have to alter them. The material limits produced by oppression create and constrain not only the type of housing you live in, but even the most intimate choices about what you do inside your home. Oppression and exploitation beget the reality and also the belief that bad health and personal failure are ineluctable facts of life.

Frantz Fanon wrote eloquently of the fatalistic hopelessness engendered by oppression in colonial Algeria. Eliminating self-destructive behaviors, like drug addiction or living in a battering relationship, requires that they be acknowledged as the subjective reflection of objective powerlessness. As Bylle Avery, director of the National Black Women's Health Project, has said, wellness and empowerment are linked. School-based birth control clinics, however necessary as part of the strategy to reduce teen pregnancy, will be ineffective as long as the social motivation for young black women to get pregnant remains unaddressed: for black women to improve their health, they must individually choose to act collectively in order to transform the social conditions which frame, constrain, and devalue their lives as black women.

TOWARD A MARXIST CONCEPTION

The ideological content of science is transparent in disease models now rejected as archaic or indisputably biased. The feudal view of disease as retribution of God and the eugenist science underlying Nazi racial hygiene clearly resonated well with the dominant politics and ideology of their respective societies. But it is far more difficult to discern the ideological content of scientific theory in one's own time and place.

Criticism of the ideology underlying existing paradigms is an important tool in undermining reactionary science. It can help us sort out the apparent riddle of the Reagan administration's embrace of "holistic" health. Such criticism also points the way toward alternative concepts. To construct a new paradigm, however, requires painstaking work. Moreover, the goal is not a "neutral" science, but one which openly acknowledges the ways in which ideology inevitably is incorporated into scientific concepts and theories. Accurate elucidation and prevention of the material and ideological components of disease processes necessitates the explicit adoption of an anti-racist and class-conscious standpoint.

We have only a hint of how a Marxist analysis of the social relations of race and class can illuminate the processes involved in the social production of disease. Such an approach has already shown that many "racial" differences in disease are actually attributable to differences in class. Similarly, the finding of some Marxist researchers that an absentee landlord, rather than race, is the best predictor of lead poisoning points to what this new science can offer in the way of prevention.

But these are small, isolated observations. Too often we are constrained by assumptions built into existing techniques and methodologies. The intimidating mathematics of multiple regression which dominate public health research cannot even contemplate an effect which becomes its own cause—such as the way in which malnutrition opens the way for infections, which cause diarrhea, which causes malnutrition. Further, existing analytic techniques cannot address phenomena like class relations or racial oppression which cannot be expressed as numbers. True, we can calculate the health effect of more or less income or education, but these are pale reflections of class relations, outcomes and not essences. Similarly, we are limited by disease definitions geared toward individual etiology. Treating the problems of substance abuse, infectious disease, infant mortality, and occupational exposure in the black community as separate maladies obscures their common social antecedent. Clearly, we need basically new approaches to understand the dialectical interpenetration of racism, class relations, and health.

Gender Bias in Health Care: A Life or Death Issue for Women with Coronary Heart Disease

CAROL JONANN BESS

INTRODUCTION

GROWING EVIDENCE in medical research suggests a gender bias against women, particularly in the area of coronary heart disease (CHD). This disparity exists at all levels of health care delivery from office visits to in-hospital care. Gender bias may result in delayed or inaccurate diagnosis, unequal medical interventions, and higher mortality for women who undergo invasive cardiac and surgical procedures. While research conducted in other areas of medical care indicate a bias against women, recent research in cardiac care presents the most worrisome evidence to date that women are dying because physicians fail to timely diagnose and treat CHD as aggressively as they do in men. . . .

Our priority in research should be to identify when it occurs, and take measures to see that it ceases. The Council on Ethical and Judicial Affairs of the American Medical Association reports, "The medical community cannot tolerate any discrepancy in the provision of care that is not based on appropriate biological or medical indications." The long-term quality of life and health of women depend on finding a solution to this problem.

I. THE SCOPE OF GENDER BIAS IN HEALTH CARE

A. A Historical Perspective

The roots of women's health issues arose from the Feminist Movement in the late 1970s and challenged the medical profession's authority over women's bodies.[1] In the midst of the Women's Movement in the late 1970s, women complained that their physical complaints were not considered by physicians as seriously as those of men. Armitage et al. were among the first researchers to examine this allegation.[2] Armitage's San Diego study suggested that men received more diagnostic services and more appropriate treatment for their complaints than did women.[3] In 1981, Verbrugge and Steiner examined the same five medical complaints as Armitage and discovered that while women actually receive more medical care than men, there were statistically significant differences between the care delivered.[4] When the complaint is chest pain, a potentially more serious condition, physicians diagnosed men differently than women. Specifically, "Men's chest pain is due to circulatory conditions (heart disease) more often; and women's, to respiratory conditions (bronchitis and pleurisy)."[5] Verbrugge attributed the apparent

CAROL JONANN BESS is a member of the class of 1995 at the University of California, Hastings College of the Law. Her credentials include the following: A.S.N., Los Medanos College, 1982; B.S.N., Graceland College, 1991; R.N., Intensive/Coronary Care, Kaiser Foundation Hospital, Martinez, California since 1982. For my father John, my mentor, my friend.

Hastings Women's Law Journal 6, 1: 41–52. Copyright 1995, University of California, Hastings College of the Law. Reprinted by permission.

contradiction in outcome from Armitage's research to the small sample in the San Diego study (n=40 patients) as compared to hers (n=46,868 visits to physician). Current literature interprets Verbrugge's study as indicating a higher morbidity among women (more acute and chronic, non-lethal conditions leading to poor health) and higher mortality among men (conditions leading to death).[6] Rodin states, "Men are sick less often, but their illnesses and injuries are more severe; men have higher rates of chronic diseases that are the leading causes of death."[7]

B. Cultural Biases Against Women Result in Gender Bias in Health Care

Researchers proposed several theories to explain the existence of gender bias in health care. In 1975, Nathanson synthesized research concerning sex differences in morbidity and utilization of physical and mental health services.[8] She employed three explanatory models previously proposed in research: "(1) women report more illness than men because it is culturally more acceptable for them to be ill—'the ethic of health is masculine'; (2) the sick role is relatively compatible with women's other role responsibilities, and incompatible with those of men; and (3) women's assigned social roles are more stressful than those of men; consequently, they have more illness."[9] Nathanson observed these studies did not differentiate between illness and illness behavior and concluded there was insufficient data using these three explanatory models to link women's higher morbidity and lower mortality to various dimensions of the feminine role."[10] Marcus and Seeman further examined the feminine role and illness and concluded inflexible role obligations contribute to differences between men and women in reporting illness; but when this variable was controlled, women reported more chronic conditions than men.[11]

In 1982, Cleary et al. studied both illness and illness behavior of men and women and con-

cluded "the consistency of sex differences found using different types of indicators and different types of data supports the notion that they reflect real differences in health."[12] Women not only reported more illness, they were actually ill more often than men. . . .

Research indicates there is no one satisfactory explanation for women's higher morbidity, but men's higher mortality. One of the most recent studies, conducted by Verbrugge in 1989,[13] examined five factors: (1) biological risks, (2) acquired risks, (3) illness behavior, (4) health-reporting symptoms, and (5) prior health care and caretakers. Verbrugge concluded of these five, acquired risks (roles and stress) account for women's poorer health.[14] Additionally, when social factors are taken into account, men still have a higher mortality than women.[15] This issue needs further research. The Council on Ethical and Judicial Affairs recognized the contradiction in the existing research, stating:

> Although biological factors account for some differences between the sexes in the provision of medical care, these studies indicate that nonbiological or nonclinical factors may affect clinical decision making. There is not enough data to identify the exact nature of nonbiological or nonclinical factors. Nevertheless, the existence of these factors is a cause for concern that the medical community needs to address.[16]

C. Female Physicians May Display Less Gender Bias than Male Physicians

Feminists placed the burden of gender bias in health care squarely in the laps of physicians. Bernstein and Kane conducted a survey to assess male and female physicians' attitudes toward female patients.[17] The results suggest that physicians perceive women as more emotionally labile than men. The more expressive a female was, the more likely the physician was to judge the female's complaints as psychosomatic.[18] When men behaved emotionally, physicians judged them similarly to expressive women.[19] Bernstein and Kane found no differences in the responses of male and female physicians.[20] This last finding may be explained by the small sample of female physicians. A total of 253 physicians participated; 225 were men, 28 were women.[21]

A recent study by Roter et al. suggests striking differences between female and male physicians, regardless of the sex of the patient.[22] In their study of 127 physicians (101 men and 26 women), they concluded that female physicians devoted more time to the clinical patient visit, talked more, and used different communication strategies than males.[23] Female physicians used patient-centered, positive, relation-building communication and provided more biomedical and psychosocial information, regardless of the sex of the patient.[24] Additionally, both male and female patients talked more with female physicians, but women especially benefited from exchanges with female physicians.[25] While this larger study of female physicians may be more reliable than earlier studies, it is difficult to compare the two studies because they do not measure the same variables. Bernstein and Kane found no differences in responses between male and female physicians' attitudes toward female patients; neither did Roter et al. The mean age of physicians studied by Bernstein and Kane was forty-one, while the mean age studied by Roter was thirty-four. This age difference, in addition to the smaller sampling of female physicians by Bernstein and Kane, suggests that younger female physicians may have different attitudes toward female patients. Additionally, ten years elapsed between studies, during which time the medical profession, as well as society, has become more sensitive to women's health issues. . . .

D. Gender Bias Affects Older Women Disproportionately

With the graying of America, the older population has become overwhelmingly female. Today women are likely to outlive men by over seven years.[26] But living longer does not mean living well. In 1986, women constituted 71% of the population entitled to both Medicare and Medicaid.[27] Older women are not only poorer than older men, but are less likely to have private health insurance or other assets. Women have "fewer personal financial resources for health care 'than older men, and these resources' must be spread out over a longer lifetime."[28]

Research suggests gender bias may be more damaging for older women, especially given women's higher morbidity rates. A recent study by Mutran and Ferraro suggests that given equal levels of disability and overall health status, older men were more likely to be hospitalized than older women.[29] Mutran and Ferraro propose that physicians' attitudes differ for three possible reasons: (1) men may be less able or less likely to care for themselves as outpatients, (2) men's self-assessments may be perceived as reflective of an actual medical problem (i.e., women are more likely to be hypochondriacs), and (3) the decision to hospitalize may be a function of the sex of the physician.[30] Regardless of the reasons, the fact that women are as ill as men, but are not hospitalized as often, constitutes discrimination based on gender. Further, this discrimination may preclude women's access to in-patient diagnostic procedures which might lead to earlier medical interventions. According to Lewis, older women's experiences with the health care system have not been positive. Lewis states:

> Their chronic diseases are often ignored or undertreated, as medicine occupies itself with more acute conditions. Physicians tend to belittle their complaints and symptoms by attributing them to "post menopausal syndrome," old age, hypochondriasis or other neurotic behaviors, "senility," or by over-prescribing tranquilizers and other medications in the belief that many physical complaints of older women are psychosomatic in origin. . . . There is little recognition of the value of older women's lifetime contributions to society. Their work is not considered part of the gross national product. Their accumulated wisdom, survival skills,

range of personality, and creativity are seldom acknowledged. It is not surprising therefore, that health care workers often reflect the larger cultural disregard and even disdain for older women.[31]

There is a fear among female medical professionals that in the current climate of soaring medical costs, the growing numbers of older patients may cause a strong incentive to ration health care based on age.[32] Age-based rationing will disproportionately affect females because there are more older women than men, and their relative impoverished state creates greater reliance on families and public insurance to meet their medical needs. Additionally, age-based rationing may signal to society that older citizens have less value and are less deserving than the young. . . .

Gender bias against women is not unique to the older woman, but is consistent with patterned inequities felt throughout the life cycle. Hess states, "Gender is less a reflection of immutable natural differences than a means of dividing people into distinct categories. The gender stratification system is a set of power relationships."[33] As women age, the inequities in medical care increase. . . .

E. The Male Model of Health Care Is the Norm

It is generally accepted that *all* medical care is based on a male model, while care of the female is "other."[34] Dr. McGoldrick stated in an editorial, "[t]ypically, the paradigm patient or research model has been the 70 kilogram man. Traditional studies on diseases which affect both sexes have characteristically used male subjects exclusively, with the results extrapolated or generalized, as if to suggest that males are the generic humans."[35] The problem with this male model is that information is extrapolated to women with effects ranging from incorrect to lethal.

Historically, drug companies have conducted clinical trials on new drugs using white males ex-clusively during all stages of testing, and physicians have prescribed these drugs to women. Indeed, women are prescribed more drugs than men, and suffer more adverse reactions.[36] Evidence in the 1970s and early 1980s suggested that women have clinically significant differences in drug metabolism and responsiveness throughout the life cycle.[37] However, the FDA and drug companies refused to use women in clinical trials because (1) testing women subjects introduces complexities due to hormonal variations (menstrual cycle, pregnancy, menopause), increasing the cost of research, and (2) drug companies fear liability from teratogenic effects.[38] Underlying these theories is the belief that information from testing young white males is applicable to women, that men and women are physiologically the same.[39]

Examples abound that extrapolation to women of a drug's effects on male research subjects is inaccurate and potentially dangerous. Even though women have a higher incidence of clinical depression, antidepressants tested only on male subjects can cause hostility and violence in women.[40] The menstrual cycle can affect antidepressant effects; a constant dose may be too high early in the cycle and too low later.[41] Menstrual variations in response to drug therapy also occur with clonidine (given for high blood pressure) and Dilantin (given for seizures).[42] Further, research suggests that oral contraceptive pills and estrogen taken for replacement during menopause may influence the metabolism of a wide variety of other drugs.[43]

Elderly women may be at higher risk for adverse drug reactions than younger women. When age bias is added to gender bias in drug therapy, the results may be lethal. According to Wolfe, "[a] lot of elderly patients have been killed or injured because extrapolations aren't valid."[44] One-third of all people over age sixty take five or more drugs simultaneously, and women take more drugs than men.[45] The U.S. Public Health Service reports that older women take sedatives, tranquilizers, hypnotic drugs,

drugs for hypertension and cardiac conditions, vitamins, analgesics, diuretics, and laxatives at two and one-half times the rate of older men.[46] The greatest danger of taking multiple medications involves the synergistic effect of one medication when taken with another; that is, drugs have a greater total effect than the sum of their individual effects. The aging process complicates the synergistic effect of medications due to delayed absorption, metabolism and excretion in the elderly.[47] For these reasons, elderly women are more likely to experience adverse drug reactions than are others, especially given the paucity of research applicable to women. . . .

NOTES

1. Karen Johnson & Laurel Dawson, "Women's Health as a Multidisciplinary Specialty: An Exploratory Proposal," 45 *J. Am. Med. Women's Assn.* 222 (1990).

2. Lois M. Verbrugge & Richard P. Steiner, "Physician Treatment of Men and Women Patients: Sex Bias or Appropriate Care?," 19 *Med. Care* 609, 632 n.1 (1981) (citing A. J. Armitage et al., "Response of Physicians to Medical Complaints in Men and Women," 241 *JAMA* 2186 (1979)).

3. Armitage, *supra* note 3, at 2190.

4. Verbrugge, *supra* note 3, at 632 n. 1.

5. *Id.* at 628. The five complaints used in both studies were fatigue, headache, vertigo/dizziness, chest pain, and back pain. Other significant differences include: (1) men complaining of fatigue receive more drug prescriptions, (2) women complaining of headache receive more diagnostic services, (3) men complaining of dizziness/vertigo get more diagnostic work-up, but women get more return appointments, (4) women with back pain receive more diagnostic, therapeutic, and follow-up care. *Id.* at 629.

6. Judith Rodin & Jeannette R. Ickovics, "Women's Health: Review and Research Agenda As We Approach the 21st Century," 45 *Am. Psychol.* 1018, 1021 (1990).

7. *Id.* at 1021 (citing Verbrugge, *infra* note 13).

8. Constance A. Nathanson, "Illness and the Feminine Role: A Theoretical Review," 9 *Soc. Sci. & Med.* 57 (1975).

9. *Id.* at 59. *See also* Council on Judicial and Ethical Affairs, "Gender Disparities in Clinical Decision Making," *Journal of the American Medical Association* 266 (1991), 559–562. (citing the following studies: W. R

Gove & J. Tudor. "Adult Sex Roles and Mental Illness," 78 *Am. J. Sociol.* 812 (1973) (concluding more women than men are mentally ill and women have more transient situational personality disorders and psychosomatic disorders); D. L. Philips & B. E. Segal, "Sexual Status and Psychiatric Symptoms" 34 *Am. Sociol. Rev.* 58 (1969) (concluding women report more symptoms because illness is stigmatizing for men, less so, for women); K. Broverman et al., "Sex-Role Stereotypes and Clinical Judgments of Mental Health," 34 *J. Consult. Clin. Psychol.* 1 (1970) (concluding concepts of mental health, held by health professionals differed depending upon the sex of the patient); W. A. Glaser, *Social Settings and Medical Organization* (1970) (concluding the sick role is more compatible with a woman's role); C. Smith-Rosenberg & C. Rosenberg, "The Female Animal: Medical and Biological Views of Woman and Her Role in 19th Century America," 60 *J. Am. Hist.* 332 (1973) (concluding woman's health is dictated by her reproductive system and disorders of this system may appear in remote areas of her body. Men suffer no parallel disability).

10. Nathanson, *supra* note 8, at 61.

11. Alfred C. Marcus & Teresa E. Seeman, "Sex Differences in Reports of Illness and Disability: A Preliminary Test of the 'Fixed Role Obligations' Hypothesis," 22 *J. Health Soc. Behav.* 174 (1981).

12. Paul D. Cleary et al., "Sex Differences in Medical Care Utilization: An Empirical Investigation," 23 *J. Health Soc. Behav.* 106, 115 (1982).

13. Lois M. Verbrugge, "The Twain Meet: Empirical Explanations of Sex Differences in Health and Mortality," 30 *J. Health Soc. Behav.* 282 (1989).

14. *Id.*

15. *Id.* at 295.

16. Council on Ethical and Judicial Affairs, *supra* note 9, at 559.

17. Bernstein & Kane, *supra* note 16, at 600.

18. *Id.* at 606.

19. *Id.*

20. *Id. See also* Stephen Colameco et al., "Sex Bias in the Assessment of Patient Complaints," 16 *J. Fam. Pract.* 1117 (1983) (concluding that female physicians as compared to male physicians do not hold more favorable attitudes toward female patients).

21. Bernstein & Kane, *supra* note 16, at 603.

22. Debra Roter, Mack Lipkin, Jr., & Audrey Korsgaard, "Sex Differences in Patients' and Physicians' Communication During Primary Care Medical Visits," 29 *Med. Care* 1083 (1991).

23. *Id.* at 1091.

24. *Id.* at 1092.

25. *Id. See also* Nicole Lurie et al., "Preventive Care For Women: Does the Sex of the Physician Matter?,"

329 *N. Eng. J. Med.* 478 (1993) (concluding women are more likely to undergo screening with PAP smears and mammograms if they see female rather than male physicians).

26. Nancy S. Jecker, "Age-Based Rationing and Women," 266 *JAMA* 3012 (1991).

27. *Id.* at 3012 (citing C. Muller, *Health Care and Gender* (1991)).

28. *Id.* at 3012 (citing Myrna Lewis, "Older Women and Health: An Overview," 10 *Women's Health* 1, 10–11 (1985)). In 1983 the median income for older women was $5,599.00 per year compared to $9,766.00 for older men. This placed women just $800.00 over the U. S. official poverty level.

29. Elizabeth Mutran & Kenneth F. Ferraro, "Medical Need and Use of Services Among Older Men and Women," 43 *J. Geront.* S162, S169 (1988).

30. *Id. But see* Marjorie Pearson et al., "Differences in Quality of Care for Hospitalized Elderly Men and Women," 268 *JAMA* 1883 (1992) (concluding the care received by men and women as in-hospital patients is more similar than different).

31. Lewis, at 12–13.

32. Jecker, *supra* note 26, at 3012.

33. Beth B. Hess, "Gender and Aging: The Demographic Parameters," 14 *Generations* 12 (1990).

34. Michelle Harrison, "Woman As Other: The Premise of Medicine," 45 *J. Am. Med. Women's Assn.* 225 (1990).

35. Kathryn E. McGoldrick, "Women's Health: Is Anatomy Still Destiny?," 45 *J. Am. Med. Women's Assn.* 211 (1990).

36. Jean Hamilton & Barbara Parry, "Sex-Related Differences in Clinical Drug Response: Implications for Women's Health," 38 *J. Am. Med. Women's Assn.* 126 (1983).

37. *Id. See* K. O'Malley et al., "Effect of Age and Sex on Human Drug Metabolism," 3 *B. Med. J.* 607 (1971); J.F. Giudicelli & J.P. Tillement, "Influence of Sex on Drug Kinetics in Man," 2 *Clin. Pharmocokinet.,* 157 (1977); S.L. Maiskiewicz et al., "Sex Differences in Absorption Kinetics of Sodium Salicylate," 31 *Clin. Pharmacol. Ther.* 30 (1982); G. Fink et al., "Sex Difference in Response to Alphaxalone Anaesthesia May Be Estrogen Dependent," 298 *Nature* 270 (1982).

38. Elizabeth L. Bowles, "The Disenfranchisement of Fertile Women in Clinical Trials: The Legal Ramifications of and Solutions for Rectifying the Knowledge Gap," 45 *V and. L. Rev.* 877 (1992). Teratogenic effects concern untoward effects of drugs on the developing fetus, causing a variety of malformations of organ systems.

39. *Id.* at 883.

40. *Id.* at 888.

41. Paul Cotton, "Is There Still Too Much Extrapolation From Date On Middle-aged White Men?," 263 *JAMA* 1049 (1990).

42. Paul Cotton, "Examples Abound of Gaps in Medical Knowledge Because of Groups Excluded From Scientific Study," 263 *JAMA* 1051 (1990).

43. Hamilton & Parry, *supra* note 43, at 128.

44. Cotton, *supra* note 42, at 1050 (quoting Sidney Wolfe, M.D., of the Public Citizens' Health Research Group, Washington, D.C.).

45. Rodin and Ickovics, *supra* note 12, at 1029.

46. *Id.* (citing U.S. Public Health Service, "Women's Health: Report of the Health Service Task Force on Women's Health Issues" (1985)).

47. Charlotte Eliopoulos. *Gerontological Nursing* 347–349 (2d ed. 1987).

The Right to Care

The Right to Health Protection

TOM H. CHRISTOFFEL

The state claims to be a state of property rights. Its purpose is to protect the people's property. Most people, however, possess nothing but their labor power, which depends entirely on their health. That is their only property and the state, therefore, has the duty to protect it and the people have the right to insist that their health, their only possession, be protected by the state.

S. Neumann*

INTRODUCTION

Garfield Park is a black ghetto on the west side of Chicago, poor and badly serviced by the city. In recent years the Northwestern University Center for Urban Affairs studied the area's health problems, focusing on causes of hospitalization. The investigators discovered that the leading cause of hospital visits was automobile accidents. Another major cause was dog bites. The area recorded ten times the number of dog bites aver-

Tom Christoffel is a professor emeritus of health policy and administration at the University of Illinois at Chicago.

*S. Neumann, *Die Offentliche Gesundheit-Spflege Und Das Eigentum* (1897), as rendered in H. Sigerist, *Medicine and Human Welfare* 95 (1941).

aged in the rest of the city. Working with a local group called the Christian Action Ministry, the Center was able to induce the city to improve street maintenance and to cooperate in a roundup of wild dogs. This episode would seem to be a model for attacking problems by attacking the causes.[1]

Over a hundred years ago Rudolf Virchow, physician and reformer, wrote that "[m]edicine is a social science, and politics is nothing else but medicine on a large scale."[2] That poor health is primarily the result of controllable factors is no longer subject to much debate.[3] That the route to improved health is, therefore, primarily political is becoming equally evident. Since health relates closely to all aspects of life, from carcinogenic food to rutted streets, efforts to assure good health and to provide effective medical care must be very broad in scope. Since health levels correlate closely with income, and because income results from political-economic and not biological factors,[4] it is also clear that poor health results in large measure from factors under human cause and control.

Thus, the concept of a right to health must incorporate the many factors affecting human

National Black Law Journal 6, nos. 2–3 (1980): 183–197. *Reprinted by permission of* The National Black Law Journal health that are under human control. Moreover, while the right to medical care is important, especially in critical situations, it is only part of the concept. Thus, the right to be treated for dog bite does nothing to stop the danger from stray dogs. Attempts to assert a right to health must begin to focus on the broader issue of health protection as part of that right. This Article introduces the right to health protection in a preliminary way, in the hope that more detailed exploration of legal strategies and mechanisms will follow.

Of course many factors that influence health levels are already addressed by the law.[3] For example, Chicago probably could not legally defend shortchanging black ghetto areas in basic city services provided to other parts of the city.[4] But it was not the courts that helped pave streets and catch loose-running dogs in Garfield Park. Rather, it was self-organization combined with the "clout" of a major university, a component of which happened to interest itself in one poor neighborhood. Clearly, therefore, successful health measures depend on more than legal rights.

HEALTH AND HEALTH STATUS

A standard dictionary definition of health is "the condition of being sound in body, mind, or spirit; *esp.* freedom from physical disease or pain."[7] *Black's Law Dictionary* includes a definition of health as the "[s]tate of being hale, sound, or whole in body, mind or soul; well being."[8] Although often criticized as too idealistic, the most cited definition of health is that of the World Health Organization, which calls it "a state of complete physical, mental and social well-being and not merely the absence of disease or infirmity."[9] Health is influenced by such varied factors as nutrition, standard and style of living, occupational satisfactions and hazards, natural and man-made environments, cultural perceptions, and the system of health-care services and delivery. Surprising though it may seem, the health

care delivery system, which is the major focus of most right-to-health discussions, has relatively little impact on health status levels.[10]

Although health is usually defined in general and idealistic terms, levels of health or the state of being healthy are subject to measurement and comparison.[11] Such measurements include productive life span, age at death, specific causes of death, morbidity, reproductive efficiency, social dysfunction, self-perception of illness, and even the very fact of being under medical care. In terms of the most basic indicator—mortality—the level of health has improved greatly over the past two centuries.[12] The must important elements underlying this change have been improved water supplies and sewage systems, more abundant food, clean-food regulations, and other preventive measures.[13] For example, in the United States, life expectancy at birth, which as recently as 1900 was 47.3 years, is now close to 72 years.[14] Almost all of this improvement results from lowered infant mortality rates, again due largely to improved sanitation and preventive measures. The exception was the period from 1936–1954 when the development of antibiotics was directly responsible for large-scale improvements in medical care. Since 1954, however, the death rate has remained relatively static,[15] and it has become increasingly evident that non-medical factors are likely to be the basis of further decline in that rate.[16]

This is not meant to disparage the role of medicine, but rather to emphasize the importance of environmental factors, including nutrition, in determining health status[17] and to underscore that any argument in behalf of a right to health must encompass more than medical care delivery. Before exploring this matter more directly, it is necessary to examine some pertinent statistics. While the 1970's offer the promise of longer and healthier lives than did the 1770's, there are important and revealing gaps.

The United States spends more on health care services than almost any other nation, both in absolute terms and in terms of health expenditures as a percent of GNP.[18] Yet, this country ranks seventh for females and nineteenth for males in life expectancy at birth.[19] Additionally infant mortality rates in the United States are almost twice that of Sweden.[20] Moreover, United States health and illness statistics continue to show a strong class of racial bias, with fewer preventive measures, poorer medical care, and more contributing causes of ill-health among those least able to afford the basics of life—a group that is disproportionately "non-White."

These variations among sub-groups of the population have been well documented,[21] and the reasons are fairly well understood. Most often they relate to those things of which poor people have less—good food, decent housing, jobs, and, in the area of medical care, preventive health-care services.

What do all these statistics mean? They indicate, first, that health status is the result of a wide variety of factors. Second, that many, if not most, of these factors are subject to human influence and control. Third, that because of the way human control over many of these factors has been exercised in the past, individual health status does not vary randomly in the population, but is closely related to socio-economic factors. And finally, that improvement in health status is possible, and so is the elimination of these nonrandom differences.[22] . . .

A RIGHT TO HEALTH PROTECTION?

Medical care focuses on *curing* disease as a means of improving health status. But effective improvement of the public's health depends even more on dealing with the cause of disease than it does on its cure.[23] This includes control of communicable diseases, regulation and improvement of the physical environment, and food and water sufficient in both quality and quantity.[24] More recently, these traditional concerns have broadened to include conditions of employment[25] and other factors involving *health protection,* which encompasses both preventive medicine (*e.g.,* immunization, screening and detection, accident

prevention) and promotion of an environment conducive to better health (*e.g.,* health education, environmental and occupational health measures, nutrition, risk-factor intervention).

The most rational government approach to the issue of a right to health is to concentrate on health protection, not only because this is the most direct and effective approach to the problem, but also because it fits most easily into the traditional role of government as a societal regulator rather than simply as a provider of funds. This concept is not new; governmental health policy carried out through administrative regulations—the "medical police"—was popular in Germany in the eighteenth century.[26]

In the United States, public health and safety measures have a long tradition.[27] No public policy is more important than the protection of the people from practices which may injure their health, and governments have traditionally exercised broad public health powers.[28] But faced today with more of a threat from contamination in the air than from that in the streets, public health measures seem to be meeting increasing resistance. This should not be surprising, for unlike controls aimed at communicable diseases and poor sanitation, environmental and occupational health measures impinge directly on private business interests. The property oriented legal system is well suited to defending property owners' "rights," even when these include poisoning and endangering the living and working environments. Thus, efforts to protect the public from health hazards cannot be expected to receive automatic judicial endorsement.[29] The key question is how to find the appropriate leverage with which to enforce health protection, and efforts toward this end have included common law, statutory and constitutional approaches.

Common law actions have played a limited role in protecting the public's health. Although the authority to abate public nuisances without compensation for property loss seems clearly available,[30] it is not often successfully used, especially by individual complainants.[31] Tort actions have not proved very successful as deterrent[32] or

preventive measures, but they hold a strong theoretical potential value for health protection.
The failure of product liability actions for smoking induced lung-cancer deaths would seem to
be discouraging, but this may represent the most
difficult extreme.[33] A recent $20 million settle-
ment payment to asbestos workers suffering
from lung cancer and asbestosis may herald similar actions. The parties agreeing to contribute to
the settlement included not only the owners of
an asbestos plant, but also government inspection agencies which had failed to inform the
workers of the health hazard they faced.[34]

The success of common law actions in protecting health will depend on the availability of
good scientific data to present to courts. This
might be an easier task than developing new
legal arguments which assert broader governmental health obligations. The task may also be
eased to the extent that courts begin to accept
risk-benefit balancing as part of their standard of
proof in health related cases.[35]

Both state and federal legislatures have recently been forced to pay more attention to regulating the general environment, and particularly
the workplace. State and federal occupational
safety, health and environmental protection
laws[36] would seem to have had their successes,[37]
though they also tend to create programs that are
understaffed, undersupported, and quite often
timid. The result is an inability to successfully
tackle some of the biggest health threats.[38]

Perhaps the greatest promise for effective
health protection lies in efforts to increase enforcement of existing statutes. Ideas and statutes
are not lacking as much as are the resources for
using them to maximum effectiveness. If more
attorneys get involved in health related litigation, and if data is more effectually compiled, it
may be possible to push existing law to its fullest
potential in much the same way that welfare and
privacy law has been aggressively developed.

A constitutional claim to a decent environment, based on due process or Ninth Amendment grounds, has won little support in the
courts,[39] since both the federal and most state
constitutions are silent regarding environmental
matters. The most meaningful exception is the
new Illinois State Constitution, which provides:

> Each person has the right to a healthful envi-
> ronment. Each person may enforce this right
> against any party, governmental or private,
> through appropriate legal proceedings subject
> to reasonable limitation and regulation as the
> General Assembly may provide by law.[40]

This provision creates standing to sue to enforce
an individual right to a healthful environment,
without requiring special damages or state action. It is not yet clear what this may mean, but it
might be used to create standing in common law
public nuisance suits or to allow courts to more
openly make environmental policy judgments.[41]
Just how effective the constitutional provision
will be in protecting health remains to be seen,
but it is an invitation to push for effective health
protection.[42]

NOTES

1. The program has received favorable comment.
See 238 J.A.M.A. 1908 (1977); The Reader, Sept. 9,
1977, at 1.

2. 1 *Die Medizinische Reform* 2 (1845), as quoted in
H. Sigerist, *Medicine and Human Welfare* 93 (1970)
[hereinafter cited as Sigerist].

3. See generally *American College of Preventive Medicine, Preventive Medicine USA* (1976) [hereinafter cited
as *Preventive Medicine*].

4. On the continuing unscientific efforts to blame
genetic factors for health and other problems, see *A.
Chase, The Legacy of Malthus* (1976).

5. See generally, *F. Grad, Public Health Law Manual*
(1976); *K. Wing, The Law and the Public's Health* (1976).

6. Cf. Hawkins v. Town of Shaw, 437 F.2d 1289
(5th Cir. 1971), aff'd on rehearing, 461 F.2d 1171 (5th
Cir. 1972), cert. denied, 426 U.S. 245 (1975). See generally Lineberry, Mandating Urban Equality: The Distribution of Municipal Public Services, 53 *Tex. L. Rev.*
26 (1974); *Clearinghouse for Civil Rights Research, The
Wrong Side of the Tracks: Measuring Inequities in
Municipal Services,* Summer, 1975.

7. *Webster's New Collegiate Dictionary* 528 (8th ed.
1975).

8. *Black's Law Dictionary* 852 (Rev. 4th ed. 1968).

9. *World Health Organization, Basic Documents* 1
(25th ed. 1976). For a criticism of such an utopian

ideal, see *R. Dubos, Man, Medicine and Environment* 67 (1968)[hereinafter cited as *Dubos*).

10. See generally, *T. McKeown, Medicine in Modern Society* (1966); *McKeown*, A Historical Appraisal of the Medical Task, in *Medical History and Medical Care* (1971); *T. McKeown, The Role of Medicine: Dream, Mirage or Nemisis?* (1976). Several critiques of the latter work are printed in *Health and Society,* Summer, 1977.

11. See, e.g., *R. Berg, Health Status Indexes* (1973); *R. Kohn & K. White, Health Care: An International Study* (1976); *D. Sullivan, Conceptual Problems in Developing an Index of Health* (Public Health Service Pub. No. 1,000, 1966); Balinsky & Berger, A Review of the Research on General Health Status Indexes, 11 *Medical Care* 523 (1973); Fanshel & Bush, A Health Status Index and Its Application to Health Services Outcomes, 18 *Operations Research* 1021 (1970); Goldsmith, The Status of Health Status Indicators, 87 *Health Service Reports* 212 (1972).

12. Between 1750 and 1850 the death rate in England and Wales fell by an estimated 50%. With few effective medical treatments to account for the improvement, the most likely cause was an increase in food supply. Between 1850 and 1900 the death rate fell 14.6% thanks to decreased mortality from certain infections. See, *J.G. Freyman, The American Health Care System* 11–15 (1974) [hereinafter cited as *Freyman*). Presumably similar trends occurred in the United States, but U.S. vital statistics before World War I are too inadequate to be definitive.

13. McKeown and Lowe conclude their historical review of health status as follows:

We are now in a position to summarize our conclusions concerning the advance in health. It began in the eighteenth century and initially appears to have been due to changes in the environment, of which the most important feature was probably an improvement in the standard of living which resulted from the opportunities for employment offered by the Industrial Revolution. About a hundred years later this influence was supported by hygienic measures—control of water, sewage, housing, etc.—introduced progressively from the mid-nineteenth century and probably effective, particularly in prevention of bowel infections, from about 1880. The third major influence was the specific measure of preventing and treating disease in the individual, which, with the exception of vaccination, became available from 1925.

> *T. McKeown & C. Lowe,*
> *An Introduction to Social Medicine* 18 (1966).

14. *U.S. Dep't of Health, Education and Welfare, Health, United States,* 1975, 227 (1976) [hereinafter cited as *Health United States*).

15. See *Freyman, supra* note 12. See also, *Preventive Medicine, supra* note 3, at 717–27.

16. See nn. 17–20.

17. The contrast, however, is hard to avoid. As Dubos puts it:

In this light, the extent of health improvement to be expected from building ultramodern hospitals with highly trained staffs and up-to-date equipment is probably trivial compared with results from the much lower cost of providing infants and children with well-balanced food, sanitary conditions, and a stimulating environment.

> *DuBos, supra* note 9, at 97.

18. In fiscal 1974 the United States spent approximately $104.2 billion on health and medical care, almost $500 per person. This amounted to 7.7% of the total GNP. See *Nat'l Center for Health Statistics, Health in the United States, 1975, A Chartbook* 6 (1975) [hereinafter cited as *Health Statistics*]. For comparative figures, see *R. Maxwell, Health Care: The Growing Dilemma* 18 (1974)[hereinafter cited as *Maxwell*].

19. *Health, United States, supra* note 14, at 221 and 223 (with figures from 35 selected countries).

20. In 1969, there were 20.7 per 1,000 live births as compared with 11.7 for Sweden. *Maxwell, supra* note 18, at 8.

21. Infant mortality rates for Blacks are almost double that for Whites: 37.6 compared to 19.5 per 1,000 live births for the period 1964–1966. *Health, United States, supra* note 14, at 353.

22. In 1972, 6.3% of the babies born to white women were of low-birth-weight; for non-white mothers the figure was 12.7%. *Health, United States, supra* note 14, at 371.

23. See note 10, *supra*. It is important to emphasize that attention to the prevention of disease must not be at the expense of medical treatment. That type of conservative distortion has been popularized by Ivan Illich and others. See *I. Illich, Medical Nemesis: The Expropriation of Health* (1976). Cf. Crawford, You Are Dangerous to Your Health: The Ideology and Politics of Victim Blaming, 7 *Int'l J. of Health Services* 663 (1977).

24. See 39A C.J.S. §§ 18–47 (1976); *G. Rosen, A History of Public Health* 428–90 (1958).

25. See Brenner, Health Costs and Benefits of Economic Policy, 7 *Int'l J. of Health Services* 581 (1977); *Report of Special Task Force to Secretary of HEW, Work in America* (1973). See also, 42 U.S.C. § 1, et. seq. concerning the U.S. Public Health Service.

26. See Rosen, *supra* note 80, at 161–67. The use of the word "police" in this context suggests an anology to crime control that holds a certain appeal. The poor, and especially the black poor, are the most frequent

and most vulnerable victims of both crime and disease. In the United States, government has always provided protection from criminal acts, although it has only recently begun to fund victim compensation programs. See, e.g., Brooks, The Case for Creating Compensation Programs to Aid Victims of Violent Crimes, 11 *Tulsa L. J.* 477 (1976); Note, Pending Crime Victim Compensation Legislation in Iowa: An Analysis, 26 *Drake L. Rev.* 838 (1977); *Md. Ann. Code* Art. 26A §§ 1–17 (1973), as amended. As regards health, the situation is reversed, i.e., various entitlement programs provide some compensation to the victims of disease, but protection from disease was until quite recently limited to sanitation and contagious disease control.

27. Id. For the modern period see *G. Rosen, Preventive Medicine in the United States 1900–1975* (1975).

28. Friedlander v. Cimino, 385 F. Supp. 1357 (S.D.N.Y. 1974), rev'd on other grounds and remanded, 520 F.2d 318 (2d Cir. 1975).

29. New challenges are being developed, however. See, *The National Defense Council, Land Use Controls in the United States: A Handbook on the Legal Rights of Citizens* (1976).

30. See Grad, *supra* note 5, at 122–33; Note, Toward Recognition of Nonsmokers' Right in Illinois, 5 *Loy. (Chi.) U.L.J.* 610. 618–22 1974; Note, Constitutionalism and Ecology, 48 *N. Dakota L. Rev.* 37, 316 (1972).

31. In one sense, the citizen suit provision of the Clean Air Act simply provides for an enhanced version of public nuisance suits. See 42 U.S.C. § 1857h-2(a) (1970).

32. Malpractice actions have served as the chief medical care quality control mechanism. See *C. Jacobs, Measuring the Quality of Patient Care* 4 (1976).

33. But see Garner, Cigarettes and Welfare Reform, 26 *Emory L.J.* 269, 295–307 (1977). See also, *Restatement (Second) of Torts § 402, Comment* b (1965).

34. See Asbestos Workers Illness—and Their Suit —May Change Health Standards, N.Y. Times, Dec. 20, 1977, at 30, col. 1; Employee's Common Law Right to a Safe Workplace Compels Employer to Eliminate Unsafe Conditions 30, *Vand. L. Rev.* 1074 (1977).

35. See, e.g., Reserve Mining Co. v. Environmental Protection Agency, 514 F.2d 492, 537 (8th Cir. 1975), noted in *Minn. L. Rev.* 893, 901 (1975).

36. See, e.g., The Occupational Safety and Health Act of 1970, 29 U.S.C. § 651 et seq.; The National Environmental Policy Act of 1969, 42 U.S.C. § 4321 et seq.; The Clean Air Act of 1970, 42 U.S.C. § 1857 et seq.; The Illinois Environmental Protection Act, *Ill. Rev. Stat.* Ch. 111 1/2 § 1001 et seq. (1975).

37. For one of the success stories, see Currie, Enforcement Under the Illinois Pollution Law, 70 *Nw. U. L. Rev.* 389 (1976).

38. See, e.g., Kraus, Environmental Carcinogenesis: Regulation on the Frontiers of Science, 7 *Envt'l L.* 83 (1976).

39. For a succinct discussion of this topic see Note, Toward Recognition of Nonsmokers' Rights in Illinois, 5 *Loy.U. (Chi.) L.J.* 610, 614–18 (1974). See also Howard, State Constitutions and the Environment, 58 *Va. L. Rev.* 193 (1972); Curran, A Constitutional Right to a Health Environment, 67 *Amer. J. of Public Health* 262 (1977). In Pickney v. Ohio Environmental Protection Agency, 375 F. Supp. 305 (N.D. Ohio, 1974), the court ruled that:

The task of defining a 'deprivation' as that term relates to the interest in a healthy environment is beyond the competence of the courts and is instead a task characteristically performed by the legislative branch. Therefore the court does not rule that an interest in a healthful environment, as alleged on the facts of this case, is an interest of such a nature that procedural due process attaches.

40. *Ill. Const.* art. 11, § 2.

41. "Where . . . [Environmental Protection Agency] regulations turn on choices of policy, on all assessment of risks, or on predictions dealing with matters on the frontiers of scientific knowledge, we will demand adequate reasons and explanations, but not 'findings' of the sort familiar from the world of adjudication." Amoco Oil Co. v. Environmental Protection Agency, 501 F.2d 722,741 (D.C. Cir. 1974).

42. Although presumably within a narrow definition of environment (i.e., not encompassing housing, employment, etc.).

No

HARRY SCHWARTZ

ABOUT A DECADE AGO, when I was writing on medical and related affairs for *The New York Times,* I received an interesting letter from a woman living in Manhattan. This woman wanted me to "expose" a particular physician as the greedy monster she felt him to be. This physician, she wrote me, had simply refused when she asked him to provide, free of charge, a psychoanalysis of herself that might last several years. This evidence was irrefutable, she felt.

I did not "expose" this physician as requested. It seemed to me then, as it does now, that physicians owe no more obligation to provide their services free of charge than do newspaper reporters, clergymen, and, yes, even ethicists. Saying this, I am of course aware that there are situations in which all of us have an implied obligation to act regardless of compensation. If I hear a person screaming because he or she is pinned in an automobile wreck, I have an obligation to try to help free that person, and if I were a physician I would have the obligation to help give emergency first aid to the victims of this accident. Nor am I opposed to charity. And, of course, physicians annually give an enormous amount of free care to patients without compensation. But what I deny is that some special duty to provide their services free to anyone who comes and requests it.

As a practical matter, the enunciation of any such obligation would be the surest way known to guarantee that areas inhabited predominantly by poor people would be denuded of physicians. How could any physician who has to support himself by his work afford to practice in an area where every patient or almost every patient could successfully demand to be treated free of charge? Medicaid payments provide the economic incentives today for physicians who practice in areas inhabited by poor people.

I can hear the charge that I am putting the physicians' desire for payment ahead of the needs of poor patients to have their lives saved. That is not true for at least three reasons.

First, I have already acknowledged physicians' responsibility to act in true emergencies, when all citizens have an obligation to act.

Second, the overwhelming majority of physician-patient meetings are for trivial reasons with little or no organic basis. Should physicians be compelled to see daily with no compensation poor people who are hypochondriacs or who have a headache or a stomachache that will go away in a few hours or who have a cold that will disappear in a few days?

Third, many of the situations in which physicians can save lives involve the use of complex diagnostic equipment, of long-term drug therapy, of major surgery, and of prolonged hospital stays. Even if a cancer surgeon were willing to operate without fee—as many do on occasion— that does not remove the huge cost of hospital stays and hospital equipment. And under present law hospitals have only a very limited obligation to provide free care.

Thus the supposed benefits of physicians giving up their fees become less impressive when we remember that the truly sick poor cannot afford to pay their hospitals. After all if hospitals don't get paid, they must close. Hospital workers—

The Hastings Center Report. *August 1983, p. 14. Reproduced by permission.* © *The Hastings Center.*

many of them poor themselves—certainly feel under no obligation to go without salary in order to permit hospitals to provide free care.

Next, let me deal with the fairness aspect of the matter. To become a physician, a man or woman has devoted many years to study and work and has usually paid large sums for college and medical education. Once in practice, a physician incurs large current expenses and must pay rent on an office, salary to assistants, tuition for courses on continuing medical education, and—last but not least—malpractice insurance. I should add here that the mere fact that a patient has been treated free of charge does not in itself prevent that very same person from turning around and suing the physician for huge sums on a malpractice charge.

Why is it fair to expect a person who has paid such large costs in the past and continues to be liable for large costs now, to place all his or her knowledge and experience at the free disposal of anyone who comes in and claims to be poor? And as we know from the depressing history of fraud in welfare, food stamps, and Medicaid, by no means all poor people who claim to be poor are actually poor.

The last desperate argument usually employed is some variant of the charge that the doctor is rich and therefore has a special obligation to help the sick poor. But by no means are all doctors rich, and in fact many medical societies have special welfare affiliates, which quietly take care of the needs of impecunious doctors unable to work because of illness or age. Besides, even

rich doctors must pay heavy taxes, thus providing money for government which has the final obligation to take care of the most disadvantaged Americans.

A market economy such as ours assumes that it is the obligation of all of us to earn our livings and then to use our earnings for what we need and want. The great majority of the population is protected against the unpredictable hazards of illness by various forms of health insurance, private or governmental, the latter including Medicaid and Medicare as well as specialized programs such as those of the Indian Health Service and of CHAMPUS, which covers dependents of members of the armed forces.

The data show clearly that for many years now the poor have seen doctors more often annually and spent more time in hospitals each year than persons with larger incomes. That is fine because many people are made poor by illness, and therefore on average the poor need more medical care than healthier and wealthier groups. Our system is not perfect and one can find the occasional unrepresentative horror story to point up its existing inadequacies. But the gaps in our medical safety net are not so huge that we need to legislate or otherwise impose upon physicians—or any other group—the positive obligation to give their time, their energy, their knowledge, and their talent free of charge to anyone who claims to be poor. After all, for most people the most vital need is food. But we do not require the grocer to give free food to every poor person who presents himself at the door.

What Are We Teaching about Indigent Patients?

STEVEN H. MILES

AN ADULT WOMAN without health insurance presented to the emergency department of a private, not-for-profit, university hospital. A male acquaintance had assaulted her and had fractured her forearm. After the assault, she impulsively took an overdose of an anticonvulsant, phenytoin. A friend brought her to the emergency department. Because a history of intravenous drug abuse had scarred the patient's peripheral veins, peripheral intravenous access was not possible. An attempt to place a catheter in her subclavian vein led to a pneumothorax and a chest tube. Intravenous access was then obtained through a jugular vein. As the overdose was an emergency, the arm was splinted and she was admitted to the medicine service on which I was the attending physician.

Two days later, she was medically stabilized. The overdose was resolved, the chest tube was pulled. A psychiatrist concluded that the overdose was in response to the stress of the assault rather than because of major depression. A counselor for battered women offered a shelter, follow-up counseling, and assistance in filing a criminal complaint, all of which the patient declined, saying that she could avoid this man. An orthopedic surgeon said the patient's arm required internal fixation to set the fracture but declined to take the patient to surgery because she did not have insurance even though she was eligible for Medicaid, which the surgeon believed would be inadequate reimbursement. When he stood firm on that decision, I spoke with the

STEVEN H. MILES, professor, center for bioethics; department of medicine, University of Minnesota Medical School

Chief of Medicine, who took it up with the Chief of Orthopedic Surgery and the hospital lawyer. The surgeons were adamant; the Medicine Department could grant "compassionate" admissions if it so desired, but this placed no obligation on surgical staff.

Embarrassed, I called the admitting physician at the county hospital to arrange a transfer. Somewhat gruffly, the County physician said that he would not take the patient in transfer. He said that she would be treated, as any other person would, if she presented to their emergency department with a broken arm after we discharged her. I pointed out that this would mean that we would have to remove (and they would have to replace) the central venous catheter whose placement had complicated the patient's stay, and he replied, "Then, get your surgeons to fix her arm."

I told the woman of my ongoing effort to get the fracture set in our hospital. She listened and opined a pessimistic view of my efforts. An hour later, while I was waiting for another call from the hospital attorney, she secretly left the hospital with the central catheter in place. She presented to the county hospital, where the intravenous access was removed and replaced. New radiographs were taken. The fracture was set.

COMMENT

This woman's treatment is neither unusual nor illegal. The hospital honored its legal and moral duty to treat the life-threatening emergency of the overdose.[1,2] Its staff refused to treat the med-

Reprinted by permission from the Journal of the American Medical Association, Vol. 268, no. 18, Nov., 1992, pp. 2561–2566. Copyright 1992, American Medical Association.

ically indigent patient when it was legally permissible to do so. The patient abetted the hospital staff's refusal to treat her by leaving the hospital after she concluded that she would not receive care.

Cases like this one are commonly and appropriately presented as anecdotes to illustrate the need for a reform to guarantee universal access to health care. Its delayed treatment and duplicated diagnostic evaluations make it an easy example of the need to reform a complex and inefficient health care system. It is saddening and, to some, infuriating. This kind of officious interpersonal encounter and disrupted medical care for such a clear and simple medical need is not something most readers would lightly tolerate in their own lives.

There is another perspective on this case that should also be highlighted. This case took place in a teaching hospital where it was part of my training of a second-year resident, two interns, and two medical students. They knew the hospital turned indigent patients away from its clinics and emergency department. They were used to the magnified consequences of untreated disease and absent primary care. Even so, they were jarred by the abrupt interruption of this woman's treatment. Surprise quickly turned to accommodation as she became yesterday's news.

This kind of case in teaching hospitals has four adverse consequences for the next generation of physicians.

First, it disrupts the transmission of a professional tradition that recognized the claim of indigent ill persons on the medical profession. The debate about indigent patient care is not new in the United States.[3] What is new is the increasing amount of medical teaching in hospitals that do not have a primary mission of serving the medically indigent. Teaching hospitals used to be places where new physicians observed, learned, and assumed medicine's final obligation to the medically indigent.[4]

Second, teaching young physicians and their patients that physicians may properly put their own advantaged financial interests ahead of their patients' immediate needs fuels cynicism on both sides of the doctor-patient relationship. There are signs that such a cynical redefinition of medical professionalism is becoming more problematic. In the last decade, medical students have become much less inclined to be primarily motivated to seek a meaningful philosophy of life and correspondingly more motivated to become financially very well off.[5] The self-indulgent sense that many house-staff physicians and medical students have of being entitled to a privileged status[6] and income[7] is reinforced when young physicians see their well-off teachers and role models refuse to care for indigent patients. It also may reinforce the stigmatizing, fatalistic attitudes that many house staff have toward poor patients.[8] It may have political consequences as well. Despite physicians' appeals to trust medical professionalism, laws on dumping and physician-owned referral facilities have been enacted. Two thirds of Americans believe that physicians are too interested in making money,[9] and the public is four times as likely as doctors to support limiting physicians' incomes to address the health care cost-access crisis.[10]

Third, teaching students to turn away from indigent patients undermines the broader, ancient message that a physician is bound by "professing" humane kindness (humanitas) and compassion (misericordia) to those in need.[11] Teaching students that we may turn away from indigent persons may have broad ramifications for the ethos of medicine, for example, to the duty to treat human immunodeficiency virus (HIV)-infected persons. From its inception in the mid-19th century, the American Medical Association (AMA) asserted the doctor's duty to assume the risk of caring for persons with infectious diseases.[12] During the brief pax-antibiotica after World War II, the AMA stressed the doctor's freedom in patient relationships against the encroaching corporatization of health care. In 1986, the AMA suggested that this contractual freedom implied that doctors were not obliged to treat HIV-infected persons.[13] In 1987, the AMA drew on its older, more profound view of the subordination of doctors' privileges to infected persons' needs.[14] Today, a third of doctors,[15] and most orthopedic surgeons,[16] see no duty to care for HIV-infected persons. Fortunately, the ingrained habits of practice with regard to HIV-infected persons are better than the asserted freedom would imply. "Medical altruism" magnifies the efficacy of education about the duty to treat HIV-infected persons.[17] A holistic ethic of medical obligation is endangered when students see their teachers turn away from a poor woman with a broken arm.

Fourth, it diminishes physicians' credibility in the debate about the essential purpose of health care. Schroeder et al[18] have noted that the impressive medical advances have more successfully met the needs of wealthy patients than they have improved the health of our society. Some propose that physicians honor patients' demands for ever more costly, and marginally effective, even futile, treatments out of respect for patient autonomy.[19] When a tertiary care teaching hospital turns away an indigent woman with a broken arm as it honors paying patients' demands for marginally effective care, it suggests that "respect for autonomy" refers to the paying customer's privilege rather than to a solemn medical obligation to essential health needs.

cial worth biases influence clinical decisions on behalf of indigent patients, or answer demands for wasteful or inefficient use of medical care. Such issues underlie 10% to 15% of all of the ethical problems that physicians identify in inpatient and outpatient settings.[21,22] These situations ask physicians to define by practice the profession's view of its virtues and duties with regard to beneficence and justice. In recognizing the ethical issues and in defining the corresponding duties and virtues summoned, many physicians choose to provide thousands of dollars of free and discounted services.[23]

Society and the medical profession are moving toward health care reform even as teaching hospitals mirror our present failure to ensure reliable universal access to basic health care. It would be ironic if this generation of American physicians-in-training were the first to practice in a universal-access health care system after being shown and taught how to turn away from sick people without money. In the United States, physician voluntarism is still the final recourse for medically indigent persons. The voluntary care of indigent persons is not a substitute for health care reform. It is a mitzvah, or good deed, by which doctors are privileged to heal a wound and acknowledge the task and person the profession is accountable to. We cannot afford to cut this class from the education of new physicians.

ADDRESSING THE NEED

Many physicians recognize that financial constraints on patient care are more than simply a feature of the practice environment but also pose fundamental ethical questions and choices to the profession.[20] Such ethical issues arise as clinicians care for persons with inadequate personal financial resources for needed services, evaluate and transfer indigent patients to other providers, respond to family proxy decision makers who appear to be motivated by what they could gain or lose if treatment is withheld or given, become sensitive to how their own so-

REFERENCES

1. Strobos J. Tightening the screw: statutory and legal supervision of inter-hospital patient transfers. *Ann Intern Med.* 1991;20:302–310.

2. Enfield LM, Sklar DP. Patient dumping in the hospital emergency department: renewed interest in an old problem. *Am J Law Med.* 1988;13:561–595.

3. Stevens R. *In Sickness and in Wealth: American Hospitals in the Twentieth Century.* New York, NY: Basic Books Inc Publishers; 1989.

4. Starr P. *The Transformation of American Medicine.* New York, NY: Basic Books Inc Publishers; 1982.

5. Colwill JM. Where have all the primary care applicants gone? *N Engl J Med.* 1992;326:387–393.

6. Dubovsky SL. Coping with entitlement in medical education. *N Engl J Med.* 1986;815:1674–1675.

7. Taylor H, Leitman R, Edwards JN. Physician's responses to their changing environment. In: Blendon RJ, Edwards JN, eds. *System in Crisis: The Case for Health Care Reform.* Washington, DC: Faulkner & Gray; 1991:168.

8. Price JH, Desmond SM, Snyder FF, Kimmel SR. Perceptions of family practice residents regarding health care and poor patients. *J Fam Pract.* 1988;27:615–621.

9. Harvey L. *Survey of Public Opinion on Health Care Issues.* Chicago, Ill: American Medical Association; 1991.

10. Blendon RJ, Edwards JN, eds. *System in Crisis: The Case for Health Care Reform.* Washington, DC: Faulkner & Gray; 1991:166, 186.

11. Pellegrino ED, Pellegrino AA. Humanism and ethics in Roman medicine: translations and commentary on a text of Scribonius Largus. *Lit Med.* 1988;7:22–38.

12. Zuger A, Miles SH. Physicians, AIDS, and occupational risks: historic traditions and ethical obligations. *JAMA.* 1987;258:1924–1928.

13. Council on Ethical and Judicial Affairs, American Medical Association. *Current Opinions.* Chicago, Ill: American Medical Association; 1986.

14. Council on Ethical and Judicial Affairs, American Medical Association. Ethical issues involved in the growing AIDS crisis. *JAMA.* 1988;259:1360–1361.

15. Gerbert B, Maguire BT, Bleecker T, Coates TJ, McPhee SJ. Primary care physicians and AIDS: attitudinal and structural barriers to care. *JAMA.* 1991;266:2837–2842.

16. Arnow PM, Pottenger LA, Stocking CB, Siegler M, DeLeeuw HW. Orthopedic surgeons' attitudes and practices concerning treatment of patients with HIV infection. *Public Health* Rep. 1989; 104:121–129.

17. Simon RIS, Weyant RJ, Asabigi KN, Zucker L, Koopman JS. Medical student attitudes toward the treatment of HIV-infected patients. AIDS *Educ Prev.* 1991;3:124–132.

18. Schroeder SA, Zones JS, Showstack JA. Academic medicine as a public trust. *JAMA.* 1989;262:803–812.

19. Singer PA, Siegler M. Advancing the cause of advance directives. *Arch Intern Med.* 1992;152:22–24.

20. Schiedermayer D, La Puma J, Miles SH. Ethics consultations masking economic dilemmas in patient care. *Arch Intern Med.* 1989;149:1303–1305.

21. Walker RM, Miles SH, Stocking CP, Siegler M. Physicians' and nurses' perceptions of ethics problems on general medical services. *J Gen Intern Med.* 1991;6:424–429.

22. Connelly JE, Campbell C. Patients who refuse treatment in medical offices. *Arch Intern Med.* 1987; 147:1829–1833.

23. Dunham NC, Kindig DA, Lastiri-Quiros S, Barham MT, Ramsay P. Uncompensated and discounted Medicaid care provided by physician group practices in Wisconsin. *JAMA.* 1991;265:2982–2986.

Access to Health Care: Position Paper

AMERICAN COLLEGE OF PHYSICIANS

EXECUTIVE SUMMARY

The American College of Physicians believes that there is an increasingly urgent need to address a growing national problem, that of many Americans lacking access to health care. Spiraling increases in health care costs are reducing access to health services, especially for those without health insurance protection or the financial means to pay. Cost containment actions are increasingly undermining the basic infrastructure on which delivery of services depends — facilities and personnel. Further, many of these cost containment actions are eroding the ability of physicians to provide optimum care for their patients.

This paper was authored by Jack A. Ginsburg and Deborah M. Prout and was developed for the Health and Public Policy Committee by the State Health Policy Subcommittee and the Health Care Professions Subcommittee. Members of the Health Care Professions Subcommittee were: F. Daniel Duffy, MD, *Chair;* Robert A. Berenson, MD; John Noble, MD; John R. Hogness, MD; Walter W. Karney, MD; Gerald E. Thompson, MD. Members of the State Health Policy Subcommittee were: Donald I. Feinstein, MD, *Chair;* Robert B. Copeland, MD; William O. McMillan Jr, MD; John T. Harrington, MD; Cecil O. Samuelson, MD; Stewart E. Dadmum, MD. Members of the Health and Public Policy Committee were: Paul F. Griner, MD, *Chair;* Thomas P. Almy, MD; Donald I. Feinstein, MD; H. Denman Scott, MD; Quentin D. Young MD; F. Daniel Duffy, MD; Lockhart B. McGuire, MD; Lynn B. Tepley, MD; Richard G. Farmer, MD; John M. Eisenberg, MD; Jerome P. Kassirer, MD; Steven A. Schroeder, MD; Sankey V. Williams, MD; Edwin P. Maynard, MD. This paper was approved by the Board of Regents on 2 February 1990.

PROBLEMS FACED BY PATIENTS AND PHYSICIANS IN THE PRESENT SYSTEM

Problem: Inadequate Access to Health Care

Lack of an adequate financing system to assure access to needed health care and lack of facilities and personnel contribute to the medical complications, unjustifiable pain and suffering, and expense that can result from failure to obtain timely diagnosis and treatment. Lack of an adequate financing system jeopardizes the nation's health care delivery system, as the cost burden of uncompensated care increases.

Problem: Inadequate Health Insurance Protection

"Health insurance," as used in this paper, is defined broadly to include private health insurance, public health benefit programs, and "insurance" protection through self-insured plans provided by many large employers and prepaid health plans, including health maintenance organizations. More than 205 million Americans, 86% of the civilian population, have some form of health

From American College of Physicians, Access to Health Care: A Proposal. *Ann Intern Med. 1990; 112: 641–661. Permission granted by the American College of Physicians.*

insurance (1). Approximately 181 million persons have private health insurance, and approximately 136 million of them obtain their insurance coverage through employment-related plans. More than 33 million persons are covered by Medicare, and about 24 million are covered by Medicaid (2). Other public health benefit programs, including those administered by the Department of Veterans Affairs (VA), the Public Health Service, and the Department of Defense, provide access to health care services for specific qualifying groups. However, health insurance coverage is neither uniform nor equitable.

Whereas many persons have overlapping and duplicative coverage, others have insufficient coverage or no protection at all. There are roughly 31 to 37 million Americans without any form of public or private health insurance. Another 50 million Americans are underinsured; that is, they have inadequate insurance protection for major hospital and medical expenses (3).

Problem: Costs Continue To Rise

Total national health care expenditures have risen from $75 billion in 1970 to approximately $600 billion in 1989. Health care costs increased at an average annual rate of 17% from 1970 to 1988; at the same time, all items of the consumer price index increased at an average annual rate of 11% (5). These dramatic increases in health care costs have generated ever greater pressures for cost containment. Efforts by employers, the government, and third-party payers to control rising costs are increasingly intruding on clinical decision making and are undermining physician-patient relationships.

Administrative costs (that is, the costs of recording, billing, reviewing, processing, auditing, and justifying medical charges) are among the fastest rising components of health care costs. Included in these expenses are the costs of insurance marketing, the profits and reserves of government and private insurance carriers, and other overhead expenses necessitated by our current health care payment mechanisms. The total costs of health care administration in the United States are estimated to be approximately 22% of all personal health care spending (6), amounting to $110 billion in 1989. Substantial additional costs are generated by the medical liability system and efforts by physicians to minimize the exposure to claims of professional malpractice. The number of professional liability cases, the size of malpractice awards, and the costs of malpractice insurance continue to rise.

Problem: A Burdensome System for Patients, Their Families, and Physicians

Current health care payment mechanisms, involving multiple public and private insurers and third-party payers, are complex, confusing, costly, wasteful, and intrusive. Health insurance coverage under private insurance plans as well as under public programs, such as Medicare and Medicaid, is generally difficult to understand and requires complex mechanisms for recording, billing, auditing, reviewing, and processing claims. Patients, their families, and physicians must complete a multitude of forms, often for several carriers, involving significant time and expense. Patients and their families are burdened with this paperwork when they are most vulnerable—worried and sick.

Physicians must also respond to demands for documentation and justification from insurance carriers and quality review organizations. These frustrating layers of review, which involve demands to justify clinical decisions, requirements for prior approval, and denials of payment, undercut provision of high-quality care for all patients by inappropriately second-guessing professional judgments and intruding into physician-patient relationships. The time and expense required to deal with these administrative burdens further limit the ability of physicians to care for patients.

CRITERIA FOR A BETTER SYSTEM

To evaluate proposals for achieving a better health care system, we identified and used the following criteria. These criteria are not intended to be all inclusive and are listed categorically rather than in order of priority.

Benefits

1. There should be a mechanism for determining the scope of benefits.

2. There should be a uniform minimum package of benefits for all.

3. Coverage decisions should be based on clinical effectiveness.

4. Coverage and benefits should be continuous and independent of place of residence or employment.

Financing

5. Financing should be adequate to eliminate financial barriers to obtaining needed care.

6. There should be mechanisms for controlling costs.

7. Administrative expenses and procedures should be minimized.

8. Professional liability costs should be minimized.

9. Existing sources of revenue should be incorporated into any new financing system.

Organization and Delivery

10. There should be an adequate infrastructure in terms of facilities and manpower to deliver optimum health care services efficiently and effectively.

11. There should be mechanisms to assure quality.

12. Innovation and improvement should be fostered.

13. The system should be flexible.

14. Incentives should be provided to encourage individuals to take responsibility for their own health, seek preventive health care, and pursue health promotion activities.

Satisfaction

15. Patients should be satisfied.

16. Physicians and other health care professionals should be satisfied.

ALTERNATIVE PROPOSALS FOR EXTENDING HEALTH INSURANCE PROTECTION

Addressing the problems of inadequate access, cost control, and excessive administrative burdens are not competing objectives. These problems can be addressed simultaneously, and solutions should not be seen as being mutually exclusive. Six major types of proposals for improving access to health care are described and evaluated against the above criteria. The proposals and our conclusions concerning their advantages and disadvantages are summarized as follows:

Proposal 1: Encourage Individuals and Employers to Purchase Private Insurance

Private insurance has been a successful financing mechanism for most Americans. However, efforts to encourage individuals to purchase insurance would not be effective in assuring protection for those lacking insurance who are unemployed, have low incomes, or have been denied coverage. Tax credits and other means of subsidizing private insurance premiums are expensive and inefficient in expanding financial access to health care.

Proposal 2: Mandate Employer Coverage

Requiring all employers to provide a package of health insurance benefits could extend insurance coverage to approximately two thirds of the uninsured population and could improve coverage for many who are underinsured. However, this approach would provide only a partial solution and would need to be coupled with other remedies. It could contribute to increased unemployment, and it would leave unaddressed the inefficiencies and inequities of current insurance mechanisms, including high overhead costs and multiple and conflicting administrative burdens for health care providers and patients. However, because of its ability to expand coverage rapidly for a significant portion of the uninsured population, this mechanism warrants consideration as a partial, short-term solution.

Proposal 3: Create Health Insurance Risk Pools

Creation of health insurance risk pools, similar to automobile insurance risk pools, would spread insurance risks for those who are in small groups or denied coverage. However, unless substantial subsidies are provided, the premiums of risk-pool members could be much higher than those of persons with comparable group insurance and would be largely unaffordable. Creation of risk pools for "uninsurable" persons could encourage greater selectivity among insurance companies, resulting in more persons being denied individual, private policies and being shifted into a risk pool.

Proposal 4: Extend Medicaid Eligibility

Expanding Medicaid eligibility might be a desirable, short-term means for improving financial access of health care services for those who are poor or nearly poor but do not qualify for public assistance. Establishing uniform, minimum eligibility standards could reduce some of the present inequities in coverage and benefits among the states. These improvements would require substantially greater amounts of federal and state funding, amounts that would be difficult to achieve at a time of budgetary constraints. Overall, this approach could serve as an interim means for improving access for low-income groups, particularly for those below the poverty level who qualify for Medicaid in some states but not in others. However, because of the social-welfare nature of the program and the low payment rates that restrict access to care, we do not advocate this approach as the primary, long-term means for increasing access to health care for all Americans.

Proposal 5: Expand Charity Care

All physicians and other health care providers should voluntarily provide care on a charitable basis to patients who are in need and lack the resources to pay customary charges. However, there are inherent risks to patients and society in a system that relies solely on benevolence for the provision of health care services. History has shown that under such a system, health care services are not equally available to all, and poor persons typically either do not receive needed care or receive services of lesser quality. Therefore, expansion of charity care does not constitute an appropriate response to the access problem.

Proposal 6: Establish a Universal Access to Health Insurance Program

Several proposals have been made that would use an insurance mechanism to spread the cost of health care services equitably on a nationwide basis among all eligible participants. Programs to establish universal access to health insurance do not require a system in which hospitals and other health facilities are owned by the national government or in which physicians and other health care workers are employed by the government.

Practically all industrialized countries except the United States have national health care programs to assure universal access. These programs take many different forms, but they share the common feature of being government programs designed to enable all citizens to obtain health care services without financial barriers. Coverage is generally universal (everyone is eligible regardless of health status) and uniform (everyone is entitled to the same benefits). Costs can be paid entirely from tax revenues or by some combination of individual and employer premiums and government subsidization.

One format is to have a single, uniform program administered at the national level, as in Sweden and France. Another format sets minimum benefits at the national level but allows programs to differ as they are administered at the provincial or state level (as in Canada and Switzerland). Another variation is to permit qualifying, nongovernment programs to operate at the local level (for example, through nonprofit sick funds and medical associations as in the Federal Republic of Germany). Still another arrangement is to have a national program administered through local councils (as in Belgium and the Netherlands). National health insurance programs can be operated solely by the government or can be structured to incorporate private health insurance.

The overall cost of a universal access program would depend on how the program were structured, the benefits provided, the extent of optional or exempted coverage, mechanisms to assure appropriate use of services, and various other considerations. The public or government share would depend on how private insurance were incorporated into the plan and the amount, if any, paid by employers and individuals.

Given the various ways in which a health insurance program could be structured, it is difficult to provide more specific analysis without an actual proposal. Physicians need not assume that payment rates under a universal access plan would be inadequate, although experience with Medicaid and Medicare gives cause for concern. There is also reason to be apprehensive that a universal access program could result in greater intervention in the practice of medicine by government or other payers, thus further diminishing physician autonomy.

A universal access plan could achieve substantial savings by reducing the amount of administrative expenses currently borne by physicians, hospitals, nursing homes, and others providing and paying for health care services. Aggregate savings could be achieved by reducing the paperwork and expenses involved in coding for services, billing and collecting payments from patients, and submitting and documenting claims to multiple insurance carriers—each with its own forms, coverage provisions, copayments and deductibles, and review and compliance requirements. Further savings could be achieved by eliminating much of the administrative overhead that health insurance carriers incur for administration, marketing, reserves, and profits.

Recent proposals (7, 8) suggest that a universal access program would shift the mix between public and private expenditures and that total expenditures would not increase at as great a rate as has been sustained in recent years. At current levels of national health care spending, each reduction of 1% in the amount of total spending for administrative costs would save $5.5 billion annually. Potential savings from reduction of administrative overhead under a national health insurance program have been estimated to be about 10% of current health care spending. Those savings might conceivably offset the costs involved in expanding access to health care (7).

Establishment of a universal access program implies that there would be some centralized planning to assure that sufficient resources are allocated to meet the nation's health care needs. Planning and financing decisions would be needed to provide appropriate health care facilities where they are most needed, to foster technologic innovation and scientific advances, and to ensure that there are sufficient numbers of appropriately trained health care professionals. Substantial investments in health services research would be required to enable the program to deliver health care services as effectively and efficiently as possible and to improve the quality of health care. Investments would also be required for research and development to permit continued achievement of advances in medical science and technology.

Financing for a universal access program could be obtained from general tax revenues, a surcharge on income taxes, payroll taxes, or income-related premiums or by various other means, including using the savings obtained by converting from the present system. Although coverage would apply equally to all, contributions could vary according to income. Contributions could also be adjusted or waived for targeted groups, such as unemployed and poor persons, children, and pregnant women. A universal health insurance program could replace the need for Medicaid and most charity care. Additional issues, such as whether to permit the purchase of coverage beyond that provided under the program and voluntary exemptions from enrollment, would require careful analysis.

Advantages of a Universal Access to Health Insurance Program

1. All persons would have access to specific health insurance benefits covering at least essential health care services. Coverage could serve as a safety net and be supplemented by private insurance.

2. Access to mainstream health care could be provided.

3. Equity would be achieved among the states, as all persons would be eligible for national insurance coverage.

4. Lower premium rates per dollar of coverage could be obtained for a uniform package of benefits than is possible under a multiplicity of plans with varying benefits and coverage.

5. Administrative overhead would be far lower than under most private-sector plans due to savings from economies of scale. Additional savings could be obtained from the reduction or elimination of costs for billing, processing claims, marketing, reserves, and profits.

6. A minimum-benefits package could be designed to include prenatal, well-child, and other primary and preventive care that could improve our nation's health status. Increased access to these and other health care services could result in better health and reduced costs for preventable illnesses.

7. Coverage could be optional for those with other insurance that is at least equivalent, and supplemental private insurance could still be purchased by those seeking additional protection.

8. The cost of expanding health insurance to uninsured persons could be broadly and equitably shared.

9. Costs would be offset to some extent by savings from increased worker productivity and resultant higher earnings and tax revenues (although such savings are difficult to measure); reduced payments for much more expensive sequelae and complications of neglected illness; elimination of expenditures for Medicaid and other programs; and diminished costs of so-called "uncompensated care" which is now ultimately shifted to private insurers, the public treasuries, and charities.

10. Health care providers would be assured of payment, thus reducing or eliminating bad debts and uncompensated care.

11. Planning and financing on a national scale could better assure that resources are allocated to provide the health care facilities and the manpower needed to deliver health care services most effectively. Adequate resources could be provided for research and development, health services research, and the education and training of needed health care professionals.

12. Administrative burdens on physicians could be reduced.

Disadvantages of a Universal Access to Health Insurance Program

1. Substantial change would be required, entailing a restructuring of health care financing mechanisms and programs.

2. Universal coverage and expansion of benefits could result in greater health care costs, thereby generating further pressures for cost containment.

3. Greater government involvement in the practice of medicine, with increasing controls on volume, utilization, costs, and quality reviews, could result in further losses of physician autonomy.

4. Governmental decisions to ration or not to pay for some procedures (for example, organ transplants) would more directly limit medical decision making and the availability of these services.

5. Centralized planning and uniform determinations of coverage and benefits could prevent development of local variations that might better meet local needs.

6. There would be a loss of clerical, administrative, and accounting jobs now required for hospitals, physicians' offices, and other health care facilities to complete and process bills and other paperwork. Employment in the insurance industry might also suffer as jobs in marketing and claims processing are lost.

7. The role of private insurance companies might be diminished and their profits reduced.

Conclusions: Establishing a Universal Access to Health Insurance Program

The primary advantage of a universal access program would be that all Americans would have specific health insurance benefits and financial access to mainstream health care. In addition to universality and portability, such a program would offer equity in benefits among the states. Substantial cost savings could be achieved compared with current aggregate health insurance costs. A single health insurance program could also alleviate much of the frustration faced by individual practitioners who must now deal with multiple insurance plans and carriers.

A universal access program could include coverage for prenatal, well-child, and other primary and preventive care that could improve the nation's health. Improvements in health could achieve additional savings from increased worker productivity and reduced payments for expenses that now arise from complications of neglected illnesses. A universal access program could alleviate the financial stress on many public hospitals that results from the provision of care to poor and indigent patients for which little or no compensation is now received.

Government administration of Medicare and Medicaid has not been a model of efficiency, nor has it given physicians, hospitals, or other health care providers reason to assume that administrative burdens would be reduced or that there would be less government interference under an expanded national program. Mechanisms would be needed to assure that the potential administrative savings from adoption of a national insurance mechanism would be allocated to improve or expand health care services.

CONCLUSIONS AND RECOMMENDATIONS

A National Program Is Needed to Assure Access

All Americans should be able to obtain appropriate health care services, irrespective of age, race, sex, financial status, or place of residence. We believe that assuring access to health care services would achieve improvements in health status, decrease incidence of morbidity and mortality, and, possibly, contribute to increased life expectancy among those groups with the least access to care and the highest, age-adjusted, disease-specific mortality rates.

A multitude of existing programs and mechanisms enables most persons to obtain the health care services that they need. Still, many persons do not have adequate health insurance protection. In addition, rising costs and increasing bureaucratic and administrative burdens of the present system require re-examination. The existing system is inefficient and expensive, and a new approach is required.

We have focused on mechanisms to increase health insurance coverage as a means of improving access to health care services. Six types of broad policy proposals have been identified; the advantages and disadvantages of each have been presented. In view of these criteria, we conclude the following:

A nationwide program is needed to assure access to health care for all Americans, and we recommend that developing such a program be adopted as a policy goal for the nation. The College believes that health insurance coverage for all persons is needed to minimize financial barriers and assure access to appropriate health care services.

Assuring access also involves issues of cost and quality. The medical profession bears responsibility to ensure that acceptable, appropriate, and cost-effective care is delivered.

A nationwide program would establish a coordinated financing mechanism that would assure access to appropriate care for all of our citizens. Public policymakers are urged to initiate action now to accomplish this goal. A national commitment to assure access to health care is essential, because the current situation is resulting in the denial of adequate care to an inordinate number of persons, cost-cutting incentives are beginning to replace medical decision making in determining use and availability of health care services, our current system has excessive administrative costs, and the infrastructure of our health care system is in jeopardy.

The Issue of Administrative Costs and Burdens Must Be Addressed

It appears that substantial savings could be obtained by reducing administrative costs, improving efficiency, and eliminating wasteful duplication of coverage. Current payment and reimbursement mechanisms in the United States necessitate large bureaucracies and enormous administrative expenses to ensure that each and every service provided by institutions, physicians, and other health care providers is attributed to a specific patient. These expenses occur in commercial and not-for-profit private insurance plans as well as in public programs. There are tremendous costs involved in identifying, billing, collecting, and reviewing payments for services. Private, competitive programs also incur costs for advertising, marketing, profits, and reserves. These administrative costs are borne not only by the insurers and public programs but also by hospitals, physicians, and others.

In contrast to private insurance costs, publicly funded programs do not include costs for profits, marketing, or premium collection. The overhead for the universal public insurance system in Canada currently averages 2.5% of program costs. Overhead costs of Medicare and Medicaid amounted to less than 3% in 1983. Today, with increased Medicare and Medicaid total outlays, these costs are closer to 2%. This figure includes costs for contractor administration, research and demonstration projects, surveys and certifications of facilities, as well as salaries for program administration (2). Additional administrative savings could be achieved under a nationwide insurance program, because there would be no need to determine income or categoric eligibility, as presently required under Medicaid.

With a gross national product (GNP) approaching $6 trillion, the amounts of money that could be saved by at least stabilizing the rate of growth in U.S. health care spending could be staggering and may indeed be enough to pay fully for the cost of a universal access to health insurance program. Each one-percentage-point reduction in the proportion of GNP now attributed to health care (which includes administrative overhead as well as other costs due to inefficiencies inherent in the system) would yield savings of almost $60 billion per year.

Criteria Must Be Used to Evaluate Proposals for Reform

The issues concerning problems of access to health care are complex. Any new program to address them on a nationwide basis will have to include consideration of the ramifications of such changes. Caution must be exercised to preserve the strengths of the existing system, such as its ability to foster innovation and achieve advances in medical science, while correcting for its deficiencies. The time has come for a re-examination of the present system and a full examination of possible new approaches. This paper is an attempt to begin that process.

We have discussed development of a comprehensive financing program as one option for assuring access to health care for all Americans. Although we recognize that consideration of this option could be controversial and divisive for the medical profession, we believe that it merits serious examination. We further recognize that there are many major policy issues that would need to be resolved before a nationwide, health insurance financing mechanism could be developed for the United States. One central task would be to define clearly the services that would be covered.

We have indicated that a new process for determining the scope of benefits would be required. Such a process must distinguish the clinical role of advising on the appropriateness of specific services from the societal role of determining the feasibility of providing such services.

The structure of the program, particularly of the financing mechanism, would be equally important. It must be designed in conformance with agreed upon criteria for a better system. We have offered criteria that might be used.

Payment rates for health care services would need to be sufficient to assure that adequate numbers are attracted to health professions careers. Likewise, sufficient financial resources would need to be devoted to supporting appropriate educational and training programs.

Planning and financing would be required to assure that facilities are kept up-to-date and are available where needed. Investments in research and development would need to be sufficient to enhance scientific knowledge and to achieve further technologic advances. Funding for health services research would be even more critical as greater emphasis would be given to improving the effectiveness and efficiency of the delivery of health care services.

Cost containment and controls to avoid excessive use of services would be necessary under a nationwide health insurance program, as under any health insurance plan. However, such efforts could be based primarily on scientifically valid determinations of medical necessity and appropriateness.

Finally, we re-emphasize the need to minimize costs and dramatically ease administrative burdens for patients, families, and physicians and other health care providers. Restructuring and reforming the professional liability system are necessary to reduce the cost of medical practice and to encourage appropriate utilization of medical services.

REFERENCES

1. Health Insurance Institute. *Source Book of Health Insurance Data.* New York: Health Insurance Institute: 1989.

2. Bureau of Data Management and Strategy. *1989 HCFA Statistics.* Baltimore: Health Care Financing Administration; 1989: publication number 03294.

3. National Leadership Commission on Health Care. *For the Health of a Nation: A Shared Responsibility.* Ann Arbor, Michigan: Health Administration Press; 1989.

4. Letsch SW, Levit KR, Waldo DR. National health expenditures, 1987, health care financing trends. *Health Care Financing Review.* 1988;10: 109–29.

5. Bureau of Labor Statistics. Consumer price index. *Soc Secur Bull.* 1990;53:57.

6. Himmelstein DU, Woolhandler S. Cost without benefit. Administrative waste in U.S. health care. *N Engl J Med.* 1986:314:441–5.

7. Himmelstein DU, Woolhandler S. A national health program for the United States. A physicians' proposal. *N Engl J Med.* 1989;320:102–8.

8. Enthoven A, Kronick R. A consumer-choice health plan for the 1990s. Universal health insurance in a system designed to promote quality and economy. *N Engl J Med.* 1989;320:29–37, 94–101.

Discrimination and Racism in Health Care

AMERICAN NURSES ASSOCIATION

SUMMARY

Discrimination and racism continue to be a part of the fabric and tradition of American society and have adversely affected minority populations, the health care system in general, and the profession of nursing. Discrimination may be based on differences due to age, ability, gender, race, ethnicity, religion, sexual orientation, or any other characteristic by which people differ. The American Nurses Association (ANA) is committed to working toward the eradication of discrimination and racism in the profession of nursing, in the education of nurses, in the practice of nursing, as well as in the organizations in which nurses work. The ANA is further committed to working toward egalitarianism and the promotion of justice in access and delivery of health care to all people.

BACKGROUND

. . . Discrimination of this nature is not always easy to prove, however its consequences are quite concrete. Prejudice, on the other hand, involves thoughts, attitudes, insensitivity, and ignorance, not actual behaviors or demonstrable denials of opportunity. Prejudice frequently leads to discrimination. A prominent and particularly negative form of prejudice in America is racism. . . . Racism has an adverse impact on the health care environment and on those receiving health care services. In the health care arena, differential access to resources limits basic and preventive health care to members of some groups. Unequal distribution of health care resources results in morbidity and mortality rates that vary substantially among racial and ethnic categories and economic classes. Health care, as a resource, must be distributed fairly and equitably. Nurses and other health care providers may be victims as well as perpetrators of racial discrimination. . . .

According to the ANA "Code For Nurses" (1985), "the nurse provides services with respect for human dignity and the uniqueness of the client unrestricted by considerations of social or economic status, personal attributes or the nature of health problems." All nurses should strive to create environments that encourage quality health care practices; all patients deserve quality care. Health care that is not sensitive to differences in race, specific health practices and needs of different groups is not quality care and can even be harmful. . . .

DIFFERENCES IN HEALTH

Despite some recent improvements in health care delivery, many problems continue for most minority populations. There are persistent and sometimes substantial differences in the health of Americans. Minorities suffer from certain diseases at up to five times the rate of white Americans. For instance, cancer is the leading cause of death for Chinese and Vietnamese. Surveillance, Epidemiologic and End Results (SEER) data from the National Cancer Institute show that Korean stomach cancer rates are five times the rate for the total population. Vietnamese women suffer from cervical cancer at nearly five times the rate of white Americans. The number of Hepatitis B cases among Asian American and Pacific Islander children is two to three times higher than for children in the United States. Compared with the general population, Hispanics have a higher incidence of cancer of the stomach, esophagus, pancreas and cervix. There is a significant problem in the Native American population with diabetes, sudden infant death syndrome and congenital malformations. Despite some improvements in health care for African Americans since the 1960's, African Americans have a life expectancy that is six years shorter than the life expectancy for white Americans.

African American men less than 45 years old have a 45% higher rate of lung cancer and ten times the likelihood of dying from hypertension than white men under age 45. Research is needed to better understand the epidemiology of these differences.

DIFFERENCES IN RESEARCH NEEDS

Efforts to address racial and ethnic disparities in health will require nurses, physicians and other health care providers to develop new approaches, in consultation with experts in minority communities, to ensure that research, treatment, and education programs for diabetes, cancer, tuberculosis, and other diseases which affect minorities disproportionately, are available in local communities and nationwide.

Every year hundreds of clinical trials for new drugs are conducted at medical centers throughout the country. . . . However, historically, minorities have been grossly underrepresented in clinical trials conducted by federally funded institutions such as the National Institutes of Health (NIH). A major impediment for minority participation is a lack of trust in the medical establishment based on past experiments such as the Tuskegee Syphilis Study and the South Dakota Hepatitis-A Vaccine Study on American-Indian babies.

The Tuskegee Syphilis Study was conducted by the U.S. Public Health Service from 1932 to 1972. This study intentionally withheld treatment from 399 poor African American men suffering from syphilis. The goal was to observe the long-term effects of syphilis. The participants were never made aware of or given treatment even though penicillin became widely available in the 1940s and later became a standard treatment for syphilis. Over three fourths of the subjects died from complications of syphilis. Many of those who survived became blind and crippled. The experiment was conducted without the benefit of the patients' informed consent.

In the South Dakota experiment, newborn Lakota Sioux Indians were injected with either an experimental hepatitis type-A vaccine or, as a control, with an approved hepatitis type-B vaccine. Indian babies were selected because many reservations, being poor, rural and crowded, experienced epidemics of hepatitis-A every five to seven years. An epidemic in 1990 and 1991 infected more than 500 people and resulted in numerous hospitalizations and one death. The goal of the program was to inject approximately 105 babies and, after studying the results, offer the vaccine to everyone. The Indian Health Service officials, who assumed responsibility for the trials, stated that Indians as a group stood to benefit from hepatitis-A vaccine. However, in a letter to doctors, the health service warned of anaphylactic reactions and such possible side effects as cancer, jaundice and death. Lawsuits filed by Indian families said the parents were not told of such potential risks when their permission to vaccinate was sought. . . .

ANA believes health care providers are professionally, morally and ethically obligated to explain the purpose, risks, potential side effects and benefits of each study before a patient agrees to participate. An informed consent document that includes all relevant information, in language the patient understands, should be thoroughly discussed with the patient, the patient's family and/or significant other. Safeguards must be put in place to ensure that prospective participants are given complete information on the nature of all research studies. . . .

DIFFERENCES IN REPRESENTATION IN THE HEALTH PROFESSION

The March 1996 Sample Survey of Registered Nurses by the U.S. Department of Health and Human Services reveals that the profession of nursing continues to be 90% white female . . . this lack of diversity in the nursing workforce is potentially harmful to the profession and the population it serves. . . . Our ability to maintain a position of global leadership depends on our willingness to recognize, stimulate, and develop capacities of all segments of society and to acknowledge the needs of those segments currently underrepresented in health careers. . . .

DIFFERENCES IN ACCESS AND PRESCRIBED TREATMENTS

Underlying some of the racial disparities in the health among Americans are differences in both need and access: minorities are more likely to need health care but are less likely to receive health care services. For example, recent studies have shown that even when minorities gain access to the health care system and even when there is a comparable ability to pay for services, they are less likely than whites to receive surgical or other therapies. ANA believes that disparities in health care based on personal characteristics such as race must be avoided. . . .

CONCLUSION

. . . ANA believes it is critically important for Americans to come to a shared understanding of the negative consequences of discrimination and racism which still pervades our society and be willing to take individual as well as collective actions to bring America closer to our ideal of equality and justice. Equality and justice must also extend to other minorities such as the aged and disabled. Health care that is individualized to the health practices and specific needs of each person and/or population group is vital to maintain and improve the health of all Americans. Nurses must work to include diversity within the health professions, processes of health care delivery, and desired patient outcomes in order to deliver the holistic care we profess is our primary goal. . . .

Minority Access and Health Reform:
A Civil Right to Health Care

SIDNEY DEAN WATSON

Whether the racial disparities in treatment decisions are caused by differences in income and education, sociocultural factors, or failures by the medical profession, they are unjustifiable and must be eliminated. Not only do the disparities violate fundamental principles of fairness, justice, and medical ethics, they may be part of the reason for the poor quality of health of [minorities] in the United States. (American Medical Association, Council on Ethical and Judicial Affairs)[1]

HEALTH CARE REFORM that includes universal coverage could lower a major barrier to care for people of color and ethnic minorities—the inability to pay for care.[2] But universal coverage alone, even with comparable fee-for-service payment or appropriately risk-adjusted capitated reimbursement,[3] will not eradicate the racial and ethnic inequities in health care delivery. Restrictive admissions practices, geographic inaccessibility, culture, racial stereotypes, and the failure to employ minority health care professionals will still create barriers to minority health care. In addition to universal financing, health care reform should include new civil rights legislation to address and reduce these noneconomic barriers to minority health care.

This article first reviews some of the recent empirical studies documenting racial and ethnic disparities in health care access and treatment. It then discusses the role of civil rights law in addressing these differences, noting the structural deficiencies of the existing health care civil rights act, namely, Title VI of the 1964 Civil Rights Act.[4] The paper concludes with a proposal for new health care civil rights legislation, which should be included in national health care reform.

RACIAL AND ETHNIC DISPARITIES IN HEALTH CARE ACCESS AND TREATMENT

Although minority Americans are generally in worse health than white Americans,[5] they have fewer doctor visits and fewer hospital admissions. African-Americans make one-third fewer visits to doctors than whites with comparable health status do.[6] A 34 percent differential exists between the percentage of Hispanics admitted for hospital inpatient care and the percentage of whites; the gap between African-Americans and whites is 9 percent.[7] African-Americans and Hispanics are less likely than whites to have private physicians,[8] and a disproportionate number of African-Americans rely on hospital emergency rooms and outpatient clinics for primary care.[9]

Some of this access differential results from America's present pay-as-you-go health care system in which health insurance is tied to employ-

SIDNEY D. WATSON is a professor of law at the Mercer University School of Law. She is also a visiting professor at the Saint Louis University Center for Law Studies.

Journal of Law, Medicine & Ethics 22 (1994): 127–137. Copyright 1994, reprinted with permission of Sidney D. Watson and American Society of Law, Medicine & Ethics. All rights reserved.

ment status.[10] Minorities are also less likely to have private health insurance and more likely to be covered by Medicaid than whites are.[11] Most important, they are more likely to be poor,[12] and more likely to be completely uninsured than white Americans are.[13]

Race also operates as a determinant of access to medical care without regard to insurance status and income level. Even when minority Americans have the same source of payment that whites do, they also visit physicians less, and have fewer hospital and nursing home admissions. When middle class African-Americans and whites are compared, African-Americans still use doctors significantly less than whites do.[14] While African-Americans account for 29 percent of the Medicaid population and 23 percent of the elderly poor, only 10 percent of Medicaid intermediate care nursing home patients are African-American and only 9 percent of Medicaid skilled nursing facilities' patients are African-American —even though elderly African-Americans have more health problems and suffer more disabilities than elderly whites do.[15] Not only do racial and ethnic disparities exist in access to medical services, but disparities also exist in medical treatment. Minorities receive different—and less —care than whites do, even when their symptoms and sources of payment are the same. Nationally, African-American patients receive only one-third (and in the Southeast, one-sixth) of the coronary artery bypass graft operations of white patients—even when their symptoms and sources of payment are the same.[16] African-Americans are also less likely to receive long-term hemodialysis, kidney transplants,[17] and potentially sight-saving treatment for glaucoma than whites.[18]

While hospitalized, minorities receive less care than whites do. African-Americans hospitalized for pneumonia are less likely than whites to receive medical services, particularly intensive care, even though their symptoms and incomes are similar.[19] African-American women receive less appropriate hospital care than white women for breast cancer,[20] and they are probably less likely to receive clinically indicated cesarian sections.[21] African-Americans are accepted less frequently for psychotherapy, assigned more often to inexperienced therapists, and seen with less intensity and for shorter periods.[22] African-American women are also less likely to receive rehabilitation and patient education instructions after a mastectomy.[23]

Finally, physicians appear to prescribe significantly fewer therapeutic treatments for their minority patients than for their white patients — even when patients' conditions are the same. African-Americans who are HIV-positive receive less antiretroviral therapy or pneumocystic carinii pneumonia prophylaxis than whites do.[24] Minorities are also less likely to receive analgesia for long-bone fractures, erythropoietin for end-stage renal disease, and treatment of alcoholism.[25]

While the exact significance of these studies of treatment differences as well as some of their methodologies are certainly subject to debate, the studies surely raise troubling questions about inequities in our health care system. The causes of these access and treatment differentials are multifaceted and complex, but geography, culture and cultural insensitivity, racial stereotyping, the lack of minority health professionals, and institutional racism all factor into the causal equation.

Some of the racial and ethnic disparity in health care treatment and access is the result of geography and lack of transportation. Minorities have difficulty obtaining care in part because of the paucity of health care providers in predominately minority neighborhoods.[26] Throughout the 1980s, hospitals that historically served the African-American community either closed, relocated to predominately white communities, or privatized.[27] Nursing homes are more likely to locate in predominately white areas than in minority neighborhoods.[28] Skimming a telephone directory of any major city or rural area reveals the dearth of physicians serving minority communities.[29]

Other barriers to care are caused by cultural differences and cultural insensitivity. Some recent immigrants are more likely to turn to folk remedies and folk healers than to traditional Western medicine.[30] Religious attitudes toward life, health, care, and treatment can cause some Asian groups to avoid seeking health care.[31] And, health care providers' cultural ignorance contributes to these barriers. Poor physician-patient communication occurs because majority providers do not understand other cultures' deferences to authority, descriptions of pain, and world-views about wellness and illness. A lack of bilingual health care providers, culturally irrelevant medical services, and diagnostic misinterpretations of the physical effects of folk medicines all inhibit access to treatment.[32]

Racial and ethnic stereotypes also play a role in the minorities' underuse of medical services. Hospital emergency room staffs more often classify African-Americans as ward patients and whites as private patients, even when they have similar sources of payment.[33] Health care professionals, like Americans in general, tend to treat Asian Pacific Islanders and Hispanics as homogenous groups, when, in fact, each is a highly diversified group of minorities with differing health statuses, health needs, and cultures.[34] This stereotyping of patients may be one of the reasons why African-Americans are less satisfied than whites with their physicians' behavior toward them.[35]

All these issues tend to be compounded by the lack of minority health providers. African-Americans make up only 3 percent of physicians, 2 percent of dentists, and 4 percent of registered nurses. Hispanics comprise only 5 percent of physicians, 3 percent of dentists, and 1 percent of registered nurses.[36] Yet, minority physicians are more likely to locate in or near minority neighborhoods and to treat minority patients.[37] They are also "more likely than white doctors to enter primary care specialties and to locate voluntarily in or near designated primary care health manpower shortage areas."[38]

Finally, a variety of hospital, nursing home, and physician practices operate to disproportionately exclude ethnic and minority Americans from care. Many standard operating procedures not aimed specifically at ethnic or racial minorities and designed to further other interests, disproportionately exclude racial and ethnic minorities. For example, many hospitals admit patients only if they have a treating physician with admitting privileges.[39] Increasingly, both hospitals and doctors refuse to deliver babies for mothers who have not received a minimum amount of prenatal care.[40] Many providers make preadmission inquiries into patients' citizenship, national origin, or immigration status; fail to make interpreters available; and fail to translate signs and forms.[41] Many hospitals and clinics have few, if any, minority physicians with admitting privileges.[42] Each of these policies and practices operates to exclude a disproportionately large number of minorities.

In sum, geography, racial and cultural insensitivity, language, a lack of minority health providers, and a host of apparently race-neutral policies and practices create circumstances that deny racial and ethnic minorities equal access to health care. Racial and ethnic disparities in health access and treatment have a long history in this country, dating from slavery and Jim Crow.[43] While intentional segregation and WHITES ONLY signs have disappeared, racial and ethnic minorities still do not have equal access to health care. Access to providers and treatments still depends to a great extent on the color of one's skin and on one's ethnic background.

THE ROLE OF CIVIL RIGHTS LAW IN REDUCING BARRIERS TO ACCESS AND TREATMENT

A host of recommendations, aimed at reducing or eliminating the disparity in minority health access and treatment, have surfaced. Universal access to health care is a crucial first step in alleviating the economic barriers so clearly connected to race and ethnicity. Training health professionals in cultural sensitivity and the special needs of minority patients will help to reduce cultural barriers. Increasing the number of minority Americans in health professional training programs should also assist in making minority health concerns more visible and in providing a pool of practitioners more likely to locate near and to treat minority patients. The use of practice parameters ought to reduce the extent to which conscious and subconscious racial stereotypes affect clinical decision making.[44]

Some professionals in the bioethics field are questioning the extent to which the traditional articulation of the principles and methods of bioethics have contributed to the inequities in minority medical access and treatment. Jorge Garcia and others critique bioethics' failure to take into account African-American and other non-European perspectives.[45] Susan Wolf advocates the need to develop a theory of process for institutional ethics committees as a check on racial, economic, and gender biases.[46]

These initiatives are important and necessary steps toward increasing minority health access. However, civil rights laws and legal remedies are also needed. The patient-provider relationship is characterized ideally as a "caregiver-patient" relationship that is both "intimate and collaborative."[47] Thus, many oppose "rights talk" when discussing the patient-caregiver association. Some fear the overlegalization of medical care, and bemoan the adversarial tone the law has introduced into the practice of medicine.[48] But, as the critical race theorists have pointed out, rights and rights talk are crucial for dealing with power inequity, even when our preference is to conceive of relationships in terms of caring and connection.[49]

Power inequity typifies the structures and practices that operate to exclude minorities from health care. Physicians, hospitals, and nursing homes may not be motivated by a desire to exclude minority patients, but, because these institutions are typically owned, managed, and staffed overwhelmingly by majority Americans, they are organized to function in ways that make them accessible, attractive, and responsive to majority Americans. The problem is that these same organizational principles and behavior patterns may also operate to disadvantage and exclude minorities who are relatively powerless given the enormity of America's health care delivery system and the meager number of minority health care professionals and health care administrators within the system.

Civil rights legislation provides a mechanism for identifying both advertent and inadvertent racial and ethnic biases within American health care. Civil rights legislation can assist in identifying and dismantling especially those policies and practices that operate silently to exclude minority Americans from health care and that result in a lesser quality and quantity of treatment for minorities than for white Americans.

In the jargon of our nation's civil rights law, much of the discrepancy in minority access and treatment results from "facially neutral policies and practices that have a disproportionate adverse racial and ethnic impact." The practices and policies that exclude minority patients are "facially neutral" because they do not mention race. The practices that result in lesser and different treatment for minorities often are not the result of a subjective intent to discriminate; that is, they are not necessarily the result of conscious, race-specific policies. Nevertheless, their impact is disproportionate because the policies hit racial and ethnic minorities harder than other groups. Their effect is especially adverse in the health care context, where such exclusionary policies can be deadly.

Health care civil rights remedies need not get caught in the maelstrom over the debate whether disproportionate adverse impact discrimination should be outlawed in the employment context. Many view the employment arena as a zero-sum game: if minorities are to make gains, then majority whites are to be disadvantaged. Some commentators, thus, argue against civil rights provisions that outlaw unintentional disparate impact as well as affirmative action remedies. Whether or not this scenario is accurate in the employment context is unimportant for our purposes, because, in the health care arena, civil rights and minority access to care and treatment are not zero-sum games. Increasing minority access to health care through civil rights remedies will not reduce the care provided to nonminorities. Civil rights remedies, in fact, may help us to develop new, more effective, more sensitive, and possibly even more cost-effective ways to deliver health services to all Americans. . . .

CONCLUSION

Health care reform needs to focus attention on minority health. Ethnic and racial minorities are generally in worse health than white Americans, but they receive fewer medical services. Empirical researchers are now documenting the disparities in minority treatment. Bioethicists are beginning to teach us about cultural differences in medical treatment and patient decision making. Civil rights law provides an additional, critically important tool for addressing racial and ethnic inequities in medical access and treatment.

Civil rights provisions should be an integral part of health care reform. Business as usual in American health care has excluded minorities. Requiring a health care provider to shown that a policy or practice which has a disproportionate racial impact is necessary to the provision of health services and cannot be achieved through less discriminatory means will begin the search for new approaches to health care delivery that increase racial and ethnic minorities' access to health care.

Race discrimination in the delivery of medical care has been a silent problem for too long. The time has come to break the silence and to expose the problem. HHS/OCR should begin collect-

ing and examining data on the utilization and treatment of minorities so that the nature of the problem can be understood better.

Civil rights statutes seek to dismantle barriers to health care access and treatment, but a larger project still remains: we need to improve the health of America's minorities, and know that we are doing so. Health care reform legislation should create, in addition to providing civil rights protections. a process by which states establish periodic goals for reducing racial and ethnic disparities in health access. One way to accomplish this is to require that states periodically prepare and implement a plan for improving access and reducing health status disparities. Mandatory collection and dissemination of data on minority access and treatment is the first step in preparing these goals and objectives. Such plans can work together with civil rights remedies and other initiatives to improve minority health care access and minority health.

ACKNOWLEDGMENTS

My thanks to Jane Perkins, Gordan Bonneyman, and the members of the National Health Law Program's Civil Rights Task Force for help in thinking about these issues. As always, my thanks to Theodore Blumoff and Linda Edwards for editing assistance. I am grateful to Bernadette Crucilla and Robert M. Lewis for research assistance and advice. I am currently advocating for collection of data on minority access and treatment as co-counsel for the plaintiffs in *Madison-Hughes v. Shalala* (C.A. 3:93 0048 (M.D. Tenn. 1993)).

REFERENCES

1. Council on Ethical and Judicial Affairs, AMA, "Black-White Disparities in Health Care, *JAMA,* 263 (1990): 2346.

2. Universal financing will not automatically ensure the end of economic discrimination. As long as programs that insure the poor contain restrictive eligibility levels, cost-sharing requirements, and low reim-

bursement rates, providers will have financial incentives to avoid treating publicly insured patients. See also Sidney D. Watson, "Health Care in the Inner City: Asking the Right Question." *N. Car. L. Rev.,* 71 (1993): 1661–63.

3. Health reform programs such as managed competition and capitated payments may create additional barriers to access for minorities, and actually reduce minority health access. Capitated patient systems can create strong incentives to serve healthier populations and to avoid sicker groups—like racial and ethnic minorities. A capitated payment rate that fails to reflect accurately the generally higher costs of treating minority patients inevitably causes providers and insurers to discriminate against minority patients in subtle, but effective, ways. For instance, plans can avoid enrolling minority consumers by defining their service areas to exclude predominately minority neighborhoods. Plans also can avoid treating minority patients by locating facilities in predominately white communities not easily accessed by the minority population. Plans that fail to hire minority physicians effectively discourage minority enrollment because minority physicians are more likely than white doctors to treat minority patients. Plans can further discourage minority enrollment by failing to have specialists who treat particular diseases, like sickle cell anemia, that affect certain racial groups. See Watson, *supra* note 2, at 1662–63.

4. 42 U.S.C. § 2000d (1988).

5. The life expectancy of Black males is almost seven years less than that for white males; for Black females it is approximately five years less than that for white females. See R.W. Johnson, *Special Report, The Foundation's Minority Medical Training Programs* (Princeton: Robert Wood Johnson Foundation, Vol. I, 1987), at 5. Blacks have higher death rates from all three of the major killers—heart disease, cancer, and stroke. See Donald H. Andersen et al., "Health Status and Medical Care Utilization," *Health Affairs,* 6 (1987): 149. Black infant mortality continues to be nearly twice that of white infants. See R.W. Johnson, *op. cit.*

6. See Howard E. Freeman et al., "Americans Report on Their Access to Health Care," *Health Affairs,* 6 (1987): 12–18. In 1986, whites in fair to poor health averaged 10.1 doctor visits, whereas the average number of visits for Blacks was only 6.8 and for Hispanics, 9.8. See *id.* at 12.

7. *Id.* at 12–13. These percentages still underestimate the discrepancy between white and minority hospital care because they do not take into account that 15.3 percent of Blacks and 19.4 percent of Hispanics surveyed were in fair to poor health as compared to only 10.6 percent of whites. *Id.*

8. Minorities are less likely to see private physicians, regardless of the patient's income level or type of insurance. Minorities are also less likely than whites to see specialists. See Institute of Medicine, *Health Care in a Context of Civil Rights* (Washington, D.C.: National Academy, 1981), at 38–39; see also Gerald D. Janes and Robin M. Williams Jr., *A Common Destiny: Blacks and American Society* (Washington, D.C.: National Academy, 1989), at 431; and U.S. Dept. of Health and Human Services, *Report of the Secretary's Task Force on Black and Minority Health, Executive Summary* (Washington, D.C.: U.S. Department of Health and Human Services, Vol. I, 1985), at 189.

9. See Karen Davis et al., "Health Care for Black Americans: The Public Sector Role," *Milbank Q.,* 65, Supp. 1 (1987): 214. In 1983, 27 percent of Blacks, but only 13 percent of whites, reported a hospital outpatient department or emergency room as their usual source of care. See Janes and Williams, *supra* note 8, at 431.

10. Jane Perkins, "Race Discrimination in America's Health Care System," *Clearinghouse Rev.,* 27 (1993): 373. See also Watson, *supra* note 2.

11. See Mark Schlesinger, "Paying the Price: Medical Care, Minorities, and the Newly Competitive Health Care System," *Milbank Q.,* 65, Supp. 2 (1987): 276.

12. The poverty rate for African-American families is three times that for white families. Woodrow Jones Jr. and Mitchell F. Rice, "Black Health Care: An Overview," in Woodrow Jones Jr. and Mitchell F. Rice, eds., *Health Care Issues in Black America* (New York: Greenwood Press, 1987), at 7.

13. Schlesinger, *supra* note 11, at 276.

14. See Paula Diehr et al., "Use of Ambulatory Care Services in Three Provider Plans: Interaction Between Patient Characteristics and Plans," *Am. J. Public Health,* 74 (1984): 49 (race was found to be correlated significantly to use in the three health care plans studied; Black use was ten percentage points less in an independent practice association (IPA), fourteen in a health maintenance organization (HMO), and twenty in a Blue Cross plan).

15. See Vernellia R. Randall, "Racist Health Care: Reforming An Unjust Health Care System to Meet the Needs of African-Americans," *Health Matrix,* 3 (1994): 155–56 (citing NAACP Legal Defense & Education Fund, Inc., "An African American Health Care Agenda: Strategies for Reforming an Unjust System, Racial Disparities in Medicaid Coverage for Nursing Home Care" (1991)). See also David Barton Smith, "The Racial Integration of Health Facilities," *Journal of Health Politics, Policy and Law,* 18 (1993): 850.

In fact, the nursing home industry has been described as America's most segregated, publicly licensed health care facility. See Cassandra Q. Butts, "The Color of Money: Barriers to Access to Private Health Care Facilities for African-Americans," *Clearinghouse Rev.*, 26 (1992): 163–64 (citing David B. Smith, *Discrimination in Access to Nursing Homes in Pennsylvania* (1991), at 5–7). Licensed nursing homes, primarily funded by the Medicaid program, serve whites; substandard boarding homes, for which Medicaid does not pay, serve Blacks. See *Linton v. Tennessee Commissioner of Health & Environment*, 779 F. Supp. 925, 932 (M.D. Tenn. 1990). Private nursing homes are more segregated than state-run homes, and when blacks do gain access to nursing homes, they are more likely to reside in nursing homes that have been cited as substandard. See David B. Smith (1993), *op. cit.*, at 857–61.

16. Kenneth C. Goldberg et al., "Racial and Community Factors Influencing Coronary Artery Bypass Graft Surgery Rates for All 1986 Medicare Patients," *JAMA*, 267 (1992): 1474 (comparing elderly Medicare patients who have comparable myocardial infarction rates.)

17. Council on Ethical and Judicial Affairs, AMA, *supra* note 1, at 2344–45.

18. See Johanna M. Seddon, "The Differential Burden of Blindness in the United States," *N. Engl. J. Med.*, 325 (1991): 1440; and Jonathan C. Javitt et al., "Undertreatment of Glaucoma Among Black Americans," *N. Engl. J. Med.*, 325 (1991): 1418.

19. Council on Ethical and Judicial Affairs, AMA, *supra* note 1, at 2345.

20. Paula Diehr et al., "Treatment Modality and Quality Differences for Black and White Breast-Cancer Patients Treated in Community Hospitals," *Medical Care*, 27 (1989): 942.

21. Council on Ethical and Judicial Affairs, AMA, *supra* note 1, at 2345.

22. *Id.*

23. See Diehr et al., *supra* note 20, at 951.

24. Richard D. Moore et al., "Racial Differences in the Use of Drug Therapy for HIV Disease in An Urban Community," *N. Engl. J. Med.*, 11 (1994): 763.

25. See Council on Ethical and Judicial Affairs, AMA, *supra* note 1, at 2345. See also Woodrow Jones Jr. and Patrick Clifford, "The Privatization of Treatment Services for Alcohol Abusers: Effect on the Black Community," *JAMA*, 82 (1990): 337.

26. See Watson, *supra* note 2, at 1649–51; see also Jane D. Lin-Fu, "Population Characteristics and Health Care Needs of Asian Pacific Americans," *Public Health Reports*, 103 (1988): 18.

27. Butts, *supra* note 15, at 161.

28. Smith (1993), *supra* note 15, at 863.

29. See Randall, *supra* note 15, at 158.

30. See Lin-Fu, *supra* note 26, at 25.

31. Laura Uba, "Cultural Barriers to Health Care for Southeast Asian Refugees," *Public Health Reports*, 107 (1992): 545. Among Southeast Asians, the belief that suffering is inevitable and that one's life span is predetermined can cause them to eschew seeking health care. *Id.*

32. *Id.*, at 546–47. See also Lin-Fu, *supra* note 26, at 24; see, generally, Pedro Ruiz, "Cultural Barriers to Effective Medical Care Among Hispanic-American Patients," *Ann. Rev. Med.*, 36 (1985): 63–71; and Gustavo M. Quesada, "Language and Communication Barriers for Health Delivery to a Minority Group," *Soc. Sci. & Med.*, 10 (1976): 324.

33. Council on Ethical and Judicial Affairs, AMA, *supra* note 1, at 2345.

34. See Lin-Fu, *supra* note 26, at 20. See also Ruiz, *supra* note 32, at 323.

35. See Randall, *supra* note 15, at 136. See also Susan M. Wolf, "Toward a Theory of Process," *Law, Medicine & Health Care*, 20 (1992): 283.

36. U.S. Department of Health and Human Services, Public Health Services, *Healthy People 2000: National Health Promotion Disease Prevention Objectives* (Washington, D.C.: U.S. Department of Health and Human Services, Sept. 1990), at 542.

37. See H.R. Rep. No. 804, 101st Cong., 2d Sess. 1990, reprinted in 1990 U.S.C.C.A.N. 3299. See also Janes and Williams, *supra* note 8, at 436–37 (75 percent of African-American physicians practice in or near African-American communities).

38. U.S. Department of Health and Human Services, Public Health Services, *supra* note 36, at 542.

39. See Stan Dorn et al., "Anti-Discrimination Provisions and Health Care Access: New Slants on Old Approaches," *Clearinghouse Rev.*, 20 (1986): 441. This policy tends to exclude minority patients because they are less likely than white patients to be treated by private physicians, regardless of their income level or types of insurance coverage. See Institute of Medicine, *supra* note 8, at 38–39; see also Janes and Williams, *supra* note 8, at 431.

40. See Dorn et al., *supra* note 39, at 441. While 79.6 percent of white women receive prenatal care during the first trimester, only 62 percent of Black women receive such care. While only 1.3 percent of white women receive no prenatal care, 4.4 percent of African-American women get no prenatal care. "Increasing Incidence of Low Birthweight—United States, 1981–1991," *MMWR*, 43 (1994): 328. In a study of low-income women, white women were eleven per-

centage points more likely than any other racial or ethnic women's group to receive prenatal care during the first trimester: White–73.9 percent; Black–60.6 percent; Hispanics–58.5 percent; Native Americans–58.8 percent; Asian and others–62.0 percent. P.H. Kim et al., "Pregnancy Nutrition Surveillance System—United States, 1979–1990," *MMWR*, 41 (1992): 31.

41. See Dorn et al., *supra* note 39, at 441.

42. *Id.* Minority physicians are more likely to treat and admit minority patients, so a failure to employ minority physicians disparately impacts on minority patients.

43. See Randall, *supra* note 15, at 127.

44. See Council for Ethical and Judicial Affairs, AMA, *supra* note 1, at 2346; and see Perkins, *supra* note 10, at 383.

45. See Jorge L.A. Garcia, African-American Perspectives, Cultural Relativism, and Normative Issues: Some Conceptual Questions," in Harley E. Flack and Edmund E. Pellegrino, eds., *African-American Perspectives on Biomedical Ethics* (Washington, D.C.: Georgetown University Press, 1992).

46. Wolf, *supra* note 35, at 283.

47. See Alexander Morgan Capron and Vicki Michel, "Law and Bioethics," *Loyola of Los Angeles L. Rev.*, 27 (1993): 36.

48. *Id.* at 36.

49. *Id.* at 37. See Patricia J. Williams. "Alchemical Notes: Reconstructing Ideals from Deconstructed Rights," *Harv. Civil Rights–Civil Liberties L. Rev.*, 22 (1987): 401.

"Her Body Her Own Worst Enemy": The Medicalization of Violence against Women

ABBY L. WILKERSON

IT HAS BECOME widely accepted that, in the past, medical conceptualizations of many diseases were based on moral norms rather than on "pure science," and that these norms were often inegalitarian. Present medical practice, particularly the interactions of female patients and male physicians, continues to promote moral norms in the guise of medical advice. Medical sociologist Kathy Davis's analysis of four hundred tapes of clinical interactions identifies frequent paternalism in the form of "general practitioners mak-

ABBY WILKERSON teaches English at George Washington University.

ing moral judgments about women's roles as wives and mothers, psychologizing women's problems, not taking their complaints seriously, massive prescription of tranquilizers, [and] usurpation of women's control over their reproduction" (1988: 22). Davis finds this kind of paternalism particularly insidious given the apparent benevolence of doctors: "It was precisely the intimate, pleasant quality of the medical encounter itself that made issues of power and control seem like something else" (ibid.).

Medicine as power and control, both within the doctor-patient relationship and in its broader social functions, depends not only on the social

From Violence Against Women: Philosophical Perspectives, *Stanley G. French, Wanda Teays, and Laura M. Purdy, eds. (Ithaca, NY: Cornell University Press, 1998). Reprinted by permission of Cornell University Press*

roles of doctor and patient, but on the social construction of science as the foundation of modern medicine. The scientific grounding of medicine provides a base of knowledge, but a deeper analysis reveals that the detached epistemology of medicine, rather than liberating it from the "tyranny of values," instead legitimizes medicine's implicit moral/political judgments. . . .

MEDICAL TREATMENT OF VIOLENCE AGAINST WOMEN

In examining this issue, I rely on certain tenets shared by activists, practitioners, and theorists associated with the women's health movement:

1. a social context of patriarchy, racism, classism, and homophobia is harmful to women's health;

2. the health care system as presently structured reflects and reinforces society's devaluation of women;[1]

3. to address these two problems adequately, not only must they be understood in relation to an inegalitarian social context, but the social structure must be transformed in many ways as well;

4. thus, health care must incorporate the goal of promoting women's interests and agency, as workers, professionals, and clients, in medical and other contexts.

These beliefs provide background for my argument that the medical treatment of violence against women reveals the harmful consequences of the narrow medical paradigm defended by Seldin. Mainstream medicine often treats the symptoms of violence while ignoring and even obscuring the causes, isolating a specific injury from the context in which it occurred and (in the case of domestic violence) is likely to recur; fails to reduce the risk of medical treatment's retraumatizing patients; and in some cases relies on conservative notions of "women's place." The paradigm Seldin defends is not only inadequate

for the needs of women, but is not altogether objective, nor free of moral norms, as it purports to be.

The clinical paradigm may conceal the nature of the injury. A 1990 *Journal of the American Medical Association* report notes that "only 5 percent of 107 victims of domestic violence at a metropolitan emergency department were identified in the physicians' records as abused" (Parsons, 1990). Similarly, Stark, Flitcraft, and Frazier show that injuries from domestic violence are likely not to be identified as such in medical care. Their study identifies features of domestic violence that clearly distinguish it from most other types of injury seen in emergency rooms, yet injuries from domestic violence are often characterized as accidents (1983: 187–88).

Unfortunately, a distinguishing feature of domestic violence is that its victims may not be in a position to explain the cause of their injuries. Debbie Burghaus, a social worker in a Chicago hospital, states, "a lot of times, the victim isn't going to offer to tell you she was beaten up, because he's waiting for her in the hall, or she's just not empowered to leave him yet" (Parsons, 1990).

Understanding the nature of domestic violence or the difficulty of pressing charges or leaving an abuser requires knowledge of patients' social and economic circumstances, such as the compounding of the effects of battering for women who face additional forms of oppression, including lesbians, women of color (Richie and Kanuha, 1993), and disabled women (Warshaw, 1994). Yet, as Dr. Carole Warshaw of Cook County Hospital states, physicians "see their job as fixing the physical problem, and they don't see the person or their life context as part of the problem, so that's not their job" (Parsons, 1990). Thus Warshaw and other feminist analysts call for a broader clinical approach that would recognize the social nature of the problem in order to facilitate prevention and intervention.

The medical paradigm pathologizes victims, obscuring structural features of medicine which perpetrate violence and hinder treatment, such as the authoritarian aspects of standard doctor-patient interactions. While women are sometimes unable to discuss battering because they fear retribution by the batterer, at other times they may actually be prevented by the doctor or other medical professional who is privileged to control communication with patients; this systemic feature of medical interactions often disadvantages battered women when they attempt to voice their concerns (Warshaw, 1994).[2] According to Lori Heise, however, "providers have found that, contrary to their expectations, women have proven quite willing to admit abuse when asked directly in a nonjudgmental way" (1994: 245).

Stark, Flitcraft, and Frazier found that many survivors seeking treatment for injuries were given "pseudopsychiatric labels in the medical records such as 'patient with multiple vague medical complaints' or multiple symptomatology with psychosomatic overlay'" (1983: 195). Yet battered women have long been known to experience the physical manifestations of chronic stress, such as "severe tension headaches, stomach ailments, high blood pressure, allergic skin reactions, and heart palpitations" (Walker, 1979: 61), along with anxiety and depression. A woman's body manifests the daily assaults on her sense of self through chronic tension and anxiety, prompting her to seek a medical remedy that may be her only safe outlet for addressing the multiple harms, medical and otherwise, that the batterer inflicts on her. Yet when she attempts to articulate her situation in "the daily language of medical discourse" (Poirier and Brauner, 1988), her perceptions can be stripped of their meaning. This aspect of medical practice undermines the social authority of women who have been battered. Moreover, psychiatric pathologization not only diverts attention from chronic, stress-related illnesses, but fails to address the real cause of the problem.

Pathologization also serves to obscure the group identity of women who are battered, perpetuating the sense that their suffering is an isolated personal problem, due to bad luck or their own inadequacy—rather than a common manifestation of relationships between men and women in this society. Many battered women have changed their lives through participation in support groups with other battered women, learning that they are not alone and that they can begin to exercise greater control over their lives. Fortunately, some hospitals do refer patients identified as battered women to such groups. But psychiatric pathologization substitutes a diagnosis for real assistance, a diagnosis that can only stigmatize, compounding the hopelessness and shame that battering often causes (Walker, 1979) by eroding women's self-regard and their identification with and regard for other women who have survived domestic violence.

Not only does the pathologization of domestic violence present an image to women of themselves as the ones with the "problem," it also serves to mask institutional responsibilities. A survivor who frequently returns to the emergency room may be labeled a chronic complainer or hypochondriac, such characterization functioning "to suppress the 'inappropriate' demands for help of those victimized elsewhere. . . . The label explains the failure of the medical paradigm and the continued suffering of the abused woman in a way that is intelligible, even acceptable, to the physician" (Stark, Flitcraft, and Frazier, 1983: 187). In fact, Stark, Flitcraft, and Frazier argue convincingly that the medical profession indirectly supports systemic violence against women by failing to acknowledge assault as such, at the same time protecting its own interests in the face of the difficulties the women present.

Failure to identify the cause of an injury may not count as misdiagnosis in the usual sense, yet if domestic violence or sexual abuse is understood as a pattern in a woman's life, rather than as discrete, unconnected incidents, a kind of misdiagnosis—and ultimately mistreatment, or inadequate treatment—does occur. Symptoms are addressed, but not their underlying causes. In my view, this failure is a result of the medical/cultural assumption that heterosexuality and marriage are biologically certified as "natural"—hence appropriate, hence safe.

This point can be understood by exploring the medical understanding of domestic violence that is acknowledged as such. Domestic violence education for the medical profession tends to rely on research on "the violent family," which obscures a widespread social problem by focusing on "an aberrant subtype" of the family rather than on problems with "the American family as such" (Stark, Flitcraft, and Frazier, 1983: 194). Clearly, the notion of "the violent family" contains an unstated norm, a belief that "the family," with heterosexuality and marriage at its core, is nonviolent, a benign institution. Here, then, is one manifestation of the set of relational norms I have alluded to in the medicalization of women's health: the belief that women belong in relationships with men, belong in "the family"—a normative assumption which denies that heterosexuality and family life constitute a context of risk for women, and implies that such risk is occasioned by aberrations from the norm, rather than being part of a continuum of various forms of violence (not necessarily physical battering) that affect all women's lives. . . .

MEDICINE, PHILOSOPHY, AND "THE UNDOING OF THE SELF"

The medical treatment of violence against women has significant implications for ongoing debates in the field of bioethics. First, the call to increase access to health care has come from many quarters—not only the philosophical literature,[3] but also from activists in the women's health, lesbian/gay/bisexual liberation, and AIDS movements, as well as from mainstream political discourse. Activists are equally concerned with injustices arising from the social power of medicine, however, including its ability to define and control people by calling them sick. If medicine does contribute significantly to the oppression of women, then simply increasing access without addressing this problem may well serve to perpetuate injustice even as it alleviates the crisis of access. Discussion must be broadened to address eradication of the oppressive aspects of the existing system.

Second, recent bioethics discussions address a broad array of questions about the role of health care in response to social group differences, and relations between individuals and communities.[4] My contention is that a biosocial understanding of human health is a necessary aspect of this analysis. I have argued that the appropriate medical treatment of women who have survived violence can only be defined, using diverse perspectives of women, in relation to a social context that shapes and influences the health status of women and our experiences of health care as well. An analysis of the medicalization of violence against women illuminates the complex relations between individual lives, the health care system, and the broader social context—exemplifying an approach that can and should be used for other specific topics in health care.

The medicalization of violence against women also requires reflection on important epistemological questions. It will be useful not only to consider this issue in the context of the critique of objectivity construed as detachment, but to consider further the relation of this episteme to "the undoing of the self" (Brison) for women.

I have discussed many problematic impacts of medical discourse and practice on violence against women: assaulting women's integrity; alienating women from our own bodies; undermining women's agency; erasing the interests of individual women as they are distinct from others'; and eroding women's self-regard, as well as our identification with and regard for other women. Paradoxically, medicine simultaneously relegates women to the category of Other as it radically individualizes us; it presents oppressive social relations as facts of nature. Medical discourse often pathologizes women, and pathology carries stigma—in this case the stigma of one's gender, a central component of identity. Experiences of violence, always enmeshed within a complex of social relations, are reduced to "female problems"—physiological or psychological inadequacies associated with *being a woman*. In a social context in which women face a variety of disadvantages, these aspects of medical care reinforce other oppressive beliefs and practices, such as the patriarchal conception of femaleness that trains the medical gaze upon the presumed disruptiveness of women's own bodies, obscuring the social forces that break those bodies, spirits, and lives.

Medicine regulates many experiences of women, enforcing its definitions of reality over women's own perceptions. Women need to be able to trust our own perceptions of our bodies and our experiences, a goal that medical theory and practice should respect and support. Along with the attack on her body, a rapist or batterer assaults a woman's sense of competence and efficacy. Standard medical conceptualizations and treatments of violence may erase or undermine women's agency and selfhood, exacerbating the "undoing of the self" that results from violence —yet it is precisely this strong sense of selfhood that is needed in order for a woman to leave a batterer and make a new life, or regain a sense of safety and control in the world again.

Women may be treated for physical injuries, while psychological injuries, which may be even deeper, are ignored, or addressed only superficially, invisible to the clinical gaze or outside its parameters, as if these subjective states of suffering, the damage to women's self-esteem and sense of agency, were insignificant.

On "the scale of the gaze," Foucault's metaphor for the epistemic principle of modern medicine, knowledge is valued for its precise quantifiability, its detachment, which is understood to render it pure, objective, and untainted by the body or the idiosyncrasy of individual consciousness. Clearly this epistemic norm does not accommodate the subjectivity of health, illness, and injury, which I have argued must be included in the construction of knowledge. At the same time, the norm functions to obscure the impact of professional (typically male) subjectivity role in oppressive power relations.

These considerations show the need for a model of knowledge that not only incorporates subjectivity, but does not radically separate epistemological questions from moral ones.[5] In the context of medicine there are distinct advantages to an epistemological perspective that incorporates egalitarian norms. My opposition to certain norms in medicine is part of a broader defense of just norms.

Yet the modern medical paradigm—the Flexnerian model defended by Seldin—defines any such moral commitments as the corruption of "pure" science with alien values. Should we therefore reject the medical gaze and refuse, for example, the diagnostic arsenal of x-rays, endoscopes, ultrasound, and magnetic resonance imaging? Some critics may indeed reject the institution of medicine altogether, or nearly so,[12] but this is not my position. Instead, I argue that the scale of the gaze, as a basis for medicine, is unnecessarily and inappropriately reductionist, excluding the inherent moral, social, and political aspects of the embodied human concerns defined as medical, even as it obscures the tacit (and often inegalitarian) moral commitments already present. What I argue for is a biosocial understanding of health.

The women's health movement and the domestic violence and rape survivors' movements have generated knowledge with the potential to correct and inform traditional medicine in two ways: through their contribution to "better science," contextually based, and thus to more accurate understandings of health, illness, and injury, which in turn provide a better basis for treatment; and through facilitating morally preferable conceptualizations and treatments of women that can help rectify some aspects of an oppressive social context. Both the institution of medicine and the discipline of bioethics can and must contribute to the survivor's remaking of the self, and to the prevention of violence, by working with these movements to transform material conditions and give women greater voice in the social definition of reality.

REFERENCES

1. Mary Daly's *Gyn/Ecology* critiques "the Gynecological Culture" and its "imposed totalitarian heterosexism" (1978: 264) and misogyny, identifying medicine as an aspect of patriarchal culture that destroys women's selfhood. . . . My approach differs from hers, however, in at least two significant ways. First, Daly posits an inherent or essential "Female Self" alienated and undermined by the external forces of patriarchy . . . [whereas] I do not identify female-ness as the core of women's identities. Second, although Daly critiques medicine as a patriarchal institution, her purpose is to offer a vision of feminism as radical lesbian separatism, rather [than] to work toward the transformation of medicine, as I am attempting to do.

2. See Bannister, 1993, and Walker, 1979, for analyses of the disadvantages battered women face in attempting to voice their concerns in the legal system.

3. Iris Young (1990a) argues that mainstream liberal philosophy is based on a "distributive paradigm" that frames the relation between health and justice in terms of access to health care. . . . For important treatments of access to health care, see Daniels, 1985, and Gauthier, 1983, whose views I critique in my forthcoming book *Diagnosis: Difference: The Moral Authority of Medicine* (Cornell).

4. See, for example, the May-June 1994 issue of the *Hastings Center Report* on these topics, as well as Dula & Goering, 1994.

5. See M. Heldke & Stephen H. Kellert, "Objectivity as Responsibility," *Metaphilosophy* 26:4 (October 1995), 360–78.

Bioethics, Public Health, and Firearm-Related Violence: Missing Links between Bioethics and Public Health

LEIGH TURNER

OPEN ANY STANDARD bioethics textbook, and therein can be found a host of subjects rang-

LEIGH TURNER is an assistant professor in the department for the study of religion, and a member of the Joint Centre for Bioethics, at the University of Toronto.

ing from the abortion rights controversy to the morality of xenographic tissue transplantation. Just as there is a wide scope to the subject matter of bioethics, its practitioners come from a multitude of disciplines, including law, medicine, nursing, theology, philosophy, sociology, and

Journal of Law, Medicine & Ethic 25(1997): 42–48. Copyright 1997. Reprinted with permission of Leigh Turner and the American Society of Law, Medicine & Ethics. All rights reserved.

anthropology. And yet, despite a rich variety of investigators and methods, bioethicists overlook numerous subjects that deserve to be addressed. In particular, they neglect issues of public health, preventive medicine, and social medicine. Although topics such as physician-assisted suicide, prenatal genetic testing, and the ethics of new reproductive technologies constitute the contemporary canon of bioethics and deserve sustained analysis, these subjects are not so significant that they should eclipse other issues. For example, gun control policies, the regulation of food additives, immunization programs, prenatal care, leave programs enabling employees to care for dying relatives, the provision of nutrition and medical care to the homeless, and the use of emergency rooms by the most impoverished citizens are all topics neglected by bioethicists. Bioethicists need to examine more critically the various assumptions that lead them to address particular themes while overlooking other significant topics.

Above, I have identified several topics that could be better addressed by bioethicists, but I will focus only on the issue of gun control and firearm-related violence. By paying particular attention to this issue, perhaps it will become more evident why bioethicists need to expand their intellectual horizons.

Absent cogent commentary from the bioethics community, the moral dimensions of firearm-related violence are explored within other disciplines. The fields of public health, social medicine, and community health sciences are not value-free, neutral fields providing little more than purely descriptive accounts about how many American citizens are wounded or killed by handguns every year. At present, these are the disciplinary settings wherein the relationships between social justice, moral health care, homelessness, gun-control, prenatal care, car safety regulations, and so forth are debated.

To select just one example, physicians at Martin Luther King, Jr. Hospital in South-Central Los Angeles are mapping the links between gun-related violence, institutional breakdown, inadequate public education in inner-city schools, racism, and the paramilitary use of police forces.[1] With 28,150 gunshot victims treated by physicians at Martin Luther King Hospital over the last fourteen years, it is not surprising that physicians from the hospital's Department of Emergency Medicine feel compelled to address these topics as moral and social issues.[2] In this setting, efforts to limit the proliferation of firearms, to reduce violence, and to improve the social and educational opportunities of the citizens of South-Central Los Angeles cannot be detached from the ethical calling of the physician to engage in acts of healing. And yet, the moral, medical, political, and social challenges addressed by these emergency room physicians are overlooked by the most prominent, "mainstream" bioethicists.

Although bioethicists dedicate enormous effort to developing principles by which to analyze ethical dilemmas, as well as to analogical methods of moral casuistry, they are less successful at exploring how, why, and when particular subjects emerge as being justifiable matters to investigate. For example, though the prominent framework of Tom Beauchamp and James Childress provides a method for developing codes, rules, and laws, it does not explain why physician-assisted suicide generates tremendous critical scrutiny whereas urban violence and human suffering are ignored by members of the bioethics community in the United States.[3] But there is every reason to think that those concerned with the "sanctity of life" or the "dignity of life" would be concerned about the current rate of firearm-related violence in the United States. The mere presence of a sophisticated set of principles or a theory of justice does not explain what scholars view as appropriate subjects for normative analysis. Bioethicists, then, need to cultivate a more reflective discipline that is critical of the manner in which topics do or do not become the focus of conferences, journal issues, and research agendas.

BIOETHICS AND FIREARM-RELATED VIOLENCE

I am perplexed why firearm-related violence is not a focal point for the consideration of bioethicists. If bioethics is defined in part by its response to the practical organization of medical care into specialties such as geriatrics, obstetrics, oncology, and neurology, then this lacuna still remains incomprehensible. Practitioners within the fields of public health, trauma care, community health services, social medicine, and emergency medicine all explore the relationships between ethics, professional responsibilities and moral obligations, firearms, violence, fear, injury, suffering, destruction, and death. Specialists in these fields provide practical programs and policy recommendations intended to alter contemporary patterns of gun-related injuries and deaths. Likewise, numerous emergency medicine physicians serve as grass roots social activists. As moral agents capable of influencing public life and the transformation of institutions and social structures, they acknowledge an obligation to respond to situations where children must pass through metal detectors to attend classes, military surgeons train at urban health care facilities to hone their skills in the treatment of traumatic "combat wounds," and gunshot victims are seen in emergency rooms so overcrowded that many such individuals are treated as outpatients. In an era of hand guns in high schools, "fortified" neighborhoods, private security corporations, devastated urban cores, and the proliferation of military weapons, bioethicists ought to speak to the suffering, fears, and terrifying practical circumstances of so many citizens.

Given that bioethicists fill important roles in developing public policies and reasoned positions concerning organ transplantation networks and state health care plans, bioethicists should be capable of developing thoughtful arguments and practical policy recommendations for social and institutional reform that could limit the number of citizens who are killed or wounded through domestic firearm-related violence. Although I suspect that many bioethicists, should they choose to enter such discussions, would support more stringent gun-control regulations, even those who oppose such measures would recognize the obligation to develop practical means to reduce the number of firearm-related deaths in the United States.

It is difficult to discern just why there is such an absence of sustained critical reflection by American bioethicists regarding firearm regulation and gun-related violence. That gun control and firearm-related violence are subjects ignored by bioethicists in a country like Japan is not surprising. There, the number of citizens killed by firearms is so low that serious attention to the subject by Japanese bioethicists would be perplexing. According to David Kopel, "The handgun murder rate is at least two hundred times higher in America than Japan."[4] A more global analysis of firearm-related violence further highlights the need for reflective moral and social analysis concerning the regulation of firearms in the United States. According to Catherine Barber et al.,

> A look at the toll of firearm violence internationally is instructive: in 1992, 38 people died in England from gun homicides, about 100 in Australia, 214 in Canada, and 17,790 in the United States. The contrast is daunting, even when the much larger population of the United States is taken into account. The U.S. total firearm death rate from suicide, homicide, or accident of 15 per 100,000 residents is over 30 times higher than that of England.[5]

It is evident why Japanese, English, Canadian, and Australian bioethicists do not discuss gun control, but the social milieu is very different in the United States. Consequently, considering why gun control and firearm-related violence is so neglected by American bioethicists helps to reveal some problematic disciplinary prejudices of American bioethicists.

Autonomy, "Fascinomas," Class Biases, and the Lure of Lucre: Why Bioethicists Neglect Public Health

Firearm-related violence is not limited to just one or two U.S. cities. The citizens of Chicago, Detroit, Los Angeles, Miami, New York, Washington, D.C., and other major urban centers all suffer from rates of gun-related violence that far exceed levels found within cities in Great Britain, Japan, Canada, and Australia. Of course, firearm-related violence is not a problem limited to U.S. urban areas. It is so pervasive that a discussion of gun control must extend to a national debate about public morality and the meaning of public health. Although the normative dimensions of firearm-related violence are not recognized by most bioethicists, they are certainly acknowledged by many members of the National Rifle Association (NRA), who often label proponents of gun control laws as communists and develop normative and legal positions based on their libertarian understanding of individual rights. Attitudes toward firearm-related violence and gun control policies are linked to substantive understandings of human flourishing, human health, civic life, and meaningful communities.

Conceivably, one reason why bioethicists fail to attend to the subject of gun-related violence and gun control is that they perceive no moral quandary requiring sustained debate and discussion. Perhaps most bioethicists think that it is not necessary to make a reasoned argument in support of stricter firearm regulations. As a citizen of Canada, where regulations surrounding the possession of firearms are much more restrictive than in the United States, I find the argument for the stringent regulation of all firearms, from handguns to assault rifles, to be compelling. Indeed, I would argue that whether the

subject is addressed through a deontological approach concerned with preserving the sanctity of human life, consequentialist reasoning that seeks minimizing personal and collective pain and suffering, or through practical reasoning concerned with fostering the public good within particular social contexts, a convincing case can be made to favor firearm regulations far more restrictive than those currently found throughout most regions of the United States. Having now lived in the United States for over four years, I am well aware that what can seem painfully self-evident to Canadians and citizens of other nations with discernible social democratic traditions needs to be bolstered by sustained reasoning and argumentation in the more atomistic (rights-oriented) U.S. milieu. Furthermore, the provision of compelling moral arguments must be accompanied by political organization and access to sizable economic resources to challenge libertarian pro-firearm organizations in the United States.

I suspect it is not a mere historical accident that so little attention is paid to urban violence and firearm regulation. To the contrary, a few important factors help to explain why bioethicists fail to develop sustained analyses of firearm-related violence, as well as other topics related to public health and social medicine.

One plausible reason why so few bioethicists contribute to discussions concerning the moral dimensions of firearm regulation in the United States is that one of the most important words in the sacred mantra of bioethicists is also dear to the members of NRA. Ever since their early focus on matters of truth telling and informed consent in medical care and research, bioethicists have placed enormous emphasis on the principle of personal autonomy. Coming from Canada, where firearm-related violence occurs at much lower rates than in the United States, I am disturbed that the very ethicists who place such an emphasis on the principle of personal autonomy neglect the many ways in which autonomy, more thoughtfully considered, can be impeded. In Los Angeles, as well as in other settings throughout the United States, the autonomy of citizens is restrained through inadequate vaccination programs, insufficient and underfunded medical care and social programs for the indigent, and haphazard prenatal programs for the poor. With regard to the accessibility of firearms in the United States, references to autonomy are often used to justify their widespread proliferation. However, autonomy can be understood to possess much richer dimensions. How, for example, is the autonomy of citizens respected when they sense that it is no longer safe to ride public transportation? How is the autonomy of children acknowledged when they cannot play in neighborhood parks even during the daytime? Perhaps as bioethicists come to realize that autonomy should not be so preeminent as to trump all other principles, rules, norms, and values, they will be able to make a more sustained contribution to the manner in which considerations of the public good and public health need to include deliberations about firearm regulation.

Anyone seeking to transform the status quo needs to grapple with the claims of powerful interest groups that challenge even mild measures to limit the proliferation of firearms. It is mystifying that, in a field such as bioethics where numerous scholars advocate communitarian conceptions of social justice, so little is raised about NRA's libertarian conception of personal autonomy. To enact more responsible legislation and to transform the pervasive character of firearm-related violence in the United States, bioethicists should craft reasoned positions that attend to the moral dimension of this subject.

Communitarian philosophers are often charged with failing to provide practical proposals for social change and merely assailing the atomism of contemporary American life. By linking their moral and social analyses of the public good to specific topics within public health, such scholars could make a more substantial contribu-

tion to American civic life. Like Robert Bellah, I, too, think it evident that the language of individualism needs to be balanced by a greater concern for the public good.[6] Although the spectrum of communities, social organizations, and ethnic groups found in many urban centers may make the establishment of a public consensus on many topics difficult to achieve, I suspect that such groups can be united around a common public concern for living in neighborhoods where citizens are not killed or wounded.

A second explanation for the lack of attention accorded to public health issues by bioethicists is found in the folklore of contemporary American biomedicine.

Perri Klass, in an account of her four years as a student at Harvard Medical School, describes the obsession medical students and physicians alike have with cases that are experienced as "fascinomas." Such cases reside outside the boundaries of everyday medical practice. They provide specialists the opportunity to utilize their most rarefied skills. Someone unfamiliar with contemporary medical education could presume that such cases would occupy just a small fraction of the time and effort of students, because most of their working lives as physicians will involve attending to the needs of patients with far more common ailments. However, Klass notes that in elite academic medicine, it is the fascinomas that attract enormous attention and effort. Klass writes:

> 'Fascinoma' is one of those hospital words. *Oma,* of course, means tumor, but 'fascinoma' is used to mean any disease remarkable chiefly for its fascination value. One-of-a-kind diseases, diseases you'll never see again, diseases unusual in this age or in this country, diseases that are for one reason or another very difficult to diagnose are fascinomas. . . . Medical students in the hospital compete for these patients.[7]

Klass amplifies the meaning of this term in her discussion of zebras. According to Klass, medical students are directed away from the mundane and the quotidian toward the exotic. She states:

> [T]his term [zebras] comes from a rather rueful joke. The idea is that when a normal person (not a medical student or doctor) hears horse beats, the first thought that comes to mind is 'Horse.' But a medical student hears hoofbeats and immediately thinks 'Zebra!' Medical students, the cliché goes, think first about the rare, unlikely diagnosis, are uninterested in common medical problems. The medical student not only expects those hoofbeats to be a zebra's, but is actually disappointed to see no exotic black and white stripes, just a plain old horse. And the fact is, the appeal of the rare and dramatic disease is built right into medical training, and the dream of someday lassoing a zebra continues to titillate many of those more advanced people who smile patronizingly at the medical students crude reflexes.[8]

Perhaps Klass somewhat exaggerates the experiences of medical students. Nonetheless, I suspect that one significant reason why bioethicists neglect firearm-related violence is that they, like many academic physicians, are often more attracted to the unfamiliar, exotic issues at the cutting edge of medicine than to critically exploring routine elements of medical care such as the provision of vaccinations, the treatment of minor illnesses of poor people and homeless individuals, and the care of the substantial number of individuals with gunshot wounds who arrive in emergency rooms. Xenographic tissue transplantation and gene therapy are topics that are just more avant garde, sexy, and intellectually satisfying than the practical matter of making neighborhoods safe. The absence of thoughtful scholarship exploring the moral dimension of firearm-related violence may in part be a product of this fascination with the arcane. As is all too often the case, issues of daily practical import are left to those found outside elite, traditional academic settings. With regard to firearm regulations and gun-related violence, the absence of at-

tention dedicated to exploring this subject is just another sign of the manner in which academics employed by prestigious institutions often avoid matters of profound import to the public good, and serve less laudable personal and institutional aims.

However, I doubt that the absence of critical reflection by bioethicists concerning gun-related violence is merely a product of a fascination with trendy, exciting issues. Instead, another possibility is that many American bioethicists live and work in settings at least somewhat removed from homeless citizens sitting beside freeways, drive-by shootings, random gunfire, and playground tragedies; and they simply prefer not to enter this world through sustained moral reflection or political activism. No one who watches the evening news can ignore the extraordinary rates of firearm-related violence, but there is a difference between casually recognizing an issue and actually becoming embroiled in its complexities. Put in more scholarly terms, the "sociology of knowledge" provides another reason why firearm-related violence is neglected by American bioethicists. Perhaps the economic and social class of most American bioethicists serves to limit their capacity to "see" the effects of gun-related violence.[9] Perhaps, most bioethicists are sufficiently wealthy and well educated that they rarely encounter citizens from neighborhoods where firearms or the signs of poverty, homelessness, and inadequate educational and social opportunities are prevalent. As members of a relatively sheltered intellectual elite, bioethicists are able psychologically to bypass these social problems just as the freeways enable them to avoid traveling through the most impoverished neighborhoods. The view of the world inculcated within Westwood and Beverly Hills differs from the view from South-Central Los Angeles.

The "local knowledge" constraining the intellectual ruminations of most bioethicists may prevent them from recognizing matters of profound social import that influence the everyday lives of the most socioeconomically disadvantaged.[10] According to Barber and her colleagues at the Massachusetts Department of Public Health,

> Media coverage of particularly grisly attacks seems to heighten fear levels in all communities, even those that haven't seen a serious assault in years. Yet an overall incidence rate of 14.5 gun assaults and 42 knife assaults for every 100,000 residents in Massachusetts masks how dramatically risk levels vary depending on one's neighborhood, demographic characteristics, and, presumably, individual risk factors. For example, an astonishing one in every 38 black male teenagers ages 15 to 19 was shot or stabbed in Boston in 1994, a figure only slightly lower than the one in 34 risk for 1992–1993. The corresponding risk for white male teenagers was one in 422. Compare these rates, however, to a weapon assault risk of one in 23,294 for elders of any ethnicity living in urban areas and one in 56,083 for white females of any age living in the suburbs. The importance of focusing discussions of risk on particular populations becomes readily apparent. Some of the state's residents are living in a virtual war zone, while others are quite removed from danger.[11]

Bioethicists need to consider more thoughtfully the extent to which their normative analyses and recommendations for institutional reform successfully incorporate the concerns and interests of citizens from impoverished, violent settings.

Conceivably, bioethicists do not recognize the magnitude of suffering tied to firearm-related violence, just as they have difficulty understanding why children are not immunized even when public programs are available or why poor people visit crowded emergency rooms for routine medical care. Perhaps bioethicists assume that firearm-related violence happens only to gang bangers, drug dealers, and other marginal or even deviant members of society, and thus do not accord the topic the attention reserved for issues that impinge on the lives of ostensibly more upright and outstanding citizens. Bioethicists,

then, fail to recognize the extent to which class-based concerns limit their ability to recognize salient health issues.[12]

This class-based blindness is evident in the obsession of many bioethicists with issues concerning overtreatment. Of course, in many instances, it is appropriate to criticize physicians for providing excessive treatment, particularly near the end of life. Bioethicists have played an important, thoughtful role in cultivating a new public sensibility that not every death need be accompanied by a prolonged display of technological wizardry. However, the emphasis on overtreatment reflects a strong middle-class bias when enormous numbers of individuals are at little risk of overtreatment for most of their lives.

Finally, bioethicists need to address better the way in which financial support for particular areas of research can lead to the neglect of significant topics. Sociologists of science recognize the way in which funding opportunities serve to channel research along particular pathways, while other topics are neglected. Though bioethicists may like to think of themselves as beyond such critiques, bioethicists benefit when their research projects receive funding. One reason why so many scholars address the ethical, legal, and social dimensions of genetics research is that this is such a well-funded area of research. Careers are made by developing research initiatives that attract such grants. I recognize the importance of addressing the moral dimensions of research in genetics, however, bioethicists need to recognize how the lure of lucre can lead them away from other worthy topics of investigation.

Clearly, institutions such as universities and independent research centers require revenue streams if they are to continue to exist. At times, as everyone working within such institutions recognizes, funds are solicited because of the need for institutional revenue, rather than because of the social significance of the proposed research. In a research climate where competition for funding from government organizations, corporations, foundations, and private donors is extremely competitive, even scholars with considerable integrity sometimes feel compelled to participate in research initiatives that neither fulfill a personal sense of responsible scholarship nor serve the public good. In an ideal research setting, worthwhile, thoughtfully crafted research projects in bioethics would receive financial support. In reality, however, the funding tail often wags the research dog, and sources of revenue play a considerable role in determining what is incorporated within research agendas. Although bioethicists are under no professional obligation to be paupers, they should take care to resist the temptation to explore only those topics where funds for research can be easily obtained. An excessive orientation to professional rewards can lead to the neglect of public matters of great concern. Bioethicists, then, need to cultivate more critical forms of moral and social analysis. When they fail to do so, they merely provide an inoculation against reflective moral analysis, by providing interlocutors with the false sense that serious attention is being accorded to significant moral issues.

CONCLUSION: TOWARD A SOCIAL BIOETHICS

Bioethicists in the United States can make an important contribution to the current debate on the regulation of firearms, just as they can contribute to a host of other moral issues falling within public health. They should not let themselves be captivated by exotic subjects of less practical import. American bioethicists need to reflect on the range of subjects that they study, and recognize that the field, as it is currently constituted, is limited by some pernicious assumptions that render bioethics far too individualistic in orientation. A greater appreciation for the implications of the language of personal autonomy

in the public discourse of groups like NRA should lead bioethicists to recognize the need to balance the principle of autonomy with other concerns for the public good. Although the many factors that produce high rates of firearm-related deaths and injuries in major American cities are complex, the social atomism of Americans described by scholars such as Bellah likely plays a significant role in exacerbating needless violence and suffering.[13] There ought to be a renegotiation of the balance between the public good and personal autonomy with regard to the regulation of firearms. American bioethicists should end their silence on this important subject, and begin contributing to public deliberations about public health, the common good, and firearm regulation.

Most disconcerting is the lack of attention paid by U.S. bioethicists to the social, educational, economic, and institutional factors that lead to the presentation of citizens with combat-like injuries in trauma centers, neonates in the neonatal intensive care units whose mothers received inadequate prenatal care, and homeless individuals in emergency wards with illnesses that could have easily been treated before reaching advanced stages. This lacuna in American bioethics was recognized twenty years ago by Gene Outka in "Social Justice and Equal Access to Health Care." There, Outka, scarcely a mainstream figure within bioethics then or now, wrote,

> Those communities committed to self-conscious moral and religious reflection about subjects in medicine have concentrated, perhaps unduly, on issues about care of individual patients (as death approaches, for instance). These issues plainly warrant the most careful consideration. One would like to see in addition, however, more attention paid to social questions in medical ethics. To attend to them is not necessarily to leave behind all of the matters which reach deeply into the human condition.[14]

These "social questions" should be central to bioethics. The exploration of what constitutes "just" forms of national health care, the rationing of medical resources, and the allocation of organs for transplantation all contain explicit social dimensions. Even so, numerous subjects that are treated as serious moral issues by physicians, nurses, social activists, religious leaders, and practitioners of public health and preventive medicine go unacknowledged by bioethicists.

I have tried to suggest how American bioethics as a discipline could be opened, unpacked, enlarged, and reframed by paying particular attention to firearm-related violence. Other topics that deserve to become subjects of debate within bioethics include the provision of prenatal care for low income families, homelessness and the use of emergency medical facilities by the indigent who have no other access to health care, and improved access to immunization programs. These are substantive issues with social and moral components that have been neglected by bioethicists. Bioethicists must enter these debates and pay more attention to ethical issues facing their colleagues in public health, social medicine, family medicine, and community health sciences. By disregarding these fields, as well as the larger community extending beyond academic institutions, bioethicists risk limiting themselves to a familiar, narrowly delineated set of well-trodden paths. American bioethicists need to recognize the practical problems in the social world around them. In so doing, they can move beyond the familiar list of standardized topics that constitutes the current canon of bioethics. Even though topics like abortion and euthanasia will continue to receive bioethicists' attention, bioethicists must recognize the important role they can play in addressing other subjects. If social medicine and public health are legitimate branches of health care, and if social ethics is an established branch of moral reasoning, then bioethicists ought to be able to craft a more attentive social bioethics that responds to these aspects of health care. By doing so, Ameri-can bioethicists can develop informed normative analyses of firearm regulation, inadequate vaccination programs, and so forth. But until this occurs, American bioethics will continue to display an individualistic ethos with a strong class bias that blinds its practitioners to profound social inequities. With such an impoverished social sensibility, bioethicists will remain able only to respond to the suffering of individuals once they present themselves as the dilemmatic individual cases so favored within current discussions.

ACKNOWLEDGMENTS

I thank my colleagues David Armstrong, Aditi Gowri, and Bill Lambert, of the School of Religion and Social Ethics at the University of Southern California, for their thoughtful readings of an earlier version of this paper. Stephen Toulmin, of the Center for Multiethnic and Transnational Studies at the University of Southern California, provided a warm milieu for discussion of this paper. Bill May, Donald Miller, John Orr, and Alison Dundes Renteln all served as sources of inspiration during my doctoral studies at the University of Southern California. Finally, I thank Eve DeVaro of the Hastings Center and Michael Vasko of this journal for reading my manuscript with such care and attention to detail.

REFERENCES

1. W. C. Shoemaker et al., "Urban Violence in Los Angeles in the Aftermath of the Riots: A Perspective from Health Care Professionals, with Implications for Social Reconstruction," *JAMA,* 270 (1993): 2833–37.

2. See *id.* at 2834.

3. T.L. Beauchamp and J.F. Childress, *Principles of Biomedical Ethics* (Oxford: Oxford University Press, 4th ed., 1994): at 25.

4. D. Kopel, "Japanese Gun Control," *Asia Pacific Law Review,* 2, no. 2 (1993): at 28.

5. C.W Barber et al., "When Bullets Don't Kill," *Public Health Reports,* 111 (1996): at 483.

6. R.N. Bellah, "Social Science as Practical Reason," *Hastings Center Report,* 12, no. 5 (1982): 32–39.

7. P. Klass, *A Not Entirely Benign Procedure* (New York: Signet, 1988): 70–71.

8. *Id.* at 68.

9. The inability of bioethicists to recognize particular moral issues receives thoughtful scrutiny from a number of scholars developing feminist scholarship in bioethics. Whereas I focus on the importance of class and class interests, they draw attention to the need for greater awareness of gender for critical social analysis. See, for example, R. Tong, *Feminist Approaches to Bioethics: Theoretical Reflections and Practical Applications* (Boulder: Westview Press, 1997); S.M. Wolf, ed., *Feminism & Bioethics: Beyond Reproduction* (Oxford: Oxford University Press, 1996); and S. Sherwin, *No Longer Patient: Feminist Ethics and Health Care* (Philadelphia: Temple University Press, 1992). For a more general consideration of the significance of gender for political and moral philosophy, see S.M. Okin, *Justice, Gender, and the Family* (New York: Basic Books, 1989).

10. For a thoughtful discussion of communal forms of common sense and variants of local knowledge that provides resources for those seeking to unveil the most pernicious assumptions current in contemporary bioethics research, see C. Geertz, *Local Knowledge: Further Essays in Interpretive Anthropology* (New York: Basic Books, 1983).

11. See Barber et al., *supra* note 5, at 488–89.

12. For a thoughtful scholarly analysis that incorporates discussions of race, ethnicity, and class within an exploration of minority access to health care, see S.D. Watson, "Minority Access and Health Reform: A Civil Right to Health Care," *Journal of Law, Medicine & Ethics,* 22 (1994): 127–37.

13. R.N. Bellah et al., *Habits of the Heart: Individualism and Commitment in American Life* (New York: Harper & Row, 1985).

14. G. Outka, "Social Justice and Equal Access to Health Care," *Journal of Religious Ethics,* 2 (1974): at 28.

Case Study Exercises

1. Should there be an age limit on rights to health care? Some countries, such as Britain, restrict certain procedures (such as organ transplants) to elderly people based on age. Is this right?

2. Should noncitizens be allowed the same access to health care as citizens? Share your reflections and note, if possible, what sorts of assumptions you hold about rights and obligations to others when it comes to health care.

3. How should we decide the balance of a parent's right to know and a child's right to privacy when it comes to drug use and drug testing?

4. A Massachusetts company, Psychemedics Corporation, announced that it was offering a service whereby parents could send a small sample of their children's hair to the company's lab and learn by mail whether a child were using marijuana, cocaine, heroin, or other drugs. (See Peter Marks, "Vexed Parents Can Now Try a Drug Test at Home," *New York Times,* 13 July 1995.)
   a. Set out the issues and concerns from at least two distinctly different perspectives (e.g., that of a parent, child, medical professional, employer, government official, civil rights advocate).
   b. Where do you think we should draw the line in trying to balance the parents' concerns about their children and the child's privacy rights?

5. Would it be right of a physician to recommend to a woman whose family has a history of breast cancer that she have both healthy breasts removed as a preventive measure? Share your reflections on this. Note also that a May 1999 Mayo Clinic survey of 572 women found that nearly 70 percent of those who had the procedure were satisfied with their decision, although 36 percent were less satisfied with their physical appearance and 20 percent of the women regretted the decision.

6. Here is a case about nuclear waste and harms to the Eskimo in Northwest Alaska:

   In 1992, a university researcher uncovered information about Project Chariot that has alarmed Alaskan Eskimos and government officials. Project Chariot was a plan to use nuclear explosives to blast a giant new harbor into the Arctic in the early 1960s as part of a U.S. Atomic Energy Commission program to find "peaceful use" of nuclear energy. Dan O'Neill, researcher at the University of Alaska, obtained documents describing how scientists buried tons of radiation-laced dirt at Cape Thompson, in Northwest Alaska in 1962. The area lies in traditional hunting and gathering grounds for the Inupiat Indians. The Eskimos suspect the buried atomic waste is the cause of a sustained and significant rise in cancer rates in the region over the last 30 years. Documents reveal that the nuclear material was first used for experiments to see how radioactive isotopes behave in an Arctic setting. In at least one test, radioactive material was allowed to drain down a creek into the sea. The buried material was not placed in any containers and no warning signs or fences were ever erected in the area. An AEC official criticized the geological survey for exceeding (by 1,000 times) 1960s standards for burying radioactive strontium 85 and cesium 137. The experiments were never publicly disclosed until O'Neill requested the project's documents under the Freedom of Information Act. (See David Hulen, "Secret Burial of A-Waste In Alaska in '62 Disclosed; Radiation: Researcher Acquires Documents Describing The Federal Project. Now, Cancer Concerns are Voiced," *Los Angeles Times* September 25, 1992.)

   a. What is our obligation now to the Eskimo villagers who may have been exposed to the buried nuclear waste?
   b. What sorts of guidelines should be put into place regarding nuclear experiments on the part of the federal government?
   c. What changes could help prevent any future situations like Project Chariot?

7. Representative Henry A. Waxman released a 1981 report written by a tobacco company executive describing how using particular blends of tobacco can raise nicotine levels in cigarettes and recommended that these be added to low-tar cigarettes. Waxman contended that this offers further evidence that tobacco industry officials have acted in a deceptive manner. Alexander W. Spears, vice chairman and CEO for Lorillard Tobacco Co., said in congressional testimony on March 25, 1994, that "we do not set nicotine levels for particular brands of cigarettes." The FDA is trying to decide if they should regulate cigarettes as drugs and the Center for Disease Control is assessing the effects of cigarette additives. The Massachusetts Assembly passed a bill in 1996 requiring tobacco companies to list all the ingredients of their cigarettes—a move met with outrage on the part of tobacco companies.
   a. In light of health risks, do consumers have the right to know cigarette ingredients?
   b. How do we balance consumer rights with tobacco companies' desire to keep trade "secrets" secret?

8. Ten percent of all births in the southwest corner of Texas (in contrast to 1.7% nationwide) are performed by midwives. It is possible for a pregnant Mexican woman to take a taxi across the international bridge and legally give birth in Texas to a U.S. citizen. In 1994, licensed Texas midwives delivered 5,530 babies to women living on both sides of the border, charging little (e.g., one charges $350 per delivery) and offering a nonthreatening environment. (See Jesse Katz, "Rio Grande Midwives Deliver Citizenship," *Los Angeles Times*, 13 June 1995.) On one hand, such incidents fuel anti-immigration sentiment. On the other hand, babies are innocents, and preventing such births would mean laws restricting pregnant women from crossing the border to visit the U.S. (which would seem draconian at best). What ought we do? Share your ideas on how we might address this issue.

9. How might HMOs address some of the disparities in health care and access of minorities to health care providers? Look in particular at the case of Latinos, who are the largest group without medical insurance. In light of the following, can you offer some recommendations to change this situation?

Despite the expansion of public insurance and managed care organizations, the rates of uninsured remain high. Latinos constitute 9.3 percent of the population yet represent almost 20 percent of the uninsured. . . . Access to care has been a long-standing problem for Latinos. Studies have demonstrated an underutilization of health services by Latinos compared with other ethnic/racial groups. While earlier studies indicated that differential access to care was explained by language use and health beliefs, recent evidence emphasizes that the lack of health insurance coverage and health systems barriers act as strong deterrents to seeking care. A recent study showed that Latinos are less likely than any other group to be linked to a regular source of care. Nevertheless, recent attempts to enroll Latinos in managed care organizations may be altering their access patterns. (See Sylvia Guendelman and Todd H Wagner, "Health services utilization among Latinos and white non-Latinos: Results from a national survey," *Journal of Health Care for the Poor and Underserved,* May 2000.)

10. In January 2000, the U.S. government publicly acknowledged that workers making nuclear weapons have been exposed to radiation and chemicals causing cancer and early death—a fact that raises the issue of compensation. (See Matthew L. Wald, "U.S. Acknowledges Radiation Killed Weapons Workers," *The New York Times,* 29 January 2000.) As noted in an earlier article, there are dangers and health risks that may be associated with defense work and weapons production, as the following case demonstrates:

Workers at an atomic weapons factory in Fernald, Ohio, who made uranium metal for nuclear bombs died at significantly younger ages and suffered more lung, intestinal, and blood cancers than other Americans, according to an analysis of their medical records. In a 1986 study by Oak Ridge Associated Universities, an Energy Department contractor in Tennessee, researchers found a trend involving unusual rates of colon cancer among Fernald workers. Dr. Gartside examined the cause of death of 1,371 Fernald workers who died from 1953 to 1991 and found much higher levels of colon, liver, and other gastrointestinal cancers, lung and respiratory cancers, and blood and lymph cancers. He also found that the median life expectancy of Fernald workers was 58 years, five years less than the median life expectancy of all Americans from 1953 to 1991. (See Keith Schneider, "Study of Nuclear Workers Finds High Cancer Rates," *New York Times,* 13 April, 1994.)

    a. What responsibility does a government have to workers in such high-risk areas as atomic weapons factories?

    b. Given that the federal government acknowledged the Fernald case in their January 2000 report, how do we assign blame and address compensation?

    c. To what extent should employers be held financially and legally responsible (e.g., for medical cost) when workers suffer occupational health risks?

11. Mickey Mantle, a baseball star who was stricken with cirrhosis of the liver through longtime alcohol abuse, received a liver transplant ahead of others who had been waiting much longer. Because his own behavior was the root of his medical problems, some argued that Mantle did not deserve to qualify for a liver transplant, especially given that demand for donated livers far exceeds the supply. In contrast, others argued against using lifestyle to disqualify Mantle, saying that by this criterion, people who have fat-laden diets would

similarly be rejected for transplants, and only the small number of those who meet some strict social criterion would "deserve" an organ transplant. Make the best case you can for or against using a lifestyle criterion (which you can set out if you wish) as a factor in allocating scarce resources such as organs.

12. Here is a different sort of love story to look at:

In October 1994, Victoria Ingram and her diabetic fiancé Randall Curlee got married knowing that Victoria had something very precious Randall wanted—her kidney. A month after their hospital wedding, Randall received a kidney from Victoria, capping off what many considered the perfect love story. However, within 6 months, he had lost his eyesight, due to the advanced diabetes, and has suffered other complications. Their marriage feeling the strain of Randall's health problems, Victoria lamented how busy she was with her own life and with being Randall's "seeing eye dog as well." (For a discussion of the case, see "In Hospital Honeymoon, Bride to Donate Kidney to Diabetic Groom," *Los Angeles Times,* October 8, 1994; and Michael Granberry, "Reality Sets In: Blindness Dims Couple's Postoperative Optimism," *Los Angeles Times,* April 6, 1995.)

Answer the following:
   a. Should there be restrictions (in the form of laws, hospital guidelines, or AMA prohibitions) against a person's being allowed to donate a kidney to his or her spouse? Set out the ethical issues and concerns.
   b. Selling or buying a kidney is against the law in this country. If Victoria Ingram-Curlee could donate her kidney to her husband, would it be qualitatively different for her to sell her kidney to the highest bidder to get money to help with her husband?
   c. Selling or buying a kidney is against the law in this country. Assuming Victoria had no second kidney to donate or was not a suitable match, would it be qualitatively different for her to buy a kidney to help her husband?

13. What rights do we have regarding organ sales and donations? Read the following and then set out your position as to whether such organ "donations" are gifts or a form of organ sales:

Starting in the year 2000, Pennsylvania will begin a program whereby families of organ donors would be paid $300 toward funeral expenses, with the amount paid directly to funeral homes. The reason for this radical departure from the norm is that the demand for human organs is vastly greater than the supply. A potential conflict is the prohibition by the National Organ Transplant Act of 1984 of organ sales. The question is whether or not Howard Nathan, member of the governor's advisory panel, is correct in his assessment that "This is absolutely not buying and selling organs." Rather, he claims, "This is about having a voluntary death benefit for a family who gave a gift." (See Sheryl Fay Stolberg, "Pennsylvania Set to Break Taboo on Reward for Organ Donations," *New York Times,* 5 May 1999.)

14. In a sting operation, the FBI confirmed suspicions of human rights violations in China— namely, an attempt to sell organs taken from the bodies of executed Chinese prisoners. Inferring that there is proof of a thriving market in body parts, the U.S. State Department deemed credible the allegations made by human rights groups and brought to the attention of the FBI by activist Harry Wu. (See Christopher Drew, "U.S. Says 2 Chinese Offered Organs from the Executed," *New York Times,* 24 February 1998.)
   a. State the case for harvesting organs from executed prisoners.
   b. State the case against harvesting organs from executed prisoners.

c. Would the situation be viewed differently if the prisoners' families were compensated? Share your reflections.

15. Share your ideas on how we should balance patient rights with recommended medical treatment in the case of Lee Lor, 15, a member of the Hmong community in Fresno, California:

The 15 year-old girl, Lee Lor, ran away from home after a Fresno judge overruled the family's desire to use a Hmong shaman to treat her ovarian cancer and ordered chemotherapy as treatment. The case struck a nerve among the tens of thousands of Hmong refugees who have settled in the San Joaquin Valley, pitting their 16th-century tribal customs against modern American medicine. Police attempting to remove the girl so she could start chemotherapy were pelted with stones. Lee's family insist that they have the right to seek herbal and spiritual remedies for their daughter before opting for Western medicine—procedures that they believe desecrate the soul and block reincarnation. To the Hmong community Lee was a prime candidate for marriage and motherhood and she would likely fetch a fine dowry; but the removal of her ovary would threaten her future marital prospects. Hospital officials pointed out that Lee needed to begin chemotherapy within weeks of her Sept. 26 cancer surgery or her chances of survival would drop from 80% to 10%. The Lors said they would never trust American doctors again, not after being told that their daughter suffered appendicitis only to discover—three days after the surgery—that one of her ovaries and a Fallopian tube were gone. Ernest Velasquez, the head of county social services which sought and won the court order forcing chemotherapy, acknowledged that officials might have done a better job communicating with Hmong leaders and the family, but claim the family was informed of the cancer right after the surgery. (Adapted from Mark Arax, "Cancer Case Ignites Culture Clash," *Los Angeles Times,* November 21, 1994.)

16. To what degree do you think culture is a factor in women's health care? After reading the following, share your thoughts on the role of culture in medical decision making:

Two recent consensus statements, one from the USA and one from France, made recommendations about clinical management of women with an inherited predisposition to breast cancer and ovarian cancer. . . . Both papers conclude that prophylactic mastectomy [the removal of a breast without evidence of cancer] and oophorectomy [the removal of ovaries] are an option for women at high risk despite incomplete evidence and documentation of cancers in some women who have had the procedures. Their approach to decision-making, however, differs substantially. The French document describes each procedure as "a mutilation . . . (which) should be envisaged for medical reasons only." Doctors should, the document continues, "oppose" prophylactic mastectomy under age 30 and prophylactic oophorectomy for women under age 35 and should consider them respectively only when the risk of breast cancer is more than 60% and the risk of ovarian cancer is more than 20%. Under French law, a physician cannot invade a patient's bodily integrity unless there is a clear therapeutic justification, even if previous permission for such invasion has been granted. . . . Thus, in France, although the patient's consent is necessary before a surgeon can proceed to prophylactic surgery, it is not sufficient in the absence of medical justification. The French document further recommends that women wait several months before considering either procedure. In the USA, valid informed consent is sufficient for procedures to take place. The US paper does not recognise the possibility of active opposition to a woman's intention of suggesting a delay. (See "Cultural basis for differences between US and French clinical recommendations for women at increased risk of breast and ovarian cancer," *The Lancet,* 13 March 1999.)

InfoTrac College Edition

1. U.S. Dept. of Health and Human Resources, "Not All Health Plan Consumers Protected Equally, Study Finds"
2. Eliot Marshall, "Panel Faults Research Consent Process"
3. Lynne Snyder, "Integrating American Indians and Alaska Natives into the Body Politic?"
4. Jon Ross, "Who Are They, Where Are They, and How Do We Talk to Them? Hispanic Americans"
5. Luisa Dillner, "Shackling Prisoners In Hospital: Contravenes International Law"
6. Michele Bloch, "A Year of Living Dangerously"
7. U.S. Dept. of Health and Human Resources Report, "Comprehensive Survey of Working Women's Health Issues"
8. Theodore H. Tulchinsky, "The Measles Tragedy Revisited"
9. Ernest Drucker, "Drug Prohibition and Public Health: 25 Years of Evidence"
10. Judith MacKay, "The Global Tobacco Epidemic: The Next 25 Years"
11. Leonard S. Miller, Xiulan Zhang, Dorothy P. Rice, and Wendy Max, "State Estimates of Total Medical Expenditures Attributable to Cigarette Smoking, 1993"
12. Virginia I. Postrel, "Fatalist Attraction: The Dubious Case against Fooling Mother Nature"
13. Elizabeth C. Kaltman, "Living Downstream: An Ecologist Looks at Cancer and the Environment"
14. Carol Browner, "Smog and Soot: Updating Air Quality Standards"
15. Marion Nestle, "The Selling of Olestra"
16. Suzette J. Middleton, "Proctor and Gamble Responds on Olestra"
17. Doug Brugge, Andrew Leong, and Zenobia Lai, "Can a Community Inject Public Health Values into Transportation Questions?"
18. Bruce C. Wolpe, "Australians Swift and Decisive on Gun Violence"

Web Connections

For links to Rights and Obligations in Health Care Web sites, articles, cases, and more exercises go to our Rights and Obligations page at philosophy.wadsworth.com/teays.purdy/rights.

Chapter 3

Medical Experimentation: Historical Considerations

THE HISTORY OF medical experimentation is a history of risk vs. benefit. One issue is who is put at risk and who stands to benefit. As we will see in this chapter, this history warrants our attention and offers us the opportunity to reflect on the individual will to live, our societal values about the nature of sacrifice for the collective good, and the values of the medical profession.

In thinking about medical experimentation, we may conjure up images of mad scientists victimizing subjects. Popular culture provides us with many such examples: the mutant clones of *Alien Resurrection,* Frankenstein's monster, the Hitler clones of *The Boys from Brazil,* and so on. Alternatively, we might picture patients struggling with a disease so far advanced that doctors offer little hope with traditional medicine. In this scenario, patients willingly undergo experimental treatment in a search for a cure or to buy more time.

At times, patients attempt extreme measures to halt the progress of their medical condition. For example, AIDS patient Jeff Getty underwent a highly experimental transplant using baboon bone marrow, actor Steve McQueen sought to cure his cancer with an experimental course of Laetrile, patient Barney Clark underwent the first human heart transplant, comedian Gilda Radner tried experimental plutonium treatments for her ovarian cancer, and newborn Baby Fae underwent an experimental heart transplant using a baboon heart in her parents' effort to save her life. Although only Jeff Getty appeared to have benefited from his experimental treatment—and even that is debatable—all serve as illustrations of potentially therapeutic medical experimentation using a human subject.

ETHICAL ISSUES AND CONCERNS IN EXPERIMENTATION

Even when patients give consent (not possible in the case of Baby Fae), ethical issues arise. These include questions about how "informed" and "voluntary" is the consent when the patient's life is on the line and the patient is also struggling with family or other pressures. There are also concerns about patients and families being harmed by false hopes and risks with low probability of success. And there are concerns about exploiting vulnerable populations such as the terminally ill in the quest for knowledge.

The stark reality is that no medical experimentation is without risk. For instance, patients seeking to alleviate their symptoms quite willingly agreed to participate in a hepatitis B experiment. Unfortunately, the experiment not only worsened the condition of some but led directly to the death of several others. All subjects of experiments incur risks, and sometimes those risks are grave. The question then becomes when, if ever, such risks are justified. What protections need to be put in place to prevent abuse or the unnecessary suffering of research subjects?

Nontherapeutic experimentation also raises questions. In this case, subjects have no hope of any direct therapeutic benefit from the experiment itself. Rather, they are being expected to make a sacrifice for the benefit of others; the hope is that helpful knowledge will be added to the scientific data base. Those used in nontherapeutic experiments may reap the rewards of appreciation on the part of others for their altruism, the satisfaction of contributing to scientific progress, or just the joy of helping others less fortunate than themselves.

Nevertheless, many see a downside to nontherapeutic medical experimentation. Some question whether the use of subjects, even with their consent, can be justified in experiments that could never directly benefit them. Others wonder how anyone in a nontherapeutic experiment, particularly when it is high-risk, can be said to give informed consent. Some raise concerns about abuse and injustice when the subjects themselves are in institutions such as prisons or nursing homes, where they are especially vulnerable to coercion and intimidation. Even despite regulatory boards and policy guidelines, medical experiments are not always closely monitored, and thus the risk of abuse is present.

We must also be alert to the possibility that researchers may be more reckless when populations, such as those in prisons or the third world, are regarded as having low social worth. For instance, one hypothesis regarding how HIV, the AIDS virus, entered the human population posits that it was through a malaria experiment conducted on prisoners: In an attempt to find a cure for malaria, researchers injected blood from mangabey monkeys into prisoner subjects. Since mangabeys carry the HIV-2 virus, this scenario might explain how humans got the disease. Even though it is a hypothesis and not a proven fact, such experiments may raise further questions.

As we will see in this chapter, medical experimentation has a long and troubled history. Medical experimentation appears to be necessary if society is to learn more about the diagnosis and treatment of disease. Supporters believe it is warranted even if some members of the society are harmed. Others raise concern about the potential for abuse and point to the extent to which human rights have been violated in the pursuit of progress, as we see in Diana Axelsen's article on Dr. Sims' gynecological experiments conducted on slave women and Paul Ramsey's article on the use of children in the Willowbrook studies.

Advocates of the use of human subjects tend to see it as a necessary evil, arguing that animal experimentation by itself would never be a sufficient research tool in addressing medical problems of human beings. They claim that animal experimentation, however valuable, can provide only a limited amount of data relevant to humans. Unfortunately, the history of medical experimentation shows that progress has sometimes come at a high price. Finding individuals willing to undertake risks on behalf of others is not always easy, and researchers have occasionally turned to captive populations such as prisoners, retarded children, the sick and dying, ethnic minorities, and soldiers for use in medical experiments. Sometimes this has been done with the subject's voluntary, if not informed, consent; sometimes not. Sometimes the experiments have potentially therapeutic value for the subjects themselves; sometimes not.

Ethical issues and concerns regarding medical experimentation include the following:

- Who should be conscripted as subjects?

- Might there be circumstances that would justify conducting an experiment without the subject's consent?

- Should society have the right to use some of its citizens, such as prisoners or soldiers, to conduct medical experiments that might benefit the society as a whole?

- Is it necessary that an independent review board or committee oversee medical experiments?

- To what degree, if at all, should researchers themselves be required to serve in an experiment?

- How do we resolve dilemmas regarding experimentation on animals, infants, fetuses, and embryos, and incompetent adults when no meaningful consent can be obtained?

In answering these questions, we are called to look at our most basic beliefs and values and ponder whether we think it morally permissible for individuals to be used or even sacrificed for the benefit of the society. We can learn by looking at the ethical issues and by examining some of the abuses that have occurred with medical experimentation. We need also to consider guidelines and codes that have been developed to shed a ray of light on the territory and help us find our way.

MEDICAL CODES AND EXPERIMENTATION

Many of the major medical codes do not address the topic of medical experimentation; the Hippocratic Oath is an early instance of such omission. The notion of patient rights was slow to achieve formal recognition—no doubt because the medical profession has been paternalistic throughout much of history. It is striking that the first AMA code, in 1847, contained more obligations on the part of patients to physicians than physicians to patients. The closest the physician has to come to informing the patient is in the promotion of consultations in difficult cases. Even then, the code itself does not require the physician to explain why such consultation is deemed necessary.

Fortunately, much has changed in this regard as medical professionals have grown to accept the patient as a necessary participant in medical decision making. That we still have a far way to go is obvious from the sorts of abuses documented here and in Chapter 4. We shall see here the significance of the Nuremberg Code and later guidelines for the use of research subjects, and the importance of abiding by strict standards in the use of research subjects.

Certainly there is a long history of the use of animals and humans in medical experiments, a history that is weighted in favor of researchers rather than subjects of experiments. One of the more egregious cases, the Nazi experiments on (mostly Jewish) prisoners during World War II, resulted in the creation of the Nuremberg Code in 1947, after the war ended. The Nuremberg Code is a formal document that puts the human subject at the center of concern: It gives individual rights and dignity precedence over any societal benefits. It mandates voluntary consent of the human subject and requires that researchers be qualified to undertake experiments. To eliminate superfluous or random experimentation, the code requires that human studies be preceded by animal studies. Furthermore, to eliminate disregard for human suffering, it requires that researchers be willing to serve as subjects in the experiment and stipulates that the expected benefits cannot take precedence over any serious risk to the human subject. Subjects must always have the right to refuse participation in the experiment and the right to withdraw at any time, and the experiment must be halted if, at any time, it becomes clear that subjects could suffer from a disabling injury or be killed.

The creation of the Nuremberg Code was an important moment in history, for the code recognizes the value of balancing risks and perceived benefits. It sets the standard that the protection of the individual subject always outweighs societal gains. Later codes, such as the Helsinki Declaration, refined, modified, and added to the Nuremberg Code and carved new ground by distinguishing therapeutic experiments from nontherapeutic experiments and addressing the issue of minors and proxy consent.

This expansion further affirmed the importance of individual rights and patient autonomy. It also made explicit the requirement that voluntary consent also be informed consent. Only this move can protect the individual liberty of human subjects, who must have a clear idea of what they are getting themselves into, be free to withdraw, and feel confident that researchers will not knowingly put them at grave risk and will stop if harm is foreseen. Without these constraints, the experiment is on tenuous ethical footing. As well, the Helsinki Declaration requires an independent review committee, a statement on the ethical considerations of the experiment, and, to minimize redundant research, publication of the results of the experiment.

ISSUES RAISED BY MEDICAL EXPERIMENTATION

Cases such as the Nazi experiments, the Tuskegee Syphilis Study on poor, black men in Alabama, and the Willowbrook Study on retarded children point to the range of concerns regarding medical experimentation. These include the following questions:

- Is the potential value sufficient to justify the experiment?

- What counts as an acceptable risk?

- Are the human subjects properly informed of risks and benefits?

- Is their informed and voluntary consent obtained before proceeding?

- Is the experiment therapeutic or nontherapeutic? Should we allow nontherapeutic experimentation when there are known nontrivial risks to the human subjects?

- Should we allow nontherapeutic experimentation when the subjects give their consent?

- Should we allow nontherapeutic experimentation without the subjects' consent when we see potential for a significant contribution to society?

- Is it right to use animals for research solely for the benefit of humans? Should there be set guidelines for the treatment of animals in medical experimentation?

- Is it morally permissible to use subjects whose consent cannot be obtained (e.g., embryos, fetuses, retarded people, the comatose)?

- Should we allow experiments with the potential for global disaster (e.g., cloning, biowarfare experiments, animal-human hybrids, xenografts)?

- How should we constitute an independent review board to oversee medical experimentation?

Most people grant the necessity of some degree of medical experimentation. Controversy arises when we turn to the issue of who, or what, will be the subjects and what is allowable in the duration, methods, and criteria used for evaluating such experiments. The decision by the Clinton administration to issue an official apology to those who participated as human subjects in the Tuskegee Syphilis Study is testimony to the ethical dimensions of medical experimentation. In apologizing for one of the most egregious medical experiments in American history, the administration recognized the lamentable role of federal officials and research scientists in violating a fundamental guideline of all legitimate experiments—informed consent.

Informed, and therefore voluntary, consent is the basis of all ethical experiments using human subjects. Where informed consent has been omitted, as in the Tuskegee case, serious questions must be asked about the ethics of the researchers themselves. Similar questions arise when the experiments take place under coercive circumstances, such as in Dr. Sims' experiments on slave women and Nazi experiments on Jewish prisoners. As a consequence, some wonder whether using the results obtained from such experiments can be morally justified, believing that the data is tainted by both the inhumanity of the research methods and the lack of any control group. In other words, they reject using the data on both human rights and scientific grounds.

A related controversy is how we should regard nontherapeutic experimentation performed without the informed consent of the subjects themselves, such as children or the incapacitated. For example, in the Willowbrook hepatitis study described in Paul Ramsey's article in this chapter, parents were asked to give consent for their mentally retarded children to be injected with the hepatitis virus. With no direct benefits to the children in the study, ethicists have debated whether such experiments could ever be justified, particularly since the parents may have felt coerced to allow their children to be used.

The readings in this chapter address a number of key issues regarding medical experimentation. The medical codes surveyed in the first section reveal the ethical foundation of the medical profession—its values, beliefs, and expectations. They help us see the degree to which medical professionals are held to a set of standards and how those standards have changed throughout the years. They also act as a catalyst for reflecting on patient rights and the standards that govern the relationships between patients and health caregivers and among members of the medical team. The readings in the first section are:

1. A Patient's Bill of Rights (American Hospital Association)

2. Patients' Bill of Rights Act of 1998, bill outline

3. Hippocratic Oath and a Christian version of the oath

4. Four versions of the AMA code (1846, 1957, 1980, and 1990)

5. The American Nurses Association Code

6. The American Physical Therapy Association Code

7. The Canadian Medical Association Code of Ethics

8. The Nuremberg Code

9. The Helsinki Declaration

10. Selections from the National Institutes of Health (NIH) guidelines for protection of human subjects

11. In the last reading in this section, Jonathan M. Eisenberg discusses the NIH guidelines with respect to women and minorities.

The second section presents philosophical and historical considerations:

1. Candace Cummins Gauthier examines the importance of patient autonomy—its significance for truth telling, informed consent, and confidentiality—drawing on the philosophers Immanuel Kant and John Stuart Mill.

2. Daniel Wikler and Jeremiah Barondess discuss what we can learn from atrocities committed by Nazi doctors that can be applied to such contemporary bioethical issues as the euthanasia debate.

3. Todd L. Savitt examines the use in the Old South of African Americans for medical experimentation and demonstration. As he details, slaves had few rights and in some cases were purchased for the sole purpose of experimentation.

4. Diana Axelsen describes Dr. J. Marion Sims' use of slave women in gynecological experiments in the mid-1800s, demonstrating his lack of concern for his subjects. By detailing how their very servitude meant their participation was involuntary, Axelsen underscores how important are the notions of voluntary and informed consent.

5. Arthur L. Caplan looks at the Tuskegee Syphilis Study, detailing how its legacy reflects on the ethical conduct of the researchers as well as raising questions about the scientific value of the experiments themselves.

6. Vanessa N. Gamble discusses the ways in which distrust of the medical profession predates the Tuskegee study and contends that it is racism that we must address before there will be any dramatic change in African-Americans' attitudes about the medical profession.

7. Paul Ramsey examines the justifications made for the use of retarded children in the Willowbrook hepatitis studies. He concludes that, in light of the abuses, we ought not allow the use of children in nontherapeutic medical experimentation.

Medical Codes

A Patient's Bill of Rights

AMERICAN HOSPITAL ASSOCIATION

A PATIENT'S BILL OF RIGHTS was first adopted by the American Hospital Association in 1973. This revision was approved by the AHA Board of Trustees on October 21, 1992.

INTRODUCTION

Effective health care requires collaboration between patients and physicians and other health care professionals. Open and honest communication, respect for personal and professional values, and sensitivity to differences are integral to optimal patient care. As the setting for the provision of health services, hospitals must provide a foundation for understanding and respecting the rights and responsibilities of patients, their families, physicians, and other caregivers. Hospitals must ensure a health care ethic that respects the role of patients in decision making about treatment choices and other aspects of their care. Hospitals must be sensitive to cultural, racial, linguistic, religious, age, gender, and other differences as well as the needs of persons with dis-

abilities. The American Hospital Association presents A Patient's Bill of Rights with the expectation that it will contribute to more effective patient care and be supported by the hospital on behalf of the institution, its medical staff, employees, and patients. The American Hospital Association encourages health care institutions to tailor this bill of rights to their patient community by translating and/or simplifying the language of this bill of rights as may be necessary to ensure that patients and their families understand their rights and responsibilities.

BILL OF RIGHTS

These rights can be exercised on the patient's behalf by a designated surrogate or proxy decision maker if the patient lacks decision-making capacity, is legally incompetent, or is a minor.

1. The patient has the right to considerate and respectful care.

2. The patient has the right to and is encouraged to obtain from physicians

and other direct caregivers relevant, current, and understandable information concerning diagnosis, treatment, and prognosis.

Except in emergencies when the patient lacks decision-making capacity and the need for treatment is urgent, the patient is entitled to the opportunity to discuss and request information related to the specific procedures and/or treatments, the risks involved, the possible length of recuperation, and the medically reasonable alternatives and their accompanying risks and benefits.

Patients have the right to know the identity of physicians, nurses, and others involved in their care, as well as when those involved are students, residents, or other trainees. The patient also has the right to know the immediate and long-term financial implications of treatment choices, insofar as they are known.

3. The patient has the right to make decisions about the plan of care prior to and during the course of treatment and to refuse a recommended treatment or plan of care to the extent permitted by law and hospital policy and to be informed of the medical consequences of this action. In case of such refusal, the patient is entitled to other appropriate care and services that the hospital provides or transfer to another hospital. The hospital should notify patients of any policy that might affect patient choice within the institution.

4. The patient has the right to have an advance directive (such as a living will, health care proxy, or durable power of attorney for health care) concerning treatment or designating a surrogate decision maker with the expectation that the hospital will honor the intent of that directive to the extent permitted by law and hospital policy.

Health care institutions must advise patients of their rights under state law and hospital policy to make informed medical choices, ask if the patient has an advance directive, and include that information in patient records. The patient has the right to timely information about hospital policy that may limit its ability to implement fully a legally valid advance directive.

5. The patient has the right to every consideration of privacy. Case discussion, consultation, examination, and treatment should be conducted so as to protect each patient's privacy.

6. The patient has the right to expect that all communications and records pertaining to his/her care will be treated as confidential by the hospital, except in cases such as suspected abuse and public health hazards when reporting is permitted or required by law. The patient has the right to expect that the hospital will emphasize the confidentiality of this information when it releases it to any other parties entitled to review information in these records.

7. The patient has the right to review the records pertaining to his/her medical care and to have the information explained or interpreted as necessary, except when restricted by law.

8. The patient has the right to expect that, within its capacity and policies, a hospital will make reasonable response to the request of a patient for appropriate and medically indicated care and services. The hospital must provide evaluation, service, and/or referral as indicated by the urgency of the case. When medically appropriate and legally permissible, or when a patient has so requested, a patient may be transferred to another facility. The institution to which the patient is to

be transferred must first have accepted the patient for transfer. The patient must also have the benefit of complete information and explanation concerning the need for, risks, benefits, and alternatives to such a transfer.

9. The patient has the right to ask and be informed of the existence of business relationships among the hospital, educational institutions, other health care providers, or payers that may influence the patient's treatment and care.

10. The patient has the right to consent to or decline to participate in proposed research studies or human experimentation affecting care and treatment or requiring direct patient involvement, and to have those studies fully explained prior to consent. A patient who declines to participate in research or experimentation is entitled to the most effective care that the hospital can otherwise provide.

11. The patient has the right to expect reasonable continuity of care when appropriate and to be informed by physicians and other caregivers of available and realistic patient care options when hospital care is no longer appropriate.

12. The patient has the right to be informed of hospital policies and practices that relate to patient care, treatment, and responsibilities. The patient has the right to be informed of available resources for resolving disputes, grievances, and conflicts, such as ethics committees, patient representatives, or other mechanisms available in the institution. The patient has the right to be informed of the hospital's charges for services and available payment methods.

The collaborative nature of health care requires that patients, or their families/surrogates, participate in their care. The effectiveness of care and patient satisfaction with the course of treatment depend, in part, on the patient fulfilling certain responsibilities. Patients are responsible for providing information about past illnesses, hospitalizations, medications, and other matters related to health status. To participate effectively in decision making, patients must be encouraged to take responsibility for requesting additional information or clarification about their health status or treatment when they do not fully understand information and instructions. Patients are also responsible for ensuring that the health care institution has a copy of their written advance directive if they have one. Patients are responsible for informing their physicians and other caregivers if they anticipate problems in following prescribed treatment.

Patients should also be aware of the hospital's obligation to be reasonably efficient and equitable in providing care to other patients and the community. The hospital's rules and regulations are designed to help the hospital meet this obligation. Patients and their families are responsible for making reasonable accommodations to the needs of the hospital, other patients, medical staff, and hospital employees. Patients are responsible for providing necessary information for insurance claims and for working with the hospital to make payment arrangements, when necessary.

A person's health depends on much more than health care services. Patients are responsible for recognizing the impact of their lifestyle on their personal health.

CONCLUSION

Hospitals have many functions to perform, including the enhancement of health status, health promotion, and the prevention and treatment of injury and disease; the immediate and ongoing care and rehabilitation of patients; the education of health professionals, patients, and the community; and research. All these activities must be conducted with an overriding concern for the values and dignity of patients.

Patients' Bill of Rights Act of 1998

BILL OUTLINE

Access to Care

Choice of Plans. Choice is one of the key components of consumer satisfaction with the health system. The Democratic bill would allow a limited point of service option (POS) for employees who are offered only a closed panel HMO. The health plan, not the employer, would be required to make the POS available, and they employer would not be required to contribute to the point of service option.

Adequacy of Provider Network. Plans must have a sufficient number, distribution, and variety of providers to ensure that all enrollees receive covered services on a timely basis.

Specialty Care. Patients with special conditions must have access to providers who have the requisite expertise to treat their problem. The Democratic bill allows for referrals for enrollees to go out of the plan's network for specialty care (at no extra cost to the enrollee) if there is no appropriate provider available in the network for covered services.

Chronic Care Referrals. For individuals who are seriously ill or require continued care by a specialist, plans must have a process for selecting a specialist as a primary care provider and for accessing necessary specialty care without impediments.

Women's Protections. The Democratic bill extends important protections for women in managed care, including direct access to ob/gyn care and services and the ability to designate their ob/gyn as a primary care provider. The proposal also includes bills regarding mastectomy length-of-stay and breast reconstruction.

Children's Protections. The Democratic bill ensures that the special needs of children are met, including access to pediatric specialists.

Continuity of Care. Patients should be protected against disruptions in care because of a change in plan or a change in a provider's network status. The Democratic bill lays out guidelines for the limited continuation of treatment in these instances. There are specific protections for pregnancy, terminal illness, and institutionalization.

Emergency Services. Individuals should be assured that if they have an emergency, those services will be covered by their plan. The Democratic bill says that individuals must have access to emergency care, without prior authorization in any situation that a "prudent lay person" would regard as an emergency.

Clinical Trials. Access to clinical trials can be the only hope left for individuals with serious and life-threatening diseases, especially when no standard treatment is effective. Plans must have a process for allowing certain enrollees to participate in a defined set of approved clinical trials and for covering the routine patient costs associated with these trials.

Drug Formularies. Prescription medications can not be one-size-fits all. For plans that use a formulary, the plan must have a process for beneficiaries to access medications that are not on the formulary when medically indicated. And, plan doctors and pharmacists must help in the formulary development.

Non-discrimination. Patients should not be discriminated against in their access to covered health care services. The Democratic bill prohibits plans from discriminating against their enrollees on a variety of factors including genetic information, sexual orientation, and disability. This provision does not affect issuance or pricing of policies.

Information

Health Plan Information. Informed decisions about health care options can only be made by consumers who have access to uniform, comparable information about health plans, plan policies, and providers. This bill requires managed care plans to provide that information.

Confidentiality. Patients need to know that their medical records are kept confidential. This bill says that health plans must have appropriate safeguards to ensure confidentiality, update records in a timely and accurate fashion, and allow patients access to their records. It does not address the broad issue of medical records confidentiality, which will require separate legislation.

Ombudsman. The health care marketplace can be confusing. The Democratic bill authorizes an ombudsman program in each state to assist consumers in understanding health insurance options, filing appeals and grievances, etc.

Quality Assurance and Improvement

Quality Assurance. In order to constantly improve the quality of health care provided, plans should be monitoring care given to their enrollees, especially with regard to at-risk or chronically ill populations. The Democratic bill requires plans to have a quality assurance program to monitor care and improve care.

Data Collection. The Democratic bill requires plans to collect data in order to monitor the quality of care provided to enrollees. Data must be in a standard format so comparisons can be made across all plans.

Advisory Board. A private/public Advisory Board would be established to advise the Secretary on the standardized minimum data set and other activities to improve health care quality.

Provider Selection. Plans should not discriminate against providers when selecting them for the network. The Democratic bill requires plans to have a written, objective process for provider selection and forbids discrimination against providers based on license, location or patient base. Plans would, however, be able to limit the number and mix of providers as needed to serve enrollees for covered benefits.

Utilization Review. When a plan is reviewing the medical decisions of its practitioners, it should do so in a fair and rational manner. The Democratic bill lays out basic criteria for a good utilization review program: physician participation in development of review criteria, administration by appropriately qualified professionals, timely decisions, and ability to appeal.

Grievance and Appeals

Internal Grievances. Patients need to be able to appeal denials of care and voice concerns about their plans. They also should have their concerns addressed in a timely manner. Plans must maintain an internal grievance process that is expedient and conducted by appropriately credentialed individuals. There also must be an expedited process for special circumstances.

External Grievances. For cases of sufficient seriousness or beyond a certain monetary threshold, individuals must have access to an external, independent body with the capability and authority to resolve these cases. In the Democratic bill, States and the Department of Labor must establish an independent external appeals process for the plans under their respective jurisdictions. The plan must pay the costs of the process, and any decision is binding on the plan. Plans may not retaliate against providers who advocate on behalf of their patients nor against patients who choose to access the appeals process.

The Hippocratic Oath

THE HIPPOCRATIC OATH

1. I swear by Apollo Physician and Asclepius and Hygieia and Panaceia and all the gods and goddesses, making them my witnesses, that I will fulfill according to my ability and judgment this oath and this covenant:

2. To hold him who has taught me this art as equal to my parents and to live my life in partnership with him, and if he is in need of money to give him a share of mine, and to regard his offspring as equal to my brothers in male lineage and to teach them this art—if they desire to learn it—without fee and covenant; to give a share of precepts and oral instruction and all the other learning to my sons and to the sons of him who has instructed me and to pupils who have signed the covenant and have taken an oath according to the medical law, but to no one else.

3. I will apply dietetic measures for the benefit of the sick according to my ability and judgment; I will keep them from harm and injustice.

4. I will neither give a deadly drug to anybody if asked for it, nor will I make a suggestion to this effect. Similarly I will not give to a woman an abortive remedy. In purity and holiness I will guard my life and my art.

5. I will not use the knife, not even on sufferers from stone, but will withdraw in favor of such men as are engaged in this work.

6. Whatever houses I may visit, I will come for the benefit of the sick, remaining free of all intentional injustice, of all mischief and in particular of sexual relations with both female and male persons, be they free or slaves.

Ludwig Edelstein, "The Hippocratic Oath: Text, Translation, and Interpretation," in Bulletin of the History of Medicine, *Supplement 1. (1943). Reprinted with permission of The Johns Hopkins Press.*

7. What I may see or hear in the course of the treatment or even outside of the treatment in regard to the life of men, which on no account one must spread abroad, I will keep to myself holding such things shameful to be spoken about.

8. If I fulfill this oath and do not violate it, may it be granted to me to enjoy life and art, being honored with fame among all men for all time to come; if I transgress it and swear falsely, may the opposite of all this be my lot.

The Oath According to Hippocrates Insofar as a Christian May Swear It

BLESSED BE GOD the Father of our Lord Jesus Christ, who is blessed for ever and ever; I lie not.

I will bring no stain upon the learning of the medical art. Neither will I give poison to anybody though asked to do so, nor will I suggest such a plan. Similarly I will not give treatment to women to cause abortion, treatment neither from above nor from below. But I will teach this art, to those who require to learn it, without grudging and without an indenture. I will use treatment to help the sick according to my ability and judgment.

And in purity and in holiness I will guard my art. Into whatsoever houses I enter, I will do so to help the sick, keeping myself free from all wrongdoing, intentional or unintentional, tending to death or to injury, and from fornication with bond or free, man or woman. Whatsoever in the course of practice I see or hear (or outside my practice in social intercourse) that ought not be published abroad, I will not divulge, but consider such things to be holy secrets.

Now if I keep this oath and break it not, may God be my helper in my life and art, and may I be honored among all men for all time. If I keep faith, well; but if I forswear myself may the opposite befall me.

From W. H. S. Jones, The Doctor's Oath: An Essay in the History of Medicine, *(1924), pp. 23–25.*
Reprinted by permission of Cambridge University Press.

Four AMA Codes of Medical Ethics

AMERICAN MEDICAL ASSOCIATION

FIRST CODE OF MEDICAL ETHICS (1847)

[The following consists of key points taken from this first code, as the original document is long and involved.]

Introduction to the Code: Medical ethics, as a branch of general ethics, must rest on the basis of religion and morality. They comprise not only the duties, but also the rights of a physician; and, in this sense, they are identical with Medical Deontology—a term introduced by a late writer, who has taken the most comprehensive view of the subject.

All persons privileged to enter the sick room, and the number ought to be very limited, are under equal obligations of reciprocal courtesy, kindness and respect.

Physicians "should have control over himself as not to betray strong emotion in the presence of his patient."

They "must be ever ready and prompt to administer professional aid to all applicants, without prior stipulation of personal advantages to themselves."

Physicians "are enabled to exhibit the close connection between hygiene and morals" and "are bound to bear emphatic testimony against quackery in all forms."

"A physician in attendance on a case should avoid expensive complications and tedious ceremonials, as being beneath the dignity of true science and embarrassing to the patient and his family, whose troubles are already great."

Code of Medical Ethics (key points)

Art. 1: Duties of Physicians to their Patients

1. A physician's mind "ought . . . to be imbued with the greatness of his mission and the responsibility he . . . incurs"

2. Treat every case with attention & humanity. Secrecy and delicacy [confidentiality] should be strictly observed.

3. Frequent visits are usually requisite, but avoid unnecessary visits.

4. "A physician should be forward to make gloomy prognostications." He "should not fail, on proper occasions, to give to the friends of the patient timely notice of danger, when it really occurs, and even to the patient himself, if absolutely necessary."

5. A physician ought not abandon a patient who is deemed incurable.

6. Promote consultations in difficult cases.

7. Promote & strengthen the good resolutions of patients—shows sincere interest in the welfare of the patient.

Art. II. Obligations of Patients to Physicians

1. Doctors have the right to expect patients to hold a sense of just duty to their physicians.

2. "The first duty of a patient is, to selection as his medical advisor one who has received a regular professional education."

3. Patients should prefer physicians whose "habits of life are regular," and they

Reprinted by permission of the American Medical Association.

should "confide the care of himself and family, as much as possible, to one physician."

4. [disclosure]: Patients should "faithfully and unreservedly communicate to their physician the supposed cause of the disease."

5. Don't weary the physician with tedious details not pertaining to the disease.

6. Obedience to prescriptions should be prompt & implicit.

7. Avoid even the "friendly visits" of a physician who is not attending them, and never send for a consulting physician without the express consent of the physician.

8. If patient wishes to dismiss his physician "common courtesy require that he should declare his reasons for so doing."

9. Patients should always, when practicable, send for their physicians in the morning, before his usual hour of going out.

10. A patient should, after his recovery, entertain a just and enduring sense of the value of the service rendered him by his physician.

PRINCIPLES OF MEDICAL ETHICS (1957)

Preamble

These principles are intended to aid physicians individually and collectively in maintaining a high level of ethical conduct. They are not laws but standards by which a physician may determine the propriety of his conduct in his relationship with patients, with colleagues, with members of allied professions, and with the public.

Section 1

The principal objective of the medical profession is to render service to humanity with full respect for the dignity of man. Physicians should merit the confidence of patients entrusted to their care, rendering to each a full measure of service and devotion.

Section 2

Physicians should strive continually to improve medical knowledge and skill, and should make available to their patients and colleagues the benefits of their professional attainments.

Section 3

A physician should practice a method of healing founded on a scientific basis; and he should not voluntarily associate professionally with anyone who violates this principle.

Section 4

The medical profession should safeguard the public and itself against physicians deficient in moral character or professional competence. Physicians should observe all laws, uphold the dignity and honor of the profession and accept its self-imposed disciplines. They should expose, without hesitation, illegal or unethical conduct of fellow members of the profession.

Section 5

A physician may choose whom he will serve. In an emergency, however, he should render service to the best of his ability. Having undertaken the care of a patient, he may not neglect him; and unless he has been discharged he may discontinue his services only after giving adequate notice. He should not solicit patients.

Section 6

A physician should not dispose of his services under terms or conditions that tend to interfere with or impair the free and complete exercise of his medical judgment and skill or tend to cause a deterioration of the quality of medical care.

Section 7

In the practice of medicine a physician should limit the source of his professional income to medical services actually rendered by him, or under his supervision, to his patients. His fee should be commensurate with the service rendered and the patient's ability to pay. He should neither pay nor receive commission for referral of patients. Drugs, remedies or appliances may be dispensed or supplied by the physician provided it is in the best interests of the patient.

Section 8

A physician should seek consultation upon request; in doubtful or difficult cases; or whenever it appears that the quality of medical service may be enhanced thereby.

Section 9

A physician may not reveal the confidences entrusted to him in the course of medical attendance, or the deficiencies he may observe in the character of patients, unless he is required to do so by law or unless it becomes necessary in order to protect the welfare of the individual or of the community.

Section 10

The honored ideals of the medical profession imply that the responsibility of the physician extend not only to the individual, but also to society, and these responsibilities deserve his interest and participation in activities that have the purpose of improving both the health and the well-being of the individual and the community.

PRINCIPLES OF MEDICAL ETHICS (1980)

Preamble

The medical profession has long subscribed to a body of ethical statements developed primarily for the benefit of the patient. As a member of this profession, a physician must recognize responsibility not only to patients, but also to society, to other health professionals, and to self. The following Principles adopted by the American Medical Association are not laws, but standards of conduct which define the essentials of honorable behavior for the physician.

Principles

I.   A physician shall be dedicated to providing competent medical service with compassion and respect for human dignity.

II. A physician shall deal honestly with patients and colleagues, and strive to expose those physicians deficient in character or competence, or who engage in fraud or deception.

III. A physician shall respect the law and also recognize a responsibility to seek changes in those requirements which are contrary to the best interests of the patient.

IV. A physician shall respect the rights of patients, of colleagues, and of other health professionals, and shall safeguard patient confidences within the constraints of the law.

V.   A physician shall continue to study, apply and advance scientific knowledge, make relevant information available to patients, colleagues, and the public, obtain consultation, and use the talents of other health professionals when indicated.

VI. A physician shall, in the provision of appropriate patient care, except in emergencies, be free to choose whom to serve, with whom to associate, and the environment in which to provide medical services.

VII. A physician shall recognize a responsibility to participate in activities contributing to an improved community.

FUNDAMENTAL ELEMENTS OF THE PATIENT-PHYSICIAN RELATIONSHIP (1990)

From ancient times, physicians have recognized that the health and well-being of patients depends upon a collaborative effort between physician and patient. Patients share with physicians the responsibility for their own health care. The patient-physician relationship is of greatest benefit to patients when they bring medical problems to the attention of their physicians in a timely fashion, provide information about their medical condition to the best of their ability, and work with their physicians in a mutually respectful alliance. Physicians can best contribute to this alliance by serving as their patients' advocate and by fostering these rights:

1. The patient has the right to receive information from physicians and to discuss the benefits, risks, and costs of appropriate treatment alternatives. Patients should receive guidance from their physicians as to the optimal course of action. Patients are also entitled to obtain copies or summaries of their medical records, to have their questions answered, to be advised of potential conflicts of interest that their physicians might have, and to receive independent professional opinions.

2. The patient has the right to make decisions regarding the health care that is recommended by his or her physician. Accordingly, patients may accept or refuse any recommended medical treatment.

3. The patient has the right to courtesy, respect, dignity, responsiveness, and timely attention to his or her needs.

4. The patient has the right to confidentiality. The physician should not reveal confidential communications or information without the consent of the patient, unless provided for by law or by the need to protect the welfare of the individual or the public interest.

5. The patient has the right to continuity of health care. The physician has an obligation to cooperate in the coordination of medically indicated care with other health care providers treating the patient. The physician may not discontinue treatment of a patient as long as further treatment is medically indicated, without giving the patient sufficient opportunity to make alternative arrangements for care.

6. The patient has a basic right to have available adequate health care. Physicians, along with the rest of society, should continue to work toward this goal. Fulfillment of this right is dependent on society providing resources so that no patient is deprived of necessary care because of an inability to pay for the care. Physicians should continue their traditional assumption of a part of the responsibility for the medical care of those who cannot afford essential health care.

Code of Ethics for Nursing (1998)

AMERICAN NURSES ASSOCIATION

1. The nurse practices with compassion and respect for the inherent dignity, worth, and uniqueness of every individual.

2. The nurse's primary commitment is to the patient, whether an individual, family or community group.

3. The nurse safeguards, promotes and advocates for the health, safety and rights of the patient.

4. The nurse is responsible and accountable for individual nursing practice.

5. The nurse owes the same duties to self as to others; this, includes the responsibility to preserve integrity, maintain competence, and continue personal and professional growth.

6. The nurse participates in the advancement of the profession through contributions to practice, education, knowledge development and/or research.

7. The nurse participates in individual and collective action to establish, maintain and improve health care environments which are conducive to the provision of quality health care, consistent with the values of the profession and supportive of ethical practice.

8. The nurse collaborates with other health professionals and with the public in promoting community, national, and international efforts to meet health needs.

9. The profession of nursing, as represented by professional associations and their members, is responsible for the articulation of nursing values, for maintaining the integrity of standards of the profession and its practice.

Reprinted with permission from ANA Position Statement on the Nonnegotiable Nature of the ANA Code with Interpretive Statements, *copyright 1985. American Nurses Publishing, American Nurses Foundation/American Nurses Association, Washington, DC.*

Code of Ethics

AMERICAN PHYSICAL THERAPY ASSOCIATION

PREAMBLE

THIS *CODE OF ETHICS* sets forth ethical principles for the physical therapy profession. Members of this profession are responsible for maintaining and promoting ethical practice. This *Code of Ethics,* adopted by the American Physical Therapy Association, shall be binding on physical therapists who are members of the Association.

Principle 1

Physical therapists respect the rights and dignity of all individuals.

Principle 2

Physical therapists comply with the laws and regulations governing the practice of physical therapy.

Principle 3

Physical therapists accept responsibility for the exercise of sound judgment.

Principle 4

Physical therapists maintain and promote high standards for physical therapy practice, education, and research.

Principle 5

Physical therapists seek remuneration for their services that is deserved and reasonable.

Principle 6

Physical therapists provide accurate information to the consumer about the profession and about those services they provide.

Principle 7

Physical therapists accept the responsibility to protect the public and the profession from unethical, incompetent, or illegal acts.

Principle 8

Physical therapists participate in efforts to address the health needs of the public.

Adopted by the House of Delegates, June 1981. Amended June 1987, June 1991.

From Physical Therapy, *Vol. 79, no. 1, January 1999. Permission granted by the American Physical Therapy Association.*

Code of Ethics, The Canadian Medical Association

PRINCIPLES OF ETHICAL BEHAVIOUR for all physicians, including those who may not be engaged directly in clinical practice.

I   Consider first the well-being of the patient.

II   Honour your profession and its traditions.

III   Recognize your limitations and the special skills of others in the prevention and treatment of disease.

IV   Protect the patient's secrets.

V   Teach and be taught.

VI   Remember that integrity and professional ability should be your best advertisement.

VII   Be responsible in setting a value on your services.

GUIDE TO THE ETHICAL BEHAVIOUR OF PHYSICIANS

A physician should be aware of the standards established by tradition and act within the general principles which have governed professional conduct.

The Oath of Hippocrates represented the desire of the members of that day to establish for themselves standards of conduct in living and in the practice of their art. Since then the principles established have been retained as our basic guidelines for ethical living with the profession of medicine.

The International Code of Ethics and the Declaration of Geneva (1948), developed and approved by the World Medical Association, have modernized the ancient codes. They have been endorsed by each member organization, including The Canadian Medical Association, as a general guide having worldwide application.

The Canadian Medical Association accepts the responsibility of delineating the standard of ethical behaviour expected of Canadian physicians.

An interpretation of these principles is developed in the following pages, as a guide for individual physicians and provincial authorities.

Responsibilities to the Patient

An Ethical Physician:

Standard of Care

1. will practise the art and science of medicine to the best of his/her ability;
2. will continue self education to improve his/her standards of medical care;

Respect for Patient

3. will practise in a fashion that is above reproach and will take neither physical, emotional nor financial advantage of the patient;

Patient's Rights

4. will recognize his/her limitations and, when indicated, recommend to the patient that additional opinions and services be obtained;

5. will recognize that a patient has the right to accept or reject any physician and any medical care recommended. The patient having chosen a physician has the right to request of that physician opinions from other physicians of the patient's choice;

6. will keep in confidence information derived from a patient or from a colleague regarding a patient, and divulge it only with the permission of the patient except when otherwise required by law;

7. when acting on behalf of a third party will ensure that the patient understands the physician's legal responsibility to the third party before proceeding with the examination;

8. will recommend only diagnostic procedures that are believed necessary to assist in the care of the patient, and therapy that is believed necessary for the well-being of the patient. The physician will recognize a responsibility in advising the patient of the findings and recommendations and will exchange such information with the patient as is necessary for the patient to reach a decision;

9. will, on a patient's request, supply the information that is required to enable the patient to receive any benefits to which the patient may be entitled;

10. will be considerate of the anxiety of the patient's next-of-kin and cooperate with them in the patient's interest;

Choice of Patient

11. will recognize the responsibility of the physician to render medical service to any person regardless of colour, religion or political belief;

12. shall, except in an emergency, have the right to refuse to accept a patient;

13. will render all possible assistance to any patient, where an urgent need for medical care exists;

14. will, when the patient is unable to give consent and an agent of the patient is unavailable to give consent, render such therapy as the physician believes to be in the patient's interest;

Continuity of Care

15. will, if absent, ensure the availability of medical care to his/her patients if possible; will, once having accepted professional responsibility for an acutely ill patient, continue to provide services until they are no longer required, or until arrangements have been made for the services of another suitable physician; may, in any other situation, withdraw from the responsibility for the care of any patient provided that the patient is given adequate notice of that intention;

Personal Morality

16. will inform the patient when personal morality or religious conscience prevent the recommendation of some form of therapy;

Clinical Research

17. will ensure that, before initiating any clinical research involving humans, such research is appraised scientifically and ethically and approved by a responsible committee and is sufficiently planned and supervised that the individuals are unlikely to suffer any harm. The physician will ascertain that previous research

and the purpose of the experiment justify this additional method of investigation. Before proceeding, the physician will obtain the consent of all involved persons or their agents, and proceed only after explaining the purpose of the clinical investigation and any possible health hazard that can be reasonably forseen;

The Dying Patient

18. will allow death to occur with dignity and comfort when death of the body appears to be inevitable;

19. may support the body when clinical death of the brain has occurred, but need not prolong life by unusual or heroic means;

Transplantation

20. may, when death of the brain has occurred, support cellular life in the body when some parts of the body might be used to prolong the life or improve the health of others;

21. will recognize a responsibility to a donor of organs to be transplanted and will give to the donor or the donor's relatives full disclosure of the intent and purpose of the procedure; in the case of a living donor, the physician will also explain the risks of the procedure;

22. will refrain from determining the time of death of the donor patient if there is a possibility of being involved as a participant in the transplant procedure, or when his/her association with the proposed recipient might improperly influence professional judgement;

23. may treat the transplant recipient subsequent to the transplant procedure in spite of having determined the time of death of the donor;

Fees to Patients

24. will consider, in determining professional fees, both the nature of the service provided and the ability of the patient to pay, and will be prepared to discuss the fee with the patient.

Responsibilities to the Profession

An Ethical Physician:

Personal Conduct

25. will recognize that the profession demands integrity from each physician and dedication to its search for truth and its service to mankind;

26. will recognize that self discipline of the profession is a privilege and that each physician has a continuing responsibility to merit the retention of this privilege;

27. will behave in a way beyond reproach and will report to the appropriate professional body any conduct by a colleague which might be generally considered as being unbecoming to the profession;

28. will behave in such a manner as to merit the respect of the public for members of the medical profession;

29. will avoid impugning the reputation of any colleague;

Contracts

30. will, when aligned in practice with other physicians, insist that the standards enunciated in this Code of Ethics and the Guide to the Ethical Behaviour of Physicians be maintained;

31. will only enter into a contract regarding professional services which allows fees derived from physicians' services to be controlled by the physician rendering the services;

32. will enter into a contract with an organization only if it will allow maintainance of professional integrity;

33. will only offer to a colleague a contract which has terms and conditions equitable to both parties;

Reporting Medical Research

34. will first communicate to colleagues, through recognized scientific channels, the results of any medical research, in order that those colleagues may establish an opinion of its merits before they are presented to the public;

Addressing the Public

35. will recognize a responsibility to give the generally held opinions of the profession when interpreting scientific knowledge to the public; when presenting an opinion which is contrary to the generally held opinion of the profession, the physician will so indicate and will avoid any attempt to enhance his/her own professional reputation;

Advertising

36. will build a professional reputation based on ability and integrity, and will only advertise professional services or make professional announcements as regulated by legislation or as permitted by the provincial medical licensing authority;

37. will avoid advocacy of any product when identified as a member of the medical profession;

38. will avoid the use of secret remedies;

Consultation

39. will request the opinion of an appropriate colleague acceptable to the patient when diagnosis or treatment is difficult or obscure, or when the patient requests it. Having requested the opinion of a colleague, the physician will make available all relevant information and indicate clearly whether the consultant is to assume the continuing care of the patient during this illness;

40. will, when consulted by a colleague, report in detail all pertinent findings and recommendations to the attending physician and may outline an opinion to the patient. The consultant will continue with the care of the patient only at the specific request of the attending physician and with the consent of the patient;

Patient Care

41. will cooperate with those individuals who, in the opinion of the physician, may assist in the care of that patient;

42. will make available to another physician, upon the request of the patient, a report of pertinent findings and treatment of that patient;

43. will provide medical services to a colleague and dependent family without fee, unless specifically requested to render an account;

44. will limit self-treatment or treatment of family members to minor or emergency services only; such treatments should be without fee;

Financial Arrangements

45. will avoid any personal profit motive in ordering drugs, appliances or diagnostic procedures from any facility in which the physician has a financial interest;

46. will refuse to accept any commission or payment, direct or indirect, for any service rendered to a patient by other persons excepting direct employees and professional colleagues with whom there is a formal partnership or similar agreement.

The Nuremberg Code

The Nuremberg Code was the work of American judges who sat in judgment in the trial of 23 Nazi physicians and scientists accused of murder and torture while conducting medical experiments.*

1. The voluntary consent of the human subject is absolutely essential. This means that the person involved should have legal capacity to give consent; should be situated as to be able to exercise free power of choice, without the intervention of any element of force, fraud, deceit, duress, over-reaching, or other ulterior form of constraint or coercion, and should have sufficient knowledge and comprehension of the elements of the subject matter involved as to enable him to make an understanding and enlightened decision. This latter element requires that before the acceptance of an affirmative decision by the experimental subject there should be made known to him the nature, duration, and purpose of the experiment; the method and means by which it is to be conducted; all inconveniences and hazards reasonably to be expected; and the effects upon his health or person which may possibly come from his participation in the experiment. The duty and responsibility for ascertaining the quality of the consent rests upon each individual who initiates, directs or engages in the experiment. It is a personal duty and responsibility which may not be delegated to another with impunity.

2. The experiment should be such as to yield fruitful results for the good of society, unprocurable by other methods or means of study, and not random and unnecessary in nature.

3. The experiment should be so designed and based on the results of animal experimentation and a knowledge of the natural history of the disease or other problem under study that the anticipated results will justify the performance of the experiment.

4. The experiment should be so conducted as to avoid all unnecessary physical and mental suffering and injury.

5. No experiment should be conducted where there is an a priori reason to believe that death or disabling injury will occur; except, perhaps, in those experiments where the experimental physicians also serve as subjects.

6. The degree of risk to be taken should never exceed that determined by the humanitarian importance of the problem to be solved by the experiment.

7. Proper preparations should be made and adequate facilities provided to protect the experimental subject against even remote possibilities of injury, disability, or death.

8. The experiment should be conducted only by scientifically qualified persons.

*For a discussion of the code's significance, see Evelynne Shuster, "The Nuremberg Code: Hippocratic ethics and human rights," *The Lancet* 1998: 351: 974–77.

Reprinted from "Trials of War Criminals before the Nuremberg Military Tribunals" (Washington, D.C.: U.S. Government Printing Office, 1948).

The highest degree of skill and care should be required through all stages of the experiment of those who conduct or engage in the experiment.

9. During the course of the experiment the human subject should be at liberty to bring the experiment to an end if he has reached the physical or mental state where continuation of the experiment seems to him to be impossible.

10. During the course of the experiment the scientist in charge must be prepared to terminate the experiment at any stage, if he has probable cause to believe, in the exercise of the good faith, superior skill and careful judgement required by him that a continuation of the experiment is likely to result in injury, disability, or death to the experimental subject.

Declaration of Helsinki:
Recommendations Guiding Medical Doctors in Biomedical Research Involving Human Subjects

INTRODUCTION

It is the mission of the physician to safeguard the health of the people. His or her knowledge and conscience are dedicated to the fulfillment of this mission. The Declaration of Geneva of the World Medical Association binds the physician with the words, "The health of my patient will be my first consideration," and the International Code of Medical Ethics declares that, "A physician shall act only in the patient's interest when providing medical care which might have the effect of weakening the physical and mental condi-

Adopted by the 18th World Medical Assembly, Helsinki, Finland, 1964, and as revised by the World Medical Assembly in Tokyo, Japan, in 1975, in Venice, Italy, in 1983, and in Hong Kong in 1989.

tion of the patient." The Purpose of biomedical research involving human subjects must be to improve diagnostic, therapeutic and prophylactic procedures and the understanding of the aetiology and patho-genesis of disease. In current medical practice most diagnostic, therapeutic or prophylactic procedures involve hazards. This applies especially to biomedical research.

Medical progress is based on research which ultimately must rest in part on experimentation involving human subjects. In the field of biomedical research a fundamental distinction must be recognized between medical research in which the aim is essentially diagnostic or therapeutic for a patient, and medical research, the essential object of which is purely scientific and without implying direct diagnostic or therapeutic value to the person subjected to the research.

Permission granted by Frontiers in Bioscience: A Journal and Virtual Library (*http://www.bioscience.org*).

Special caution must be exercised in the conduct of research which may affect the environment, and the welfare of animals used for research must be respected.

Because it is essential that the results of laboratory experiments be applied to human beings to further scientific knowledge and to help suffering humanity, the World Medical Association has prepared the following recommendations as a guide to every physician in biomedical research involving human subjects. They should be kept under review in the future. It must be stressed that the standards as drafted are only a guide to physicians all over the world. Physicians are not relieved from criminal, civil and ethical responsibilities under the laws of their own countries.

I. BASIC PRINCIPLES

1. Biomedical research involving human subjects must conform to generally accepted scientific principles and should be based on adequately performed laboratory and animal experimentation and on a thorough knowledge of the scientific literature.

2. The design and performance of each experimental procedure involving human subjects should be clearly formulated in an experimental protocol which should be transmitted for consideration, comment and guidance to a specially appointed committee independent of the investigator and the sponsor provided that this independent committee is in conformity with the laws and regulations of the country in which the research experiment is performed.

3. Biomedical research involving human subjects should be conducted only by scientifically qualified persons and under the supervision of a clinically competent medical person. The responsibility for the human subject must always rest with a medically qualified person and never rest

on the subject of the research, even though the subject has given his or her consent.

4. Biomedical research involving human subjects cannot legitimately be carried out unless the importance of the objective is in proportion to the inherent risk to the subject.

5. Every biomedical research project involving human subjects should be preceded by careful assessment of predictable risks in comparison with foreseeable benefits to the subject or to others. Concern for the interests of the subject must always prevail over the interests of science and society.

6. The right of the research subject to safeguard his or her integrity must always be respected. Every precaution should be taken to respect the privacy of the subject and to minimize the impact of the study on the subject's physical and mental integrity and on the personality of the subject.

7. Physicians should abstain from engaging in research projects involving human subjects unless they are satisfied that the hazards involved are believed to be predictable. Physicians should cease any investigation if the hazards are found to outweigh the potential benefits.

8. In publication of the results of his or her research, the physician is obliged to preserve the accuracy of the results. Reports of experimentation not in accordance with the principles laid down in this Declaration should not be accepted for publication.

9. In any research on human beings, each potential subject must be adequately informed of the aims, methods, anticipated benefits and potential hazards of the study and the discomfort it may entail. He or she should be informed that

he or she is at liberty to abstain from participation in the study and that he or she is free to withdraw his or her consent to participation at any time. The physician should then obtain the subject's freely-given informed consent, preferably in writing.

10. When obtaining informed consent for the research project the physician should be particularly cautious if the subject is in a dependent relationship to him or her or may consent under duress. In that case the informed consent should be obtained by a physician who is not engaged in the investigation and who is completely independent of this official relationship.

11. In case of legal incompetence, informed consent should be obtained from the legal guardian in accordance with national legislation. Where physical or mental incapacity makes it impossible to obtain informed consent, or when the subject is a minor, permission from the responsible relative replaces that of the subject in accordance with national legislation. Whenever the minor child is in fact able to give a consent, the minor's consent must be obtained in addition to the consent of the minor's legal guardian.

12. The research protocol should always contain a statement of the ethical considerations involved and should indicate that the principles enunciated in the present Declaration are complied with.

II. MEDICAL RESEARCH COMBINED WITH PROFESSIONAL CARE (CLINICAL RESEARCH)

1. In the treatment of the sick person, the physician must be free to use a new diagnostic and therapeutic measure, if in his or her judgment it offers hope of saving life, reestablishing health or alleviating suffering.

2. The potential benefits, hazards and discomfort of a new method should be weighed against the advantages of the best current diagnostic and therapeutic methods.

3. In any medical study, every patient—including those of a control group, if any—should be assured of the best proven diagnostic and therapeutic method.

4. The refusal of the patient to participate in a study must never interfere with the physician-patient relationship.

5. If the physician considers it essential not to obtain informed consent, the specific reasons for this proposal should be stated in the experimental protocol for transmission to the independent committee.

6. The physician can combine medical research with professional care, the objective being the acquisition of new medical knowledge, only to the extent that medical research is justified by its potential diagnostic or therapeutic value for the patient.

III. NON-THERAPEUTIC BIOMEDICAL RESEARCH INVOLVING HUMAN SUBJECTS (NON-CLINICAL BIOMEDICAL RESEARCH)

1. In the purely scientific application of medical research carried out on a human being, it is the duty of the physician to remain the protector of the life and health of that person on whom biomedical research is being carried out.

2. The subjects should be volunteers—either healthy persons or patients for whom the

experimental design is not related to the patient's illness.

3. The investigator or the investigating team should discontinue the research if in his/her or their judgment it may, if continued, be harmful to the individual.

4. In research on man, the interest of science and society should never take precedence over considerations related to the well-being of the subject.

Protection of Human Subjects Guidelines

NATIONAL INSTITUTES OF HEALTH, OFFICE FOR PROTECTION FROM RESEARCH RISKS

46.111 CRITERIA FOR IRB APPROVAL OF RESEARCH

a. In order to approve research covered by this policy the IRB shall determine that all of the following requirements are satisfied:

1. Risks to subjects are minimized: (i) by using procedures which are consistent with sound research design and which do not unnecessarily expose subjects to risk, and (ii) whenever appropriate, by using procedures already being performed on the subjects for diagnostic or treatment purposes.

2. Risks to subjects are reasonable in relation to anticipated benefits, if any, to subjects, and the importance of the knowledge that may reasonably be expected to result. . . .

3. Selection of subjects is equitable. In making this assessment the IRB should take into account the purposes of the research and the setting in which the research will be conducted and should be particularly cognizant of the special problems of research involving vulnerable populations, such as children, prisoners, pregnant women, mentally disabled persons, or economically or educationally disadvantaged persons.

4. Informed consent will be sought from each prospective subject or the subject's legally authorized representative. . . .

5. Informed consent will be appropriately documented. . . .

6. When appropriate, the research plan makes adequate provision for monitoring the data collected to ensure the safety of subjects.

7. When appropriate, there are adequate provisions to protect the privacy of

Revised June 18, 1991.

Reprinted by permission of the National Institutes of Health.

subjects and to maintain the confidentiality of data.

b. When some or all of the subjects are likely to be vulnerable to coercion or undue influence, such as children, prisoners, pregnant women, mentally disabled persons, or economically or educationally disadvantaged persons, additional safeguards have been included in the study to protect the rights and welfare of these subjects.

. . . .

46.116   GENERAL REQUIREMENTS FOR INFORMED CONSENT

Except as provided elsewhere in this policy, no investigator may involve a human being as a subject in research covered by this policy unless the investigator has obtained the legally effective informed consent of the subject or the subject's legally authorized representative. An investigator shall seek such consent only under circumstances that provide the prospective subject or the representative sufficient opportunity to consider whether or not to participate and that minimize the possibility of coercion or undue influence. The information that is given to the subject or the representative shall be in language understandable to the subject or the representative. No informed consent, whether oral or written, may include any exculpatory language through which the subject or the representative is made to waive or appear to waive any of the subject's legal rights, or releases or appears to release the investigator, the sponsor, the institution or its agents from liability for negligence.

a. Basic elements of informed consent.
    Except as provided in paragraph (c) or (d)

of this section, in seeking informed consent the following information shall be provided to each subject:

1. a statement that the study involves research, an explanation of the purposes of the research and the expected duration of the subject's participation, a description of the procedures to be followed, and identification of any procedures which are experimental;

2. a description of any reasonably foreseeable risks or discomforts to the subject;

3. a description of any benefits to the subject or to others which may reasonably be expected from the research;

4. a disclosure of appropriate alternative procedures or courses of treatment, if any, that might be advantageous to the subject;

5. a statement describing the extent, if any, to which confidentiality of records identifying the subject will be maintained;

6. for research involving more than minimal risk, an explanation as to whether any compensation and an explanation as to whether any medical treatments are available if injury occurs and, if so, what they consist of, or where further information may be obtained;

7. an explanation of whom to contact for answers to pertinent questions about the research and research subjects' rights, and whom to contact in the event of a research-related injury to the subject; and

8. a statement that participation is voluntary, refusal to participate will involve no penalty or loss of benefits to which the subject is otherwise entitled, and the subject may discontinue participation at any time . . .

46.207 ACTIVITIES DIRECTED TOWARD PREGNANT WOMEN AS SUBJECTS

a. No pregnant woman may be involved as a subject in an activity covered by this subpart unless:

   1. the purpose of the activity is to meet the health needs of the mother and the fetus will be placed at risk only to the minimum extent necessary to meet such needs, or
   2. the risk to the fetus is minimal.

b. An activity permitted under paragraph (a) of this section may be conducted only if the mother and father are legally competent and have given their informed consent after having been fully informed regarding possible impact on the fetus, except that the father's informed consent need not be secured if:

   1. the purpose of the activity is to meet the health needs of the mother;
   2. his identity or whereabouts cannot reasonably be ascertained;
   3. he is not reasonably available; or
   4. the pregnancy resulted from rape.

46.208 ACTIVITIES DIRECTED TOWARD FETUSES *IN UTERO* AS SUBJECTS

a. No fetus *in utero* may be involved as a subject in any activity covered by this subpart unless:

   1. the purpose of the activity is to meet the health needs of the particular fetus and the fetus will be placed at risk only to the minimum extent necessary to meet such needs, or

   2. the risk to the fetus imposed by the research is minimal and the purpose of the activity is the development of important biomedical knowledge which cannot be obtained by other means.

b. An activity permitted under paragraph (a) of this section may be conducted only if the mother and father are legally competent and have given their informed consent, except that the father's consent need not be secured if:

   1. his identity or whereabouts cannot reasonably be ascertained,
   2. he is not reasonably available, or
   3. the pregnancy resulted from rape.

46.209 ACTIVITIES DIRECTED TOWARD FETUSES *EX UTERO*, INCLUDING NONVIABLE FETUSES, AS SUBJECTS

a. Until it has been ascertained whether or not a fetus *ex utero* is viable, a fetus *ex utero* may not be involved as a subject in an activity covered by this subpart unless:

   1. there will be no added risk to the fetus resulting from the activity, and the purpose of the activity is the development of important biomedical knowledge which cannot be obtained by other means, or
   2. the purpose of the activity is to enhance the possibility of survival of the particular fetus to the point of viability.

b. No nonviable fetus may be involved as a subject in an activity covered by this subpart unless:

1. vital functions of the fetus will not be artificially maintained,
2. experimental activities which of themselves would terminate the heartbeat or respiration of the fetus will not be employed, and
3. the purpose of the activity is the development of important biomedical knowledge which cannot be obtained by other means.

46.210   ACTIVITIES INVOLVING THE DEAD FETUS, FETAL MATERIAL, OR THE PLACENTA

Activities involving the dead fetus, mascerated fetal material, or cells, tissue, or organs excised from a dead fetus shall be conducted only in accordance with any applicable State or local laws regarding such activities. . . .

NIH Promulgates New Guidelines for the Inclusion of Women and Minorities in Medical Research

JONATHAN M. EISENBERG

SOME MEDICINES, such as penicillin, seem to benefit humans regardless of gender, race, or other demographic factors. However, other medicines and treatments have varying effects on people of different demographic groups. For example, we know that certain diet pills increase women's, but not men's, blood pressure; and that white people require larger doses of lithium to control mania than do African Americans.[1]

If human-subject medical research (or "clinical research") is conducted on people of one de-

mographic group, such as white males, then the results may be applicable only to that group of people. For this medical research consistently to produce information useful for the prevention and treatment of all people's health problems, it must take into account all relevant demographic factors.

The National Institutes of Health ("NIH"), part of the Department of Health and Human Services, is the main biomedical research agency of the federal government; the NIH also provides support for government-funded medical research done at private sites.[2] In March 1994, the NIH announced guidelines—applicable to all NIH-funded researchers—that demand the

DR. JONATHAN M. EISENBERG, M.D., is administrator for the Agency for Health Care Policy and Research.

Berkeley Women's Law Journal 10 (1995): 183–189. Copyright 1995, by Berkeley Women's Law Journal. Reprinted by permission.

inclusion of "women and minorities" as subjects in clinical research.[3] The publication of these guidelines, in conjunction with 1990 guidelines, represents a significant step toward making medical research more effective at improving the health of all people.

However, the NIH may not have gone far enough. Specifically, it should have expressly insisted on the inclusion of *female* minorities as subjects in clinical research. Women's health statistics sometimes vary by ethnic group or by other demographic distinctions. For example, female breast cancer death rates vary tremendously based on ethnicity.[4] The prevalence of overweight women also differs by ethnic group, as well as by socioeconomic status.[5] The NIH's guidelines should acknowledge these differences among women and require medical researchers to study people with varying demographic factors to obtain more accurate and more widely applicable results.

I. HISTORY

For several decades, feminists have criticized the medical research community for ignoring women's health problems.[6] Indeed, many "clinical trials"[7]—important types of clinical research—excluded female subjects on one or several of the following grounds:

- men are considered to be easier to use in medical studies because their sex hormones do not vary cyclically to the same degree as women's;

- in certain diseases, such as coronary heart disease, where the frequency of occurrence may be lower for women than for men, the number of female subjects under study must be greater (as fewer women exhibit the disease), thereby increasing costs;

- women of childbearing ages may become pregnant during the course of studies and

subject their fetuses to dangerous drugs or devices leading to birth defects (as was the case in the tests of Thalidomide and DES in the 1950s and '60s); and

- men, particularly white men, are said to be easier to recruit as subjects for studies.[8]

Regardless of the validity of these justifications for gender discrimination in clinical research, the result has been "startling gaps" in our knowledge of women's health, according to Bernadine Healy, M.D., former director of the NIH.[9]

By the mid-1980s, the NIH was aware of this problem, but the initial commitment to change was debatable.[10] Beginning in 1990, feminist activists and female members of Congress increased pressure on the NIH. In response, the NIH made several new efforts in women's health,[11] including promulgating its first set of guidelines for the use of women and minorities as clinical research subjects.[12] In 1994 the NIH revised these guidelines.

II. THE NEW GUIDELINES

In the NIH Revitalization Act of 1993,[13] Congress required the NIH to include "women and minorities" as subjects in clinical research. The new guidelines were effective upon publication[14] and contain the following major provisions:

- the NIH must ensure the inclusion of "women and members of minority groups and their subpopulations"—where "subpopulations" does not expressly include minority women[15]—in all NIH-funded, human-subject research, including clinical trials;

- the NIH will fund only those medical research projects that include women and minorities and members of their subpopulations—or that give an express scientific justification for the exclusion of these people;

- "[c]ost is not an acceptable reason for exclusion except when the study would duplicate data from other sources";
- "[w]omen of childbearing potential should not be routinely excluded from participation in clinical research";
- "[t]his policy applies to research subjects of all ages"; and
- the NIH must initiate "programs and support for outreach efforts to recruit these groups into clinical studies."[16]

Dr. Belinda M. Seto, an NIH senior advisor who is partially responsible for developing the guidelines, summarized the new guidelines' purpose: "Ultimately, we want researchers to do what is scientifically appropriate. We want them to ask the questions: Is there impact on women? On minorities? Think of them as additional parameters, like age."[17]

On the whole, the new guidelines seem quite similar to the 1990 guidelines, although the new guidelines claim to "supersede and strengthen the previous policies."[18] New items include: (1) the mention of minority subpopulations; (2) the statements dismissing arguments for exclusion of women or minorities based on costs; (3) the statement about including subjects of all ages; and (4) the mandated outreach efforts.[19]

Indeed, the two sets of guidelines are so similar that Seto estimates that the medical researchers receiving NIH funding exhibited greater than ninety percent compliance with the new guidelines even before they were published because this community was already in compliance with the old guidelines.[20] But ninety percent compliance does not mean that ninety percent of NIH-funded medical research projects actually include women and people of color as subjects. Rather, it means that ninety percent of these projects in their applications for NIH funding addressed the questions of inclusion of women and minorities as subjects.

However, if the researchers can justify the exclusion of women and people of color in a clini-

cal trial to an NIH review board[21] on scientific grounds they can still obtain funding. According to Seto, an example of a scientifically valid reason for excluding women and minorities from clinical research is that information about women and minorities with respect to the disease or drug being studied already is known, and it would be unnecessarily duplicative to conduct an inclusive study that would generate the same information.[22] This example seems reasonable.

III. CRITICISM OF THE NEW GUIDELINES

The NIH accepted public comments and criticisms about the guidelines for one year.[23] At the time of this writing, the one-year period had not expired, but the NIH had received few comments and none that would prompt voluntary changes in the guidelines.[24]

Those comments that have been received can be grouped into three categories:

1. Geography: Some researchers in states with ethnically homogeneous populations, such as New Hampshire and Oregon, complain of the unfeasibility of recruiting minorities to be participants in clinical trials.

2. Size: Researchers argue that they should not have to seek a gender and ethnic mix in their small-scale, exploratory studies, but only in subsequent large-scale studies based on the smaller studies.

3. Costs: Researchers continue to complain that the inclusion of women in clinical trials would greatly increase the costs of the studies.[25]

Only the "geography" argument seems strong. Researchers in locations with ethnically homogeneous populations will indeed have a difficult time constructing ethnically diverse study populations. Perhaps the answer to such a researcher's dilemma is that she be given NIH grants to study only (1) diseases or drugs that seem to affect all people similarly, or (2) diseases specific to the single ethnic group in the local population—and that she be denied funding to study diseases that affect people across the demographic spectrum. It is an unfortunate truth that such a researcher, because of her location, often will not be able to produce test results usable in the prevention and treatment of all people's health problems.

The "size" argument seems particularly weak. How can a researcher reach an accurate preliminary understanding of a disease's effects if she initially looks only at how these effects are manifested in a single demographic group? Additionally, how can a researcher be sure that she has designed a sound, large-scale clinical trial, involving diverse study populations, if the small-scale, preparatory work is based on a homogeneous study population?

The "cost" argument falls flat, too. If there exists any possibility that a disease or a medicine affects men and women differently, then the disease or medicine *has* to be studied with respect to both men and women. If a study is done of men only, then the results will be applicable to men only. A second study of women will be necessary. This is what happened with the 1980s study of the effect that regularly taking aspirin had on a person's risk for a heart attack. Only men were studied; the result, that aspirin intake did cut the risk for a heart attack, was valid only for men.[26] Another study was needed to conclude that women also benefited from regular aspirin intake.[27] Two separate studies, one of men and the other of women, inevitably will cost more than a single study involving people of both genders.

An additional concern centers on the wording of the new guidelines. While the guidelines mention "women and minorities," they do not expressly mention "women minorities." Because women's health statistics sometimes vary by ethnic group,[28] the guidelines should explicitly state that NIH-funded clinical research must give particular, overt attention to women of color.

Asked about this omission, Seto answered that the term "women and minorities" includes by implication women of color; moreover, she said, the review boards that determine which NIH grant applications receive funding ensure that research proposals "reflect disease demographics" of all sorts, including gender, race, age, and socioeconomic status.[29] Of course, if the review boards already function to ensure that all research proposals take into account relevant disease demographics, as Seto claims, one wonders why the guidelines needed to be written at all.

Dr. Marvin Kalt, director of external programs at the National Cancer Institute, is an NIH official listed on the new NIH guidelines as a contact person.[30] When asked if the guidelines should list more groups of people than "women and minorities," such as low-income people or lesbians, Kalt responded that "you can't get to the point of micromanaging research."[31] Nonetheless, it is scientifically appropriate for researchers to consider additional demographic parameters when they design experiments. When they refrain from doing so, the NIH ought to play a larger oversight role to improve the research.

IV. CONCLUSION

The new guidelines represent a step in the right direction for medical science because they close some of the loopholes left by the 1990 guidelines through which researchers could continue excluding (white) women and minorities as subjects in clinical research. Now, neither additional costs of recruiting and using women and minorities in clinical trials nor women's condition of pregnancy will justify the exclusion of these groups.

The next step is for human-subject medical research to take account systematically of all relevant demographic factors. This step must be taken, guided by either the force of government intervention or the medical research community's own initiative, for only then will clinical research consistently produce information useful in the maintenance and improvement of all people's health.

NOTES

1. *At Last, Women, Minorities Count in Medical Research, USA Today,* Mar. 11, 1994, at A12; Shari Roan, *Sex, Ethnic Bias in Medical Research Raises Questions, L.A. Times,* Aug. 3, 1990, at A1.

2 *See* Office of the Federal Register, National Archives and Records Administration, *The United States Government Manual* 1994/95, at 313 (1994). The government sponsors more than 90% of the medical research done in this country. In 1991, the latest year for which figures are available, there was $12.5 billion in medical research done in the United States, and the government funded nearly $11.7 billion of it. Researchers at private hospitals and universities often are funded through NIH grants. *Statistical Abstract of the United States 1994: The National Data Book* 110 (U.S. Dep't of Commerce, Economics and Statistics Administration, Bureau of the Census 1994). Meanwhile, medical research done by the NIH itself accounts for about 10% of all medical research done in this country. Philip J. Hilts, *National Health Institutes to Revamp Criticized Research Program, N.Y. Times,* May 5, 1994, at B11.

3. NIH Guidelines on the Inclusion of Women and Minorities as Subjects in Clinical Research, 59 Fed. Reg. 14,508 (1994).

4. *National Center for Health Statistics, U.S. Dep't of Health and Human Services, Healthy People 2000 Review,* 1993, at 171 (1994).

5. Henry S. Kahn, et al., *Race and Weight Change in US Women: The Roles of Socioeconomic and Marital Status,* 81 *Am. J. Pub. Health* 319 (March 1991).

6. For an overview of this history, *see* Judith H. LaRosa & Vivian W. Pinn, *Gender Bias in Biomedical Research,* 48 *J. Am. Med. Women's Ass'n* 146–49 (1993). For an 18-year-old example of the feminist criticism,

see Gena Corea, *The Hidden Malpractice: How American Medicine Treats Women as Patients and Professionals* 232 (1977). Finally, for one medical doctor's contrary view, *see* Andrew G. Kadar, *The Truth About Sexist Medicine: Do Women Receive Inferior Medical Care? Absolutely Not, Says an M.D., Atlanta Const.,* Aug. 7, 1994, at C1.

7. "A 'clinical trial' is a broadly based . . . clinical investigation, usually involving several hundred or more human subjects, for the purpose of evaluating an experimental intervention in comparison with a standard or control intervention or comparing two or more existing treatments." 59 Fed. Reg. 14,511.

8. LaRosa & Pinn, *supra* note 6, at 146; Harry Schwartz, *Medicine Should Come First, USA Today,* Mar. 11, 1994, at A12.

9. Bernadine Healy, *Foreword* to *Report of the National Institutes of Health Opportunities for Research on Women's Health* (1992).

10. *See* Ruth L. Kirschstein, *Research on Women's Health,* 81 *Am. J. Pub. Health* 291–93 (March 1991); LaRosa & Pinn, *supra* note 6, at 148.

11. These efforts included the creation of the Office of Research on Women's Health within the Office of the Director of the NIH, and the launching of the Women's Health Initiative, a long-term, large-scale clinical study of mostly post-menopausal women. *Nat'l Inst. of Health, Overview: Office of Research on Women's Health* (1994); *Nat'l Inst. of Health, Women's Health Initiative Overview Statement* (1994).

12. LaRosa & Pinn, *supra* note 6, at 148–49.

13. 42 U.S.C. § 289a-2 (1994).

14. 59 Fed. Reg. 14,510.

15. The guidelines' definition of minority subpopulations includes the following elements "[e]ach minority group contains subpopulations which are delimited by geographic origins, national origins and/or cultural differences." For example, the minority group "Hispanic" includes people of "Mexican, Puerto Rican, Cuban, Central or South American or other Spanish culture or origin, regardless of race." Also, "[a]ttention to subpopulations also applies to individuals of mixed racial and/or ethnic parentage. 59 Fed. Reg. 14,511.

16. *Id.* at 14,508–14,511. To advance the outreach efforts, in August 1994 the NIH published a 37-page "Outreach Notebook" for researchers that explains, among other things, how to determine the extent to which women and minorities should be included in a clinical study and how to resolve ethical issues surrounding recruiting and retaining participants in studies. Some African Americans refuse to participate in government-sponsored clinical trials because of the

memory of the horrifying "studies" of the sexually transmitted disease syphilis conducted in Tuskegee, Alabama, in the 1930s. There, researchers gave African-American men placebos rather than penicillin, a known cure for syphilis, to observe the long-term debilitating effects of this disease. *See generally* James H. Jones, *Bad Blood: The Tuskegee Syphilis Experiment* (1981). Conceivably, further ethical issues would arise if the government offered to pay people of color to participate in clinical studies.

17. Telephone interview with Dr. Belinda M. Seto, senior NIH employee (Jan. 17, 1995).

18. 59 Fed. Reg. 14,508.

19. *Id.*

20. Telephone interview with Seto, *supra* note 17.

21. These review boards are composed of independent medical scientists, not NIH scientists, but they award NIH funds. Telephone interview with Dr. Marvin Kalt, senior employee at the National Cancer Institute, an NIH institute (Jan. 18, 1995).

22. Telephone interview with Seto, *supra* note 17.

23. 59 Fed. Reg. 14,510.

24. *Id.*

25. Telephone interview with Seto, *supra* note 17.

26. *See* Susan Okie, *Study: NIH Slow to Include Women in Disease Research, Wash. Post,* June 19, 1990, at A10.

27. *See* Janny Scott, *Aspirin Lowers Heart Attack Risk to Women, L.A. Times,* Mar. 16, 1991, at A1.

28. *See supra* notes 4 and 5 and accompanying text.

29. Telephone interview with Seto, *supra* note 17.

30. 59 Fed. Reg. 14,513.

31. Telephone interview with Kalt, *supra* note 21.

Philosophical and Historical Considerations

Philosophical Foundations of Respect for Autonomy

CANDACE CUMMINS GAUTHIER

ABSTRACT. Understanding the philosophical foundations of the principle of respect for autonomy is essential for its proper application within medical ethics. The foundations provided by Immanuel Kant's principle of humanity and John Stuart Mill's principle of liberty share substantial areas of agreement including: the grounding of respect for autonomy in the capacity for rational agency, the restriction of this principle to rational agents, and the important distinction between influence and control. Their work helps to clarify the scope and role of the principle of respect for autonomy in health care delivery; its implications for truth telling, informed consent, and confidentiality; and its relationship to other moral principles, such as beneficence and distributive justice.

CANDACE CUMMINS GAUTHIER is associate professor of philosophy and religion, clinical assistant professor, School of Medicine, University of North Carolina at Chapel Hill.

RESPECT FOR AUTONOMY IN HEALTH CARE DECISIONS

The principle of respect for autonomy, which requires that persons with the capacity for rational agency be allowed and encouraged to exercise that capacity through self-determination, has gained increasing importance in medical ethics.

Medical decisions ultimately affect the patient in ways fundamentally different from their effect on the provider. The patient's bodily integrity, life-style, work and recreation, and personal relationships, and even life, itself, are all at stake. The personal nature and impact of these decisions make it important to respect the patient's own wishes concerning treatment. However, the traditional beneficence-based values of the medical profession motivate the health care provider to act on what is perceived to be the patient's best interests in terms of health, relief of suffering, and the preservation of life. Moreover, the natural vulnerability and dependence of the patient in this relationship make it easy to elicit patients' agreement to treatments they may not otherwise

Kennedy Institute of Ethics Journal 3, no. 1(1993): 21–38. Copyright 1993. Reprinted by permission of The Johns Hopkins University Press.

wish to undergo. The moral requirement of respect for patient autonomy can restore a measure of balance to this relationship by allowing and encouraging competent patients to be the ultimate decision makers regarding their oven medical treatment.

The principle of respect for autonomy in medical care requires health care providers to allow and encourage fully competent patients to make decisions about their own lives and medical treatment without attempting to control those decisions. This formulation of the principle links the idea of respect for autonomy to the activity of medical decision making; emphasizes the obligations of the health care provider rather than the rights of the patient; and includes the limiting factor of competence, which may discourage some of the overextension of the principle to which Childress refers.

PHILOSOPHICAL FOUNDATIONS

An understanding of the philosophical foundations of the principle of respect for autonomy is essential for its proper application to medical ethics and helps to prevent the types of misuse that have led to attacks from those who see this principle as a threat to the traditional medical value of beneficence or in conflict with social justice. The clearest philosophical sources for this principle are found in the ethical theory of Immanuel Kant and the social and political philosophy of John Stuart Mill.

The Kantian Concept of Autonomy

Kant's ethical theory is based on the concept of autonomy or freedom of the will. According to Kant ([1785] 1964a, p. 114) this is the capacity that rational beings have for both acting independently of cause and effect in the form of natural law and acting on moral principles provided by reason

alone. This capacity for rational agency or self-determination is shared neither by things that exist in nature and are non-rational nor by objects that are manufactured by humans. Such things are always subject to the laws of nature and are, therefore, not free (Kant [1785] 1964a, pp. 96, 114).

Kant's conception of respect for autonomy is found in his principle of humanity, which, as one of the formulations of the Categorical Imperative, provides a moral standard for the treatment of persons. The principle of humanity states, "Act in such a way that you always treat humanity, whether in your own person or in the person of any other, never simply as a means, but always at the same time as an end" (Kant [1785] 1964a, p. 96). The last phrase of this principle appears to be a shortened form of ". . . but always at the same time as an end in itself." While it is fairly clear what it would mean to treat another person simply as a means to our own end, it is often difficult to see how we can treat another as an end. It is precisely here, however, that the idea of respect for autonomy is found. Kant means that the humanity or, more precisely, the rational nature ([1785] 1964a, pp. 96, 138–39) of others should always be treated as an end in itself, or as intrinsically valuable, rather than solely as a means or an instrument for our own purposes. When we treat another person as an end in himself or herself, we respect that person's dignity and intrinsic value as a rational and autonomous being. We recognize that as a free and rational being the other has the capacity to choose his or her own goals and projects on the basis of moral principles known by reason and, thus, to act on a personal conception of what is right. Only when we respect and do not interfere with others' goals, projects, and actions, chosen on their own conception of what is right, are we respecting their autonomy as rational agents.

Of course, we must interact with others and have relationships with them, which often necessarily involve treating them as a means to attaining our own goals and ends. Yet, Kant allows for this necessity. He writes that we should treat human beings ". . . never *simply* as a means, but always *at the same time* as an end." This is accomplished in our interactions with others by allowing them and, even further, encouraging them to exercise their own capacity for moral choice in projects that involve or affect them.

Mill's Concept of Liberty

The clearest and best developed conception of respect for the autonomy of others appears in John Stuart Mill's essay, *On Liberty*. Although Mill does not use the word "autonomy" in this essay, referring instead to "liberty" or "independence," in a letter to a French correspondent ([1871] 1972, pp. 1831–32), he describes the central theme of the work as the principle of "l'autonomie de l'individu."

In *On Liberty*, Mill ([1859] 1977, p. 217) states that he plans to establish the limits of legitimate control that can be exercised by the state and by the members of a society over the individual. However, his primary concern is the immense power of the majority in a society to impose its beliefs, attitudes, and values on the others through public opinion rather than the power of the government exercised through laws and legal sanctions ([1859] 1977, p. 219). Thus, Mill proposes and defends a " . . . limit to the legitimate interference of collective opinion with individual independence . . ." ([1859] 1977, p. 220). Mill formulates this principle of liberty in the following way: ". . . the only purpose for which power can be rightfully exercised over any member of a civilized community, against his will, is to prevent harm to others. His own good, either physical or moral, is not a sufficient warrant" ([1859] 1977, p. 223).

Although Mill defends three spheres of liberty, the liberty of tastes and pursuits is the most relevant to a concept of respect for autonomy in health care decisions. He describes this more fully as the liberty ". . . of framing the plan of our life to suit our own character; of doing as we

like, subject to such consequences as may follow: without impediment from our fellow-creatures, so long as what we do does not harm them, even though they should think our conduct foolish, perverse, or wrong" ([1859] 1977, p. 226). Mill also refers to this liberty as the freedom to act on one's opinions ([1859] 1977, p. 260). His primary argument for this freedom is its necessity for the development of individuality, which he believes is essential for human well-being. It is, in Mill's words, ". . . one of the principal ingredients of human happiness, and quite the chief ingredient of individual and social progress" ([1859] 1977, p. 261).

Mill's argument, then, is based primarily on consequentialist reasoning. Allowing each person in society to act on his or her opinion of what is right is necessary for both human development and happiness. The individuality that results from respecting this type of liberty is good both for each member of a society and for the society as a whole.

However, Mill also defends liberty of action on the basis of the rational nature of human beings. He writes:

> The human faculties of perception, judgment, discriminative feeling, mental activity, and even moral preference, are exercised only in making a choice. He who lets the world, or his own portion of it, choose his plan of life for him; has no need of any other faculty than the ape-like one of imitation. He who chooses his plan for himself, employs all his faculties. He must use observation to see, reasoning and judgment to foresee, activity to gather materials for decision, discrimination to decide, and when he has decided, firmness and self-control to hold to his deliberate decision. ([1859] 1977, pp. 262–63)

Mill considers the exercise of these faculties to be essential to the strengthening of reason. He is saying, then, that only by respecting the liberty of others do we allow them to exercise, develop, and employ the rational faculties essential for individuality.

Thus, on a deeper level, Mill's arguments are also based on the rational nature of human beings. It is only because humans are beings with the faculties of judgment, discrimination, mental activity, and moral preference that respect for liberty has the consequences that Mill characterizes as desirable. It is precisely because humans are rational that liberty of choice and action result in individuality and, ultimately, personal well-being and happiness for both the individual and society. If humans did not possess the capacity for rational activity, respect for their liberty could not have these consequences.

Of course, the freedom to act on one's opinions cannot be unlimited, and Mill is careful to define the domain of self-regarding behavior in which both legal and social freedom is to be absolute. It is ". . . . when a person's conduct affects the interests of no persons besides himself, or needs not affect them unless they like . . ." ([1859] 1977, p. 276). To clarify the distinction between self-regarding and other-regarding behavior, Mill notes that when a ". . . person is led to violate a distinct and assignable obligation to any other person or persons, the case is taken out of the self-regarding class . . . ," and the sanctions of the law or public opinion may be used to force the behavior that would meet those obligations ([1859] 1977, p. 281).

Many of the criticisms of the principle of respect for autonomy as applied to health care have come from those who suppose it to undermine care and concern for others. A careful reading of Mill, however, shows that this is not necessarily the case. Mill ([1859] 1977, pp. 276–77) argues that respect for the liberty of others in self-regarding conduct is not selfish or indifferent. Indeed, we may, and should, attempt to influence others for their own benefit. We may use encouragement, advice, instruction, and persuasion for this purpose but not compulsion through the force of legal sanctions or the control of public opinion ([1859] 1977, pp. 277, 292).

Mill ([1859] 1977, p. 277) provides three arguments for the limits he places on the authority of society over the individual. He argues that individuals are the ones most interested in their own well-being and they are the most knowledgeable about their own feelings and circumstances. He also notes that the general presumptions about what is best that society would use to dictate the self-regarding actions of individuals might themselves be wrong or at least inapplicable in particular cases.

Again, while these are consequentialist arguments, they do refer to the capacity of competent and rational human beings to make decisions about self-regarding conduct based on knowledge and judgment. Mill, then, seems ultimately to base his arguments for liberty on the capacity of rational beings both to make choices and to act on a personal conception of what is right.

APPLICATIONS IN THE DELIVERY OF HEALTH CARE

Both Kant and Mill provide powerful reasons for health care providers to respect the autonomy of their patients in medical decision making. Kant argues that only when we treat others as ends in themselves do we treat them as persons, respecting their freedom or capacity to choose based on moral principles recognized by reason. Mill argues that human beings will only be able to develop and exercise their rational faculties if they are permitted full liberty in self-regarding decisions and actions. Moreover, this development and exercise is essential for individual happiness and well-being as well as for social progress.

Paternalism in health care, following the Hippocratic tradition, has generally been defended on the basis of a consequentialist argument. Although paternalism is directed toward the good of an individual patient rather than the good for society as a whole, it is nevertheless supposedly justified by the balance of positive over negative consequences for that patient. However, as suggested above, a careful reading of Mill indicates that in his version of utilitarianism even a net balance of positive over negative consequences cannot justify an act that violates an individual's rights, including security from wrongful interference with freedom.

If a health care professional attempts to control or manipulate a patient's decisions to further interests of the professional that are not shared by the patient, the patient is being treated simply as a means and not at the same time as an end. Health care providers generally may assume that patients desire health and continued life, but patients must still be permitted to agree to a recommended treatment or to reject it based on their own perceptions of their goals and how best to meet them. It is important to emphasize that patients may not always share the specific goals of health care providers.

While patient and provider may well agree that the general goals of medical care are patient health and well being, they may disagree over specific meanings attached to these goals. There also may be disagreement about what life style changes or amount of inconvenience or suffering would be tolerable to meet even fully shared goals. Jay Katz (1984, p. 98) has argued that physicians' reluctance to engage patients in conversation has been based on the dangerous and incorrect idea, ". . . that physicians and patients have an identity of interest in medical matters." Since the goals of health and cure rarely can be completely attained and can be sought in alternative ways, each with attendant risks and benefits, Katz (1984, p. 98) concludes that ". . . health turns out to be an ambiguous state about which doctors and patients may have conflicting expectations." His recommendation is that open and honest conversation between patient and physician can develop the mutual trust that is essential to respect for physicians' and patients' humanity (Katz 1984, pp. 100–103). Thus, patients should be encouraged to assess their own goals in relation to health care, and a frank discussion of the treatment goals of both the provider and the patient should be a part of the patient-provider relationship.

It is also the case that medical treatment decisions are most often self-regarding. Thus, they generally fall into the class of actions that ought to be free from force and control, according to Mill. As long as these decisions do not lead to a breach of specific duties to others or otherwise cause harm to others, they are self-regarding and are clearly in the sphere of absolute liberty. Exceptions may arise in cases involving third parties, for example, when a parent's death from the refusal of a blood transfusion would leave small children without needed care.

Mill's discussion also provides an idea of what the health care professional may do in an effort to influence a patient's self-regarding behavior in medical decision making. The professional may, and certainly should, offer information on relevant considerations such as the short and long-term consequences of various treatment options and of treatment refusal. In addition, she may give advice, instruction, or encouragement, and even employ persuasion as long as it does not constitute force or control.

The line between persuasion and coercion is difficult to draw and raises questions about what sorts of persuasion are allowable. However, Kant's principle of humanity can help to clarify the distinction. Both withholding relevant information, or misrepresenting the available treatment options, in order to control the patient's decision, and emotional manipulation through guilt or fear would treat the patient simply as a means and not at the same time as an end. However, methods of persuasion that allow patients to make decisions based on what they think is right, by providing truthful, relevant information, including the provider's own judgment about what is best, treat patients as ends in themselves. In general, methods of persuasion that appeal to patients' rational capacities, specifically the ability to choose based on information relevant to their own goals and their own application of moral principles, will be morally permissible while methods that by-pass or interfere with patients' use of their rational faculties will be proscribed.

Both Kant and Mill also provide guidelines applicable to determining whose autonomy should be respected in a health care setting. Since Kantian respect for autonomy is respect for a capacity possessed by rational beings, it must be understood to apply only to the treatment of those who are capable of reason. Kant ([1797] 1964b, p. 122) allows paternalistic beneficence toward young children and the insane, presumably based on their lack of rational capacities. Therefore, those who are too young to have fully developed their rational faculties and those whose mental or neurological condition precludes reasoning would not be asked or expected to make their own treatment decisions. It should be noted, however, that decisions made on the basis of the advance directive of a formerly competent patient can be understood as respecting that patient's autonomy.

It is important to recognize that this capacity is not a matter of the rationality of any specific medical decision, as judged by others, it is simply a matter of the patient being capable of rational decision making. Thus an adult who has this capacity but chooses to forego life-sustaining treatment based on all relevant information cannot be considered irrational simply because health care professionals disagree with the decision or even believe it to be "irrational." The determination of a patient's capacity for rational decision making should be made independently of any specific health care decision.[1]

Similarly, Mill limits respect for the liberty of self-regarding behavior to those capable of taking care of themselves or acting on their own behalf. Qualifying the principle of liberty, he writes, ". . . this doctrine is meant to apply only to human beings in the maturity of their faculties" ([1859] 1977, p. 224) thereby excluding children and young persons who still require care by others. In another work ([1848] 1965, p. 803), Mill discusses ". . . the doctrine that individuals are the proper guardians of their own interests, and that government owes nothing to them but to save them from being interfered with by other people. . . ." Explaining that this doctrine

". . . can never be applicable to any persons but those who are capable of acting in their own behalf," he mentions infants, lunatics, and those who have fallen into imbecility, as specific exceptions. In the health care setting this would exclude not only children, but also adults who are mentally or neurologically unable to make treatment decisions for themselves. It should not be interpreted, however, as excluding mentally competent adults who require total physical care. Mill, himself, emphasizes that this limitation must not be used to control the actions or decisions of those who are capable of taking care of themselves, but are judged by others as not doing so properly ([1859] 1977, p. 282). Thus, health care providers must not rely on a treatment decision made by an apparently competent adult, which they judge as wrong, as proof that the patient is not mentally competent and thus not entitled to respect for liberty.[2]

RESPECT FOR AUTONOMY IN TRUTH TELLING, INFORMED CONSENT, AND CONFIDENTIALITY

Additional evidence for the importance of the principle of respect for autonomy comes from the fact that this principle provides one possible basis for the moral requirements of truth telling, informed consent, and confidentiality for competent patients within the patient-provider relationship. True and complete information about the patient's condition and the available treatment options is necessary for the exercise of patient autonomy, if autonomy is understood to involve the full use of one's rational faculties in decision making. Even when there is no immediate treatment decision to be made, patients may need the information that physicians have gained from physical examinations and diagnostic tests to make other important decisions in their lives. If patients have sought medical attention and submitted to examinations and tests, it should be assumed that they want and need this information for planning their lives and their activities, unless they have specifically stated otherwise. Withholding or distorting information for any purpose, even for "the patient's own good," interferes with the use of these faculties and treats competent patients as incompetent to make decisions about their lives and their medical treatment. It also treats a patient merely as a means to whatever purpose the provider has in withholding or misrepresenting this information.

The legal and moral requirement of informed consent for medical treatment is clearly based on respect for patient autonomy. Morally valid consent must be based on true and complete information that is provided by a health care professional and, equally importantly, is understood by the patient. Without an adequate comprehension of the relevant information, competent patients cannot exercise their rational faculties in making treatment choices based on that information. Consent also must not be the result of coercion, manipulation, or undue pressure. Using these methods to obtain consent obviously violates the principle of respect for autonomy. These methods attempt to control the patient's decision in order to attain a goal of the health care provider, one that the patient presumably does not share, since if the goal were shared such methods would be unnecessary. As such, they interfere with the patient's liberty of action and treat the patient merely as a means to this goal.

The moral requirement of confidentiality also respects the competent patient's autonomy, or self-determination, in an important but often unrecognized way. Confidentiality within the patient-provider relationship allows patients to determine who has access to specific information about them. When confidentiality is violated, the patient's decision to share certain information exclusively with a chosen professional is being overridden without the patient's awareness or consent. Ideally, patients should be notified when confidential information is disclosed to others in consultation or support services. How-

ever, even unauthorized disclosure is justified when it is necessary to prevent substantial harm or injury to another person, as suggested by the limit Mill places on the exercise of liberty based on harm to others.

The requirements of truth telling and confidentiality apply to incompetent patients to the extent that they are capable of participating in a relationship with their physician even if treatment decisions are ultimately made by a guardian or proxy decision maker. Children, for example, cannot be expected to develop the rational capacity for making decisions about themselves on the basis of available information if they are routinely given false information, nor can they form a conception of their own personhood and ability to be self-determining if they are treated as objects rather than developing persons. Some mentally impaired adults may still retain the capacity to process information even if they cannot employ that information to make decisions on their own behalf. Lying to these patients would appear to deny them whatever minimal use of the human faculties they retain.

The concept of a relationship between patient and health care provider might also be enlarged in these cases to include the incompetent patient's primary care-giver. If so, a justification could be provided for confidentiality within these relationships based on respect for the autonomy of the person responsible for the patient. Parents, spouses, and adult children are the ones who seek medical care from a specific provider for their incompetent charges and are most often the ones providing information about the patient as well as their own lives and family relationships. Unauthorized disclosure of information about the patient, then, would violate the autonomy of this additional participant in the patient-provider relationship.

NOTES

1. Charles Culver and Bernard Gert in "The Inadequacy of Incompetence" (1990) support this point. Yet

they provide persuasive arguments to justify overruling clearly irrational treatment decisions by competent patients in certain cases.

2. Here, Culver and Gert would disagree, permitting physicians to override a competent patient's refusal judged to be irrational in the sense of "dangerous to self without compensating benefit" (1990, pp. 640–41).

REFERENCES

Clements, Colleen D., and Sider, Roger C. 1987. Medical Ethics' Assault Upon Medical Values. In *Bioethics: Readings and Cases,* ed. Baruch A. Brody and H. Tristram Engelhardt, Jr., pp. 109–13. Englewood Cliffs, NJ: Prentice-Hall, Inc.

Childress, James F. 1990. The Place of Autonomy in Bioethics. *Hastings Center Report* 20 (1): 12–17.

Culver, Charles, and Gert, Bernard. 1990. The Inadequacy of Incompetence. *The Milbank Quarterly* 68: 619–43.

Danis, Marion, and Churchill, Larry R. 1991. Autonomy and the Common Weal. *Hastings Center Report* 21 (1): 25–31.

Dworkin, Gerald. 1971. Paternalism. In *Morality and the Law,* ed. Richard A. Wasserstrom, pp. 107–26. Belmont, CA: Wadsworth Publishing Company, Inc.

Engelhardt, Jr., H. Tristram. 1986. *The Foundations of Bioethics.* New York: Oxford University Press.

Hill, Jr., Thomas E. 1989. Kant's Theory of Practical Reason. *Monist* 72: 363–83.

Kant, Immanuel. [1785] 1964a. *Groundwork of the Metaphysic of Morals,* trans. H. J. Paton. New York: Harper and Row, Publishers.

———. [1797] 1964b. *The Doctrine of Virtue,* trans. Mary J. Gregor. Philadelphia: University of Pennsylvania Press.

Katz, Jay. 1984. *The Silent World of Doctor and Patient.* New York: The Free Press.

Mill, John Stuart. [1848] 1965. *Principles of Political Economy.* In *Collected Works of John Stuart Mill,* vol. III, ed. J. M. Robson. Toronto: Toronto University Press.

———. [1859] 1977. *On Liberty.* In *Collected Works of John Stuart Mill,* vol. XVIII, ed. J. M. Robson. Toronto: Toronto University Press.

———. [1861] 1969. *Utilitarianism.* In *Collected Works of John Stuart Mill,* vol. X, ed. J. M. Robson. Toronto: Toronto University Press.

———. [1871] 1972. Letter to Emile Acollas. In *Collected Works of John Stuart Mill,* vol. XVII, ed. Francis E. Mineka and Dwight N. Lindley. Toronto: Toronto University Press.

O'Neill, Onora. 1985. Between Consenting Adults. *Philosophy and Public Affairs* 14: 252–77.

———. 1989. Universal Laws and Ends-In-Themselves. *Monist* 72: 341–61.

Reiman, Jeffrey H. 1976. Privacy, Intimacy, and Personhood. *Philosophy and Public Affairs* 6: 26–44.

Tomlinson, Tom, and Brody, Howard. 1990. Futility and the Ethics of Resuscitation. *Journal of the American Medical Association* 264: 1276–80.

Bioethics and Anti-Bioethics in Light of Nazi Medicine: What Must We Remember?

DANIEL WIKLER and JEREMIAH BARONDESS

ABSTRACT. Only recently have historians explored in depth the role of the medical profession in Nazi Germany. Several recent works reveal that physicians joined the Nazi party in disproportionate numbers and lent both their efforts and their authority to Nazi eugenic and racist programs. While the crimes of the physician Mengele and a few others are well known, recent research points to a much broader involvement by the profession, even in its everyday clinical work. Analogous activities existed in the German legal and industrial communities; disruption of the medical ethic thus sprang from the broader social contexts of Nazi Germany. The new United States Holocaust Memorial Museum, now opening on the Mall in Washington, D.C., will have an opportunity to educate the public about both the great crimes at Auschwitz and other camps, and the gradual but thorough degradation of ethics in the German medical profession. From this presentation, contemporary bioethics can ponder the proper use of the Nazi analogy in bioethical debate.

DANIEL WIKLER is currently on leave from the University of Wisconsin-Madison and is a senior staff ethicist at the World Health Organization in Geneva, Switzerland. While at the University of Wisconsin-Madison he is a professor in the program in medical ethics in the department of history of medicine, and in the department of philosophy.

DR. JEREMIAH BARONDESS is President of the New York Academy of Medicine.

INTRODUCTION

Over the half century since the fall of the Third Reich, our interest in the Holocaust, its antecedents, and its sequelae continues unabated. Despite its obvious importance for bioethics, however, the role of German doctors during the Nazi era received relatively little attention after the conclusion of the Nuremberg trials.[1] Now these terrible events are receiving the attention they deserve. . . .

While the main events in Nazi medicine have been thoroughly chronicled, there is little agreement on their explanation and meaning. Moreover, we must learn how to discern and apply the lessons of this history in a responsible way. In the literature of bioethics, references to the Nazi period have become a standard method of argumentation. In particular, when bioethicists warn of a slippery slope, the Third Reich lies at its bottom. Despite the obvious importance of the Nazi analogy, this argument has become something of a loose cannon, intended as an unanswerable caution against particular clinical measures and even used to forestall entire lines of research. Ironically, this weapon has recently been used against bioethics itself, as we discuss below. In this article, we provide personal perspectives on the interpretation of that era.

Kennedy Institute of Ethics Journal 3, no. 1(1993): 39–55. Copyright 1993. Reprinted by permission of The Johns Hopkins University Press.

HALLMARKS OF NAZI MEDICINE

For the educated public, the term "Nazi Doctor" undoubtedly brings to mind Josef Mengele and his partners in crime. At Auschwitz and elsewhere, thousands of unconsenting subjects were subjected to scientific or pseudo-scientific investigations and experiments which routinely led to suffering and death. The scale and inhumanity of these abuses shocked the world and led directly, via the Nuremberg Code (Annas and Grodin 1992), to today's elaborate regulation and review of medical research involving human subjects.

Less well-known, even to bioethicists, is the central role played by physicians in the camp's overall extermination process. Robert J. Lifton, who has studied the psychology of the physicians involved, observes that

> In Auschwitz, Nazi doctors presided over the murder of most of the one million victims of that camp. Doctors performed selections. . . . Doctors supervised the killing in the gas chambers and decided when the victims were dead. Doctors conducted a murderous epidemiology, sending to the gas chamber groups of people with contagious diseases. . . . Doctors ordered and supervised, and at times carried out, direct killing of debilitated patients on the medical blocks by means of phenol injections into the bloodstream or the heart. . . . Doctors consulted actively on how best to keep selections running smoothly; on how many people to permit to remain alive to fill the slave labor requirements of the I. G. Farben enterprise at Auschwitz; and how to burn the enormous numbers of bodies that strained the facilities of the crematoria . . . As one survivor . . . put the matter, "Auschwitz was like a medical operation," and "the killing program was led by doctors from beginning to end." (1986, p. 18)

Of course, the involvement of physicians did not stop there. The mass killings of Jews and others during the war years were preceded by a huge program of exterminating the disabled. "Aktion T-4," so-called because of the Berlin address (Tiergartenstrasse 4) of its headquarters, involved a national sorting of Germans of all faiths into the categories of the fit and the unfit, of the productive and the "useless eaters." A parallel program extended to children. More than 200,000 of those identified as defective were collected in institutions that had once provided care, and murdered (Gallagher 1990). The very term "euthanasia," inappropriately and cynically chosen by the Nazi regime in keeping with its cover story, was stained forever.

These unspeakable acts of crime and betrayal, supervised at all times by physicians sworn to act in the interests of the sick, helped to prepare the way for the events known as the Holocaust.

NAZISM AS BIOMEDICAL POLITICS: THE IDEOLOGICAL SETTING

Eugenic thinking was at its zenith at the time of Hitler's rise to power. The prospect of bettering humankind by improving its genetic endowment appealed to thinkers across the political spectrum, including many humanitarians. The office of one of the authors of this article lies literally in the shadow of Van Hise Hall, named for an honored leader of the Wisconsin Progressives and president of the state university—who called publicly for sterilization of the mentally handicapped.

It is a commonplace that in Nazi Germany eugenics ran amok, discrediting its program for the indefinite future. The recent spate of scholarly publications on Nazi medicine and politics, however, has shown that eugenic thinking in Germany had far greater implications. It provided a lens through which the Nazi program, not just regarding the sick and the disabled but in its entire ambition, could be portrayed as a healing mission. The centrality of medicine to the Nazi era follows as a matter of course.

Twentieth-century eugenics was not essentially racist, though after 1933 German eugenics took on a uniform racist coloring. In either form, however, it was susceptible to a world-view in which the basic unit of biology was something larger than the individual. Whether that unit, the "patient," was the race, the nation, or mankind as a whole, the "defective" individual would be viewed as a diseased part, harming the larger organism through its contributions to the latter's gene pool and impairing its functioning by its inability to contribute usefully to the work done by others.

The Nazis made eugenics an official state ideology, but, as Müller-Hill (1988), Proctor (1988), and others have shown, the ground had been well-plowed before 1933. As Proctor (p. 38) observes, "One often hears that National Socialists distorted science . . . but . . . it was largely medical scientists who *invented* racial hygiene in the first place. Many of the leading institutes and courses on *Rassenhygiene* and *Rassenkunde* were established at German universities long before the Nazi rise to power. And by 1932 it is fair to say that racial hygiene had become a scientific orthodoxy in the German medical community." . . .

ORDINARY MEDICINE
IN THE THIRD REICH

The sad and terrible fact is that physicians, as a group, were enthusiastic supporters of and participants in Nazism. Almost half were members of the Nazi party, a much higher percentage than any other profession (Kater 1989; Proctor 1988; Gallagher 1990); two-thirds were Nazi-affiliated in some way (Kater 1989). Physicians were seven times more likely to join the SS than were other German males (Proctor 1988). The Nazi Party's enthusiasm for the medical model of politics

paid physicians great homage, and the doctors returned the favor.

The contribution of German doctors to Nazi policies, however, went beyond personal conviction and support of Party power. Many of the principal Nazi initiatives and programs, ranging from eugenics to anti-Semitism, drew on contributions in ways large and small from thousands of doctors.

German doctors participated in the persecution of the Jews with little complaint. Their first victims were fellow physicians of Jewish ancestry. Gallagher (1990) reports that

> . . . on what was called "Boycott Day" in Berlin on April 1, 1933, members of the German Physicians' League in the early hours of the morning broke into the apartments and homes of Jewish and socialist doctors. They were dragged from the beds, beaten, and then hauled off to an area near the Berlin Lehrter. There, stripped of their clothes, they were forced to run laps about the track as they were subjected to hazing, pistol shots, and beatings with sticks. Many of them were then taken to the cellars of the Hedemannstrasse jail, where they were tortured further before being released. (p. 190; see also Kater 1989, p. 184)

As the decade progressed, Jewish physicians were, in stages, removed from positions of responsibility, forbidden to treat non-Jewish patients, and then evicted from the profession altogether. Not only was there hardly any protest; these acts were planned and carried out by the leaders of the profession themselves (Kater 1989; Proctor 1988). Nor did the rank and file show any hesitancy in seizing the opportunities left open by the removal of their Jewish competition. Some physicians grew impatient and in 1935 complained to the government of an inability to attract patients from their Jewish colleagues; they were obliged by exhortations to German patients to find non-Jewish doctors (Kater 1989, p. 189). The eventual murder of the Jewish physicians drew no more protest from their colleagues than did the fate of the German Jews from their fellow citizens generally. . . .

THE CONTEMPORARY RELEVANCE OF NAZI BIOETHICS

If we can avoid repeating the wrongs of the past only if we remember them, what precisely are we to remember and thus avoid? Nearly all historians of Nazi medicine agree that the worst atrocities committed by doctors were an outgrowth of earlier developments. Simply resolving not to repeat the crimes would be pointless if they become inevitable once the root causes, such as ideological or institutional trends, are put in motion. The descent into moral degradation must be blocked at the top of the slippery slope.

Our task is thus to diagnose the moral disease. But there are many more explanations for Nazi medical misbehavior than there are historians examining it. Was the root cause the conception of medicine as a purely "scientific" world without values (Müller-Hill 1988; Kater 1989)? The frustration of not being able to ameliorate hereditary chronic disabilities (Gallagher 1990)? Emphasis of nature over nurture in explaining social problems (Proctor 1988)? The specific legacy of racism? The eugenic ideal? The continued uncertainty over what led Germany astray leaves contemporary observers free to interpret the bearing of the German experience on our own era through the lens of their distinctive outlook and interests. Although abortion was virtually banned in the Third Reich, the Right to Life movement compares the millions of abortions each year to the mass murders of the Holocaust. The American Medical Association's executive vice-president sounded a familiar AMA theme in commenting on the Berlin *Ärztekammer*'s exhibit, which the AMA co-sponsored: "The great concern of American physicians is the Government increasingly interfering with the doctor-patient relationship"[2] (Leary 1992).

Whether one agrees or disagrees with these interpretations, however, it is plain that the Nazi medical experience looms large over the central bioethical uncertainties of our time:

- As the United States inches toward a "right to die," are we flirting with disaster? A key question is an historical one: does the Nazi era show that desensitizing doctors to causing deaths is a calamitous move? Or that the problem was the conception of "euthanasia" as a prerogative of the state rather than a right of the individual?

- Should the Nazi record make us wary of the enhanced scope of genetic screening and genetic engineering expected to result from advances in molecular biology and the human genome project? Does a eugenic impulse lie at the heart of these programs — and need we fear that if we avoid the racism and quackery of Nazi eugenics and limit our interventions to enhancing the choices of prospective parents?

- Is community welfare an illegitimate consideration in weighing patient benefit against cost? Must the specter of Aktion T-4 dissuade us from encouraging the public to consider the interests of the next generation as they incur huge medical expenses during the last months of life?

Contemplation of the Nazi era in medicine has immediate practical utility. Its bearing on the issues of euthanasia, the uses of genetic information, and on cost-containment is so direct and important that these debates must be carried out in the context of a continuing and searching attempt to interpret and explain the historical record of the Third Reich. Universities, and in particular their medical schools, should have access to teaching materials for their students, to enable them to make sense of the constant references to these Nazi practices in the bioethical debates. The public, moreover, needs familiarity with the German record so that it can learn what to ask of its physicians, its lawmakers, and even its philosophers — and what not to ask. Here the degradation of ordinary medical practice is of even greater significance than the atrocities at Auschwitz.

Exhibits and other forms of education about Nazi medicine could also use the occasion to make Americans aware of our own history, both good and bad. Relatively few know the troubling story of American eugenics, including a vigorous program of involuntary sterilization, from which the Nazi theoreticians learned a great deal. The record of occasional abuse of human subjects of medical experimentation is largely unknown; in the case of the Tuskegee syphilis study, our past sins also had a racist coloring. The public should also have a greater familiarity with the elaborate safeguards that have since been put in place, such as the laws and regulations forbidding involuntary bodily intrusions, and the Institutional Review Boards which must approve medical research protocols. Presentation of these protections in the light of the Nazi record would provide an effective reminder of why they were enacted and why their continued functioning is important to every citizen.

A DANGEROUS SUBJECT?

Nowhere has the discussion of bioethics in light of the Nazi era roused such strong feelings as in Germany and Austria, the lands of the Nazi Reich. The passion of these arguments is of course understandable. In the past three years, however, the course of the debate has taken a surprising turn: numerous participants have decided that the lesson of the Nazi experience for bioethics is that bioethics should not be discussed at all. Bioethics, in their view, is itself a slippery slope.

The story of this controversy, which has been recounted in many German publications and in the English-speaking press as well (Schöne-Seifert and Rippe 1991; Singer 1991), dates back to the summer of 1989. The Australian philosopher Peter Singer, co-editor of the British journal *Bioethics* and a figure of considerable reputation in Anglophone moral philosophy, was invited to give a lecture at a conference called "Bioengineering, Ethics, and Mental Retardation," to be held in Marburg, Germany; he also accepted an invitation to give a public lecture at the University of Dortmund. Singer (1987) had defended in his book *Practical Ethics,* the prerogative of parents of seriously defective newborns, such as anencephalics, to decide whether their offspring should live or die.[3] A coalition of anti-biotechnology and disability-rights groups labeled Singer as an advocate of policies that would rekindle the Nazi's "euthanasia" program of the handicapped, and warned that if he were allowed to appear they would disrupt the proceedings (Schöne-Seifert and Rippe 1991). Singer received a letter rescinding his invitation to speak at Marburg. The letter distinguished between discussions "behind closed doors with critical scientists who want to convince you that your attitude infringes human rights" and promotion of Singer's views "in public" (Singer 1991).

This challenge quickly developed into a movement, one aimed at preventing Singer or others thought to be like him from giving any lectures at all. Entire conferences were shut down because of threats, protests and disruption. An invited address by Singer was shouted down with the chant, "Singer Raus!" ("Singer Out") and Singer was manhandled at the speaker's podium (Singer 1991). (Singer, three of whose grandparents were murdered in the Holocaust, recalled the "Juden Raus" slogan of sixty years ago.)

Soon the target extended beyond public occasions; university courses were cancelled and academic careers threatened because of the association with these "dangerous" ideas. Moreover, the target widened: where once only Peter Singer's views on euthanasia for defective newborns was the target, now all of bioethics, and even the whole of Anglo-American philosophy, came under attack. Bioethics was condemned as a "public relations department of the new biotechnologies" (Schöne-Seifert and Rippe 1991),[4] a kind of stalking-horse for the medical-industrial complex. The campaign soon caught the press's attention. *Der Spiegel,* the newsmagazine, published a long article by one of the protesters, Franz Christoph (1989), accompanied by photographs depicting the Nazi horrors; it refused, however, to publish a reply by Singer, the object of the attacks (Singer 1991).

For the American observer, sympathy for the anti-bioethics movement is difficult. As Singer himself observed, "There is . . . a peculiar tone of fanaticism . . . that goes beyond normal opposition to Nazism, and instead begins to seem like the very mentality that made Nazism possible." The protesters are careless in selecting targets (Schöne-Seifert and Rippe 1991). Indeed, the anti-bioethics movement builds on a recent history of protests that are difficult to comprehend. Protesters blocked the gates of the Max Planck Institute for Breeding Research in Cologne to prevent the planting of pink petunias, saying that the genetic alteration revived memories of Nazi racial experiments in concentration camps ("West German Scientists . . ." 1990). Benno Müller-Hill, a pioneer researcher on Nazi medical atrocities and also a geneticist, reports that his genetics department has been firebombed twice in recent years, as has the department at Heidelberg (see Meyer 1989).

It is noteworthy that these acts have been committed only in German-speaking Europe. There has been little echo elsewhere on the Continent, and none in the United States.[5] The lack of an academic commitment to free speech and open inquiry in those countries is worrisome. Might one not take comfort, however, from the fact that at least some people in Germany and Austria care so passionately about preventing a

return of Nazi thinking? And might it not be dangerous for questions of euthanasia and eugenics to be debated calmly and dispassionately on ground which had proven to be fertile soil for inhumanity? After all, the anti-bioethics furor in Germany and Austria followed closely on the recent publication of the historical works documenting the Nazi medical atrocities; some of the writers were in the forefront of the protesters (Schöne-Seifert and Rippe 1991). Did they not best know whereof they spoke?

The answer might be "yes" if we accept the premise that the best, or even the only, way to prevent the fall down the slippery slope is to prevent the issues from being debated at all. This premise will win few followers here; nor should it. The implication of the Nazi era for contemporary bioethics, with which we are here concerned, cannot be discussed if we refuse to discuss bioethics. And it is ludicrous to suppose that academic discussions of this sort will lead to a new Auschwitz.

But the German protesters' challenge raises, in our opinion, an important issue, in view of our argument that the most important Nazi-era phenomenon for contemporary bioethics was the moral degradation of ordinary medicine. The German protesters do not want a public debate, they say, because despicable and dangerous views are made respectable merely by being debated; this occurs, they say, even if these views are fully rebutted. That is why their response is not to enter the debate but to prevent it. As the new history of Nazi medicine has shown, the misbehavior of the ordinary German physician was possible in large part because abhorrent ideas became commonplace and respectable. When German doctors lost their moral instincts, their ability to notice evil and to recoil from it, their sins of omission and commission came easily.

Discussion of the meaning of Nazi medicine for contemporary bioeothics will therefore be a hazardous enterprise in German-speaking Europe. As the Nazis' opponent, the United States is in a less difficult position as it contemplates these events. Nevertheless, we cannot be complacent. As mentioned above, the Nazis acknowledged us as their teachers in instituting eugenic programs of forced sterilization. Our own misdeeds in human experimentation, though not at all comparable to Mengele's, are the occasion for humility. And the integrity of physicians' ethics is constantly endangered. Recently, for example, Illinois passed a law (over the protests of the AMA) requiring that two physicians be present when executions by lethal injection are carried out (Ill. Rev. Stat. ch. 38, par. 119-5 (1992)). The law promises participating physicians anonymity and a cash payment. Germany is not the only country with ghosts in its medical closet (though it has by far the worst ones), or with present-day moral lapses. Continuing reflection on the events in Germany 1933–1945, and reinterpretation of their implications, will be necessary not only in resolving bioethical disputes, but as a precondition for bioethics itself.

We would like to thank Irving Ishado for research assistance.

NOTES

1. Michael Kater (1989) reports that a German chronicle of these events a few years after the war was effectively suppressed.

2. Warren E. Leary (1992) suggests that the Nazi horrors stemmed in part from the state's role in ensuring access to care, even in Weimar, Germany. This suggestion was rebutted in a letter published shortly thereafter (Landsberger 1992).

3. This position is a standard, though not universal, view in the bioethics literature in English. On other issues, ranging from aid to the poor to education for the disabled, Singer has favored redistribution from the fortunate to the unfortunate. In the United States, Singer is best known for his book *Animal Liberation* (1975, second edition 1990) which was instrumental in launching the last decade's movement for humane treatment of animals.

4. Quoting and translating E. Klee, *"Durch Zyankali erlöst": Sterbehilfe und Euthanasie heute*. Frankfurt: M. Fischer, 1990, p. 81.

5. One of the conferences shut down by protesters in Germany was simply moved to nearby Netherlands, where it proceeded without incident (Singer 1991). At a recent Congress of the International Association of Bioethics, with delegates from 37 countries, Singer was elected president. However, his associate, Helga Kuhse, was shouted down at a talk in Bielefeld, Germany, the week before, and another speaker was spattered with green paint (personal communications).

REFERENCES

Annas, George J., and Grodin, Michael A. 1992. *The Nazi Doctors and the Nuremberg Code: Human Rights in Human Experimentation*. Oxford: Oxford University Press.

Caplan, Arthur L., ed. 1992. *When Medicine Went Mad: Bioethics and the Holocaust*. Totowa, NJ: Humana Press.

Christoph, Franz. 1989. (K)ein Diskurs Uber 'lebensunwertes Leben.' *Der Spiegel* (5 June) no. 23.

Eley, Geoff. 1991. Dealing with the Past: Nazism and other Continuities. *Michigan Quarterly Review* 30: 488–505.

Gallagher, Hugh G. 1990. *By Trust Betrayed*. New York: Henry Holt.

Kater, Michael H. 1989. *Doctors Under Hitler*. Chapel Hill: University of North Carolina Press.

Landsberger, Henry A. 1992. Don't Tie Weimar Clinics to Nazi Horrors. *New York Times* (29 November): E10.

Lifton, Robert J. 1986. *The Nazi Doctors*. New York: Basic Books.

Meyer, Ernie. 1989. When Ethics Fall Prey to 'Thrill of Science.' *Jerusalem Post* (12 May).

Müller-Hill, Benno. 1988. *Murderous Science*. Oxford: Oxford University Press.

Proctor, Robert. 1988. *Racial Hygiene*. Cambridge: Harvard University Press.

Schöne-Seifert, Bettina, and Rippe, Klaus-Peter. 1991. Silencing the Singer: Antibioethics in Germany. *Hastings Center Report* 21 (6): 20–27.

Singer, Peter. 1975. *Animal Liberation*. (2d ed. 1990). New York: Random House.

———. 1991. On Being Silenced in Germany. *New York Review of Books* (15 August): 36–42.

———. 1987. *Practical Ethics*. Oxford: Oxford University Press/Clarendon Press.

West German Scientists Plant Genetically Altered Flowers. 1990. *Reuters* (14 May).

The Use of Blacks for Medical Experimentation and Demonstration in the Old South

TODD L. SAVITT

"AN ABUNDANCE OF MATERIALS in the southern medical journals reveals that slaves had a fairly significant role in medical education and in experimental and radical medical and surgical practice of the antebellum South," remarked J. Walter Fisher in a 1968 article describing some of the medical uses to which slaves were put in the Old South.[1] Further investigation into this subject indicates that southern white medical educators and researchers relied greatly on the availability of Negro patients for various purposes. Black bodies often found their way to dissecting tables, operating amphitheaters, classroom or bedside demonstrations, and experimental facilities. This is not to deny that white bodies were similarly used.[2] In northern cities and in southern port towns such as New Orleans, Louisville, Memphis, Charleston, and Mobile, where poor, transient whites were abundant, seamen, European immigrants, and white indigents undoubtedly joined blacks in fulfilling the "clinical material" needs of the medical profession. But blacks were particularly easy targets, given their positions as voiceless slaves or "free persons of color" in a society sensitive to and separated by race. This open and deliberate use of blacks for medical research and demonstration well illustrates the racial attitudes of antebellum white southerners.

Interestingly, people generally assumed that information gained from observation of Negro

bodies was applicable to Caucasians. Despite the political rhetoric then current in the Old South about a separate medicine for blacks and for whites,[3] the research and teaching reflected, in fact, the opposite. Negroes did not seem to differ enough from Caucasians to exclude them from extensive use in southern medical schools and in research activities.[4]

Use of blacks for medical experimentation and demonstration was not the result of a conscious organized plan on the part of white southerners to learn more about the differences between the races or even how better to care for their black charges. The examples related in this article reflect the actions of individual researchers and medical institutions. Taken together, however, a pattern emerges. Blacks were considered more available and more accessible in this white-dominated society: they were rendered physically visible by their skin color but were legally invisible because of their slave status.

Throughout history medicine has required bodies for teaching purposes. Students had to learn anatomy, recognize and diagnose diseases, and treat conditions requiring surgery; researchers had to try out their ideas and new techniques; and practitioners had to perform autopsies to confirm their diagnoses and to understand the effects of diseases on the human body. The need for human specimens became more recognized and more emphasized in America during the first half of the nineteenth century as the ideas of the French school of hospital medicine reached this country.[5] Bedside experience,

TODD L. SAVITT is a historian of medicine who teaches history and medical ethics at the East Carolina University School of Medicine.

Journal of Southern History XLVIII, no. 3 (August 1982): 331–348. Copyright © 1982 by the Southern Historical Association. Reprinted by permission of the Managing Editor.

clinical-pathological correlations, and statistical studies became increasingly important. And medical schools throughout the United States, including those in the South, attempted to meet the new demands of students for a modern education. Clinics, infirmaries, and hospitals were opened in conjunction with those colleges; patients, however, were not always willing to enter. To fill beds it became essential to use the poor and the enslaved. Medicine thus capitalized on the need of the indigent and the helpless for medical care. In the South white attitudes toward blacks ensured the selection of patients of this group as specimens, though some whites were also used.

Competition for students among southern medical schools was fierce during the thirty years preceding the Civil War, which led each institution to publicize the positive aspects of its program in newspapers, medical journals, circulars, and magazines. One of the major requisites of any school was an abundant supply of clinical material—living patients for medical and surgical demonstrations as well as cadavers for anatomical dissections and pathological examinations. Institutional reputations were made and broken on the basis of the availability of teaching specimens. The Transylvania University Medical Department in Lexington, Kentucky, serves as a case in point. One of the causes for its decline from eminence during the 1830s was its purported difficulty in procuring bodies for clinical teaching. . . . On the other hand, a medical school was established in nearby Louisville (Louisville Medical Institute) in 1837, owing in part to the presence of a large black (as well as transient white) population, well suited to the needs of teaching institutions.[6] . . . There,

> "An intelligent nurse and faithful servant will be in constant attendance." No mention of the presence of medical students was necessary. The boarding fee was reasonable (fifteen cents per day), and the doctor's fee was waived if the case turned out to be incurable and the slave had to be sent home.[7] . . .

In Georgia, Kentucky, Alabama, South Carolina, Virginia, and presumably in other southern states the patients used for the education of students were frequently black. Newspaper advertisements by the Atlanta Medical College, for example, encouraged owners to send their sick and injured slaves to the infirmary for treatment.

. . . Probably typical of patient use for demonstrations at the Atlanta Medical College Infirmary was what a professor of materia medica termed "An interesting case of Hepatic Abscess in a negro man" who "was subject to the examination of the Students for several weeks during the course of lectures, and was lectured upon and prescribed for in presence of the Class." Similarly, he wrote that a black woman suffering from tuberculosis "had been under our occasional observation for a year previously."[8]

South Carolina medical institutions were even more explicit in their public requests for black patients. In the late 1830s both Charleston medical schools operated infirmaries during the regular teaching sessions from November to March, and both catered to the large black population resident in the city and surrounding area. The hospital of the Medical College of the State of South Carolina admitted slaves, poor whites, and free blacks. As an inducement to lure patients from the competing medical-school hospital, infirmary officials made owners of slaves liable for no professional charges, the only account rendered being that for food and nursing. This was so, they explained, because "The sole object of the Faculty . . . [is] to promote the interest of Medical education within their native State and City."[9] The surgery established by the faculty of the other school, the Medical College of South Carolina, admitted slaves and free blacks only. An advertisement placed in the Charleston *Courier* requested planters with servants "laboring under Surgical diseases," local physicians with slave patients requiring surgical intervention, and "Such [free] persons of color as may not be able to pay for Medical advice . . . ," to call at the hospital. "The object of the Faculty . . . ," the announcement continued, "is to collect as many interesting cases, as possible, for the benefit and instruction of their pupils."[10]

By 1841 the Medical College of the State of South Carolina had established a permanent year-round hospital with large wards for black and white patients. College officials claimed that they had little trouble filling beds at this new infirmary, because "the slave population of the city, and neighboring plantations, is capable of furnishing ample materials for clinical instruction." Students at the school saw not only "all the common diseases of the climate" but also a variety of operative procedures, owing to the presence of a slave population "peculiarly liable to surgical diseases requiring operations for their relief."[11] The medical college continued to use black patients for surgical demonstrations throughout the antebellum years. During the late 1850s, for instance, surgical cases occurring among blacks while school was in session were admitted to the "Coloured Wards" of a newly constructed public hospital and were reserved for the exclusive use of student doctors.[12]

The use of black patients for medical-school training was not confined to the lower South. The Hampden-Sydney College Medical Department (called the Medical College of Virginia after 1854) located in Richmond employed many of the same techniques as the South Carolina and Georgia institutions to attract Negroes into its infirmary wards. Faculty physicians announced in an 1853 publication that "The number of negroes employed in our factories will furnish materials for the support of an extensive hospital, and afford to the student that great desideratum—clinical instruction." They placed ads in country editions of Richmond newspapers informing rural slaveholders of the infirmary's facilities, charged lower rates for blacks, and attempted (unsuccessfully) to establish first a slave hospital, then a free hospital for all indigents and for slaves.[13] Though none of the infirmary's records are extant, evidence from case histories in the local medical journals indicates that a majority of the patients were black.[14]

Neither whites nor blacks held hospitals in high esteem during the antebellum period. Not only did patients object to having medical students and doctors touching and poking them and discussing their illnesses and the merits or problems of particular modes of treatment in their presence, but they also feared that experiments might be performed on them and that they would be permitted to die so autopsies could be undertaken.[15] Nor were medical school announcements, circulated to attract students, calculated to encourage the sickly to request hospital admission. A Transylvania University Medical Department advertisement for the 1846–1847 session, though perhaps more wishful than accurate, was typical: "Clinical instructions fully equal to the wants of the class, are given at the hospital. Experience during the last session fully attested, that there were always patients sufficiently numerous for all useful purposes. Valuable opportunities are here presented for the study of the physical signs of Thoracic Diseases."[16] Illiterate slaves did not have to read such circulars to learn about medical-school hospitals; their reputations preceded them.

Though fears about mistreatment in southern hospitals were generally unfounded (doctors and students appeared, usually, to do their best to cure patients on the wards), concerns regarding the use made of deceased patients were real. Autopsies and anatomical dissections were (and are) integral and important aspects of a medical education, but people expressed great aversion to the prospect of having their bodies minutely investigated after death. Complained one Georgia physician: "There is a superstitious prejudice existing in reference to them [autopsies], and it is seldom we can secure a case, except where the light of science has made headway."[17] In 1861 a resident doctor at Charleston's Roper Hospital made the following entry in his case book after one of his white patients died: "No autopsy could be held in this case, as his friends by some accident heard of his death immediately on its taking place, and forthwith came for the body."[18] The result was that physicians and students had to resort to grave robbing, hurried dissections before bodies were claimed, and deception to obtain ca-davers for autopsy and anatomical investigations.

The attitudes of white southerners both to-ward the use of human bodies in medical educa-tion and toward blacks were silently but clearly revealed in the medical profession's heavy re-liance on Negro cadavers. Human anatomical dissection was illegal in many states during the antebellum period,[19] although medical schools continued to teach anatomy. Unless approached by angry relatives or friends of deceased persons city authorities rarely questioned medical educa-tors as to the sources of their anatomical speci-mens. Southern blacks, because of their helpless legal and inconsequential social positions, thus became prime candidates for medical-school dis-sections. Physicians usually found it much more convenient to obtain black specimens than white. "In Baltimore," commented Harriet Mar-tineau after an 1834 visit, "the bodies of coloured people exclusively are taken for dissection, 'be-cause the whites do not like it, and the coloured people cannot resist.'"[20] Dr. Henry M. Dowling of Leesburg, Virginia, had little difficulty receiv-ing permission for an autopsy on a twelve-year-old slave girl with a suspected case of worms be-cause the victim's owner was "a gentleman of intelligence, and unaffected by the vulgar preju-dices entertained on this subject . . ." by others.[21]

When it came to obtaining Caucasian bodies for postmortem examinations, however, even "gentlemen of intelligence" found ways to refuse physicians. For example, of twenty-four individ-ual autopsies reported by white southern physi-cians in the *Transylvania Journal of Medicine and the Associate Sciences* (1828–1839) and the *Transyl-vania Medical Journal* (1849–1851) nineteen were performed on blacks and only five on whites, in a state where the white population far exceeded the black. Also indicative of the race differential is an article that appeared in the *Transactions of the Medical Association of the State of Alabama* de-scribing an 1853 typhoid-fever epidemic in the vicinity of Sumterville. Of the approximately forty-five blacks and twenty whites who con-tracted the disease, it killed a young white physi-

cian and his sister as well as ten other persons of both races. The three autopsies the reporting physician performed, however, were all on slaves.[22]

Bondsmen were not entirely voiceless in the matter of autopsies. Some masters honored the wishes of deceased slaves' relatives or friends and refused permission for postmortem examina-tions. Colonel S. B. Stevens of Quincy, Florida, objected when Dr. Richard Jarrot proposed to perform an autopsy on the body of 102-year-old Moses, dead of what appeared to be acute pleuri-tis.[23] The master of a large Lowndes County, Al-abama, plantation released for postmortem ex-amination the body of only one of eight slave children who had died during a violent dysentery outbreak in 1851 despite the request of the attend-ing physicians for other cadavers.[24] And a Vir-ginia slaveowner, "unwilling to do violence to his [slave's] prejudices and feelings," withheld as-sent when a physician requested an autopsy on the bondsman's wife.[25]

Occasionally, the prevailing attitude of whites —that dissection was acceptable when confined to the black population—was expressed in print. A correspondent to the Milledgeville, Georgia, *Statesman and Patriot* in 1828 agreed that it was necessary to dissect corpses to learn anatomy but opposed the use of whites for such a procedure. He endorsed a proposal then before the state leg-islature that permitted local authorities to release bodies of executed black felons to medical soci-eties for the purpose of dissection, assuring the safety of white corpses. "The *bodies of colored* per-sons, whose execution is necessary to public se-curity, may, we think, be with equity appropri-ated for the benefit of a science on which so many lives depend, while the measure would in a great degree secure the sepulchral repose of those who go down into the grave amidst the lamenta-tions of friends and the reverence of society."[26]

The Kentucky House of Representatives seri-ously considered a similar proposal. It rejected by the narrow margin of seven votes a bill "to au-thorize and require the Judges of the different Circuit Courts of this state to adjudge and award the corpses of negroes, executed by sentences of said judges, to the Faculties of the different chartered Colleges in this state, for dissection and experiment."[27] In Virginia the vast majority of cadavers obtained for dissection at the five antebellum medical schools were those of Negroes.[28] The faculty of the Medical College of Georgia in Augusta hired, between 1834 and 1852, several slaves to act as intermediaries in the purchase of bodies from masters in the surrounding plantation country. In 1852 it purchased Grandison Harris in Charleston to obtain cadavers and to perform janitorial duties. He robbed graves and also bought black bodies for the next fifty years or so.[29] And the Medical College of South Carolina openly acknowledged in its circular of 1831 that it obtained "Subjects . . . for every purpose" from the black rather than the white population of Charleston so as to carry on "proper dissections . . . without offending any individuals. . . ."[30] This undisguised use of Negroes for dissection in Charleston continued into the postwar era.[31]

Blacks usually knew full well how the bodies of their friends and relatives were being used, and they were both offended and frightened. The Reverend Robert Wilson of Charleston in 1856 overheard one aged Negro woman exclaim to her friend as they passed a building housing the city's medical school, "Please Gawd, when I dead, I hope I wi' dead in de summah time."[32] Classes ran only from November to March, the cold months when bodies did not decompose rapidly. A former slave, Charlie Grant, recalled many years after the event how, as an adolescent boy near Florence, South Carolina, he was paid two dollars by a local doctor to dig up and carry to his office the body of a one- or two-year-old slave child who had just been buried. Though Grant did not let on, he knew what was happening: "Dr. Johnson want to cut dat child open. Dat what he want wid it."[33] Black fear of medical schools and dissection inevitably carried over into the postbellum period, when whites, as a means of maintaining control over freedmen, reinforced the idea of "night-doctors" who stole,

killed, and then dissected blacks.[34] The accuracy of the belief that whites actually killed blacks for use in dissection is hard to verify.[35] But the fear blacks harbored was well known, as illustrated by four of the nine verses of the following poem, probably written by a white in black dialect in the late nineteenth or early twentieth century. It poked fun at these very real concerns of blacks:

THE DISSECTING HALL

Yuh see dat house? Dat great brick house?
Way yonder down de street?
Dey used to take dead folks een dar
Wrapped een a long white sheet.

An' sometimes we'en a nigger'd stop,
A-wondering who was dead,
Dem stujent men would take a club
An' bat 'im on de head.

An' drag dat poor dead nigger chile
Right een dat 'sectin hall
To vestigate 'is liver—lights—
His gizzard an' 'is gall.

Tek off dat nigger's han's an' feet—
His eyes, his head, an' all,
An' w'en dem stujent finish
Dey was nothin' left at all.[36]

The abolitionist Theodore Dwight Weld was not exaggerating when he claimed in his 1839 polemical work, *American Slavery as It Is:* "'Public opinion' would tolerate surgical experiments, operations, processes, performed upon them [slaves], which it would execrate if performed upon their master or other whites."[37]

. . . There was little fear of retribution, and as long as death or debility attributable to the new technique did not result the cost was negligible. Blacks, therefore, did have reason for fearing misuse at the hands of southern white physicians.

Generally speaking, in the era prior to acceptance of the germ theory there was only a fine line between seeking an appropriate treatment and engaging in actual experimentation.[38] A physician confronted with sick patients administered whatever treatments he had found efficacious from previous experience without really understanding their actual operation within the body.

If the standard remedy failed another compound was tried, regardless of its "scientific" merit. Few practitioners attempted to perform controlled experiments to determine the properties and effects of the drugs they used or to establish basic physiological or surgical principles that would serve as guides for the medical profession. Medical practice at this time was basically empirical, as southern white doctors indicated in their journal articles. And here blacks often served as the test subjects for new remedies. . . .

Empirical trials of remedies on patients were not unusual in the practice of medicine anywhere in antebellum America, but outright experimentation upon living humans may have occurred more openly and perhaps more often in the South owing to the nature of the slave society. No studies of human experimentation and use of white medical specimens in the North or South presently exist to substantiate this claim. Comparative statistics of this nature are difficult to obtain. Certainly, the indigent and socially voiceless were used by medical people for their own ends in the North and, as Ronald Leslie Numbers has pointed out in a recent article, in Europe at that time. The social status of Dr. William Beaumont's experimental subject, a poor French-Canadian trapper named Alexis St. Martin, is illustrative of this attitude. Beaumont induced St. Martin by force and by various legal and financial means to submit to some nine years (1824–1833) of intermittent experimentation on the physiological activity of his stomach, part of which had been permanently exposed in a gunshot accident. The ethics of human experimentation were not established at this time—people generally accepted the research of Beaumont and others without questioning their ethics or the patient's rights.[39] It did not seem odd or unusual then to use blacks as a number of physicians in the South did. Some whites took advantage of southern blacks by testing new techniques or remedies in the name of medical progress. In several instances physicians purchased blacks for the sole purpose of experimentation; in others the doctors used free blacks and slaves owned by others. Though white subjects were included in one or two cases of experimentation, blacks always made up the overwhelming majority of patients. A few major medical breakthroughs did result from the research performed upon Negroes, for which the physicians involved received fame and glory. The slaves, identified, if at all, by first name only, are unknown now to their descendants and to the general public.

A tale passed down by residents of the Alabama Black Belt illustrates the inclination of some southern whites to use blacks for experimental purposes and to discount the worth of slave lives in their society. When the region around Marion was first being settled people were unsure of its healthfulness. They feared the mists, swamp gases, and miasmata that rose from the low ground. According to tradition, a number of farmers purchased a slave, set him up in a hut with tools, supplies, and food, and left him there for a period of time to see if he could survive. Finding him still healthy when they returned, the settlers moved in, and the area grew rapidly.[40] Whether true or not, the story describes some southern whites' attitudes toward using blacks in experiments.

A number of doctors had similar inclinations. Dr. T. Stillman of Charleston, for example, operated a private infirmary in the 1830s that specialized in the treatment of skin diseases, although he also cared for patients with a variety of other disorders. During the month of October 1838 Stillman concluded his usual lengthy advertisement in the Charleston *Mercury* with an offer to purchase from slaveowners any chronically diseased slaves they might wish to "dispose of." He would pay "The highest cash price" for fifty blacks "affected with scrofula or king's evil, confirmed hypochondriasm, apoplexy, diseases of the liver, kidneys, spleen, stomach and intestines, bladder and its appendages, diarrhea, dysentery, &c."[41] It was obvious from the wording of the advertisement that Dr. Stillman planned to test newly formulated remedies on these fifty chronically ill blacks for the benefit of medical science, as well, no doubt, as for personal gain.

In a few instances actual discussions of the kinds of experiments to which slaves were subjected are available, both from the point of view of the patients and the physicians. There lived in Clinton, seat of Jones County, Georgia, during the 1820s and early 1830s, a physician-planter who was attempting to discover the best remedies for heat stroke. This man, Dr. Thomas Hamilton, borrowed the slave Fed from a grateful patient in order to test some of his medications on a human subject. He had a hole dug in the ground which he then had heated with fire to a high temperature. Fed sat naked on a stool on a platform placed within this ovenlike pit with only his head above ground level. To retain the heat Hamilton fastened wet blankets over the hole. Fed took a different medicine each of the five or six times he entered the pit over a period of two or three weeks, so that Hamilton could determine which preparation best enabled the slave to withstand high temperatures. Fed fainted each time from the heat and from exhaustion (he had put in a full day's work before each experiment). According to Fed's account of the proceedings the doctor found cayenne pepper to be the most effective preparation. Experimentation did not end here, however. Fed claimed, in a book written in London some years after his escape from slavery, that Hamilton came to his master's farm to perform other experiments on him for nine months, after which time "I had become so weak, that I was no longer able to work in the fields." . . . Other aspects of Fed's narrative also bear up under historical scrutiny.[42]

Hamilton's crude experiments did little to advance medical knowledge. The same cannot be said for Dr. James Marion Sims's use of slave women to develop a cure for vesico-vaginal fistula. . . . Once Sims had conceived of a way to operate on patients with vesico-vaginal fistula he set about putting his ideas into practice with the cooperation of his slave subjects. He never disguised the fact that what he was doing was entirely experimental. . . .

It is significant that all the subjects in Sims's experiments were black. When he decided to pursue his idea of curing vesico-vaginal fistula he "ransacked the country for [Negro] cases" and found enough to warrant enlarging his eight-bed slave infirmary. . . .

Other examples can be offered of the white southern physician's bias toward the use of black subjects in medical experimentation. Dr. Ephraim McDowell of Danville, Kentucky, revered in American medical history as the first to perform successfully an ovariotomy (removal of an ovary), operated initially upon a white woman, Mrs. Jane Todd Crawford, in 1809. Little known is the fact that McDowell's subsequent four ovariotomies, during which he improved his technique, were all performed on black women — again, this in Kentucky, a state with a relatively small black population.[43] . . .

A final example of the usefulness of blacks to physicians in a slave society was the performance of Caesarean operations on pregnant women. Attempts at delivering children abdominally when they could not pass through the mother's contracted or occluded pelvis had been generally unsuccessful throughout history. Doctors in antebellum America continued to perform this procedure and occasionally met with success. The racial statistics, derived from compilations of the Philadelphia physician Dr. Robert P. Harris in the 1870s and early 1880s, are revealing: of fifteen northern women whose race was reported, thirteen were white, one black, and one Mexican (California); in the South, twenty-nine of thirty-six cases were black.[44] This trend continued throughout the nineteenth century. . . .

It is to be expected in a slave society that the subjugated will be exploited. Such was the case in the American South where blacks acted not only as servants and laborers but also as medical specimens. Some medical scientists living in that society took advantage of the slaves' helplessness to utilize them in demonstrations, autopsies, dissections, and experiments, situations distasteful to whites and rejected by them. Some whites, usually the poor and the friendless, found themselves in the same position as blacks. But given the racial attitudes of that time and place, blacks were particularly vulnerable to abuse or mishandling at the hands of researchers, medical teachers, or students.

NOTES

1. Fisher, "Physicians and Slavery in the Antebellum Southern Medical Journal," *Journal of the History of Medicine and Allied Sciences,* XXIII (January 1968), 45. W. Montague Cobb discussed a similar theme in "Surgery and the Negro Physician: Some Parallels in Background," National Medical Association, *Journal,* XLIII (May 1951), 145–52, especially 147–48.

2. David C. Humphrey, "Dissection and Discrimination: The Social Origins of Cadavers in America, 1760–1915," New York Academy of Medicine, *Bulletin,* XLIX (September 1973), 819–27; John B. Blake, "Anatomy," in Ronald L. Numbers, ed., *The Education of American Physicians: Historical Essays* (Berkeley, Los Angeles, and London, 1980), 34–35, 37.

3. John Duffy, "A Note on Ante-Bellum Southern Nationalism and Medical Practice," *Journal of Southern History,* XXXIV (May 1968), 274–76; John S. Haller, Jr., "The Negro and the Southern Physicians: A Study of Medical and Racial Attitudes, 1800–1860," *Medical History,* XVI (July 1972), 247–51; Todd L. Savitt, *Medicine and Slavery: The Diseases and Health Care of Blacks in Antebellum Virginia* (Urbana, Chicago, and London, 1978), 7–17.

4. Commenting on this irony, the anatomist W. Montague Cobb, himself black, wrote in 1951, ". . . our [white] colleagues recognized in the Negro [on the dissecting table] a perfection in human structure which they were unwilling to concede when that structure was animated by the vital spark." Cobb, "Surgery and the Negro Physician," 148.

5. On the ideas and importance of the Paris school of hospital medicine see Erwin H. Ackerknecht, *Medicine at the Paris Hospital, 1794–1848* (Baltimore, 1967); Michel Foucault, *The Birth of the Clinic: An Archaeology of Medical Perception* (New York, 1973). On the influence of the Paris school on American medicine see Richard H. Shryock, *The Development of Modern Medicine: An Interpretation of the Social and Scientific Factors Involved* (New York, 1947), 170–91; Gerald N. Grob, *Edward Jarvis and the Medical World of Nineteenth-Century America* (Knoxville, Tenn., 1978), 37–38.

6. Robert Peter, *The History of the Medical Department of Transylvania University* (Louisville, 1905), 61; catalogues of the Medical Department of Transylvania University, 1829–1855, in the library at Transylvania College, Lexington, Kentucky; "Preamble and Resolutions of the Dissecting Class [of Transylvania Medical College, 1837/38]," Appendix to Thomas D. Mitchell,

"Transylvania Catalogue of Medical Graduates, with an Appendix, Containing a Concise History of the School from Its Commencement to the Present Time," *Transylvania Journal of Medicine and Associate Sciences,* XI (January–March 1838), 229-30. For a discussion of the history of anatomy in antebellum Kentucky see Wayne C. Williams, "The Teachers and Teaching of Anatomy in the Medical Department of Transylvania University, 1799–1857" (unpublished paper in author's and Savitt's possession), 7–16. Mr. Williams is Director of the Audiovisual Dept., East Carolina University School of Medicine. See also John H. Ellis, *Medicine in Kentucky* (Lexington, Ky., 1977), 13.

7. Quoted in Franklin M. Garrett, *Atlanta and Environs: A Chronicle of Its People and Events* (2 vols., Athens, Ga., 1954), I, 395–96 (quotation on p. 395), from Atlanta *Weekly Intelligencer,* October 12, 1855. See also Gerald L. Cates, "Medical Schools in Ante-Bellum Georgia" (unpublished M.A. thesis, University of Georgia, 1969), 92–93.

8. J. G. Westmoreland, "Report of Medical Clinic, Continued," *Atlanta Medical and Surgical Journal,* 1 (February 1856), 329 (first two quotations), 331 (third quotation). On the use of blacks and indigent whites in Alabama see W. Taylor, "Annual Oration," Medical Association of the State of Alabama, *Transactions,* VIII (February 1855), 121.

9. Charleston *Courier,* November 14, 1837.

10. *Ibid.,* November 16, 1837.

11. *Annual Circular of the Trustees and Faculty of the Medical College of the State of South Carolina . . . Session of 1840–41* (Charleston, 1840), 5–6.

12. "A Plan of Organization for the Roper Hospital. Adopted by the Medical Society, Jan. 3, 1846," *Rules and Regulations for the Government of the Trustees and Officers of the Roper Hospital* (Charleston, 1861), 11–12; *Annual Circular of the Trustees and Faculty of the Medical College of the State of South Carolina . . . Session of 1857–58* (Charleston, 1858), 17. See also Joseph I. Waring, *A History of Medicine in South Carolina, 1825–1900* (Columbia, S. C., 1967), 75–76, 79n.

13. "An Address to the Public in Regard to the Affairs of the Medical Department of Hampden-Sydney College, by Several Physicians of the City of Richmond, 1853," quoted in Wyndham B. Blanton, *Medicine in Virginia in the Nineteenth Century* (Richmond, 1933), 38–39 (quotation); Richmond *Enquirer,* May 8, 1860; "Notes of the Hampden-Sydney Medical Department Minutes," in William T. Sanger, *Medical College of Virginia Before 1925, and University College of Medicine 1893–1913* (Richmond, 1973), 8; editorial, "A State General Hospital," *Virginia Medical and Surgical Journal,* 1 (April 1853), 173–74; editorial, "The Virginia Free Hospital," *ibid.,* III (June 1854), 273–75. For more

descriptive details see Savitt, *Medicine and Slavery,* 262–86.

14. Of 109 patients mentioned in Richmond medical journals between 1851 and 1860, 63.3 percent (69) were black. For a listing of the pertinent journal articles see Savitt, *Medicine and Slavery,* 286.

15. See for example Richmond *Daily Dispatch,* July 21, 1854; William W. Brown, *Clotel; or The President's Daughter* (London, 1853), 123–24, cited in Gladys-Marie Fry, *Night Riders in Black Folk History* (Knoxville, Tenn., 1975), 175–76; Keith A. Winsell, "Black Identity: The Southern Negro, 1830–1895" (unpublished Ph.D. dissertation, University of California at Los Angeles, 1971), 188.

16. *Circular of the Transylvania University Medical Department, Session of 1846–47,* p. 4. For a vivid description of the popular image of distasteful hospital life see Thomas Jefferson to James C. Cabell, May 16, 1824, in [Nathaniel F. Cabell, ed.], *Early History of the University of Virginia as Contained in the Letters of Thomas Jefferson and Joseph C. Cabell* (Richmond, 1856), 310.

17. Henry A. Ramsay, "Gastro-Enteritis of Twelve Months Duration, Exhibiting in Autopsy an Entire Absence of the Spleen, and Calcareous Depositions in Both Lungs," *Charleston Medical Journal and Review,* V (November 1850), 728–32 (quotation on p. 732).

18. Roper Hospital Case Book #2, 1858–62, p. 432, in possession of Dr. Robert Jordan, Sanford, North Carolina (microfilm copy at Waring Historical Library, Medical University of South Carolina, Charleston). See also, Walter Brice, "Typhoid Fever, as It Prevailed in Fairfield District, South Carolina," *Charleston Medical Journal and Review,* VI (September 1851). 671.

19. George B. Jenkins, "The Legal Status of Dissecting," *Anatomical Record,* VII (November 1913), 387–88; John B. Blake, "The Development of American Anatomy Acts," *Journal of Medical Education,* XXX (August 1955), 434.

20. Harriet Martineau, *Retrospect of Western Travel* (2 vols., London and New York, 1838), I, 140, quoted in Humphrey, "Dissection and Discrimination," 819.

21. Dowling, "Case of Verminose Disease," *Transylvania Journal of Medicine and the Associate Sciences,* II (May 1829), 250.

22. L. H. Anderson, "Report on the Diseases of Sumterville and Vicinity," Medical Association of the State of Alabama, *Transactions,* VII (January 1854), 61–66.

23. Jarrot, "Amputation for Gangrene of the Foot, Successfully Performed on a Negro, at the Advanced Age of One Hundred and Two Years," *Charleston Medical Journal and Review,* IV (May 1849), 301–303.

24. P. N. Cilley, "Diseases of Lowndesboro and Vicinity," Medical Association of the State of Alabama, *Proceedings,* V (December 1851), 91–95.

25. A Young Practitioner, "Report of a Case of Disease Supposed to be Peritonitis," *Monthly Stethoscope and Medical Reporter,* 1 (June 1856), 364.

26. Milledgeville *Statesman and Patriot,* August 16, 1826. The author wishes to thank Professor Larry Morrison, History Department, Virginia Polytechnic Institute and State University, for bringing this newspaper article to his attention.

27. *Journal of the House of Representatives of the Commonwealth of Kentucky . . .* (Frankfort, Ky., 1833), 107 (quotation), 122–23, 177–78. See also John D. Wright, Jr., "Robert Peter and Early Science in Kentucky" (unpublished Ph.D. dissertation, Columbia University, 1955), 61, 70; F. Garvin Davenport, *Ante-Bellum Kentucky: A Social History, 1800–1860* (Oxford, Ohio, 1943), 23.

28. Savitt, *Medicine and Slavery,* 290–93; James O. Breeden, "Body Snatchers and Anatomy Professors: Medical Education in Nineteenth-Century Virginia," *Virginia Magazine of History and Biography,* LXXXIII (July 1975), 321–45.

29. Lane Allen, "Grandison Harris, Sr.: Slave, Resurrectionist and Judge," Georgia Academy of Science, *Bulletin,* XXXIV (April 1976), 192–99.

30. Fry, *Night Riders,* 173–74.

31. Faculty Minutes, Medical College of the State of South Carolina, May 8, 1876 (Waring Historical Library). For reference to similar attitudes at the Medical College of Georgia in Augusta see Cates, "Medical Schools in Ante-Bellum Georgia," 32. On the use of blacks for dissection in an Alabama medical school see Howard L. Holley, "Dr. Phillip Madison Shepard and His Medical School," *De Historia Medicinae,* II (February 1958), 1–5. For an instance in Kentucky see the "Autobiography of Dr. Charles A. Hentz" (typescript), X, 108, Hentz Family Papers (Southern Historical Collection, University of North Carolina, Chapel Hill, N. C.).

32. Robert Wilson, "Their Shadowy Influence Still Hovers About Medical College," Charleston *Sunday News Courier,* April 13, 1913. The author wishes to thank Mrs. Anne Donato of the Waring Historical Library, Medical University of South Carolina, Charleston, for bringing this article to his attention.

33. George P. Rawick, ed., *The American Slave: A Composite Autobiography* (19 vols., Westport, Conn., 1972, II: *South Carolina Narratives,* Part 2, pp. 175–76 (quotation on p. 176).

34. Fry, *Night Riders,* 170–211.

35. There is evidence to indicate that black bodies from the South were regularly shipped to northern medical schools during the post-Civil War era. See Frederick C. Waite, "Grave Robbing in New England," Medical Library Association, *Bulletin,* XXXIII (July 1945), 283–84; Cobb, "Surgery and the Negro Physician," 148.

36. *Scribe*, I (December 1951), 17. The author is again indebted to Mrs. Anne Donato for this reference.

37. Weld, *American Slavery as It Is: Testimony of a Thousand Witnesses* (New York, 1839), 170.

38. For a broad overview of this subject see Richard H. Shryock, "Empiricism Versus Rationalism in American Medicine, 1650–1950," American Antiquarian Society, *Proceedings*, N.S., LXXIX, Part 1 (April 15, 1969), 99–150.

39. Numbers, "William Beaumont and the Ethics of Human Experimentation," *Journal of the History of Biology*, XII (Spring 1979), 113–35. See also Chester R. Burns, "Medical Ethics in the United States Before the Civil War" (unpublished Ph.D. dissertation, Johns Hopkins University, 1969), 83. For an early expression of this attitude toward blacks as experimental subjects in South Carolina see Edmund Berkeley and Dorothy S. Berkeley, *Dr. Alexander Gorden of Charles Town* (Chapel Hill, N. C., 1969), 95–96. For a full description of Beaumont's work see James T. Flexner, *Doctors on Horseback: Pioneers of American Medicine* (New York, 1937), 237–89.

40. Weymouth T. Jordan, *Ante-Bellum Alabama: Town and Country* (Tallahassee, Fla., 1957), 34–35.

41. Charleston *Mercury*, October 12, 1838, reprinted in Weld, *Slavery as It Is*, 171.

42. Louis A. Chamerovzow, ed., *Slave Life in Georgia: A Narrative of the Life, Sufferings, and Escape of John Brown, a Fugitive Slave, Now in England* (London, 1855), 45–48, cited in F. Nash Boney, "Doctor Thomas Hamilton: Two Views of a Gentleman of the Old South," *Phylon*, XXVIII (Fall 1967), 288–92 (quotation on page 291).

43. Samuel D. Gross, "Report of the Committee on Surgery," Kentucky State Medical Association, *Transactions*, II (October 1852), 104–106; Cobb, "Surgery and the Negro Physician," 148.

44. Robert P. Harris, "The Operation of Gastro-Hysterotomy (true Caesarian Section) . . . ," *American Journal of the Medical Sciences*, N.S., LXXV (April 1878), 336–39. For more detail on Caesarean section cases in Virginia see Savitt, *Medicine and Slavery*, 118–19.

Race, Gender, and Medical Experimentation: J. Marion Sims' Surgery on Slave Women, 1845–1850

DIANA AXELSEN

Sims, James Marion (1813–1883). American surgeon and pioneer in gynecology. Born in Southern Carolina and graduated from Jefferson Medical College in Philadelphia, he is known chiefly for the semiprone position and the curved speculum that are named after him, and that contributed to his success in operating for vesicovaginal fistula. He established the State Hospital for Women in New York, and was president of the American Medical Association and honorary president of the International Medical Congress.

Miller-Keane Encyclopedia and Dictionary of Medicine, Nursing, and Allied Health, 1992[1]

DIANA E. AXELSEN has taught philosophy and women's studies for 23 years at Spelman College in Atlanta and California Lutheran University. She currently is a senior books production editor at Sage Publications.

As THE 21ST CENTURY draws near, we are far more aware of the moral hazards posed by ex-

Reprinted by permission of Diana E. Axelsen. Black Women in American History: From Colonial Times through the Nineteenth Century, *ed. Darlene Clark Hine.*

perimentation with human subjects than were the people of the mid-19th century. J. Marion Sims did not practice medicine in a world with hospital ethics committees, review boards, and a federal Food and Drug Administration. Nor did he have the advantage of almost instant access to research being done in his field throughout the world, or the country, or even of the South. Although it is important to learn about this horrifying part of medical history in the United States, the aim of this chapter is not to vilify Sims. Certainly the racism and exploitation of human subjects needs to be known. More important, however, we need to understand how the very actions that led to his being celebrated as the "father of gynecology" could exemplify a shocking disregard for the personhood of African American women. Most important of all, we need to see the story of J. Marion Sims in the context of a culture in which race and gender still play a crucial role in a health care system that continues to affect women of color in profoundly negative ways.

When I first began research on Sims' experimental surgery with slave women in the 1970s, bioethics was still a relatively new field. The moral implications of experimentation with human subjects were among the most central concerns, and the horror of the Tuskegee experiments on African American men with syphilis was getting a lot of attention. Experimentation on LSD with members of the U.S. Army and the use of prison inmates as experimental subjects were being challenged. Feminists were calling attention to the injustice of using Third World women as subjects in experiments with contraceptives. New bioethics textbooks included accounts of other violations of the rights of experimental subjects.

Now, 25 years later, racism and sexism, as well as discrimination based on socioeconomic status, continue to affect the health status of non-whites and of all women, especially women of color. And J. Marion Sims continues to be celebrated as a pioneer in gynecology, while little attention is given to the ways the in-

stitution of slavery made those contributions possible. A new book edited by Marcia Bayne-Smith, *Race, Gender, and Health* (1996), provides a current analysis of how discrimination based on race, gender, and class continues to jeopardize the health status of four groups of women in the United States today: African Americans, Asian/Pacific Islander women, American Indian and Alaskan Native women, and Latinas.[2] The problems she identifies make it clear that we need to look again at the story of Anarcha, Betsy, and Lucy, three of our forgotten foremothers.[3]

THE STATUS OF HEALTH CARE FOR SLAVES

First, we shall look at the status of health care for slaves in the 19th-century culture in which Sims practiced. In *Black Culture and Black Consciousness,*[4] Lawrence Levine describes the importance of folk remedies among slaves and notes that slaves resisted attempts by their masters to interfere with these traditional medical practices. Many of these remedies were of African origin, and the medical lore was preserved and transmitted in this country by grandparents born in Africa. Levine also notes that "a number of slave practitioners won considerable renown for their skills."[5] Indeed, white patients of one Tennessee slave petitioned the state legislature to allow him to practice medicine formally. Also, white, black, and Native American populations shared folk practices and learned from one another.

On the other hand, Western medicine was gaining a firm foothold in the South. The Alabama Medical Association was organized in 1846, and there were significant numbers of physicians in Alabama. Ten years later, the Alabama legislature passed an act authorizing the Medical College of Alabama by the Alabama General Assembly on January 30, 1860.[6] According to Eugene Genovese, "Most slaveholders provided physicians' services for their slaves at an average cost of three dollars per slave per year, and many spent large numbers—ten dollars to more than a hundred—to provide medical care for slaves."[7] However, because not all slaveholders offered even minimal care, because Western medicine was often dangerous and even deadly rather than helpful, and because it is difficult to assess the overall contribution of folk medicine to the slave community, the actual health status of slaves remains a matter of controversy.

The environment in which J. Marion Sims practiced medicine, then, was one in which slaves had some access both to traditional folk medicine and to some of the resources of Western medicine. Provision of the latter, however, was an economic investment by slaveholders in the health of their slaves.

THE LIFE STORY OF J. MARION SIMS

Sims' Autobiography

Until 1950, the primary source of information about Sims' work was his own autobiography, *The Story of My Life*,[8] although there were some medical biographies in the early 1900s, including one by his son-in-law.[9] Sources that refer to Sims often quote from his autobiography, especially to his descriptions of his bout with malaria. He is known as a pioneer in the treatment of clubfoot, as well as in "women's medicine." His early years of practice included surgery on the mouth and jaw. His role in founding the Women's Hospital in New York, where for many years he was chief surgeon, is the focus of attention with respect to his career outside the South.

Woman's Surgeon

In 1950, Seale Harris published a biography of Sims, *Woman's Surgeon,* which is one of the most important sources of information concerning Sims's life and work. Harris reports that colleagues and medical historians praise celebrate Sims as "the father of American gynecology."[10] Harris regards Sims's most notable surgical con-

tribution to be his development of the technique for repair of vesicovaginal fistula, that is, a tear in the vaginal wall resulting in chronic leakage from the bladder. Although today this condition occurs primarily as a congenital defect and occasionally as a result of accident or in unattended childbirth, tears in the vaginal wall were not uncommon results of childbirth in Sims' time. Sims is known for his development of the speculum and pioneered in the use of wire sutures. He also introduced the lateral recumbent "Sims position" for pelvic examinations, childbirth, and surgery, though today this has for the most part been superseded by the lithotomy position (patient lying on her back with hips and knees fully flexed and feet in stirrups). Sims's attention to sanitary procedures is noteworthy because it preceded Listerism and probably accounts for his unusually low mortality rate during surgery (he lost no patients during the period we are considering).

Horrors of the Half-Known Life

The first book to point out the abuse of slave women in Sims' surgery was not published until 1976. British historian Graham Barker-Benfield devotes a chapter of his book, *Horrors of the Half-Known Life: Male Attitudes Toward Women and Sexuality in 19th-Century America,* to Sims.[11] I am not aware of any published analysis of this important historical instance of the abuse of women prior to Barker-Benfield's work.[12]

J. MARION SIMS, SURGEON

The Early Years

James Marion Sims was born in South Carolina in 1813 and graduated from Jefferson Medical College in Philadelphia in 1835. That fall, he moved to Mount Meigs, in Montgomery County, Alabama, where he set up practice. In 1840, he moved into the town of Montgomery. Though from the beginning of his career Sims displayed an interest in innovative surgical techniques, he did not intend to enter women's medicine, and in fact he had a deep distaste for the treatment of "women's diseases." This distaste was apparently overcome by his competitiveness with men in the development of new surgical techniques and by his desire for superiority and recognition in the male medical world of the 19th century. He saw surgery as a way of proving himself, and he regarded unsuccessful surgery as a personal failure. Sims also paved the way for an emphasis on invasive surgery as a treatment of preference for many "female disorders."[13] Moreover, Sims saw women as defined in large part by their capacity for reproduction; this attitude is reflected in his later preoccupation with problems of infertility in women.[14]

In 1845, Sims saw his first patient with vesicovaginal fistula. She was a slave woman known to us only as Anarcha. Sims had been asked to deliver her baby with forceps after she had endured three days of labor, and he reluctantly agreed. When he later saw Anarcha and was asked to consider doing surgery to repair the vaginal injuries she had sustained, resulting in both vesicovaginal fistula and rectovaginal fistula, he pronounced treatment impossible. In the next two months, he saw two other slave women, Betsy and Lucy, who were also suffering from vesicovaginal fistula. He insisted that neither woman could be treated successfully.

Sims as a Medical Pioneer

Sims changed his mind about the possibility of treating Anarcha, Betsy, and Lucy as a result of his using atmospheric pressure to distend the uterus while manually treating a woman whose uterus had been displaced in an accident. He realized that he might be able to use atmospheric pressure to his advantage in surgery on the three women. Aware of the need for an instrument to aid in the process, he developed a forerunner of the modern speculum, using a pewter spoon and an elaborate arrangement of mirrors and lighting.[15] Convinced now of the possibility of successful surgery, he made inquiries around the countryside and found that, indeed, there were other slave women who had been hidden away for years, suffering from vesicovaginal fistula. Sims had found subjects who could be used to explore the possibilities of this new surgical procedure.

SLAVE WOMEN AS EXPERIMENTAL SUBJECTS

According to Harris, women suffering from vesicovaginal fistula were unable to take any part in normal life, although their condition was not a direct cause of death. However, Sims tells us, those afflicted allegedly lived on year after year in misery and ostracism, wishing for death and sometimes committing suicide.[16] Exploring the surgical procedure that now seemed possible to Sims is portrayed by Harris as not only a surgical breakthrough but a "cure" for the psychological woes of women with this condition.

The Surgical Procedures

In 1845, Sims planned surgery for Lucy, Anarcha, and Betsy, as well as for nine other slave women whom he agreed to support, except for the provision that their masters would pay taxes on them and provide their clothing. In the first surgical procedures, Sims succeeded in closing the fistulas, but small perforations remained after healing, leakage continued, and infection of the sutures was a continuing problem. These difficulties were finally eliminated after he began using wire rather than silk sutures. The slave women endured operation after operation between 1845 and 1849 as Sims refined his surgical technique. Finally, in May, 1849, the 30th operation of Anarcha was successful.[17]

The Issue of Anesthesia

The history of anesthesia during this period is important in our analysis of Sims's work. He had performed all his surgery on the slave women without any anesthesia other than occasional use of opium, which was ineffective and tended to produce nausea and constipation.[18] Sims and Harris praised the endurance and stoicism of the slave women. After the successful operation on Anarcha, many white women came to Sims for treatment of vesicovaginal fistula. However, none was able to endure a single operation.[19]

Although Crawford Long had used inhaled ether as an anesthetic as early as 1842, Sims was unaware of Long's work in the adjoining state of Georgia. Long had apparently gotten the idea of using ether by observing that he and others sustained cuts, bruises, and other injuries during the "ether frolics" of the time, but did not feel any pain when at the time of injury. Long, however, apparently failed to realize the significance of the use of ether, or he had used it only in cases that he regarded as inadequate tests of its overall effectiveness.[20] Also, it appears that Long may have simply substituted ether for whiskey in emergencies when liquor was not available. Long first read about W. T. G. Morton's work with ether in December, 1846, but Long himself did not publish an account of his own use of it until 1849.[21] Thus, it is understandable that Sims was apparently unaware of Long's work.

Less understandable, however, is Sims' continued failure to use ether or to seek out current research in the area of anesthesiology. After G. Q. Colton used nitrous oxide or "laughing gas" as an entertainment in an 1844 demonstration in Hartford, Connecticut, Horace Wells used nitrous oxide in surgery. Wells is credited by some historians with developing the idea of anesthesia by inhalation. He continued his work with nitrous oxide in Boston in 1845. In 1846, also in Boston, W. T. G. Morton demonstrated the use of inhaled ether as an anesthetic.[22] The first published report of the discovery of surgical anesthesia in the United States appears in the November 28, 1846 issue of *The Boston Medical and Surgical Journal.*[23] From 1846 onward, the use of ether spread throughout America and Europe. Charles Jackson, a chemist, is also credited with the use of ether in Plymouth, Massachusetts, in 1842. Jackson may have suggested to

Morton the substitution of ether for nitrous oxide, because chemists knew that ether had similar effects as nitrous oxide and could be used in amounts large enough to be effective as an anesthetic—something not possible with nitrous oxide.[24]

Sims developed an interest in anesthesia and in Long's part in its history sometime after 1850, and he published an article on its history in an 1877 issue of the *Virginia Medical Monthly.*[25] However, Sims seemed unaware of the experimentation done in this area prior to 1850. This fact is especially striking because, according to Harris, Sims was given to "diligent reading of the medical journals."[26] Obviously, Sims's slave patients were in no position to demand that he search for an effective anesthetic. Moreover, slave women rarely used alcohol, seldom drank to excess, and did not use opium or other narcotics in use among some upper-class white women. Thus, it is unlikely that the slave women requested any of these substances. Even after his unsuccessful attempt to operate on white women demonstrated the pain associated with surgery, apparently Sims continued to ignore the issue of pain control for at least a year. This aspect of his work reflects the dehumanizing and insensitive way in which Sims treated his patients.

Moreover, both Harris and Sims overemphasized the severity of the condition Sims was treating. Although certainly a source of chronic discomfort and possible secondary irritation, and although obviously embarrassing in many situations, vesicovaginal fistula is not a disorder involving chronic or severe pain. As we noted above, Harris suggests that some slave women found their condition so unbearable that it drove them to suicide; however, this claim seems simply to be part of the unjustified exaggeration with which both Sims and Harris portrayed the condition. According to Genovese, there was a low incidence of suicide among the slave population generally; most slaves, he says, "seem to have resorted to suicide to escape capture after having run away or to avoid punishment after sale."[27] In any case, the discomfort of vesicovaginal fistula, in comparison to the effects of excessive beatings, chronic malnutrition, and other forms of physical and psychological aggression, hardly constitutes a plausible motive for suicide. Moreover, that slave women would have been allowed to retreat as invalids because of this condition is unlikely, given the general insistence that work takes priority.

THE RELATIONSHIP BETWEEN SIMS AND SLAVE WOMEN

Sims's attitude toward pain management and his exaggeration of the severity of his patients' condition are striking dimensions of the larger issue of the control he had over his patients. Obviously, the powerlessness of the slaves in seeking alternative medical care or in objecting to any aspect of Sims' practice must be seen as central to the coercive nature of this surgery. According to Barker-Benfield, Sims bought slaves to use as experimental subjects.[28] Harris does not mention this, but he does state that temporary control over the first twelve slaves to be operated on was given to Sims by the women's masters, with the provision that the masters pay the taxes and provide clothing.[29] Because these women had no opportunity to refuse the surgery, describing them as "cooperative" is meaningless. Sims failed utterly to recognize his patients as autonomous persons, and his insensitivity, heightened by his own personal drive for success, cannot be minimized, especially as a balance to the enormous amount of praise accorded Sims for this work and for subsequent applications of the techniques developed in Montgomery. Harris describes the numerous memorials to Sims, in Montgomery and elsewhere, and adds,

> Montgomery has not forgotten the heroic roles of the three slaves, Anarcha, Lucy, and Betsy, who suffered, not only that they themselves

might be cured, but that women injured at childbirth in future generations might be saved from lives of misery and invalidism. A movement has been begun, sponsored by leading women in Montgomery, to establish a memorial to the three slave heroines.[30]

Thus, Harris perpetuated a view of these slave women not only as choosing freely to participate in their own treatment but also as volunteers for experimental surgery intended to help future generations. It is obvious that these women, admirable though they may be, could not have made such choices because they were not free to choose or to refuse participation.

Sims, however, was very much a product of his own professional training and of his culture. His surgery occurred in the 19th century South, where racial, sexual, political, and economic power structures were uniquely suited to provide an opportunity for an abuse of human subjects such as those of Sims. A society in which being white and male was a general source of power, and in which being a physician carried special prestige, explains much of Sims's behavior. In this period, too, stoic acceptance of pain was seen as "natural" for women in childbirth and was also attributed to slaves generally. Sims' work should be understood not only as an expression of his own values, but, more broadly, as an example of the ways in which social values can deprive whole groups of persons of the right to participate in decisions concerning their own health. Today, the medical issues are different, but the need to look closely at the impact of societal values on the treatment of women in medicine remains. There is still a need to be on guard against invasive surgery, including Caesarean sections and hysterectomies, and against various forms of experiments with both contraception and reproduction.[31] As in Sims' time, poor and non-white women are especially vulnerable. Only when all women are free to choose whether to participate in research, and only when all are free to choose from the best forms of gynecological and obstetric care, will we have used the lessons of the 19th century to free women from male-controlled research and practice in "women's medicine." A real societal commitment to the health of African American women and of all women of color will require a major change in the values that underlie the entire system of health care in the United States.

NOTES

1. *Miller-Keane Encyclopedia and Dictionary of Medicine, Nursing, And Allied Health.* 1992.

2: Marcia Bayne-Smith, Ed., *Race, Gender, and Health* (Thousand Oaks, CA: Sage Publications, 1996).

3. See Diane Adams, Ed., *Health Issues for Women of Color* (Thousand Oaks, CA: Sage Publications, 1996) for a discussion of the impact of race and gender on health care for these and other ethnic groups in the United States.

4. Lawrence W. Levine, *Black Culture and Black Consciousness* (New York: Oxford University Press, 1977), p. 64.

5. Levine, pp. 64–65.

6. Lucille Griffith, *History of Alabama* (Northport, Alabama: Colonial Press, 1962), p. 146, and Saffold Bernay, *Handbook of Alabama* (Birmingham: Roberts and Son, 1892), p. 211. See also Lucille Griffith, *Alabama: a Documentary History to 1900* (Tuscaloosa, AL: University of Alabama Press, 1972).

7. Eugene Genovese, *Roll, Jordan, Roll: The World of Slaves Made* (New York: Pantheon, 1974), p. 62.

8. J. Marion Sims, *The Story of My Life.* Edited by H. Marion-Sims. (New York: Appleton, 1884, 1885, 1888). [Incomplete]

9. John Allan Wyeth, *With Sabre and Scalpel* (New York: Harper and Brothers, 1914).

10. Seale Harris, *Woman's Surgeon* (New York: Macmillan, 1950), pp. 374, 392.

11. G. J. Barker-Benfield, *The Horrors of the Half-Known Life: Male Attitudes Toward Women and Sexuality in 19th-Century America* (New York: Harper and Row, 1976).

12. For one more recent discussion of Sims' experimental surgery, see Robert S. Mendelsohn, *Male Practice: New Doctors Manipulate Women* (Chicago: Contemporary Books, 1981).

13. Harris, p. 82; Barker-Benfield, pp. 92–94.

14. Barker-Benfield, pp. 117–119.

15. Harris, pp. 82–86.

16. Harris, p. 87.

17. Harris, pp. 100–102.

18. Harris, pp. 100–102, 108–109.

19. Harris, p. 109.

20. Harris, pp. 312–313.

21. Victor Robinson, *Victory Over Pain: A History of Anesthesia* (New York: Henry Schuman, 1946), pp. 90–91.

22. Howard Riley Raper, *Man Against Pain: The Epic of Anesthesia* (New York: Prentice-Hall, 1945), pp. 151–154. See also Raper, pp. 142–154, and Robinson, pp. 83–140.

23. Smithsonian Institute, Museum of History and Technology, Medical History Section (Washington, D.C.).

24. Robinson, p. 109.

25. Harris, pp. 311–315. Sims' article, titled "The Discovery of Anesthesia," appeared in the *Virginia Medical Monthly,* 4:81–109, 1877. The point of the article was to establish the priority of the role of Sims' fellow Southerner, Crawford Long, as the discoverer of anesthesia.

26. Harris, p. 81.

27. Genovese, p. 639.

28. Barker-Benfield, p. 101.

29. Harris, p. 87.

30. Harris, pp. 375–376.

31. For a discussion of 20th-century values relating to obstetrical care, see Jeanne Guillemin, "Babies by Cesarean: Who Chooses, Who Controls?" in *The Hastings Center Report,* 11 (June, 1981), pp. 15–18.

Twenty Years After:
The Legacy of the Tuskegee Syphilis Study

ARTHUR L. CAPLAN

This year [1992] marks the twentieth anniversary of the end of the Tuskegee syphilis study, one of the more notorious episodes in the history of human subjects research in the United States. Begun in 1932, the study was purportedly designed to determine the natural history of untreated syphilis in a population of some 400 black men in Tuskegee, Alabama. The research subjects, all of whom had syphilis at the time they were enrolled in the study, were matched against 200 uninfected controls.

Though the subjects had received the standard heavy metals therapy available in 1932, they were denied antibiotic therapy when it became clear in the 1940s that penicillin was a safe and effective treatment for the disease. Subjects were recruited with misleading promises of "special free treatment" (actually spinal taps done without anesthesia to study the neurological effects of syphilis), and were enrolled without their informed consent. Disclosure of the ongoing research in the popular media in 1972 led to the termination of the study and ultimately to the National Research Act of 1974, which mandates institutional review board (IRB) approval of all federally funded proposed research with human subjects.

As final payments are being made under the agreement that settled a class action lawsuit brought on behalf of the subjects of the Tuskegee study, the articles that follow look at

ARTHUR CAPLAN is director of the center for bioethics and trustee professor of bioethics, University of Pennsylvania, 1994 to present; professor of molecular and cellular engineering and professor of philosophy; chief, division of bioethics, University of Pennsylvania Medical Center.

different facets of Tuskegee's legacy. Should the results of an immorally conducted study continue to serve as the "gold standard" in our clinical understanding of syphilis? How shall we strike a balance between protecting vulnerable classes of subjects already discriminated against and seeing that minorities are adequately represented in—and reap the benefits of—clinical trials? What lingering meanings does Tuskegee have in the African American community, and how do those meanings affect current efforts not only to conduct biomedical research, but also to provide effective health care in the community? And finally, what messages do race, or other kinds of difference, carry in our culture?
—Bette-Jean Crigger

WHEN EVIL INTRUDES

Twenty years ago Peter Buxtun, a public health official working for the United States Public Health Service, complained to a reporter for the Associated Press that he was deeply concerned about the morality of an ongoing study being sponsored by the Public Health Service—a study compiling information about the course and effects of syphilis in human beings based upon medical examinations of poor black men in Macon County, Alabama. The men, or more accurately, those still living, had been coming in for annual examinations for forty years. They were not receiving standard therapy for syphilis. In late July of 1972 the *Washington Star* and the

Arthur L. Caplan, "When Evil Intrudes," Hastings Center Report 22, no. 6 (1992): 29–32. Reprinted with permission of the author.

Syphilis Victims Got No Therapy

The experiment, called the Tuskegee Study, began in 1932 with about 600 black men, mostly poor and uneducated, from Tuskegee, Ala., an area that had the highest syphilis rate in the nation at the time. . . .

As incentives to enter the program, the men were promised free transportation to and from hospitals, free hot lunches, free medicine for any disease other than syphilis and free burial after autopsies were performed. . . .

Of the decision not to give penicillin to the untreated syphilitics once it became widely available, Dr. Miller [chief of the venereal disease branch of the Centers for Disease Control in 1972] said, "I doubt that it was a one-man decision. These things rarely are. Whoever was director of the VD section at that time, in 1946 or 1947, would be the most logical candidate if you had to pin it down."

New York Times, 26 July 1972

New York Times ran front-page stories based on Buxtun's concerns about what has been called the longest running "nontherapeutic experiment" on human beings in medical history and "the most notorious case of prolonged and knowing violation of subject's rights"—the Tuskegee study.[1]

Buxtun went public with his ethical concerns after years of complaining to officials from the Centers for Disease Control and the Public Health Service with no apparent effect. His decision to blow the whistle led to a series of sensational congressional hearings chaired by Senator Edward Kennedy in February and March of 1973. Legislators and federal officials expressed outrage over the immorality of a study in which poor, illiterate men had been deceived and given placebo treatment rather than standard therapy so that more could be learned about syphilis. Americans found it hard to believe that the Public Health Service had intentionally and sys-

tematically duped men with a disease as serious as syphilis—contagious, disabling, and life-threatening—for more than forty years.

The level of outrage about the Tuskegee study was enormous. One CDC official labeled the experiment akin to "genocide."[2] As a result of public anger over the immorality of the study, Congress created an ad hoc blue ribbon panel to review both the Tuskegee study and the adequacy of existing protections for subjects in all federally sponsored research. Even though the panel did not receive all the information about the study that the government had available,[3] they were still concerned enough about what had taken place to recommend the creation of a national board with the resources to reexamine all aspects of human experimentation in the United States. Congress, in 1974, created the National Commission for the Protection of Human Subjects of Biomedical and Behavioral Research which, in its seventeen reports and numerous appendix volumes, laid the foundation for the ethical requirements that govern the conduct of research on human subjects in the United States to this day.

Syphilis continues to challenge America's and the world's medical, public health, and moral resources. While there are a variety of antibiotics available to treat the disease, it has proven to be a stubborn and resilient foe. The Centers for Disease Control has found steady and alarming increases in the incidence of primary and secondary syphilis over the past decade. It is still a major public health problem in the United States today, especially among young black males.

The rise in the incidence of the disease has ensured that writings about the diagnosis, management, and treatment of syphilis are prominently featured in the professional literature of public health and biomedicine as well as in standard textbooks about venereal and infectious diseases. Ongoing concern about syphilis has led physicians and public health officials to draw upon as much information as they can about the course of the disease. One of the bitter if generally unacknowledged ironies of the Tuskegee study is that, while it now occupies a special place of shame in the annals of human experimentation, its findings are still widely cited by the contemporary biomedical community.

In looking at instances of scientific misconduct and moral malfeasance with respect to research it is quite common to find the position advanced that good science is incompatible with bad ethics. When one wrestles with the horror of the medical abuse of vulnerable human beings it is somewhat comforting to believe that those who engage in such abuse could not produce anything of real value to medicine. Yet the continuing invocation of the findings of the Tuskegee study by those who diagnose, study, or treat syphilis shows that it is sometimes impossible to avoid a confrontation with the question of the ethics of relying on knowledge obtained in the course of immoral research.

The "bad ethics, therefore bad science" argument actually has two distinct components. One part of the argument holds that researchers engaged in obvious immoral conduct with their subjects could not generate useful or valid scientific findings. The second part holds that when the ethical conduct of research is egregiously immoral then any findings obtained ought not to be admitted into the body of scientific knowledge. While it may often be true that it is difficult to trust findings obtained using subjects who were abused or harmed (as was the case in Nazi concentration camp studies),[4] this part of the argument is not always true. Even a cursory glance through the literature of health care reveals that the Tuskegee study was and remains a key source of information about the diagnosis, signs, symptoms, and course of syphilis. No effort has been made to impugn its findings, and the biomedical community has relied upon them for decades.

James Jones, in his landmark book on the Tuskegee study, *Bad Blood,* notes that no researcher involved in the study ever published a single, comprehensive summary of its findings.

The absence of such a review paper may have fostered the impression that no substantive findings of any real significance were obtained. But Jones also notes in the appendix to his book that Public Health Service scientists, physicians, and nurses associated with the study published a total of thirteen articles between 1936 and 1973 based solely upon its findings. These papers appeared in a wide variety of peer-reviewed journals, including *Public Health Reports, Milbank Fund Memorial Quarterly, Journal of Chronic Diseases,* and *Archives of Internal Medicine.*

It is a relatively simple matter to establish the importance assigned to the findings of the Tuskegee study by the contemporary biomedical community. The computerization on large data bases of the majority of the world's professional biomedical journals allows searches to be conducted to see which, if any, recent journal articles cite any of the thirteen papers presenting the findings of the Tuskegee study. An initial database search for the period January 1985 to February 1991 produced twenty such citations from a wide spectrum of journals, including American, British, and German publications. The twenty citations make reference to seven of the original thirteen papers.

A visit to any large medical library will also quickly reveal the importance assigned to the findings of the Tuskegee study in recent years. An informal random selection of twenty medical textbooks on sexually transmitted diseases, infectious disease, human sexuality, and public health published after 1984 turned up four books that made explicit reference to the study and cited at least one of the same thirteen articles. Three textbooks were published in the United States, one in England.

The range of journals in which contemporary articles on syphilis, venereal disease, and dementia directly cite the papers reporting the findings of the Tuskegee study is quite large. Direct citations of the Tuskegee study papers appear in articles in the *Journal of Family Practice* (1986), *The Lancet* (1986), *British Heart Journal* (1987), *New England Journal of Medicine* (1987), *Journal of the*

American Geriatrics Society (1989), *The American Journal of Medicine* (1989), *American Journal of Public Health* (1989), and *Medical Clinics of North America* (1990), among others.

Nearly all the references in both the periodical literature and the medical textbooks use the Tuskegee study to describe the natural history of the disease. A recent review article on cardiovascular syphilis is typical of the way in which the Tuskegee study and its findings are cited:

> In 1932, the United States Public Health Service initiated the Tuskegee Study to delineate further the natural history of untreated syphilis. A total of 412 men with untreated syphilis and 204 uninfected matched controls were followed prospectively. Vonderlehr (15), reviewing the autopsy material from the first years of the study, noted that only one-fourth of the untreated patients were without evidence of any form of tertiary syphilis after 15 years of infection. Moreover, cardiovascular involvement was the most frequently detected abnormality. Peters (16) analyzed the autopsy data from the first 20 years of the study. He found that 50% of patients who had been infected for 10 years had demonstrable cardiovascular involvement. Of the 40% of syphilitic patients who died during this period, the primary causes of death were cardiovascular or central nervous system syphilis (16). Of the 41% of survivors at 30 years of follow-up, 12% had clinical evidence of late, predominantly cardiovascular syphilis (17). Most of these patients had evidence of cardiovascular syphilis at the 15-year analysis (17). These data . . . indicate that . . . complications are usually evident 10 to 20 years after primary infection, and cardiovascular syphilis is the predominant cause of demise in those patients who die as a direct result of syphilis.[5]

The reference numbers 15, 16, and 17 in the excerpt are to three of the thirteen papers reporting the findings of the Tuskegee study.

Yet another representative example from the contemporary periodical literature of health care invoking the findings of the Tuskegee study appears in a review of neurosyphilis and dementia:

> Neurosyphilis is rare as a manifestation of syphilis. Tertiary and late latent syphilis have been decreasing in incidence since the 1950s. There have been two studies of untreated syphilis: in the Oslo study neurosyphilis eventually developed in 7% of the patients, and in the Tuskegee study, syphilitic involvement of the cardiovascular system or the central nervous system was the primary cause of death in 30% of the infected patients, with cardiovascular involvement being much more common than neurosyphilis.[6]

Textbook references are quite similar to those that appear in the periodical literature. In giving an overview of the natural course of untreated syphilis one recent text states:

> A prospective study involving 431 black men with seropositive latent syphilis of 3 or more years' duration was undertaken in 1932 (the Tuskegee study, 1932–1962) (16). This study showed that hypertension in syphilitic black men 25–50 years of age was 17 percent more common than in nonsyphilitics. Cardiovascular complications including hypertension were more common than neurologic complications were, and both were increased over control populations. Anatomic evidence of aortitis was found to be 25–35 percent more common in autopsied syphilitics, while evidence of central nervous system syphilis was found in 4 percent of the patients.[7]

Reference number 16 is to one of the thirteen papers in which the Tuskegee findings were presented.

These examples clearly illustrate the continuing importance assigned to the Tuskegee study by those concerned with understanding and treating syphilis. The case for the study's importance could be further bolstered by tracking down secondary and tertiary references to its findings. There can be no disputing the fact that contemporary medicine has accepted the findings as valid and continues to rely on them as a key source of knowledge about the natural history of the disease.

The acceptance of the Tuskegee study findings as valid refutes the argument that bad ethics is always incompatible with valid science, but the question still remains as to whether the data of the Tuskegee study should continue to be utilized. It may make sense in some situations to argue that data obtained by immoral means should not be used purely on ethical grounds. But even if it were wrong to cite data acquired by immoral means there is simply no way to purge the knowledge gained in the Tuskegee study from biomedicine. Too much of what is known about the natural history of syphilis is based upon the study, and that knowledge has become so deeply embedded that it could not be removed.

Still, the view that the study was immoral and therefore worthless has flourished. This is a cause for concern, because the belief that not much of value came from the Tuskegee study allows both medicine and bioethics to avoid examining such troubling questions as how immoral research could be conducted by reputable scientists under the sponsorship of the American government for forty years, how such research could be allowed to continue long after the promulgation of the Nuremberg and Helsinki Codes, and what the moral duties and responsibilities are of those in biomedicine who continue to cite the study's findings today.

While one of the textbooks that discusses the Tuskegee study does make reference to the ethical shadow hanging over the findings,[8] none of the others and none of the articles in the peer-reviewed periodical literature that directly cite the papers based on the study do so. Should the results of the Tuskegee study continue to be invoked in review articles and texts without some accompanying discussion of the manner in which the findings were obtained and the ethical impact that the study had on the subsequent responsibilities of researchers? Given that the study played a crucial role in causing Americans to rethink the ethics of human experimentation, it would seem morally incumbent upon those who discuss its findings in the context of textbooks and review articles to allot some space for a discussion of the ethical problems associated with it.

There are obvious limits to the extent to which anyone writing a scientific paper or book can review the circumstances and conditions under which scientific knowledge was obtained. The history of medicine is replete with examples of research, certainly considered immoral by contemporary standards, that generate findings still widely accepted and cited. Not every article in a scientific journal can be used as a vehicle for educating the reader about the morality of human experimentation.

But there are obvious forums in biomedicine, such as textbooks and review articles, where it makes sense for authors to include some discussion of the ethical circumstances surrounding morally dubious or blatantly immoral research. The obvious immorality of research methods should not blind us to the importance of noting and discussing them. If no place is made for discussions of the morality of studies such as Tuskegee, the research community may become complacent about the importance of its responsibilities toward human subjects at the same time as the public comes to believe that good science cannot emerge from immoral research.

REFERENCES

1. Stephen B. Thomas and Sandra C. Quinn, "The Tuskegee Syphilis Study, 1932 to 1972: Implications for HIV Education and AIDS Risk Education Programs in the Black Community," *American Journal of Public Health* 81, no. 11 (1991): 1498–1505, at 1501; Ruth Faden and Tom Beauchamp, *A History and Theory of Informed Consent* (New York: Oxford, 1986), p. 165.

2. James H. Jones, *Bad Blood: The Tuskegee Syphilis Experiment* (New York: Free Press, 1981), p. 207.

3. Jay Katz, personal communication, 1991.

4. See Arthur Caplan, ed., *When Medicine Went Mad* (New York: Humana, 1992).

5. J. D. Jackson and J. D. Radolf, "Cardiovascular Syphilis," *The American Journal of Medicine* 87 (October 1989): 428–29.

6. J. A. Rhymes, C. Woodson, R. Sparage-Sachs, and C. K. Cassel, "Nonmedical Complications of Diagnostic Workup for Dementia: University of Chicago Grand Rounds," *Journal of the American Geriatrics Society* 37, no. 12 (1989): 1157–64, at 1160.

7. G. L. Mandell, R. G. Douglas, Jr., and J. E. Bennett, eds., *Principles and Practice of Infectious Diseases,* 3rd ed. (New York: Churchill Livingstone, 1990), p. 1797.

8. K. K. Holmes, P. Mardh, P F. Sparling, and P. J. Wiesner, *Sexually Transmitted Diseases,* 2nd ed. (New York: McGraw-Hill, 1990).

Under the Shadow of Tuskegee: African Americans and Health Care

VANESSA NORTHINGTON GAMBLE

INTRODUCTION

On May 16, 1997, in a White House ceremony, President Bill Clinton apologized for the Tuskegee Syphilis Study, the 40-year government study (1932 to 1972) in which 399 Black men from Macon County, Alabama, were deliberately denied effective treatment for syphilis in order to document the natural history of the disease.[1] "The legacy of the study at Tuskegee," the president remarked, "has reached far and deep, in ways that hurt our progress and divide our nation. We cannot be one America when a whole segment of our nation has no trust in America."[2]

VANESSA N. GAMBLE is an associate professor of history of medicine and family medicine at the University of Wisconsin Madison Medical School. She is also the director of the center for the study of race and ethnicity in medicine.

The president's comments underscore that in the 25 years since its public disclosure, the study has moved from being a singular historical event to a powerful metaphor. It has come to symbolize racism in medicine, misconduct in human research, the arrogance of physicians, and government abuse of Black people.

The continuing shadow cast by the Tuskegee Syphilis Study on efforts to improve the health status of Black Americans provided an impetus for the campaign for a presidential apology.[3] Numerous articles, in both the professional and popular press, have pointed out that the study predisposed many African Americans to distrust medical and public health authorities and has led to critically low Black participation in clinical trials and organ donation.[4]

The specter of Tuskegee has also been raised with respect to HIV/AIDS prevention and treatment programs. Health education researchers Dr

The American Journal of Public Health *87, no. 11 (Nov. 1997): 1773–1778. Copyright 1997 by the American* Public Health Association. *Reprinted by permission.*

Stephen B. Thomas and Dr Sandra Crouse Quinn have written extensively on the impact of the Tuskegee Syphilis Study on these programs.[5] They argue that "the legacy of this experiment, with its failure to educate the study participants and treat them adequately, laid the foundation for today's pervasive sense of black distrust of public health authorities."[6] The syphilis study has also been used to explain why many African Americans oppose needle exchange programs. Needle exchange programs provoke the image of the syphilis study and Black fears about genocide. These programs are not viewed as mechanisms to stop the spread of HIV/AIDS but rather as fodder for the drug epidemic that has devastated so many Black neighborhoods.[7] Fears that they will be used as guinea pigs like the men in the syphilis study have also led some African Americans with AIDS to refuse treatment with protease inhibitors.[8]

The Tuskegee Syphilis Study is frequently described as the singular reason behind African-American distrust of the institutions of medicine and public health. Such an interpretation neglects a critical historical point: the mistrust predated public revelations about the Tuskegee study. Furthermore, the narrowness of such a representation places emphasis on a single historical event to explain deeply entrenched and complex attitudes within the Black community. An examination of the syphilis study within a broader historical and social context makes plain that several factors have influenced, and continue to influence, African Americans' attitudes toward the biomedical community.

Black Americans' fears about exploitation by the medical profession date back to the antebellum period and the use of slaves and free Black people as subjects for dissection and medical experimentation.[9] Although physicians also used poor Whites as subjects, they used Black people far more often. During an 1835 trip to the United States, French visitor Harriet Martineau found that Black people lacked the power even to protect the graves of their dead. "In Baltimore the bodies of coloured people exclusively are taken for dissection," she remarked, "because the Whites do not like it, and the coloured people cannot resist."[10] Four years later, abolitionist Theodore Dwight Weld echoed Martineau's sentiment. "Public opinion," he wrote, "would tolerate surgical experiments, operations, processes, performed upon them [slaves], which it would execrate if performed upon their master or other whites."[11] Slaves found themselves as subjects of medical experiments because physicians needed bodies and because the state considered them property and denied them the legal right to refuse to participate.

Two antebellum experiments, one carried out in Georgia and the other in Alabama, illustrate the abuse that some slaves encountered at the hands of physicians. In the first, Georgia physician Thomas Hamilton conducted a series of brutal experiments on a slave to test remedies for heatstroke. The subject of these investigations, Fed, had been loaned to Hamilton as repayment for a debt owed by his owner. Hamilton forced Fed to sit naked on a stool placed on a platform in a pit that had been heated to a high temperature. Only the man's head was above ground. Over a period of 2 to 3 weeks, Hamilton placed Fed in the pit five or six times and gave him various medications to determine which enabled him best to withstand the heat. Each ordeal ended when Fed fainted and had to be revived. But note that Fed was not the only victim in this experiment; its whole purpose was to make it possible for masters to force slaves to work still longer hours on the hottest of days.[12]

In the second experiment, Dr J. Marion Sims, the so-called father of modern gynecology, used three Alabama slave women to develop an operation to repair vesicovaginal fistulas. Between 1845 and 1849, the three slave women on whom Sims operated each underwent up to 30 painful operations. The physician himself described the agony associated with some of the experiments:[13] "The first patient I operated on was Lucy. . . . That was before the days of anaesthetics, and the poor girl, on her knees, bore the operation with great hero-ism and bravery." This operation was not success-ful, and Sims later attempted to repair the defect by placing a sponge in the bladder. This experi-ment, too, ended in failure. He noted:

> The whole urethra and the neck of the bladder were in a high state of inflammation, which came from the foreign substance. It had to come away, and there was nothing to do but to pull it away by main force. Lucy's agony was extreme. She was much prostrated, and I thought that she was going to die; but by irri-gating the parts of the bladder she recovered with great rapidity.

Sims finally did perfect his technique and ulti-mately repaired the fistulas. Only after his exper-imentation with the slave women proved suc-cessful did the physician attempt the procedure, with anesthesia, on White women volunteers.

EXPLOITATION AFTER THE CIVIL WAR

It is not known to what extent African Ameri-cans continued to be used as unwilling subjects for experimentation and dissection in the years after emancipation. However, an examination of African-American folklore at the turn of the cen-tury makes it clear that Black people believed that such practices persisted. Folktales are replete with references to night doctors, also called stu-dent doctors and Ku Klux doctors. In her book, *Night Riders in Black Folk History,* anthropologist Gladys-Marie Fry writes, "The term 'night doc-tor' (derived from the fact that victims were sought only at night) applies both to students of medicine, who supposedly stole cadavers from which to learn about body processes, and [to] professional thieves, who sold stolen bodies—living and dead—to physicians for medical re-search."[14] According to folk belief, these sinister characters would kidnap Black people, usually at

night and in urban areas, and take them to hospi-tals to be killed and used in experiments. An 1889 *Boston Herald* article vividly captured the fears that African Americans in South Carolina had of night doctors. The report read, in part:

> The negroes of Clarendon, Williamsburg, and Sumter counties have for several weeks past been in a state of fear and trembling. They claim that there is a white man, a doctor, who at will can make himself invisible, and who then approaches some unsuspecting darkey, and having rendered him or her insensible with chloroform, proceeds to fill up a bucket with the victim's blood, for the purpose of making medicine. After having drained the last drop of blood from the victim, the body is dumped into some secret place where it is impossible for any person to find it. The colored women are so worked up over this phantom that they will not venture out at night, or in the daytime in any sequestered place.[15]

Fry did not find any documented evidence of the existence of night riders. However, she demonstrated through extensive interviews that many African Americans expressed genuine fears that they would be kidnapped by night doctors and used for medical experimentation. Fry con-cludes that two factors explain this paradox. She argues that Whites, especially those in the rural South, deliberately spread rumors about night doctors in order to maintain psychological con-trol over Blacks and to discourage their migration to the North so as to maintain a source of cheap labor. In addition, Fry asserts that the experiences of many African Americans as victims of medical experiments during slavery fostered their belief in the existence of night doctors.[16] It should also be added that, given the nation's racial and political climate, Black people recognized their inability to refuse to participate in medical experiments.

Reports about the medical exploitation of Black people in the name of medicine after the end of the Civil War were not restricted to the realm of folklore. Until it was exposed in 1882, a grave robbing ring operated in Philadelphia and provided bodies for the city's medical schools by plundering the graves at a Black cemetery. According to historian David C. Humphrey, southern grave robbers regularly sent bodies of southern Blacks to northern medical schools for use as anatomy cadavers.[17]

During the early 20th century, African-American medical leaders protested the abuse of Black people by the White-dominated medical profession and used their concerns about experimentation to press for the establishment of Black-controlled hospitals.[18] Dr Daniel Hale Williams, the founder of Chicago's Provident Hospital (1891), the nation's first Black-controlled hospital, contended that White physicians, especially in the South, frequently used Black patients as guinea pigs.[19] Dr Nathan Francis Mossell, the founder of Philadelphia's Frederick Douglass Memorial Hospital (1895), described the "fears and prejudices" of Black people, especially those from the South, as "almost proverbial."[20] He attributed such attitudes to southern medical practices in which Black people, "when forced to accept hospital attention, got only the poorest care, being placed in inferior wards set apart for them, suffering the brunt of all that is experimental in treatment, and all this is the sequence of their race variety and abject helplessness."[21] The founders of Black hospitals claimed that only Black physicians possessed the skills required to treat Black patients optimally and that Black hospitals provided these patients with the best possible care.[22]

Fears about the exploitation of African Americans by White physicians played a role in the establishment of a Black veterans hospital in Tuskegee, Ala. In 1923, 9 years before the initiation of the Tuskegee Syphilis Study, racial tensions had erupted in the town over control of the hospital. The federal government had pledged that the facility, an institution designed exclusively for Black patients, would be run by a Black professional staff. But many Whites in the area, including members of the Ku Klux Klan, did not want a Black-operated federal facility in the heart of Dixie, even though it would serve only Black people.[23]

Black Americans sought control of the veterans hospital, in part because they believed that the ex-soldiers would receive the best possible care from Black physicians and nurses, who would be more caring and sympathetic to the veterans' needs. Some Black newspapers even warned that White southerners wanted command of the hospital as part of a racist plot to kill and sterilize African-American men and to establish an "experiment station" for mediocre White physicians.[24] Black physicians did eventually gain the right to operate the hospital, yet this did not stop the hospital from becoming an experiment station for Black men. The veterans hospital was one of the facilities used by the United States Public Health Service in the syphilis study.

During the 1920s and 1930s, Black physicians pushed for additional measures that would battle medical racism and advance their professional needs. Dr Charles Garvin, a prominent Cleveland physician and a member of the editorial board of the Black medical publication The *Journal of the National Medical Association,* urged his colleagues to engage in research in order to protect Black patients. He called for more research on diseases such as tuberculosis and pellagra that allegedly affected African Americans disproportionately or idiosyncratically. Garvin insisted that Black physicians investigate these racial diseases because "heretofore in literature, as in medicine, the Negro has been written about, exploited and experimented upon sometimes not to his physical betterment or to the advancement of science, but the advancement of the Nordic investigator." Moreover, he charged that "in the past, men of other races have for the large part interpreted our diseases, often tinctured with inborn prejudices."[25]

FEARS OF GENOCIDE

These historical examples clearly demonstrate that African Americans' distrust of the medical profession has a longer history than the public revelations of the Tuskegee Syphilis Study. There is a collective memory among African Americans about their exploitation by the medical establishment. The Tuskegee Syphilis Study has emerged as the most prominent example of medical racism because it confirms, if not authenticates, long-held and deeply entrenched beliefs within the Black community. To be sure, the Tuskegee Syphilis Study does cast a long shadow. After the study had been exposed, charges surfaced that the experiment was part of a governmental plot to exterminate Black people.[26] Many Black people agreed with the charge that the study represented "nothing less than an official, premeditated policy of genocide."[27] Furthermore, this was not the first or last time that allegations of genocide have been launched against the government and the medical profession. The sickle cell anemia screening programs of the 1970s and birth control programs have also provoked such allegations.[28]

In recent years, links have been made between Tuskegee, AIDS, and genocide. In September 1990, the article "AIDS: Is It Genocide?" appeared in *Essence,* a Black woman's magazine. The author noted: "As an increasing number of African-Americans continue to sicken and die and as no cure for AIDS has been found some of us are beginning to think the unthinkable: Could AIDS be a virus that was manufactured to erase large numbers of us? Are they trying to kill us with this disease?"[29] In other words, some members of the Black community see AIDS as part of a conspiracy to exterminate African Americans.

Beliefs about the connection between AIDS and the purposeful destruction of African Americans should not be cavalierly dismissed as bizarre and paranoid. They are held by a significant number of Black people. For example, a 1990 survey conducted by the Southern Christian Leadership Conference found that 35% of the 1056 Black church members who responded believed that AIDS was a form of genocide.[30] A

New York Times/WCBS TV News poll conducted the same year found that 10% of Black Americans thought that the AIDS virus had been created in a laboratory in order to infect Black people. Another 20% believed that it could be true.[31]

African Americans frequently point to the Tuskegee Syphilis Study as evidence to support their views about genocide, perhaps, in part, because many believe that the men in the study were actually injected with syphilis. Harlon Dalton, a Yale Law School professor and a former member of the National Commission on AIDS, wrote, in a 1989 article titled, "AIDS in Black Face," that "the government [had] purposefully exposed Black men to syphilis."[32] Six years later, Dr Eleanor Walker, a Detroit radiation oncologist, offered an explanation as to why few African Americans become bone marrow donors. "The biggest fear, she claimed, is that they will become victims of some misfeasance, like the Tuskegee incident where Black men were infected with syphilis and left untreated to die from the disease."[33] The January 25, 1996, episode of "New York Undercover," a Fox Network police drama that is one of the top shows in Black households, also reinforced the rumor that the US Public Health Service physicians injected the men with syphilis.[34] The myth about deliberate infection is not limited to the Black community. On April 8, 1997, news anchor Tom Brokaw, on "NBC Nightly News," announced that the men had been infected by the government.[35]

Folklorist Patricia A. Turner, in her book *I Heard It through the Grapevine: Rumor and Resistance in African-American Culture,* underscores why it is important not to ridicule but to pay attention to these strongly held theories about genocide.[36] She argues that these rumors reveal much about what African Americans believe to be the state of their lives in this country. She contends that such views reflect Black beliefs that White Americans have historically been, and continue to be, ambivalent and perhaps hostile to the existence of Black people. Consequently, African-American attitudes toward biomedical research are not influenced solely by the Tus-kegee Syphilis Study. African Americans' opinions about the value White society has attached to their lives should not be discounted. As Reverend Floyd Tompkins of Stanford University Memorial Church has said, "There is a sense in our community, and I think it shall be proved out, that if you are poor or you're a person of color, you were the guinea pig, and you continue to be the guinea pigs, and there is the fundamental belief that Black life is not valued like White life or like any other life in America."[37]

NOT JUST PARANOIA

Lorene Cary, in a cogent essay in *Newsweek,* expands on Reverend Tompkins' point. In an essay titled "Why It's Not Just Paranoia," she writes:

> We Americans continue to value the lives and humanity of some groups more than the lives and humanity of others. That is not paranoia. It is our historical legacy and a present fact; it influences domestic and foreign policy and the daily interaction of millions of Americans. It influences the way we spend our public money and explains how we can read the staggering statistics on Black Americans' infant mortality, youth mortality, mortality in middle and old age, and not be moved to action.[38]

African Americans' beliefs that their lives are devalued by White society also influence their relationships with the medical profession. They perceive, at times correctly, that they are treated differently in the health care system solely because of their race, and such perceptions fuel mistrust of the medical profession. For example, a national telephone survey conducted in 1986 revealed that African Americans were more likely than Whites to report that their physicians did not inquire sufficiently about their pain, did not tell them how long it would take for prescribed medicine to work, did not explain the seriousness of their illness or injury, and did not discuss

test and examination findings.[39] A 1994 study published in the *American Journal of Public Health* found that physicians were less likely to give pregnant Black women information about the hazards of smoking and drinking during pregnancy.[40]

The powerful legacy of the Tuskegee Syphilis Study endures, in part, because the racism and disrespect for Black lives that it entailed mirror Black people's contemporary experiences with the medical profession. The anger and frustration that many African Americans feel when they encounter the health care system can be heard in the words of Alicia Georges, a professor of nursing at Lehman College and a former president of the National Black Nurses Association, as she recalled an emergency room experience. "Back a few years ago, I was having excruciating abdominal pain, and I wound up at a hospital in my area," she recalled. "The first thing that they began to ask me was how many sexual partners I'd had. I was married and owned my own house. But immediately, in looking at me, they said, 'Oh, she just has pelvic inflammatory disease.'"[41] Perhaps because of her nursing background, Georges recognized the implications of the questioning. She had come face to face with the stereotype of Black women as sexually promiscuous. Similarly, the following story from the *Los Angeles Times* shows how racism can affect the practice of medicine:

> When Althea Alexander broke her arm, the attending resident at Los Angeles County-USC Medical Center told her to "hold your arm like you usually hold your can of beer on Saturday night." Alexander who is Black, exploded. "What are you talking about? Do you think I'm a welfare mother?" The White resident shrugged: "Well aren't you?" Turned out she was an administrator at USC medical school.

This example graphically illustrates that health care providers are not immune to the beliefs and misconceptions of the wider community. They carry with them stereotypes about various groups of people.[42]

BEYOND TUSKEGEE

There is also a growing body of medical research that vividly illustrates why discussions of the relationship of African Americans and the medical profession must go beyond the Tuskegee Syphilis Study. These studies demonstrate racial inequities in access to particular technologies and raise critical questions about the role of racism in medical decision making. For example, in 1989 The *Journal of the American Medical Association* published a report that demonstrated racial inequities in the treatment of heart disease. In this study, White and Black patients had similar rates of hospitalization for chest pain, but the White patients were one third more likely to undergo coronary angiography and more than twice as likely to be treated with bypass surgery or angioplasty. The racial disparities persisted even after adjustments were made for differences in income.[43] Three years later, another study appearing in that journal reinforced these findings. It revealed that older Black patients on Medicare received coronary artery bypass grafts only about a fourth as often as comparable White patients. Disparities were greatest in the rural South, where White patients had the surgery seven times as often as Black patients. Medical factors did not fully explain the differences. This study suggests that an already-existing national health insurance program does not solve the access problems of African Americans.[44] Additional studies have confirmed the persistence of such inequities.[45]

Why the racial disparities? Possible explanations include health problems that precluded the use of procedures, patient unwillingness to accept medical advice or to undergo surgery, and differences in severity of illness. However, the role of racial bias cannot be discounted, as the American Medical Association's Council on Ethical and Judicial Affairs has recognized. In a 1990 report on Black-White disparities in health care, the council asserted:

> Because racial disparities may be occurring despite the lack of any intent or purposeful efforts to treat patients differently on the basis of race, physicians should examine their own practices to ensure that inappropriate considerations do not affect their clinical judgment. In addition, the profession should help increase the awareness of its members of racial disparities in medical treatment decisions by engaging in open and broad discussions about the issue. Such discussions should take place as part of the medical school curriculum, in medical journals, at professional conferences, and as part of professional peer review activities.[46]

The council's recommendation is a strong acknowledgment that racism can influence the practice of medicine.

After the public disclosures of the Tuskegee Syphilis Study, Congress passed the National Research Act of 1974. This act, established to protect subjects in human experimentation, mandates institutional review board approval of all federally funded research with human subjects. However, recent revelations about a measles vaccine study financed by the Centers for Disease Control and Prevention (CDC) demonstrate the inadequacies of these safeguards and illustrate why African Americans' historically based fears of medical research persist. In 1989, in the midst of a measles epidemic in Los Angeles, the CDC, in collaboration with Kaiser Permanente and the Los Angeles County Health Department, began a study to test whether the experimental Edmonston-Zagreb vaccine could be used to immunize children too young for the standard Moraten vaccine. By 1991, approximately 900 infants, mostly Black and Latino, had received the vaccine without difficulties. (Apparently, 1 infant died for reasons not related to the inoculations.) But the infants' parents had not been informed that the vaccine was not licensed in the United States or that it had been associated with an increase in death rates in

Africa. The 1996 disclosure of the study prompted charges of medical racism and of the continued exploitation of minority communities by medical professionals.[47]

The Tuskegee Syphilis Study continues to cast its shadow over the lives of African Americans. For many Black people, it has come to represent the racism that pervades American institutions and the disdain in which Black lives are often held. But despite its significance, it cannot be the only prism we use to examine the relationship of African Americans with the medical and public health communities. The problem we must face is not just the shadow of Tuskegee but the shadow of racism that so profoundly affects the lives and beliefs of all people in this country.

REFERENCES AND NOTES

1. The most comprehensive history of the study is James H. Jones, *Bad Blood,* new and expanded edition (New York: Free Press, 1993).

2. "Remarks by the President in Apology for Study Done in Tuskegee," Press Release, the White House, Office of the Press Secretary, 16 May 1997.

3. "Final Report of the Tuskegee Syphilis Study Legacy Committee," Vanessa Northington Gamble, chair, and John C. Fletcher, co-chair, 20 May 1996.

4. Vanessa Northington Gamble, "A Legacy of Distrust: African Americans and Medical Research," *American Journal of Preventive Medicine* 9 (1993): 35–38; Shari Roan, "A Medical Imbalance," *Los Angeles Times,* 1 November 1994; Carol Stevens, "Research: Distrust Runs Deep; Medical Community Seeks Solution," *The Detroit News,* 10 December 1995; Lini S. Kadaba, "Minorities in Research," *Chicago Tribune,* 13 September 1993; Robert Steinbrook, "AIDS Trials Short-change Minorities and Drug Users," *Los Angeles Times,* 25 September 1989; Mark D. Smith, "Zidovudine: Does It Work for Everyone?" *Journal of the American Medical Association* 266 (1991): 2750–2751; Charlise Lyles, "Blacks Hesitant to Donate; Cultural Beliefs, Misinformation, Mistrust Make It a Difficult Decision," *The Virginian-Pilot,* 15 August 1994; Jeanni Wong, "Mistrust Leaves Some Blacks Reluctant to Donate Organs," *Sacramento Bee,* 17 February 1993; "Nightline," ABC News, 6 April 1994; Patrice Gaines, "Armed with the Truth in a Fight for Lives," *Washington Post,* 10 April 1994; Fran Henry, "Encouraging Organ Donation from Blacks," *Cleveland Plain Dealer,*

23 April 1994; G. Marie Swanson and Amy J. Ward, "Recruiting Minorities into Clinical Trials: Toward a Participant-Friendly System," *Journal of the National Cancer Institute* 87 (1995): 1747–1759; Dewayne Wickham, "Why Blacks Are Wary of White MDs," *The Tennessean,* 21 May 1997, 13A.

5. For example, see Stephen B. Thomas and Sandra Crouse Quinn, "The Tuskegee Syphilis Study, 1932 to 1972: Implications for HIV Education and AIDS Risk Education Programs in the Black Community," *American Journal of Public Health* 81 (1991): 1498–1505; Stephen B. Thomas and Sandra Crouse Quinn, "Understanding the Attitudes of Black Americans," in *Dimensions of HIV Prevention. Needle Exchange,* ed. Jeff Stryker and Mark D. Smith (Menlo Park, Calif.: Henry J. Kaiser Family Foundation, 1993), 99–128; and Stephen B. Thomas and Sandra Crouse Quinn, "The AIDS Epidemic and the African-American Community: Toward an Ethical Framework for Service Delivery," in "It Just Ain't Fair": *The Ethics of Health Care for African Americans,* ed. Annette Dula and Sara Goering (Westport, Conn.: Praeger, 1994), 75–88.

6. Thomas and Quinn, "The AIDS Epidemic and the African-American Community," 83.

7. Thomas and Quinn, "Understanding the Attitudes of Black Americans," 108–109; David L. Kirp and Ronald Bayer, "Needles and Races," *Atlantic,* July 1993, 38–42.

8. Lynda Richardson, "An Old Experiment's Legacy: Distrust of AIDS Treatment," *New York Times,* 21 April 1997, A1, A7.

9. Todd L. Savitt, "The Use of Blacks for Medical Experimentation and Demonstration in the Old South," *Journal of Southern History* 48 (1982): 331–348; David C. Humphrey, "Dissection and Discrimination: The Social Origins of Cadavers in America, 1760–1915," *Bulletin of the New York Academy of Medicine* 49 (1973): 819–827.

10. Harriet Martineau, *Retrospect of Western Travel,* vol. 1 (London: Saunders &amp [sic]; Ottley; New York: Harpers and Brothers; 1838), 140, quoted in Humphrey, "Dissection and Discrimination," 819.

11. Theodore Dwight Weld, *American Slavery As It Is: Testimony of a Thousand Witnesses* (New York: American Anti-Slavery Society, 1839), 170, quoted in Savitt, "The Use of Blacks," 341.

12. F. N. Boney, "Doctor Thomas Hamilton: Two Views of a Gentleman of the Old South," *Phylon* 28 (1967): 288–292.

13. J. Marion Sims, *The Story of My Life* (New York: Appleton, 1889), 236–237.

14. Gladys-Marie Fry, *Night Riders in Black Folk History* (Knoxville: University of Tennessee Press, 1984), 171.

244   CHAPTER 3: MEDICAL EXPERIMENTATION

15. "Concerning Negro Sorcery in the United States," *Journal of American Folk-Lore* 3 (1890): 285.

16. Ibid., 210.

17. Humphrey, "Dissection and Discrimination," 822–823.

18. A detailed examination of the campaign to establish Black hospitals can be found in Vanessa Northington Gamble, *Making a Place for Ourselves: The Black Hospital Movement, 1920–1945* (New York: Oxford University Press, 1995).

19. Eugene P. Link, "The Civil Rights Activities of Three Great Negro Physicians (1840–1940)," *Journal of Negro History* 52 (July 1969): 177.

20. Mossell graduated, with honors, from Penn in 1882 and founded the hospital in 1895.

21. "Seventh Annual Report of the Frederick Douglass Memorial Hospital and Training School" (Philadelphia, Pa.: 1902), 17.

22. H. M. Green, "A More or Less Critical Review of the Hospital Situation among Negroes in the United States" (n.d., circa 1930), 4–5.

23. For more in-depth discussions of the history of the Tuskegee Veterans Hospital, see Gamble, *Making a Place for Ourselves,* 70–104; Pete Daniel, "Black Power in the 1920's: The Case of Tuskegee Veterans Hospital," *Journal of Southern History* 36 (1970): 368–388; and Raymond Wolters, *The New Negro on Campus: Black College Rebellions of the 1920s* (Princeton, NJ: Princeton University Press, 1975), 137–191.

24. "Klan Halts March on Tuskegee," *Chicago Defender,* 4 August 1923.

25. Charles H. Garvin, "The 'New Negro' Physician," unpublished manuscript, n.d., box 1, Charles H. Garvin Papers, Western Reserve Historical Society Library, Cleveland, Ohio.

26. Ronald A. Taylor, "Conspiracy Theories Widely Accepted in U.S. Black Circles," *Washington Times,* 10 December 1991, A1; Frances Cress Welsing, *The Isis Papers: The Keys to the Colors* (Chicago: Third World Press, 1991), 298–299. Although she is not very well known outside of the African-American community, Welsing, a physician, is a popular figure within it. *The Isis Papers* headed for several weeks the best-seller list maintained by Black bookstores.

27. Jones, *Bad Blood,* 12.

28. For discussions of allegations of genocide in the implementation of these programs, see Robert G. Weisbord, "Birth Control and the Black American: A Matter of Genocide?" *Demography* 10 (1973): 571–590; Alex S. Jones, "Editorial Linking Blacks, Contraceptives Stirs Debate at Philadelphia Paper," *Arizona Daily Star,* 23 December 1990, F4; Doris Y. Wilkinson, "For Whose Benefit? Politics and Sickle Cell," *The Black Scholar* 5 (1974):26–31.

29. Karen Grisby Bates, "Is It Genocide?" *Essence,* September 1990, 76.

30. Thomas and Quinn, "The Tuskegee Syphilis Study," 1499.

31. "The AIDS 'Plot' against Blacks," *New York Times,* 12 May 1992, A22.

32. Harlon L. Dalton, "AIDS in Blackface," *Daedalus* 118 (Summer 1989): 220–221.

33. Rhonda Bates-Rudd, "State Campaign Encourages African Americans to Offer Others Gift of Bone Marrow," *Detroit News,* 7 December 1995.

34. From September 1995 to December 1995, New York Undercover was the top-ranked show in Black households. It ranked 122nd in White households. David Zurawik, "Poll: TV's Race Gap Growing," *Capital Times* (Madison, Wis), 14 May 1996, 5D.

35. Transcript, "NBC Nightly News," 8 April 1997.

36. Patricia A. Turner, *I Heard It through the Grapevine: Rumor in African-American Culture* (Berkeley: University of California Press, 1993).

37. "Fear Creates Lack of Donor Organs among Blacks," Weekend Edition, National Public Radio, 13 March 1994.

38. Lorene Cary, "Why It's Not Just Paranoia: An American History of 'Plans' for Blacks," *Newsweek,* 6 April 1992, 23.

39. Robert J. Blendon, "Access to Medical Care for Black and White Americans: A Matter of Continuing Concern," *Journal of the American Medical Association* 261 (1989): 278–281.

40. M. D. Rogan et al., "Racial Disparities in Reported Prenatal Care Advice from Health Care Providers," *American Journal of Public Health* 84 (1994): 82–88.

41. Julie Johnson et al., "Why Do Blacks Die Young?" *Time,* 16 September 1991, 52.

42. Sonia Nazario, "Treating Doctors for Prejudice: Medical Schools Are Trying to Sensitize Students to 'Bedside Bias.'" *Los Angeles Times,* 20 December 1990.

43. Mark B. Wenneker and Arnold M. Epstein, "Racial Inequities in the Use of Procedures for Patients with Ischemic Heart Disease in Massachusetts," *Journal of the American Medical Association* 261 (1989): 253–257.

44. Kenneth C. Goldberg et al., "Racial and Community Factors Influencing Coronary Artery Bypass Graft Surgery Rates for All 1986 Medicare Patients," *Journal of the American Medical Association* 267 (1992): 1473–1477.

45. John D. Ayanian, "Heart Disease in Black and White," *New England Journal of Medicine* 329 (1993): 656–658; J. Whittle et al., "Racial Differences in the Use of Invasive Cardiovascular Procedures in the

Department of Veterans Affairs Medical System," *New England Journal of Medicine* 329 (1993): 621–627; Eric D. Peterson et al., "Racial Variation in Cardiac Procedure Use and Survival following Acute Myocardial Infarction in the Department of Veterans Affairs," *Journal of the American Medical Association* 271 (1994): 1175–1180; Ronnie D. Homer et al., "Theories Explaining Racial Differences in the Utilization of Diagnostic and Therapeutic Procedures for Cerebrovascular Disease," *Milbank Quarterly* 73 (1995): 443–462; Richard D. Moore et al., "Racial Differences in the Use of

Drug Therapy for HIV Disease in an Urban Community," *New England Journal of Medicine* 350 (1994): 763–768.

46. Council on Ethical and Judicial Affairs, "Black-White Disparities in Health Care," *Journal of the American Medical Association* 263 (1990): 2346.

47. Marlene Cimons, "CDC Says It Erred in Measles Study," *Los Angeles Times,* 17 June 1996, A 11; Beth Glenn, "Bad Blood Once Again," *St. Petersburg Times,* 21 July 1996, 5D.

Judgment on Willowbrook

PAUL RAMSEY

IN 1958 AND 1959 the *New England Journal of Medicine* reported a series of experiments performed upon patients and new admittees to the Willowbrook State School, a home for retarded children in Staten Island, New York.[1] These experiments were described as "an attempt to control the high prevalence of infectious hepatitis in an institution for mentally defective patients." The experiments were said to be justified because, under conditions of an existing controlled outbreak of hepatitis in the institution, "knowledge obtained from a series of suitable studies could well lead to its control." In actuality, the experiments were designed to duplicate and confirm the efficacy of gamma globulin in immunization against hepatitis, to develop and improve or improve upon that inoculum, and to learn more about infectious hepatitis in general.

The experiments were justified—doubtless, after a great deal of soul searching—for the fol-

lowing reasons: there was a smoldering epidemic throughout the institution and "it was apparent that most of the patients at Willowbrook were naturally exposed to hepatitis virus"; infectious hepatitis is a much milder disease in children; the strain at Willowbrook was especially mild; only the strain or strains of the virus already disseminated at Willowbrook were used; and only those small and incompetent patients whose parents gave consent were used.

The patient population at Willowbrook was 4478, growing at a rate of one patient a day over a three-year span, or from 10 to 15 new admissions per week. In the first trial the existing population was divided into two groups: one group served as uninoculated controls, and the other group was inoculated with 0.01 ml. of gamma globulin per pound of body weight. Then for a second trial new admittees and those left uninoculated before were again divided: one group

From Paul Ramsey, The Patient as a Person *(New Haven, CT: Yale University Press, 1970), pp. 47–53.*
Reprinted by permission of Yale University Press.

served as uninoculated controls and the other was inoculated with 0.06 ml. of gamma globulin per pound of body weight. This proved that Stokes et al. had correctly demonstrated that the larger amount would give significant immunity for up to seven or eight months.[2]

Serious ethical questions may be raised about the trials so far described. No mention is made of any attempt to enlist the adult personnel of the institution, numbering nearly 1,000 including nearly 600 attendants on ward duty, and new additions to the staff, in these studies whose excusing reason was that almost everyone was "naturally" exposed to the Willowbrook virus. Nothing requires that major research into the natural history of hepatitis be first undertaken in children. Experiments have been carried out in the military and with prisoners as subjects. There have been fatalities from the experiments; but surely in all these cases the consent of the volunteers was as valid or better than the proxy consent of these children's "representatives." There would have been no question of the understanding consent that might have been given by the adult personnel at Willowbrook, if significant benefits were expected from studying that virus.

Second, nothing is said that would warrant withholding an inoculation of some degree of known efficacy from part of the population, or for withholding in the first trial less than the full amount of gamma globulin that had served to immunize in previous tests, except the need to test, confirm, and improve the inoculum. That, of course, was a desirable goal; but it does not seem possible to warrant withholding gamma globulin for the reason that is often said to justify controlled trials, namely, that one procedure is *as likely* to succeed as the other.

Third, nothing is said about attempts to control or defeat the low-grade epidemic at Willowbrook by more ordinary, if more costly and less experimental, procedures. Nor is anything said about admitting no more patients until this goal had been accomplished. This was not a massive urban hospital whose teeming population would have to be turned out into the streets, with resulting dangers to themselves and to public health, in order to sanitize the place. Instead, between 200 and 250 patients were housed in each of 18 buildings over approximately 400 acres in a semirural setting of fields, woods, and well-kept, spacious lawns. Clearly it would have been possible to secure other accommodation for new admissions away from the infection, while eradicating the infection at Willowbrook building by building. This might have cost money, and it would certainly have required astute detective work to discover the source of the infection. The doctors determined that the new patients likely were not carrying the infection upon admission, and that it did not arise from the procedures and routine inoculations given them at the time of admission. Why not go further in the search for the source of the epidemic? If this had been an orphanage for normal children or a floor of private patients, instead of a school for mentally defective children, one wonders whether the doctors would so readily have accepted the hepatitis as a "natural" occurrence and even as an opportunity for study.

The next step was to attempt to induce "passive-active immunity" by feeding the virus to patients already protected by gamma globulin. In this attempt to improve the inoculum, permission was obtained from the parents of children from 5 to 10 years of age newly admitted to Willowbrook, who were then isolated from contact with the rest of the institution. All were inoculated with gamma globulin and then divided into two groups: one served as controls while the other group of new patients were fed the Willowbrook virus, obtained from feces, in doses having 50 percent infectivity, i.e., in concentrations estimated to produce hepatitis with jaundice in half the subjects tested. Then twice the 50 percent infectivity was tried. This proved, among other things, that hepatitis has an "alimentary-tract phase" in which it can be transmitted from one person to another while still "inapparent" in the first person. This, doubtless, is exceedingly important information in learning how to control epidemics of infectious hepatitis. The second of the two articles mentioned above describes studies of the incubation period of the virus and of whether pooled serum remained infectious when aged and frozen. Still the small, mentally defective patients who were deliberately fed infectious hepatitis are described as having suffered mildly in most cases: "The liver became enlarged in the majority, occasionally a week or two before the onset of jaundice. Vomiting and anorexia usually lasted only a few days. Most of the children gained weight during the course of hepatitis."

That mild description of what happened to the children who were fed hepatitis (and who continued to be introduced into the unaltered environment of Willowbrook) is itself alarming, since it is now definitely known that cirrhosis of the liver results from infectious hepatitis more frequently than from excessive consumption of alcohol! Now, or in 1958 and 1959, no one knows what may be other serious consequences of contracting infectious hepatitis. Understanding human volunteers were then and are now needed in the study of this disease, although a South American monkey has now successfully been given a form of hepatitis, and can henceforth serve as our ally in its conquest. But not children who cannot consent knowingly. If Peace Corps workers are regularly given gamma globulin before going abroad as a guard against their contracting hepatitis, and are inoculated at intervals thereafter, it seems that this is the least we should do for mentally defective children before they "go abroad" to Willowbrook or other institutions set up for their care.

Discussions pro and con of the Willowbrook experiments that have come to my attention serve only to reinforce the ethical objections that can be raised against what was done simply from a careful analysis of the original articles reporting the research design and findings. In an address at the 1968 Ross Conference on Pediatric Research, Dr. Saul Krugman raised the question, Should vaccine trials be carried out in adult volunteers before subjecting children to similar tests?[3] He answered this question in the negative. The reason adduced was simply that "a vaccine virus trial may be a more hazardous procedure for adults than for children." Medical researchers, of course, are required to minimize the hazards, but not by moving from consenting to unconsenting subjects. This apology clearly shows that adults and children have become interchangeable in face of the overriding importance of obtaining the research goal. This means that the special moral claims of children for care and protection are forgotten, and especially the claims of children who are most weak and vulnerable. (Krugman's reference to the measles vaccine trials is not to the point.)

The *Medical Tribune* explains that the 16-bed isolation unit set up at Willowbrook served "to protect the study subjects from Willowbrook's other endemic diseases—such as shigellosis, measles, rubella and respiratory and parasitic infections—while exposing them to hepatitis."[4] This presumably compensated for the infection they were given. It is not convincingly shown that the children could by no means, however costly, have been protected from the epidemic of hepatitis. The statement that Willowbrook "had endemic infectious hepatitis and a sufficiently open population so that the disease could never be quieted by exhausting the supply of susceptibles" is at best enigmatic.

Oddly, physicians defending the propriety of the Willowbrook hepatitis project soon began talking like poorly instructed "natural lawyers"! Dr. Louis Lasagna and Dr. Geoffrey Edsall, for example, find these experiments unobjectionable —both, for the reason stated by Edsall: "the children would apparently incur no greater risk than they were likely to run by nature." In any case, Edsall's example of parents consenting with a son 17 years of age for him to go to war, and society's agreements with minors that they can drive cars and hurt themselves were entirely beside the point. Dr. David D. Rutstein adheres to a stricter standard in regard to research on infectious hepatitis: "It is not ethical to use human subjects for the growth of a virus for any purpose."[5]

The latter sweeping verdict may depend on knowledge of the effects of viruses on chromosomal difficulties, mongolism, etc., that was not available to the Willowbrook group when their researches were begun thirteen years ago. If so, this is a telling point against appeal to "no discernible risks" as the sole standard applicable to the use of children in medical experimentation. That would lend support to the proposition that we always know that there are unknown and undiscerned risks in the case of an invasion of the fortress of the body—which then can be consented to by an adult in behalf of a child only if it is in the child's behalf medically.

When asked what she told the parents of the subject-children at Willowbrook, Dr. Joan Giles replied, "I explain that there is no vaccine against infectious hepatitis. . . . I also tell them that we can modify the disease with gamma globulin but we can't provide lasting immunity without letting them get the disease."[6] Obviously vaccines giving "lasting immunity" are not the only kinds of vaccine to be used in caring for patients.

Doubtless the studies at Willowbrook resulted in improvement in the vaccine, to the benefit of present and future patients. In September 1966, "a routine program of GG [gamma globulin] administration to every new patient at Willowbrook" was begun. This cut the incidence of icteric hepatitis 80 to 85 percent. Then follows a significant statement in the *Medical Tribune* article: "A similar reduction in the icteric form of the disease has been accomplished among the employees, who began getting routine GG earlier in the study."[7] Not only did the research team (so far as these reports show) fail to consider and adopt the alternative that new admittees to the staff be asked to become volunteers for an investigation that might improve the vaccine against the strain of infectious hepatitis to which they as well as the children were exposed. Instead, the staff was routinely protected earlier than the inmates were! And, as we have seen, there was evidence from the beginning that gamma globulin provided at least some protection. A "modification" of the disease was still an inoculum, even if

this provided no lasting immunization and had to be repeated. It is axiomatic to medical ethics that a known remedy or protection—even if not perfect or even if the best exact administration of it has not been proved—should not be withheld from individual patients. It seems to a layman that from the beginning various trials at immunization of all new admittees might have been made, and controlled observation made of their different degrees of effectiveness against "nature" at Willowbrook. This would doubtless have been a longer way round, namely, the "anecdotal" method of investigative treatment that comes off second best in comparison with controlled trials. Yet this seems to be the alternative dictated by our received medical ethics, and the only one expressive of minimal care of the primary patients themselves.

Finally, except for one episode, the obtaining of parental consent (on the premise that this is ethically valid) seems to have been very well handled. Wards of the state were not used, though by law the administrator at Willowbrook could have signed consent for them. Only new admittees whose parents were available were entered by proxy consent into the project. Explanation was made to groups of these parents, and they were given time to think about it and consult with their own family physicians. Then late in 1964 Willowbrook was closed to all new admissions because of overcrowding. What then happened can most impartially be described in the words of an article defending the Willowbrook project on medical and ethical grounds:

> Parents who applied for their children to get in were sent a form letter over Dr. Hammond's signature saying that there was no space for new admissions and that their name was being put on a waiting list.
>
> But the hepatitis program, occupying its own space in the institution, continued to admit new patients as each new study group began. "Where do you find new admissions except by canvassing the people who have applied for admission?" Dr. Hammond asked.

So a new batch of form letters went out, saying that there were a few vacancies in the hepatitis research unit if the parents cared to consider volunteering their child for that. In some instances the second form letter apparently was received as closely as a week after the first letter arrived.[8]

Granting—as I do not—the validity of parental consent to research upon children not in their behalf medically, what sort of consent was that? Surely, the duress upon these parents with children so defective as to require institutionalization was far greater than the duress on prisoners given tobacco or paid or promised parole for their cooperation! I grant that the timing of these events was inadvertent. Since, however, ethics is a matter of criticizing institutions and not only of exculpating or making culprits of individual men, the inadvertence does not matter. This is the strongest possible argument for saying that even if parents have the right to consent to submit the children who are directly and continuously in their care to nonbeneficial medical experimentation, this should not be the rule of practice governing institutions set up for their care.

Such use of captive populations of children for purely experimental purposes ought to be made legally impossible. My view is that this should be stopped by legal acknowledgement of the moral invalidity of parental or legal proxy consent for the child to procedures having no relation to a child's own diagnosis or treatment. If this is not done, canons of loyalty require that the rule of practice (by law, or otherwise) be that children in institutions and not directly under the care of parents or relatives should *never* be used in medical investigations having present pain or discomfort and unknown present and future risks to them, and promising future possible benefits only for others.

NOTES

1. Robert Ward, Saul Krugman, Joan P. Giles, A. Milton Jacobs, and Oscar Bodansky, "Infectious Hepatitis: Studies of Its Natural History and Preven-

tion," *New England Journal of Medicine* 258, no. 9 (February 27, 1958): 407–16; Saul Krugman, Robert Ward, Joan P. Giles, Oscar Bodansky, and A. Milton Jacobs, "Infectious Hepatitis: Detection of the Virus during the Incubation Period and in Clinically Inapparent Infection," *New England Journal of Medicine* 261, no. 15 (October 8, 1959): 729–34. The following account and unannotated quotations are taken from these articles.

2. J. Stokes, Jr., et al., "Infectious Hepatitis: Length of Protection by Immune Serum Globulin (Gamma Globulin) during Epidemics," *Journal of the American Medical Association* 147 (1951): 714–19. Since the half-life of gamma globulin is three weeks, no one knows exactly why it immunizes for so long a period. The "highly significant protection against hepatitis obtained by the use of gamma globulin," however, had been confirmed as early as 1945 (see Edward B. Grossman, Sloan G. Stewart, and Joseph Stokes, "Post-Transfusion Hepatitis in Battle Casualties," *Journal of the American Medical Association* 129, no. 15 [December 8, 1945]: 991–94). The inoculation *withheld* in the Willowbrook experiments had, therefore, proved valuable.

3. Saul Krugman, "Reflections on Pediatric Clinical Investigations," in *Problems of Drug Evaluation in Infants and Children*, Report of the Fifty-eighth Ross Conference on Pediatric Research, Dorado Beach, Puerto Rico, May 5–7, 1968 (Columbus: Ross Laboratories), pp. 41–42.

4. "Studies with Children Backed on Medical, Ethical Grounds," *Medical Tribune and Medical News* 8, no. 19 (February, 20, 1967): 1, 23.

5. *Daedalus,* Spring 1969, pp 471–72, 529. See also pp. 458, 470–72. Since it is the proper business of an ethicist to uphold the proposition that only retrogression in civility can result from bad moral reasoning and the use of inept examples, however innocent, it is fair to point out the startling comparison between Edsall's "argument" and the statement of Dr. Karl Brandt, plenipotentiary in charge of all medical activities in the Nazi Reich: "Do you think that one can obtain any worthwhile, fundamental results without a definite toll of lives? The same goes for technological development. You cannot build a great bridge, a gigantic building—you cannot establish a speed record without deaths!" (quoted by Leo Alexander, "War Crimes: Their Social-Psychological Aspects," *American Journal of Psychiatry* 105, no. 3 [September 1948]:172). Casualties to progress, or injuries accepted in setting speed limits, are morally quite different from death or maiming or even only risks, or unknown risks, directly and deliberately imposed upon an unconsenting human being.

6. *Medical Tribune,* February 20, 1967, p. 23.

7. *Medical Tribune,* February 20, 1967, p. 23.

8. *Medical Tribune,* February 20, 1967, p. 23.

Case Study Exercises

1. Do you see common concerns or any pattern in the experiments discussed in this chapter (e.g., on slaves, the Tuskegee study, the Willowbrook study)?

2. Eponyms—such as *Alzheimer's* disease and *Parkinson's* disease—are a form of homage to the person being recognized. Do you think it is ethically sound to name a medical condition after someone who has behaved despicably? Set out your position after considering the following case:

   . . . a common condition of unknown cause that affects the joints, eyes, urethra and skin and is known as Reiter's syndrome, named after a German doctor, Hans Conrad Reiter, who reported a case in a military officer in 1916. The eponym was adopted in English language journals in the early 1940's. But by then Dr. Reiter had become an early disciple of Hitler. And now, new attention to his career shows that his involvement in Nazi atrocities was deeper than previously known. Two arthritis experts at the University of California at Los Angeles have added further evidence of Dr. Reiter's role as a Nazi who helped plan and approve "human experiments" in concentration camps. Writing in the current issue of *The Journal of Clinical Rheumatology,* Dr. Daniel J. Wallace and Dr. Michael Weisman renewed calls made over the last quarter of a century to drop Dr. Reiter's name from the syndrome. Dr. Reiter may have earned the highest marks for his teaching and service to the community, the doctors said. But, they asked, "Should a war criminal be rewarded with eponymous distinction?" (See Lawrence K. Altman, M.D., "The Doctor's World: Experts Re-examine Dr. Reiter, His Syndrome and His Nazi Past," *The New York Times,* 7 March 2000.)

3. Do you think scientists should use the data obtained from the Nazi experiments and the Tuskegee Syphilis Study? Share your thoughts on using results obtained by means, as we saw in these two cases, that seriously violate human rights.

4. How should we respond to the issues raised by Vanessa M. Gamble regarding African Americans' distrust of the medical profession? What steps might be taken to minimize prejudice and discrimination on the part of medical professionals and researchers?

5. In an article on 18th century medical ethics and the work of John Gregory on ethical issues in British medicine, Laurence B. McCullough discusses some of the unjust practices. He remarks on "sporting" with patients in the Royal Infirmary by using experiments as the first line of treatment. What lessons do you think we should learn from the following:

   The Royal Infirmary was established to care for the deserving, working poor, who received free care. The sick had first to obtain a ticket of admission from one of the benefactors of the Infirmary and then pass screening by the lay managers of the institution, who selected against patients with "fever" or any other sign of life-threatening illness, to keep mortality rates down. Thus, a not-for-profit institution invented market segmentation for the purpose of advancing institutional self-interest. The lay managers exerted strict control of resources and complained regularly of the overuse of resources and high mortality rates on the teaching ward.

   There were regular accusations of callousness made against the physicians of the Infirmary, who were appointed by the benefactors and served without recompense. Physicians, Gregory says, abused the label "incurable" by applying it too quickly, so as to rationalize the use of experiments as the first line of treatment. (See Laurence B. McCullough, "Bioethics in the Twenty-First Century: Why We Should Pay Attention to Eighteenth-Century Medical Ethics," in *Kennedy Institute of Ethics Journal* 6 (4) 1996.)

6. In the Advisory Committee on Human Radiation Experiments (ACHRE) report, one chapter dealt with the use of children in nontherapeutic medical experimentation. Discuss the ethical concerns raised by the following and set out your recommendations:

[T]he availability of certain persons, not able to consent personally, may constitute a strategic resource in terms of time or location not otherwise obtainable. It must be remembered, however, that the Nazis hid behind this rationalization in explaining certain highly questionable or clandestine medical experiments. Such justification should not even be considered except in dire circumstances. . . . As part of the Committee's Ethics Oral History Project, we interviewed two pediatricians who were beginning their careers in academic medicine in the late 1940s. One of these respondents, Dr. Henry Seidel, had some research experience with institutionalized children. He noted that "we got access [to the children] very easily," and although his research was merely observational, it was "not hard to imagine" that experimental research with these children could have been conducted. When asked about the studies conducted by Dr. Saul Krugman on institutionalized children at the Willowbrook State School . . . Seidel observed, "I didn't have any problem imagining that possibility. In retrospect, I'm sure it could happen, you know. There was something about those reports that rang true. . . ." William Silverman, the other pediatrician interviewed . . . recalled that, in the 1950s, many pediatricians, including himself, believed that it was not necessary to obtain the permission of parents before using a pediatric patient as a subject in research—even if the research was nontherapeutic (he has since become a strong proponent of the parental permission requirement in pediatric research). He also asserted that performing nontherapeutic experiments on children without authorization from parents was part of a broader "ethos of the time" in which "everyone was a draftee" in a national war on disease. (See Chapter 7 of the ACHRE report for further discussion.)

7. Do you think the Patients' Bill of Rights covers all your concerns as a patient? Looking over any of our narratives in this text, do you see any concerns raised by patients or families that are omitted or not sufficiently recognized in this document? Do you think the oaths and codes adequately address issues of justice and oppression (related to race and ethnicity, gender, class, disability, etc.)?

8. How do we balance patient autonomy with protecting the public? To what degree should we consider cosmetic surgery to be medical experimentation and set down strict regulations? Should we require long-term studies before allowing a drug or procedure to be marketed? Share what questions you think ought to be asked before permitting women access to breast implants. If possible, draw from at least one of the codes in the first section of this chapter.

9. Read the following and answer the questions below:

In 1988 an Oxford University researcher, Dr. Charles Gilks, proposed that AIDS might have entered the human population because of a series of little-known malaria experiments in which people were inoculated with fresh blood from monkeys and chimpanzees. He postulated that this blood may have infected humans with primate viruses that were the ancestors of the AIDS virus. Here's the evidence: Many AIDS researchers believe the human AIDS virus originated in monkeys and chimpanzees. One monkey (the sooty mangabey) is often infected with a virus very close to HIV 2, which caused AIDS in West Africa. At least one chimpanzee has been found to be infected with a virus almost identical to HIV 1, the virus that causes AIDS in the U.S. and Europe.

From 1922 into the 1950's researchers inoculated themselves or others (including prisoners) with fresh blood from chimps or mangabeys. They were studying malaria and the purpose of these experiments was to see if malaria parasites that infect primates could infect humans. These studies involved 34 people who were injected with blood from chimps and 33 people who were injected with blood from people who received chimpanzee blood. Also, 2 people were given blood from mangabeys and 3 others got blood from macaques that had been injected with mangabey blood. (See Gina Kolata, "New Theory Ties AIDS to Malaria Experiments," *The New York Times,* 27 Nov 88.)

Share your thoughts on the following:
a. What issues and concerns are raised by these experiments?
b. Do you think Dr. Gilks, the Oxford researcher, has enough evidence to support his hypothesis (that AIDS entered the human population because of these experiments in which blood from primates was injected into human subjects)?

10. As you can see in the case discussed in question 9, scientists have also subjected themselves to risk as participants in experimental studies. A premise of the Nuremberg Code was that a requirement that scientists be willing to be subjects in an experiment of their design would be a deterrent for scientific abuse or excess. Discuss the wisdom of such a requirement.

11. In an alternative theory about the origin of AIDS, journalist Edward Hooper hypothesizes that the AIDS virus was transmitted to humans because of polio vaccines. Hooper argues that

. . . the deadly HIV virus may have been unleashed more than 30 years ago by well-meaning Western doctors giving experimental polio vaccines to African children. . . . Hooper says an oral vaccine given to about a million people in central Africa from 1957 to 1960 was cultured from the cells of primates. Scientists have concluded in recent years that AIDS originated in a primate: the chimpanzee. . . . He reasons that although Africans have been killing and eating the meat of primates for centuries, the earliest known sample of the human AIDS virus is from 1959 — after the polio vaccine had been administered. He writes that areas in which the polio vaccine was administered later became the epicenter of the African AIDS epidemic. And he says the researchers giving out the polio vaccine were also engaged in medical experiments on several hundred chimps in an African camp. "It is, in short, not unreasonable to propose that some of the vaccine batches fed in Central Africa between 1957 and 1960 could have been prepared in chimp tissue, and that some of this tissue may have been infected with the . . . precursor of HIV," he writes. (See Marlene Cimons, "Lessons Sought in the Origin of AIDS," *Los Angeles Times,* 23 December 1999.)

a. Do you think this theory has merit and deserves investigation?
b. What should we do when we have competing theories such as Hooper's (above) and Gilks's (set out in exercise 9)?

12. What has come to light about the use of female slaves for experimental surgery and medical experimentation raises a number of questions:
a. To what extent should this history of using slave women in medical experimentation be recognized (e.g., in history and medical texts)?
b. Assuming there are still segments of the population that are similarly vulnerable to medical exploitation, what steps could be taken to make sure that we, as a society, minimize injustice and abuse at the hands of researchers and members of the medical profession?

13. What do you think ought to be done to recognize the individual and collective harm done by the Willowbrook studies? Set out your ideas after reading the following:

Twenty-five years after the patients of the infamous Willowbrook State School won a class-action lawsuit that led to the widespread deinstitutionalization of the mentally retarded, lawyers, doctors, administrators and some class members themselves gathered to celebrate the settlement, called the Willowbrook Consent Judgment—and to criticize its aftermath. The conference . . . was called "Social Justice Has Prevailed." But many of the 450 present said it had not: There are still mentally retarded people institutionalized; care still needs improvement, even in group homes; the state is not meeting the promises it made in the settlement, and no reparations, or even apologies, have been made.

. . . Several of the participants, including William Bronston, one of the Willowbrook doctors who helped organize the parents who filed the lawsuit, returned to the site for the first time since the 70's. During one panel discussion, he called for an apology to be issued to those who suffered. "The parents," Dr. Bronston said privately during a lunchtime presentation of awards and speeches, "have never been acknowledged as Holocaust survivors, American-style." (See Shaila K. Dwan, "Recalling a Victory for the Disabled," *The New York Times,* 3 May 2000.)

14. In 1992 it was disclosed that the CIA funded mind control experiments back in the 1950s— yet another unsavory bit of Cold War history. As noted:

In the 50's psychiatric experiments were conducted in Canada, in part financed by the Central Intelligence Agency (CIA). These experiments began after some soldiers held as prisoners returned from the Korean War brainwashed, and Western intelligence agencies began experiments on the possibility of mind control. McGill University in Montreal, Canada was one of the centers where such experiments were carried out. In 1992 the Canadian government, after previously refusing to compensate victims, agreed to pay $80,000 to each of the 80 or so patients who underwent the so-called "psychic driving" treatment in Montreal, intended to wipe the brain clear of all trauma. It was reported that the patients were put into a drugged sleep for weeks or months, subjected to electroshock therapy until they were "depatterned," and forced to listen repeatedly to recorded messages broadcast from speakers on the wall or under their pillows. Despite the decision to pay compensation, the Canadian government has not acknowledged legal responsibility. (See Clyde H. Farnsworth, "Canada Will Pay 50's Test Victims," *The New York Times,* 19 November 1962.)

 a. To what degree do you think a government should be held responsible when they finance or otherwise participate in experiments such as this mind control study?
 b. Using the Internet or other sorts of research, can you see if there have been any similar kinds of experiments in the last decade?

15. Theodore Kaczynksi (alias "the Unabomber") was said to have been the subject of some rather bizarre and brutalizing psychological experiments while a student at Harvard University stating in 1958. (See Alston Chase, "Harvard and the Making of the Unabomber," *The Atlantic Monthly,* June 2000.) Do you think universities should allow the use of use their own students in nontherapeutic experiments?

16. Discuss the strengths and weakness of the Nuremberg Code. Do you think the Helsinki Declaration has sufficiently addressed the weaknesses or omissions of the Nuremberg Code?

17. What do you see as the major legacy of the Nazi experiments? Is this the same as for the Tuskegee study? What do you think we should learn from the sorts of egregious cases of medical experimentation discussed here in this chapter?

18. How do the medical codes reveal the values and beliefs of the medical profession? What sorts of omissions do you see? If you were to suggest changes or modifications to any of the codes, what would you recommend?

19. In the movie *Outbreak,* a monkey infected with an Ebola-like virus is loose in the wooded property behind a house in which a young girl who has befriended the monkey lives (the

monkey will come to her to get food). The researchers ask that the child be sent outside to lure the monkey out of the woods so they can capture it, although doing so clearly puts her at risk. The parents agree. At that moment utilitarian values prevailed. Applying this to medical experimentation we might ask:

a. Is nontherapeutic experimentation of children, as Paul Ramsey argues, always to be avoided?

b. Could you conceive of any circumstance where a child or children should be put at risk in an experiment, even though it holds no direct benefit for them? When, if ever, might such sacrifice for others be asked of a child?

InfoTrac College Edition

1. Jonathan D. Moreno, "The Dilemmas of Experimenting on People. (Striking a Balance Between Human Rights and Medical Progress)"
2. Jochen Vollmann and Rolf Winau, " Informed Consent in Human Experimentation before the Nuremberg Code"
3. *British Medical Journal,* "The Nuremberg Code (1947). (reprinted from *Doctors of Infamy: The Story of the Nazi Medical Crimes*)"
4. Jennifer Leaning, "War Crimes and Medical Science: Not Unique to One Place or Time; They Could Happen Here"
5. Robert W. Kestling, " Blacks under the Swastika: A Research Note"
6. Daniel J. Nolan, "100 Years of X Rays: They Turned Medicine Inside Out"
7. *Jet,* "Journal Editorial Blasts HIV Testing on Poor in Third World Countries; Compares to Tuskegee Study"
8. *Jet,* "Black Caucus Urges U.S. to Apologize for Deceiving Syphilis Victims 60 Years Ago. (Tuskegee Syphilis Study)"
9. *Weekly Compilation of Presidential Documents,* "Remarks in Apology to African-Americans on the Tuskegee Experiment. (Bill Clinton Speech)"
10. *Weekly Compilation of Presidential Documents,* "Memorandum on Protections for Human Subjects of Classified Research"
11. Constance Holden, "Draft Research Code Raises Hackles (New Code of Research Ethics in Canada)"

Web Connections

For links to Medical Experimentation: Historical Considerations Web sites, articles, cases, and more exercises, go to our Medical Experimentation page at philosophy.wadsworth.com/ teays.purdy/experimentation

Chapter 4

Contemporary Issues in Informed Consent

IT WOULD BE NICE to think that abuses of research subjects were past history, that the sorts of cases we examined in the last chapter would not or could not be repeated. It would be nice to think the various codes designed to protect human and animal subjects would be respected. But that is not the case. As we will see in this chapter, some of the injustices committed in the various historical cases are not behind us. In addition, advances in research techniques and technology have given rise to new concerns.

We now face issues unimaginable in earlier days; such as the use of embryos and fetuses in experimentation and transplantation. Other sorts of transplantation issues also face us. For instance, what sorts of ethical concerns arise from the transplanting of human organs and body parts? Is it morally wise of us to allow animal organs to be transplanted into other animals or into humans? What risks might we be running and who should decide if they are worth taking? Decisions in this area have wide-ranging consequences. In January 1998 the Food and Drug Administration (FDA) said it would set out guidelines for xenotransplants, in spite of concerns that deadly viruses could potentially be transferred across species, resulting in AIDS-like epidemics. Virologist Jonathan S. Allan, quoted in a report in *The Chronicle of Higher Education,* said the FDA should at least distinguish between nonhuman primates and pigs, since primates such as baboons are far more dangerous to human health than are pigs. Moreover, scientists admit that the level of risk in xenotransplants is unknown. Issues such as these have enormous impact, and illustrate just how significant are the ethical issues facing us in medical research.

Lest we think informed consent is now an established principle governing experimentation and therapy, and thus that patient autonomy (so long as there is no economic incentive) is secure, we need to consider recent history: for example, government radiation studies (discovered by Eileen Welsome, a journalist at the *Albuquerque Tribune,* and later officially investigated by a President's Commission led by Ruth

Faden), the use of biowarfare vaccines without consent of servicemen and -women in the Gulf War, the easing of consent requirements for use of experimental vaccines and experimental research by the Pentagon, and AIDS experiments in third world countries. Such cases show how fragile, yet important, ethical safeguards are.

There are also recent issues regarding experimentation that have a potentially global impact and cry out for an international bioethics tribunal or overseer to guide such decision making. Countries are doing experiments on biological and chemical weapons and have even begun stockpiling biowarfare supplies. The Pentagon recently proceeded with anthrax vaccinations, and, as we know from the Gulf War, earlier vaccinated troops without their consent against the threat of biowarfare from Iraq. This has implications for the use of human subjects, because the vaccines had not previously been used in combination and thus had unclear health consequences.

As well, questions arise about whether or not it is wise, on moral and other grounds, to keep supplies of the smallpox virus now that it has been virtually eradicated from the face of the earth. Plus, there are any number of global issues related to nuclear technology. As our look at the report on the Human Radiation Experiments will show, numerous human rights abuses have spanned decades. Not only were military personnel used as unwitting guinea pigs, but so were terminally ill patients, children, and the populations of entire cities. For example, evidently an aboveground nuclear test in Nevada in 1965 was timed to go off when the winds would carry the fallout over Los Angeles so its effect on such a large population could be studied.

Such studies not only blatantly ignored the moral requirement to get the informed consent of the subjects, but also lacked even a pretense of therapeutic value for the participants. The Nuremberg Code and more recent codes had no effect on those undertaking these experiments; and we have paid for this ever since. For example, the human radiation studies were similarly undertaken without obtaining the consent of the experimental subjects.

As biological experimentation grows ever bolder, new issues will continue to confront us. The recent explosive proliferation of cloning experiments, including the creation of part-human, part-cow embryonic stem cells, provoked a public outcry that led President Clinton to direct the National Bioethics Advisory Commission to investigate the implications of the research. Further work on the justifiable limits of medical experimentation clearly is needed. As the readings in this chapter demonstrate, the territory is wide—and keeps getting wider.

The ethical issues regarding medical experimentation are both global and local. Some apply on an international scale, some raise significant environmental concerns, and some apply to individual research subjects—such as when individuals, as consumers, become possibly unknowing objects of experimentation. For example, because of the paucity of research on breast implants and the limited number of animal studies prior to their introduction on the market, we could conclude that women who got breast implants served as subjects in experiments. There is reason to believe that the manufacturer of the upholstery foam used in earlier implants called "la Même" (French for "the same," as in "same as your breast") had no knowledge that this material was used in creating a product designed to be placed inside a human body. Moreover, there appeared to be no long-range studies before breast implants were put on the market, and most of the studies that were done used beagles—dogs—as subjects. Even if we consider the information obtained in such studies applicable to humans, those studies lasted no longer than five years in duration. In light of the difficulty of finding information on the effects of silicone in the human body, it seems as though silicone itself was not studied much, if at all, before its use in breast implants. The related ethical concerns deserve closer study. The sheer number of American women alone (over one million) who got breast implants makes this story particularly disturbing.

Women are not the only ones used on a grand scale in consumer-focused medical research. Look at sports. Performance-enhancing drugs like steroids, androstenedione, creatine, and erythropoietin (EPO) are widely used by athletes to boost their endurance, build strength and stamina, and speed of recovery from injury. Nevertheless, athletes who use such drugs and over-the-counter supplements are effectively subjects in a medical experiment with unknown long-term risks and little or no follow-up. Few, if any, studies have been conducted on the effects of some of these performance-enhancing drugs on women and teenage boys and girls (most such experiments have been conducted on men and, even then, have not been long-term studies). As we will see in the readings in this chapter, there are serious concerns about the health risks of such drugs and supplements. Like breast implants, these substances warrant further attention because of the large numbers of athletes, professional as well as amateur, that are effectively research subjects.

These are not the only cases that call for scrutiny. Issues have been raised about the ethical conduct of researchers who use third world subjects (e.g., in the AIDS trials) or conduct psychiatric research. The use of animals in research raises concerns as well: Ethicists and others have questioned the enormous numbers of animals sacrificed for unnecessary or redundant research, have questioned the lack of attention to minimizing suffering, and have raised concerns about potential abuses using animal hybrids and animal-to-animal and animal-to-human transplants.

All of these practices demand a close look at the standards we expect of researchers and medical caregivers participating in medical research. Furthermore, we need a clear definition of what we mean by informed consent, for it is of fundamental importance in examining all of these contemporary cases. In some cases, the participation is willing, as with athletes who use creatine, though it could hardly be called "informed." In some cases, subjects had some knowledge of risks, as do women and girls who have recently chosen to get breast implants. In other cases, such as the Gulf War veterans and subjects of radiation experiments, the subjects had no knowledge whatsoever that they were participating in an experiment and, consequently, could not either agree to participate or choose to withdraw. Thus, when we look at informed consent issues, it helps to have some familiarity with the ways in which the concept of "informed" has evolved.

LEGAL HISTORY OF INFORMED CONSENT

If we examine the history of informed consent, we see that it is a relatively recent concept. This is due to the fact that the history of Western medicine is a history of paternalism—and this paternalistic approach has shifted only recently, in response to the emphasis on patient autonomy. The 1914 decision *Schloendorff v. Society of NY Hospitals* carved a line in the sand of medical decision making by affirming that every human being of adult years and sound mind has a right to determine what happens to his or her own body.

Subsequent decisions, such as *Canterbury v. Spence, Berkey v. Anderson,* and *Cobbs v. Grant* expanded and refined the idea that for consent to be meaningful it must be informed. Attention then focused on what it means to be informed; eventually, being informed entailed being told of even low-probability risks and of possible alternative treatments. With the *Cobbs* decision, the physician was seen to have a fiduciary requirement to reveal to the patient any known risks. Because of the various codes and legal opinions in the area of medical decision making, we have seen an expansion of patient autonomy.

However, the 1990 case of *Moore v. the Regents of University of California* has drawn limits around self-determination, particularly with regard to commercial rights connected with medical research. John Moore, who recovered from hairy-cell leukemia apparently because of the unique properties of his own blood, became an unwitting participant in the creation of a cell line and biological products aimed at curing viral-caused diseases. Although he started treatment for his condition in 1976 and had vast amounts of blood, sperm, and bone marrow removed for research purposes, it wasn't until 1984 that he was asked to sign a consent form. Even then he was not told about the cell line that was developed using his blood and tissues. When asked to relinquish any rights to possible products based on his tissues, Moore became suspicious. He then sued on thirteen causes of action, but lost on all except for violation of his informed consent.

In a rather curious decision, the Supreme Court of California ruled that Moore did not have the right to profit from any discoveries or products derived from his blood or tissues. The Court argued, for instance, that, having given consent to the splenectomy, Moore agreed to the "disposal" of his spleen. "Disposal," in the Court's loose reading, was equivalent to "donation," and so could allow its use for research, including its use in creating biological products for commercial purposes. It remains to be seen what the consequences of the *Moore* decision will be in the area of medical experimentation and in the development and commercialization of biotechnology.

These cases, or selections from the decisions, can be accessed by going to our Web site. It is helpful to read the decisions and get an overview of the way in which the notions of "self-determination," "patient autonomy," "extraordinary" medical treatment (vs. "ordinary" medical treatment), and "informed consent" have been examined and developed in the various rulings related to bioethics and the law. In the case of "informed consent," our understanding of the concept and our expectations as to what it covers have grown over the years, basically moving from a broad notion of whether or not consent was even granted for a medical procedure or treatment, to one in which knowledge of even low-probability risks must be disclosed. In other words, justices realized that, for consent to be "informed," patients must have had all the relevant information—however insignificant it may seem—made known to them before any effective decision making could take place.

This chapter gives us an overview of these wide-ranging concerns. The readings in the first section look at individual decision making in informed consent.

1. Leonard H. Glantz, George J. Annas, Michael A. Grodin, and Wendy K. Mariner cast a critical eye on medical research in developing countries, arguing that care must be taken to make sure such experimentation is truly therapeutic in kind.

2. Nicholas Regush raises concerns and criticisms about the use of breast implants, focusing on the case of the Même (foam-covered) implant and the potential harms suffered by those women who used them.

3. Wanda Teays examines the ethical issues in the use of performance-enhancing drugs, looking at the extent of the problem and the factions (such as coaches, sponsor-advertisers, peers) pressuring athletes to use drugs and "nutritional" supplements. She argues that these athletes have, effectively, been subjects of a vast experiment without being fully cognizant of the risks.

4. Gail Geller, Misha Strauss, Barbara A. Bernhardt, and Neil A. Holtzman look at the process of giving informed consent and offer recommendations for patients and providers alike.

In the second section we look at a variety of issues raised in treating the body as property.

1. Looking at the growing market in organs, Karen Wright details the extent to which organs and body tissues are in demand and explores some of the ethical issues that arise from this highly profitable enterprise.

2. Dorothy Nelkin and Lori Andrews discuss the commercialization of the body made possible by biotechnology, pointing out some crucial issues, particularly in light of the *Moore* case.

3. Ellen Wright Clayton examines ethical issues raised in the use of human embryos, using the *Davis v. Davis* case, which centered on the question of which party of a divorced couple should be granted "custody" of the woman's frozen embryos; she wanted to use them to attempt to have a child and the man wished to destroy them. Clayton argues that the ruling in this case will apply to issues regarding in vitro fertilization (IVF).

4. Also examining fetal transplantation and experimentation, Wanda Teays focuses on the issues of commercial rights. She gives an overview of the various positions regarding moral authority in decision making and looks at some economic and moral ramifications surrounding the creation of biological products derived from fetal tissue.

5. Arthur L. Caplan looks at the public policy concerns regarding organ-harvesting of dead people. He argues that the transplant community should not attempt to change existing standards without both public and professional discussion of the issue.

6. Janet Radcliffe-Richards et al. set out the case for allowing kidney sales.

7. James Lindemann Nelson examines transplants of animal organs in humans and argues that we need to look more carefully at the moral standing of animals, such as baboons, that are harvested for organs. He contends that we need to rethink the line we draw between human beings and the rest of creation.

The third section focuses on societal and environmental issues concerning medical experiment.

1. The final report of the Advisory Committee on Human Radiation Experiments (chaired by Ruth Faden) describes the extent of the problem.

2. In light of the reports on the Human Radiation Experiments, Jonathan D. Moreno discusses issues raised by the Department of Defense's guidelines set out in the 1950s. He details some of the ethical disagreements that erupted and gives us a look into reactions to a paper by Dr. Robert Stone on the use of humans in radiation studies.

3. Gary E. Varner looks at the debate over the use of animals in research and attempts to find a commonality of concerns and the possibility for closing some of the distance between the two sides.

Individual Decision Making

Research in Developing Countries: Taking "Benefit" Seriously

LEONARD H. GLANTZ, GEORGE J. ANNAS,
MICHAEL A. GRODIN, and WENDY K. MARINER

AN APRIL 1998 *New York Times Magazine* article described Ronald Munger's efforts to obtain blood samples from a group of extremely impoverished people in the Philippine island of Cebu.[1] Munger sought the blood to study whether there was a genetic cause for this group's unusually high incidence of cleft lip and palate. One of many obstacles to the research project was the need to obtain the cooperation of the local health officer. It was not clear to Munger, or the reader, whether the health officer had a bona fide

LEONARD H. GLANTZ is an Associate Professor of Public Health at the Boston University School of Public Health and Medicine. GEORGE J. ANNAS is the Edward R. Utley Professor and Chair, Health Law Dept, Boston University School of Public Health. MICHAEL A. GRODIN is Director of the Law, Medicine, and Ethics Program and Professor of Health Law, Health Law Dept., Boston University Schools of Public Health and Medicine. WENDY K. MARINER is a Professor specializing in Health Law at the Boston University School of Public Health.

interest in protecting the populace or was looking for a bribe. The health officer asked Munger a few perfunctory questions about informed consent and the study's ethical review in the United States, which Munger answered. Munger also explained the benefits that mothers and children would derive from participating in the research. The mothers would learn their blood types (which they apparently desired) and whether they were anemic. If they were anemic, they would be given iron pills. Lunch would be served, and raffles arranged so that families could win simple toys and other small items.

Munger told the health officer that if his hypotheses were correct, the research would benefit the population of Cebu: if the research shows that increased folate and vitamin B6 reduces the risk of cleft lip and palate, families could reduce the risk of facial deformities in their future offspring. The reporter noted that the health officer "laughs aloud at the suggestion that much of

The Hastings Center Report *(Nov–Dec 1998): 38–42. Reprinted by permission of Leonard H. Glantz, George J. Annas, Michael A. Grodin, Wendy K. Mariner, and The Hastings Center. Copyright 1998, The Hastings Center.*

what is being discovered in American laboratories will make it back to Cebu any time soon." Reflecting on his experience with another simple intervention, iodized salt, the health officer said that when salt was iodized, the price rose three-fold "so those who need it couldn't afford it and those who didn't need it are the only ones who could afford it."

The simple blood collecting mission to Cebu illustrates almost all the issues presented by research in developing countries. First is the threshold question of the goal of the research and its importance to the population represented by the research subjects. Next is the quality of informed consent, including whether the potential subjects thought that participation in the research was related to free surgical care that was offered in the same facility (although it clearly was not) and whether one could adequately explain genetic hypotheses to an uneducated populace. Finally, there is the question whether the population from which subjects were drawn could benefit from the research. This research intervention is very low risk—the collection of 10 drops of blood from affected people and their family members. The risk of job or insurance discrimination that genetic research poses in this country did not exist for the Cebu population; ironically, they were protected from the risk of economic discrimination by the profound poverty in which they lived.

Even this simple study raises the most fundamental question: "Why is it acceptable for researchers in developed countries to use citizens of developing countries as research subjects?" A cautionary approach to permitting research with human subjects in underdeveloped countries has been recommended because of the risk of their inadvertent or deliberate exploitation by researchers from developed countries. This cautionary approach generally is invoked when researchers propose to use what are considered "vulnerable populations," such as prisoners and children, as research subjects.[2] Vulnerable populations are those that are less able to protect themselves, either because they are not capable of making their own decisions or because they are particularly susceptible to mistreatment.[3] For example, children may be incapable of giving informed consent or of standing up to adult authority, while prisoners are especially vulnerable to being coerced into becoming subjects. Citizens of developing countries are often in vulnerable situations because of their lack of political power, lack of education, unfamiliarity with medical interventions, extreme poverty, or dire need for health care and nutrition. It is the dire need of these populations that may make them both appropriate subjects of research and especially vulnerable to exploitation. This combination of need and vulnerability has led to the development of guidelines for the use of citizens of developing countries as research subjects.

CIOMS GUIDELINES

In 1992, the Council for International Organizations of Medical Sciences (CIOMS), in collaboration with the World Health Organization, published guidelines for the appropriate use of research subjects from "underdeveloped communities."[4]

Like other human research codes, the CIOMS guidelines combine the protection of subjects' rights with protection of their welfare; as subjects become less able to protect their own rights (and therefore become more vulnerable), researchers and reviewers must increase their efforts to protect the welfare of subjects.[5] Perhaps the most important statement in these guidelines is what appears to be the injunction against using subjects in developing countries if the research could be carried out reasonably well in developed countries. Commentary to guideline 8 notes, for example, that there are diseases that rarely or never occur in economically developed countries, and that prevention and treatment research therefore needs to be conducted in the countries at risk for those diseases. The conclusion to be drawn from the substance of these guidelines is that in order for research to be ethically conducted, it must offer the potential of actual benefit to the inhabitants of that developing country.

In order for underdeveloped communities to derive potential benefit from research, they must have access to the fruits of such research. The CIOMS commentary to guideline 8 states that, "as a general rule, the sponsoring agency should ensure that, at the completion of successful testing, any product developed *will* be made reasonably available to inhabitants of the underdeveloped community in which the research was carried out: exceptions to this general requirement should be justified, and agreed to by all concerned parties before the research is begun."[6] This statement is directed at minimizing exploitation of the underdeveloped community that provides the research subjects. If developed countries use inhabitants of underdeveloped countries to create new products that would be beneficial to both the developed and the underdeveloped country, but the underdeveloped country cannot gain access to the product because of expense, then the subjects in the underdeveloped countries have been grossly exploited. As written, however, this CIOMS guideline is not strong or specific enough to prevent exploitation. Exemplifying this problem are recent short course zidovudine (AZT) studies in Africa that were approved and conducted despite the existence of the CIOMS guidelines.[7]

THE AFRICAN MATERNAL-FETAL HIV TRANSMISSION STUDIES

The goal of the short course AZT studies was to see if lower doses of the drug AZT than those used in the United States could reduce the rate of maternal-child transmission of HIV. It was well established that doses of AZT that cost $800 (not taking into account screening and other related costs) reduced maternal-fetal transmission of HIV by as much as two-thirds in the United States.[8,9] If the developed countries had been willing to subsidize the cost of this regimen in Africa, no additional research would have been needed. But because many African countries could not afford this expense, the decision was made to attempt to see if lower (and therefore cheaper) doses would prevent maternal-fetal HIV transmission. Several impoverished countries were chosen as research sites. The justification for conducting research in those countries was not that they suffered from a disease that did not afflict people in developed countries, and not because no treatment existed, but because their impoverishment made an existing therapy unavailable to them (as long as developed countries refused to subsidize the costs).[10]

The issue, as always, is to determine the ethical acceptability of the proposed research *before* it is conducted. In a case like this, where the researchable problem exists *solely* because of economic reasons, the research hypothesis must contain an economic component. The research question should be formulated as follows:

1. We know that a given regimen of AZT will reduce the rate of maternal-child transmission of HIV.

2. Maternal-child transmission of HIV in many African countries is a serious problem but the effective AZT regimen is not available because it is too expensive.

3. If an effective AZT regimen costs $X, then it will be made available in the country in which it is to be studied.

4. Therefore, we will conduct trials in certain African countries to see if $X worth of AZT will effectively reduce maternal-child transmission of HIV in those countries.

The most important part of the development of this research question is number 3. Without knowing what dollar amount X actually represents, it is impossible to formulate a research question that can lead to any benefit to the citizens of the country in which the research is to be conducted. There is no way to determine what $X represents in the absence of committed funding. Therefore, an essential prerequisite to designing ethical research in underdeveloped countries is identifying the source and amount of funding for providing the fruits of the research to the people of the developing country in which it is to be studied as a condition of the research being approved.

If a study found, for example, that $50 worth of AZT has the same effect as $800 worth of AZT, it would greatly benefit the developed world. Developed countries, which currently spend $800 per case on drugs alone, could pay substantially less for this preventive measure, and, because the research was conducted elsewhere, none of their citizens would have been put at any risk. At the same time, if the underdeveloped country could not afford to spend $50 any more than it could spend $800, then it could not possibly derive information that would be of any benefit to its population. This is the definition of exploitation.[11]

It is only now that an effort is being made to determine how to raise the money to actually provide AZT to prevent maternal-child HIV transmission (as well as the other costly services that go with the appropriate administration of the drug) to the impoverished African countries that provided the human subjects.[12] These efforts began after parallel studies conducted in Thailand reported that lower doses of AZT reduced maternal-fetal transmission of HIV.[13] The Thai government had committed to providing the AZT before its trials began. In the African trials, however, no one "ensured" that at the completion of successful testing the product would be made reasonably available, thereby violating the CIOMS guidelines.[14] The guidelines say that there can be exceptions to this general requirement, but that exceptions must be "justified" and "agreed to by all concerned parties." It is not clear to whom the exception must be "justified"

or on what grounds. Moreover, if the "concerned parties" are the sponsor and/or the investigator and the host country, they may not adequately represent the interests of the research subjects. The fact that representatives of the research community and officials of the host countries agree to exploit the population does not make the research any less exploitive.[15]

RULES FOR ETHICAL RESEARCH IN DEVELOPING COUNTRIES

We believe the standards for research in developing countries should include the following.

There should be a rebuttable presumption that researchers from developed countries will not conduct research in developing countries unless it can be shown that a direct benefit *will* be bestowed upon the residents of that country if the research proves to be successful. The person or entities proposing to conduct the study must demonstrate that there is a realistic plan, which includes identified funding, to provide the newly proven intervention to the population from which the potential pool of research subjects is to be recruited. In the absence of a realistic plan and identified funding, the population from which the research subjects will be drawn cannot derive benefit from the research. Therefore, the benefits cannot outweigh the risks, because there are, and will be, no benefits. Only by having committed funding and a plan to make a successful intervention available can it be determined that there will be sufficient benefit to justify conducting research on the target population. The distribution plan must be realistic. Where the health care infrastructure is so undeveloped that it would be impossible to deliver the intervention even if it were free, research would be unjustified in the absence of a plan to improve that country's health care delivery capabilities.

Some might argue that this standard is too strict and that it would reduce the amount of research that could be conducted in certain countries. The answer, of course, is that if the benefits of the research are not made available to the inhabitants of that country, they have lost nothing by the lack of such research. Others might argue that research in underdeveloped countries is justified if it might benefit the individual research subjects, even if it will not benefit anyone else in the population. However, research is, by definition, designed to create generalizable knowledge, and is legitimate in a developing country only if its purpose is to create generalizable knowledge that will benefit the citizens of that country. If the research only has the potential to benefit the limited number of individuals who participate in the study, it cannot offer the benefit to the underdeveloped country that legitimizes the use of its citizens as research subjects. It should be emphasized that research whose goal is to prevent or treat large populations is fundamentally public health research, and public health research makes no sense (and thus should not be done) if its benefits are limited to the small population of research subjects.

It might be argued that there is no requirement that such a plan be devised prior to conducting research in the United States, and, therefore, that by adopting such a requirement we would be imposing a higher standard for research conducted in developing countries than we do for research conducted in the United States.

This argument only further demonstrates the differences between wealthy and poor countries. The reality in the United States is that regardless of the very significant gaps in insurance and Medicaid coverage and the health care discrepancies between the rich and poor, medical interventions are relatively widely available, especially when compared to developing countries. Upon the successful completion of the research that demonstrated the effectiveness of the 076 regimen in reducing maternal-child transmission, the primary beneficiaries of this new preventive intervention in the United States were poor women and their newborns. Unlike the United States, absent a plan to pay for a new interven-

tion and lacking the infrastructure to deliver an intervention, it is virtually guaranteed that the intervention will not be generally available in a developing country.

The more accurate analogy to the African AIDS trials would be if investigators proposed the 076 protocol in the United States knowing that only poor women would be recruited as research subjects and that, if successful, the intervention would not be made generally available to poor women. Such research would be clearly unethical. Not only would this be a gross violation of the ethical principle of distributive justice, it would be a violation of the regulatory obligation of the equitable selection of subjects.[16]

A further objection is that one cannot always trust what a government or another potential funder promises. What is to prevent the promisor from reneging? The answer is, nothing. One can try to expose the funder to embarrassment and other pressures that might cause it to live up to the promise upon which researchers and subjects relied. However, the potential unethical behavior in the future by the funder is no excuse for not having a realistic plan at the outset. Furthermore, if we take this obligation seriously, this should only occur once per funder. After reneging once, they cannot be relied upon again to justify research in the future.

An additional objection to our position is that it will restrict access to new interventions because once a new intervention is developed, the price will come down and therefore the intervention will become available to the people of the impoverished country. The answer is to ask those who control the pricing of interventions if this will be the case in any particular instance. One could have asked Glaxo if it would reduce its price once it was shown that lower doses of AZT were effective. If the answer is yes, one can proceed. If the answer is no, or "we have not decided," there seems to be no justification to proceed if the current price would significantly restrict availability. There is nothing magical about pricing. Pricing is in the absolute control of manufacturers and there is no need to guess or speculate about what will happen to price. Indeed, this objection to our argument would justify conducting the full 076 trial itself in developing countries. The price *might* come down enough so that determining the efficacy of short course AZT regimens might not be needed at all. Such speculation should not be sufficient to put subjects at risk.

Finally, it might be argued that there are diseases that only affect people in developing countries for which there are no effective treatments, but that the treatments that might be discovered could be expensive. The argument continues that it is not right to fail to develop treatments that could benefit some affected people because it will not be available to most affected people. This objection raises quite a different issue from the one addressed in this article. The impetus for such research is the absence of effective treatment and not the absence of economic resources. We have discussed research intended to determine whether effective but unaffordable interventions would work if used in lower, less expensive dosages. The researchable issue arises from an economic circumstance. The only way such research could offer any benefit is by "curing" the economic problem by establishing that the less expensive form of the intervention will be affordable and available. Absent knowledge of financial resources, one might well be creating a new unaffordable, and therefore useless, intervention. In contrast, in the case in which one is developing a new intervention, not because of poverty, but because no known effective intervention exists, and the disease is prevalent in a particular geographic area, the issue is quite different. In such a case one is not conducting research to try to "cure" the effects of poverty but rather because of the need to create new knowledge to treat a currently untreatable disease. However, even this case may raise problems similar to the ones addressed here. If one were to try to develop an intervention for such a condition and chose research subjects from impoverished segments of a society, knowing that only the

richest segment of that society could benefit from that intervention, such subject selection would be unethical for many of the reasons we have discussed.

Our proposal to require researchers and their funders to develop realistic plans to make their interventions available to the relevant population of the developing country in which the research is proposed should not be controversial. It is well accepted in principle not only by groups like CIOMS, but by the funders of many of the African HIV trials, including the Centers for Disease Control and Prevention and the National Institutes of Health.[17] The principle is often honored in the breach, however. Research funders who hope that their studies will yield beneficial knowledge may neglect the steps necessary to ensure that the benefits will be made available. Ethical codes have not been sufficiently specific or enforceable to protect research subjects from exploitation. It is essential to replace vague promises with realistic plans that must be reviewed and approved before the research commences.

In at least one other instance it has been suggested that economic issues be addressed in the review of proposed research projects. The U.S. National Research Council's Committee on Human Genome Diversity recommended that "Arrangements regarding financial interests in the products or outcomes of the research should be negotiated as *part of the original project review* and informed-consent process."[18]

It is essential that the wealthier countries of the world use their resources, both financial and technological, to help resolve the health problems that afflict the poor of the world. Doing so will undoubtedly require research. But research is a means to solving health problems, not an end in itself. The goal must be to create interventions that will benefit the people of the countries in which the research is conducted. They will benefit only if the knowledge gained produces interventions that are affordable and accessible. This needs to be determined as a condition of approval before research is conducted so that limited research funds are not wasted, and research subjects are not drawn from populations that will not be able to benefit from the research.

REFERENCES

1. Lisa Belkin, "The Clues Are in the Blood," *New York Times Magazine,* 26 April 1998.

2. Michael Grodin and Leonard Glantz, eds., *Children as Research Subjects: Science, Ethics, and Law* (New York: Oxford University Press, 1994).

3. Wendy K. Mariner, "Distinguishing 'Exploitable' from 'Vulnerable' Populations: When Consent Is Not the Issue," in *Ethics and Research on Human Subjects: Proceedings,* ed. Zbigniew Bankowski and Robert J. Levine (Geneva: CIOMS, 1993), pp. 44–55.

4. Zbigniew Bankowski and Robert J. Levine, eds., *Ethics and Research on Human Subjects: International Guidelines* (Geneva: CIOMS, 1993), pp. 25–32, 43–46.

5. Sharon Perley, Sev S. Fluss, Zbigniew Bankowski, and Francoise Simon, "The Nuremberg Code: An International Overview," in *The Nazi Doctors and the Nuremberg Code,* ed. George J. Annas and Michael A. Grodin (New York: Oxford University Press, 1992), pp. 149–73.

6. Bankowski and Levine, *Ethics and Research,* p. 26. Emphasis added.

7. George Annas and Michael Grodin, "Human Rights and Maternal-Fetal HIV Transmission Prevention Trials in Africa," *American Journal of Public Health* 88, no. 4 (1998): 560–63.

8. Edward Connor, Rhoda Sperling Richard Gelber et al., "Reduction of Maternal-Infant Transmission of Human Immunodeficiency Virus Type 1 with Zidovudine Treatment," *NEJM* 331 (1994): 1173–80.

9. "Recommendation of the U.S. Public Health Service Task Force on the Use of Zidovudine to Reduce Prenatal Transmission of Human Immunodeficiency Virus," *MMWR Morbidity and Mortality Weekly Reports* 43 (1994): 1–20.

10. Harold Varmus and David Satcher, "Ethical Complexities of Conducting Research in Developing Countries," *NEJM* 337 (1997): 1003–1005.

11. The per capita health care expenditures of most of the African countries involved in mother-to-child HIV transmission prevention trials range from $5 to $22 U.S. *World Bank Sector Strategy Health Nutrition and Population,* 1997.

12. M. Bunce, "Chirac Seeks Worldwide Relief for AIDS in Africa," *Boston Globe,* 8 December 1997.

13. "Administration of Zidovudine During Late Pregnancy and Delivery to Prevent Perinatal HIV Transmission—Thailand 1996–1998," *MMWR Morbidity and Mortality Weekly Reports* 47, no. 8 (1998): 151–54. The editorial note states that "to implement these findings, ministries of health, donor agencies, and other interested agents *should* develop policies and practices to strengthen access to prenatal care, testing and counseling for HIV infections, and provision of ZDV for HIV-infected pregnant woman."

14. Bankowski and Levine, *Ethics and Research,* p. 45.

15. As the National Research Council's Committee on Human Genome Diversity properly put it, in the context of research on human subjects, "[s]ensitivity to the special practices and beliefs of a community cannot be used as a justification for violating universal human rights." Committee on Human Genetic Diversity, *Evaluating Human Genetic Diversity* (Washington, D.C.: National Academy Press, 1997), p. 65.

16. 45 CFR 46.111(a)(3).

17. Varmus and Satcher, "Ethical Complexities of Conducting Research in Developing Countries."

18. *Evaluating Human Genetic Diversity,* at pp. 55–68. Emphasis added.

Toxic Breasts

NICHOLAS REGUSH

WHEN SYBIL NIDEN GOLDRICH was diagnosed with breast cancer in 1983, she blamed herself. Her body had failed her. It was embarrassing. No one but her family had to know. "I was certain that everyone would think that my cancer was due to an inability to handle stress," says Goldrich, now fifty-two. She resolved that she would wear falsies after her double mastectomy until she could find the best plastic surgeon around to reconstruct her breasts. And then she would go on with her life.

There seemed to be no reason not to have new breasts. Would any surgeon amputate an arm or a leg and not offer a replacement? "This is why I thought it would be easy to be reconstructed and complete my cancer process," Goldrich says. She discovered that at least twenty thousand women each year were having their breasts reconstructed with silicone-gel implants following cancer surgery, and another eighty thousand were electing to have implants for cosmetic reasons. Goldrich interviewed three reputable plastic surgeons before settling on Dr. Kurt Wagner; each assured her that the procedure would be simple with very little risk involved. "My surgeon seemed confident, so I too was confident," she says.

But immediately after Wagner inserted the foam-covered implants in July 1983, Goldrich developed an infection. When her bandages were removed over two months later, she had her first good look at herself in the bathroom mirror. "My heart sank," Goldrich says. "There were two baseball-shaped protrusions from my chest wall and a small red scar clearly visible two inches below them. Those were breasts? They were hard as rocks. Nothing like the milky, flesh-toned breasts that I had expected."

Desolate, she put on her shirt and curled up into a ball on her bed. "I thought of myself as a two-time loser," she says. "First cancer, and now this. My body had obviously rejected the implant." Two years later, after five surgeries and countless days of pain and suffering, Goldrich had a different idea of what had gone wrong. By then, news had trickled out about the dangers of breast implants: they hardened, they ruptured, they blocked a mammogram's ability to screen for cancer. Goldrich already had to live with fears about a recurrence of her breast cancer, but now she has a new worry. There is reason to believe that the leakage of silicone and a chemical from the implants' foam could itself cause increased risks of inflammatory diseases or cancer.

Breast implants, of course, are not the only form of plastic surgery that has gained popularity in recent years. The numbers of face-lifts, tummy tucks, liposuctions, nose jobs, and lip implants have all skyrocketed over the last decade, as has the number of doctors who perform them. "Everywhere you look, there are impossible and conflicting images of women," says Robin Lakoff, coauthor of *Face Value: The Politics of Beauty*. "Women are made to believe that love

NICHOLAS REGUSH is an award-winning journalist specializing in medical and scientific issues.

Mother Jones *magazine (Jan/Feb 1992): 25–31.* © *1992, Foundation for National Progress. Permission granted by* Mother Jones *magazine.*

and approval from men are dependent on the right image. That desperation will continue until women become looked upon as full people rather than just body parts."

About 750,000 women a year elect to have cosmetic surgery, spurred on by ubiquitous images of the body beautiful, by husbands or boyfriends, and by doctors' newspaper ads that make nip-and-tuck look as easy as highlighting one's hair. In Houston last March, plastic surgeon Dr. Franklin Rose took out an ad in the *Houston Chronicle,* explaining that the "cultural influence is such in this city that for a woman to feel attractive usually includes a Mercedes, a gold Rolex, and three or four operations—nose, breasts, liposuctions. It's just part of living in this city in a certain way, in a certain socioeconomic strata." The ad ends like this: "The Texas woman is a combination of many things, not the least of which is a surgeon's scalpel."

But breasts, more than thin thighs or a smooth brow, are most potent as a symbol of women's sexual self-worth. So it's not surprising that over 2 million women have had breast implants, and 130,000 more seek them each year. Breast augmentation is a $450-million-a-year business, as the American Society of Plastic and Reconstructive Surgeons, Inc., a lobbying group of 4,500 doctors, is well aware: During a "practice enhancement" campaign in the early eighties, the group issued a memo to the FDA, asserting, "There is a substantial and enlarging body of medical information and opinion to the effect that these deformities [small breasts] are really a disease" that, left uncorrected, results in a "total lack of well-being."

Among the most popular "cures" for this "disease" over the last decade has been the Même implant, a silicone-gel sac with a unique polyurethane foam cover that was supposed to prevent breast hardening. Since its development in 1982, the Même has captured over a quarter of the current implant market; over 200,000 women carry the Même in their bodies. But in spite of the large numbers of women opting for the "im-

proved" implant, the foam used for its cover—originally manufactured for use in such things as furniture upholstery, oil filters, and carburetors—went almost completely unmonitored for eight years.

It wasn't until last April that the Food and Drug Administration released a report showing that, in conditions similar to those in the body, the foam can release the chemical 2,4–toluenediamine (TDA), which causes liver cancer in rats and is a suspected human carcinogen. Days after the announcement, the Même's manufacturer, Bristol-Myers Squibb, pulled the implant from the market and, in September, the company closed down its plastic-surgery unit that produced the Même.

Most of the Même's recipients thought that they were making a relatively risk-free decision to augment their breasts. They were never warned of the implants' potential dangers. There are now several dozen injury suits against the three successive manufacturers of the Même. In one recent case, a New York jury awarded a woman $4.45 million (the case is under appeal); in another, a California woman settled out of court for $450,000. A class-action suit against Bristol-Myers Squibb is being prepared in Canada.

Some lawyers are predicting that these suits, along with the several hundred in process against the makers of other types of breast implants, will eventually rival the multibillion-dollar litigation fight against A.H. Robins, which manufactured the Dalkon Shield IUD. But as with the Robins suit, financial reparations won't change this simple fact for many women: They were told the Même implant was safe, that it wouldn't hurt them, by manufacturers and doctors who should have known better—and the dangers were then ignored by the government agencies that were supposed to protect them.

It is early morning in Ottawa. Pierre Blais, a private consultant on medical products, is in the basement laboratory of his home. As the Canadian government scientist who blew the whistle on the Même in January 1989, Blais has been inundated with requests from former implant users and their doctors and lawyers. Sets of damaged Même implants and other silicone-gel types without the foam arrive by courier almost daily from different parts of the United States and Canada, along with medical records and mammogram results. The packages are beginning to pile up in the living room upstairs.

Among the eighty or so sets of damaged implants he's received so far, Blais says that ones with broken covers are the most common. The gel released from the silicone sacs has often seeped into armpits and lymph nodes. In one typical case, an implant deflated, and leakage on both sides began to erode the user's ribs. Some of the women who have contacted Blais have also complained of symptoms ranging from sharp pain in their breasts and pelvic regions to inflammation and severe fatigue. "I'm not only worried about the potential of the implants to cause cancer," says Blais, a small, wiry fifty-one-year-old, "but also that their chemical constituents may wreak havoc in the body over the long term."

Right now, Blais is examining two Même implants. Only they don't look much like implants. The two buckets on his desk that are holding the products are filled with greenish gel. That is what is left of fifty-two-year-old Janie Cruise's surgically implanted breasts. It took almost seven hours on March 1, 1990, for doctors at the University of California Medical Center in Los Angeles to make unexpectedly large incisions under Cruise's breasts and then scrape out the seemingly endless amounts of infected green ooze from her chest wall. The smell of the infection was so bad that the chief surgeon became ill.

While Cruise's case may be extreme, Blais says that her history is all too typical. Cruise, then forty-four, was living in Southern California when she decided to get implants. Her seven-year marriage had just fallen apart, and she was facing re-entry into the singles scene. Encouraged by a close friend—"Janie, you'll look flaw-less!"—Cruise handed over a few thousand dollars for what seemed like a miracle cure for her sagging self-confidence. "My girlfriend planted the seed and it started growing," Cruise says. "I especially wanted to look nice in a bathing suit."

Cruise's plastic surgeon, Dr. Howard Sterling of Fullerton, California, assured her that the Même, a new implant, would keep her breasts soft and give her a "happy surgery." The doctor was known to brag that his own wife was a pleased Même user.

Within a couple of days after her surgery on November 22, 1983, Cruise felt severe pain in her left breast, but Sterling shrugged it off. "He said his wife had similar pain, and he called us both big babies," Cruise recalls. "So I never bothered going back to him."

The following year, Cruise quit her job as a regional sales manager for a piano distributorship and moved from California to Florida, hoping to start a new life. The breast pain journeyed with her. Then came the severe headaches, fatigue, muscle and joint pain, numbness in her right hand, bronchitis, and gastrointestinal ailments; often, when she would wake up in the morning, her chest felt like someone was sleeping on it. All of these symptoms and more, she says, "sort of evolved over a period of a year and a half."

She visited one medical specialist after another—about two dozen all told. She took medication for her pain, enrolled in pain clinics, tried biofeedback, and talked with a psychologist. Nothing helped. "There was not one single suspicion voiced that my symptoms might be linked to the implants," she says. Cruise began blaming her medical problems on the damp Florida weather. Now she is waiting for Blais's evaluation of the evidence: Did her implants break because of design, or because of the use of substandard raw materials?

Blais believes that most, if not all, of these products will fail in time. He says women who assumed that their doctors could be counted on to give them safe and effective breast implants misplaced their trust. "Plastic surgeons have been putting in a lot of junk that has been very poorly manufactured," he says. "It's never been made to last, and that means a lot of women are going to have broken implants and leaking gel and other chemicals and debris moving through their bodies. I'm very fearful that the health problems we are seeing today with all the implants are merely a hint of the disaster to come."

Dr. Howard Sterling doesn't much remember Janie Cruise, one of his earliest Même recipients. Didn't she once send him porno-type pinups? No, wait. That was someone else. Oh, so Cruise had some problems. A lot of pain? Really? "Well, she never reported any of them to me," he says, ending that topic of discussion.

But Sterling, who intermittently clears his throat and speaks very quickly into the phone, does want to talk about the Même. In fact, he boasts that he is "probably one of the plastic surgeons who has implanted the most Mêmes in the whole damn U.S. of A."—roughly 670 sets of the implants. Though he's never formally studied his Même patients, Sterling volunteers that most of them, including his wife, two daughters, and "girls" in his office, have had "beautiful experiences." His complication rate runs about 15 to 20 percent, but he says that's mostly because some of the implants harden.

Sterling did have some fleeting concerns about the Même in 1983, the same year that Cruise had her surgery. Some of his patients were developing blood blisters between the implant's foam layer and the inner silicone-gel bag. The accumulation of blood made the implants heavier. "When I took the Mêmes out, I could see that parts had a shiny surface, indicating that there was little or no adhesion there to the foam," he explains.

Why did he continue implanting the Même? "Because it didn't make breasts harden to the same extent as other implants did, and it was the best thing available at the time," he replies. And by 1984, his cases of blood blisters had dropped dramatically, perhaps partly because Sterling had

stopped giving his patients an anti-inflammatory drug for infection control that was linked to blood-clot formation.

Sterling also believed that the Même had a long history of safety because it was similar to the Natural-Y, a foam-covered implant developed for mastectomy patients. One of that implant's developers in the late sixties was Sterling's mentor, Dr. Franklin Ashley, who headed the plastic-surgery department at the University of California at Los Angeles. The other was Harold Markham, who became president of Natural-Y Surgical Specialties, Inc., and eventually masterminded the development of the Même. Schooled in advertising and marketing, Markham was previously a medical-device salesman and consultant.

Ashley's published claims of good test results initially generated only sporadic clinical interest in the Natural-Y. Some doctors reported difficulties in removing the Natural-Y cleanly when hardening or infection developed. They said that the foam got entangled with breast tissue. In spite of that, by the late seventies, the implant had gained the faithful support of a small group of plastic surgeons, and Natural-Y, Inc., began work on a lighter, more-streamlined foam-covered implant, primarily for cosmetic purposes—the Même. "Because the Même was supposedly an improved design, we [plastic surgeons] assumed it was probably safe," Sterling says. "The company said it was. All we really knew is what the company told us."

The company couldn't have provided Sterling with much in the way of clinical trial data on the Même. For example, it had sponsored a small, uncontrolled study, which followed only eighty-one Même recipients over eighteen months. Dr. Steven Herman, the New York City plastic surgeon who published the study in 1984, claimed excellent results for the implant. However, there was something Herman didn't mention: according to a detailed 1986 deposition, which includes a description of cutting checks, Markham claims that Herman undertook the study in exchange for a royalty on Même sales. (Herman continues to deny receiving any compensation from the company.)

Early animal studies on the Même, which the company cited to plastic surgeons as further proof of the implant's safety, were of the shortcut variety, according to Pierre Blais. As senior scientific advisor to Canada's Health Protection Branch, an agency similar to the FDA, Blais reviewed numerous types of implants, and a colleague had brought the Même to his attention. "Their approach [to testing] was rudimentary," he says. "Sorely lacking was toxicological testing for the presence of chemical by-products of the foam in the body over the short and long term. Concerns had been raised by biomaterials scientists since the early sixties about the potential of some polyurethane foams to release toxic substances, if not carcinogens. But this issue was apparently not a priority for the company."

Blais would later learn that, until June 1988, the Même's manufacturer had incomplete knowledge about the foam's chemical structure and the way the foam was produced. Instead of scientific study, the company relied heavily on promotional literature to sell the Même, including numerous testimonials from plastic surgeons about the "excellent results" they were getting with the implant. The anecdotes were packaged in the form of information bulletins by Markham's daughter, Jacqueline, who had a master's degree in fine arts. In a September 1986 bulletin, she stated emphatically that "there is absolutely no theoretical or factual basis for concerns about cancer with our foam."

From 1987 until the implant was pulled from the market in April 1991, the right to manufacture the Même was sold twice: once to Cooper Surgical, part of the Cooper Companies, Inc., of New York, which primarily manufactures optical products, and then to Surgitek, a division of Bristol-Myers Squibb. In its grab for the implant market, Surgitek trumpeted the success of an Atlanta plastic surgeon, Dr. T. Roderick Hester, whose enthusiasm for the Même was such that he had implanted it in about twelve hundred women, almost doubling Sterling's mark. Like Sterling, Hester did not run a controlled study on his patients. But he did publish some data in *Perspectives in Plastic Surgery* in 1988, claiming that the Même was performing very well indeed; he was later forced to admit that his research was not carried out in a particularly rigorous manner. Meanwhile, he was paid a thousand dollars a crack on at least four occasions to speak at conferences on behalf of the Même; once, Surgitek paid his travel expenses to California so he could "explain clinical stuff" to company employees. "It's standard practice among surgeons to receive a small honorarium in exchange for their time," Hester says.

The FDA has long been empowered to require more rigorous studies on breast implants. The agency could easily have directed manufacturers to conduct detailed studies on every aspect of the Même, especially its foam cover. But again and again, over two decades, FDA officials bowed to the interests of plastic surgeons and manufacturers and turned their backs on the women who used breast implants.

In 1976, Congress passed amendments to the Federal Food, Drug, and Cosmetic Act, enabling the FDA to regulate the use of medical devices, including breast implants. But it wasn't until 1982 that the agency showed signs of making a move. With an eye on the lobbying by plastic surgeons, who were represented on its medical-device advisory panel, the FDA declined to take strong regulatory action. Instead, it only proposed that implants be placed in a category indicating that there was insufficient evidence to provide reasonable assurance of their safety and efficacy. It took another six years, during which time approximately half a million women received implants, for the FDA to notify manufacturers that they would be required to submit safety and efficacy data on their products for review. And it wasn't until last

April—another thirty months and approximately 330,000 implants after the notice—that the ruling was finalized.

According to investigations by the Human Resources and Inter-Governmental Relations Subcommittee, headed by Manhattan Democrat Ted Weiss, the concerns of FDA scientists about breast implants were blocked by higher-level agency officials for fifteen years. The FDA's press office says that the agency had more important regulatory priorities in mind, such as heart valves and AIDS drugs. But an independent federal report on the workings of the agency, conducted last May, places matters in much broader perspective. Various congressional assessments of the FDA also paint a picture of an agency severely cannibalized in the eighties by the Reagan administration's deregulatory philosophy and stingy funding, an agency that increasingly became more protective of business than of consumers. "FDA's inaction on breast implants was typical," says Weiss. "Unfortunately, the ruling philosophy has been 'Let the buyer beware!'"

It was only in late 1987, after several women had filed personal-injury suits against Natural-Y and more than ten thousand Mêmes had been put in, that someone at Cooper Surgical began to take notice of the incomplete information available on the Même's foam. In one court case, University of Florida biochemist Chris Batich testified that he had demonstrated how the foam could release cancer-causing TDA under harsh, chemical conditions. After reviewing that testimony, Tom Powell, a Cooper Surgical vice-president, called chemist Ed Griffiths, product manager at Scotfoam Corporation, the foam's manufacturer. Griffiths confirmed that the product could release at least a small amount of the chemical.

Griffiths had assumed that Cooper Surgical was using the foam for an industrial application. "My eyes popped out when Powell explained his company was buying the foam from a jobber in Los Angeles and using it as a covering for a breast implant," he recalls. "They had been using our foam for many years, and it was the first time that I or anyone else at the company had heard about it." Griffiths then advised Powell that Scotfoam didn't recommend such use in implants due to a lack of long-term data on the foam's suitability and health effects. "I wanted him to know that we had no expertise in determining the suitability of the foam in medical applications and that it was his—the end user's—responsibility."

Cooper Surgical apparently got the message, although there was no attempt to pull the Même from the market. In a series of letters exchanged between the two companies, dated from January 11, 1988, to August 3, 1988, the Même's manufacturer expressed the desire to conduct basic studies on the foam, which would characterize its chemical stability. To that end, Scotfoam provided Cooper Surgical with its formula and ingredient lists for the foam under an "absolute secrecy agreement."

By year's end, a new, eight-month animal study sponsored by Cooper Surgical had been concluded at the Veterans Administration Medical Center in Nashville, Tennessee. Its purpose was to determine what happened to miniature polyurethane-coated breast implants at the site of implantation in rats. In one test, pathologist Steven Woodward found that the foam size decreased at least 50 percent in two to eight months. Woodward concluded that the lost foam was strong evidence that the material broke down after implantation. "The logical extension was more detailed site studies and a look at the breakdown products [of the foam]," Woodward says now.

Cooper Surgical appeared interested in following up on Woodward's findings. Documents show that the company initiated studies in 1988 to examine the chemistry of the foam and its breakdown products. But in December of that year, Cooper Surgical sold the Même production plant to Surgitek, a subsidiary of Bristol-Myers Squibb—which decided not to fund the studies after all. Jonathan Weisberg, a spokesman for

Bristol-Myers, would later say that further studies weren't warranted. Instead, Weisberg pointed
to another study, one of ten explanted Mêmes,
that Bristol-Myers had sponsored, which
showed that the "lost" foam in Woodward's
study was simply entwined appropriately with
tissue. After reviewing that data, Woodward
would stick by his own study.

Besides facing giant holes in its scientific data
base on the Même, Surgitek was legally ordered
to clean up unsanitary conditions in its newly
acquired manufacturing plant. Several months
before the company acquired the Même, the
FDA, reacting to outside pressure, had launched
an inspection of the manufacturing facilities that
had been expanded from a garage.

Over a sixteen-day period, beginning on July
11, 1988, FDA agents turned up serious violations
of the Federal Food, Drug, and Cosmetic Act,
including deficiencies in the process that was
used to determine whether the implants were
sterile and the lack of an adequate quality-
assurance program. The company also had not
been training its employees properly. Some were
observed blowing into each breast-implant shell
for inflation during inflation testing. Inspectors
were unable to recover records both of the raw
materials used and the established specifications
for the implants. But they did find eleven
recorded cases of medical problems associated
with breast implants, including the Même,
which the company had never reported to the
FDA as required. The problems included infection, gel leakage, and separation of the foam covering from the shell. Between that inspection and
the closing of the plant three years later, about
120,000 additional women received the Même.

In June 1988, Sybil Niden Goldrich published a
short article about her experiences with breast
implants in *Ms.* magazine. She described how,
after her final reconstructive surgery, she was

determined to find out why she had been a
"breast-implant failure." Goldrich had called the
FDA for information on breast implants and was
informed that every plastic surgeon was provided with a concise manufacturer's warning listing potential complications from and caveats
about implants. It was up to the surgeon to
properly inform his patient about the pros and
cons. She then obtained samples of implant
package inserts and was floored by the list of
complications mentioned, including leakage of
gel, breast hardening, rupture of the implant's
shell, infection, blood clots, fluid accumulation,
skin decay, and loss of nipple sensation. "I naturally wondered, when I wrote the article, how
many other women were out there with breast
implants, who had not been advised of the
potential risks," she says.

Within weeks after her article was published,
Goldrich began receiving long-distance calls
from women around the country who had
thought they were alone with their breast-
implant problems. Almost all of the callers mentioned how little information about the dangers
of implants they had received from their doctors.
Then the FDA called. Faced with mounting consumer complaints about breast implants in general, the agency had scheduled a public meeting
of its medical-device advisory panel for November to help determine the types of safety and efficacy studies that manufacturers of breast implants would be required to submit for review.
Would Goldrich attend to present a consumer's
viewpoint?

By the time Goldrich arrived in Washington,
breast implants were hot news. Only days before
the meeting, the Washington-based Public Citizen Health Research Group released internal
data from Dow Corning, showing that injections
of silicone caused malignant tumors in over 23
percent of rats tested. The consumer group also
released evidence that FDA scientists were concerned about the manufacturer's experimental
findings and that at least one of the reviewers at
the agency wanted an alert to be issued immedi-

ately to the public, warning of the potential long-term cancer risk of breast implants. One internal FDA memo had stated: "While there is no direct proof that silicone causes cancers in humans, there is considerable reason to suspect that it can do so."

The FDA's advisory panel took note of the Dow Corning Corp.'s rat study during its deliberations and concluded that the available data did not warrant removal of breast implants from the market. But it did ask the FDA to establish a national information program on the devices so as to assure that patients received balanced information about the surgery. The recommendation pleased Goldrich, who had used up most of her allotted speaking time on that very subject.

Pierre Blais had realized that the Même's foam was actually intended for industrial use back in 1989 as part of his job at Canada's Health Protection Branch. After evaluating available data, Blais concluded there was a possibility that "women with the Même faced a double cancer threat, one from the silicone gel in the implant and another from its foam." In January of that year, he fired off a memo to David Johnson, a higher-level official, warning that the Même was "unfit for implantation," partly because its chemical products could be released in the body. In a four-page technical report, Blais termed the foam coating a "packaging and general-purpose foam." And he further questioned whether an expert on this type of material "would consider, recommend, or approve the use of such a foam on a device designed to be implanted permanently in a disease-prone area such as the female breast."

Johnson edited the documents, and Blais was ordered by his immediate boss to eliminate all references to his certainty that the Même was unfit. He complied, but wrote back in a memo, "In my opinion, the content of the original documents is significantly altered." Several days later, Blais was ordered to destroy his original memos and technical report on the Même. The follow-

ing July, Blais was fired for his insistence that the Même be withdrawn from the market—and for being the likely source of leaks to the media. He was eventually rehired after filing a wrongful-termination suit, but resigned in December 1989.

One month after his firing, Blais began work with a researcher at Laval University in Quebec City. The research verified under conditions more closely approximating those in the human body that the Même's foam could release TDA. "It was becoming pretty clear that this foam was unstable," he says. Blais reported his progress to scientists, who, after the FDA advisory panel met in December, conducted their own studies. That data, which confirmed Blais's research, was made public one week before Surgitek "voluntarily" withdrew the implant from the market. By that time a total of 200,000 women had the Même.

Bristol-Myers Squibb closed Surgitek's plastic-surgery unit last September, but that was not an admission of guilt. Surgitek said that its data on the safety and effectiveness of its other product line—silicone-gel breast implants without foam—was deemed insufficient by the FDA, and that, rather than appeal the decision, it was quitting the breast-implant business. In its announcement, Bristol-Myers Squibb said that it remained "committed to completing appropriate research to resolve all outstanding scientific issues" associated with the Même.

Nearly a decade after the implant's introduction, discovering exactly how much TDA is released by the Même's foam into the body has become a top research priority. Last June, the FDA ordered Surgitek to find out how much TDA might be in the blood, urine, and breast milk of women with the Même. But a dispute over methodology in the studies means that there will likely be a continuing controversy over the issue for years to come, no matter what the findings show.

The issue of how to quantify the Même's cancer risk is not likely to be settled very soon either.

Surgitek claims, on the basis of a recent study it sponsored, that, if there is a cancer risk associated with the Même, it is insignificant, certainly no worse than about one in several million. That would mean, at most, one woman would be affected. The FDA's official worst-case scenario is that the figure may be one in twelve thousand but is far more likely to be one in about a million—which would mean that between one and seventeen women with breast implants are in danger. On that basis, the agency is informing women with the Même that the risks associated with the removal of the implant are likely to be far greater than any cancer risk. But some FDA scientists, as well as Pierre Blais, argue that the cancer risk may actually be between one in 50 and one in 200. According to that estimate, between 1,000 and 4,000 women could contract cancer because of their implants.

"The FDA is taking absolutely the most conservative stance possible and is, for example, excluding from the risk analysis some early animal studies that show implanted foam similar to the one used in the Même is a strong chemical inducer of tumors," Blais says. "Unfortunately in this case, it appears that time will tell, and this is totally unacceptable. What a time to begin addressing the scientific issues! Thousands of women are waiting for more definitive answers."

Meanwhile, there is little sign that manufacturers or plastic surgeons feel remorseful about the current dilemma women face. Both Surgitek and Dow Corning insist that what's carcinogenic to rodents is not necessarily translatable to humans. Some doctors, like Hester and Sterling, blame the media for stirring things up: "I might not have implanted quite so many [Mêmes] had I known what I know now," Sterling says, "but I want you to know that my wife and daughters are still doing well." Hester admits that "the controversy will let us get more definitive about the TDA." Even so, he recently published an article that championed the idea of implanting two sets of Mêmes—he called it "stacking"—to achieve a better effect in certain patients.

As for the American Society of Plastic and Reconstructive Surgeons, the group that referred to small breasts as a disease, it recently voted to collect $1,050 from each of its thirty-seven hundred certified members to finance a campaign to counter bad news about silicone-gel breast implants. Garry Brody, a Los Angeles plastic surgeon and high-profile member of the group, hints at what lies ahead in the controversy when he says, "The whole process [of removing implants from the market] has destroyed the right [of women] to choose."

Back home in Los Angeles, Sybil Goldrich hopes she can answer that challenge. She is concerned that the four-million-dollar publicity campaign will convince consumer groups to rally around the principle of having access to breast implants—even if they are not proven safe and effective. At the FDA meeting that she attended recently in Washington, a number of women spoke angrily against the idea of removing all implants from the market. "The emotions were pretty high," she says, "especially from those women representing cancer groups." And she adds, "This is something that I understand, but I also don't believe that a breast-cancer patient would knowingly accept a product that might be defective." The FDA subsequently decided to allow breast implants to remain on the market at current availability levels, but will re-evaluate this decision after monitoring recipients for the next year.

Goldrich recently wrote a letter to Dr. David Kessler, the FDA commissioner, to say how wonderful it would have been if some of that vast amount of money being collected by the plastic surgeons had been designated for independent research to produce a safe and effective breast implant for women who have had breast-cancer surgery.

She also suggested to Kessler that whatever decision is made about the remaining breast implants on the market, it should be based on science and science alone.

The Ethics of Performance-Enhancing Drugs

WANDA TEAYS

IN THIS ARTICLE, I want to look at the use of performance-enhancing treatments and drugs in sports. It's one of those cases of truth being stranger than fiction. And it's an issue that affects all sports. Statistics reveal a widespread problem. Doctors writing in the *Journal of the AMA* report that more than 1 million elite and recreational athletes,[1] as well as an estimated 2 million non-athletes use performance-enhancing drugs. Data from the 23rd Olympic games in Los Angeles revealed that there was 1.7% positive test results on the drug testing of athletes.[2] It has been estimated that 50% of the 9000 athletes who competed in the 1988 Olympics used steroids at some time during their training[3] and 5–10% of female college athletes use steroids.[4]

The picture then is this: the use of steroids and other performance-enhancing drugs is NOT a minor problem. And with such incentives as awards, money, and fame, it's not a problem that is likely to go away. Rather, with the use of performance-enhancing drugs in epidemic proportions and the range of choices, including such things as anabolic steroids, human growth hormones, testosterone, EPO, blood doping, and surgery it's an issue that we need to examine. Look at some of recent cases where the issue of drugs arose:

1. American shot-putter Randy Barnes and sprinter Dennis Mitchell were both suspended indefinitely after testing positive for drugs.[5]

2. The U.S. Olympic Committee seeks to retroactively award or upgrade medals to American swimmers who lost to German swimmers in the 1960s and 1970s because of supposed steroid use by the East German team.[6]

3. Pro cyclists in the Tour de France were said to have undergone surgery to have their iliac artery enlarged to increase blood flow and some were taking a blood thickening drug, EPO (erythropoietin). Supposedly they then slept with heart-rate monitors to alert them if their pulse dropped below 25 beats a minute.[7] The Swiss Cycling Federation handed down eight-month bans to three cyclists who were expelled from the Tour de France in the summer of 1998 for using performance-enhancing drugs.[8]

4. In 1999 we saw the friendly competition of two ball players, Mark McGwire and Sammy Sosa, both said to be users of dietary supplement, creatine,[9] and McGwire a user of androstenedione, a precursor to testosterone banned by other professional sporting associations including the International Olympic Committee, but not professional baseball organizations.

Both McGwire and Sosa broke the record of most home-runs in a season set by Roger Maris in 1961. In setting the new record, Mark McGwire was the hero of the moment. Without knowing the role played by the supplements, it isn't clear whether he deserves to be celebrated for a job well done or publicly shamed. The question then is: Does the fact he took performance-enhancing drugs negate the accomplishment, even though he did nothing technically illegal? To answer that, we

WANDA TEAYS is Professor of Philosophy and Philosophy Department Chair at Mount St. Mary's College, Los Angeles.

need to decide how much weight to put on what is legally versus morally permissible. In other words, where do we draw lines around moral permissibility when it comes to performance-enhancing drugs? What I'd like us to look at is how to assign moral responsibility and accountability. There are two central concerns: the individual athlete and the enablers in the form of coaches, doctors, and team sponsors, and the society at large. Both have a role to play here.

In a recent survey of 195 top athletes, over 50% said they would take a prohibited performance-enhancing drug that would bring about their death from side effects if they could be assured of winning every competition for the next five years without being caught.[10] This brings to mind Faustian bargains where people sell their souls to the devil and attest to how powerful is the desire for victory.

International Olympic Committee vice president Anita DeFrantz recognized that Mark McGwire was able to stand there with balls coming at him at 90 or 100 miles an hour—and did not say his home-run record was tainted by the fact he used androstenedione. But she did raise concerns about the consequences for his health and his future. As she put it, "The scary part is we don't know what it does to you."[11]

Androstenedione, first synthesized around 1930 and, in the form of a nasal spray, was used as a performance-enhancing drug in the '70s and '80s in East Germany. There is some concern about the use of something that can temporarily triple normal testosterone levels.[12] Athletes like McGwire who consume performance-enhancing drugs could be seen as human subjects in one vast medical experiment. And unless we see athletes as disposable, this should alarm us. One issue this brings up is informed consent. Athletes who take performance-enhancing drugs are, presumably, willing. However, peer pressure, coaches, and competition play a coercive role, as we will examine shortly. But it is important for athletes to know what risks they are taking.

Graham Richardson, Director of the 2000 Sydney Olympic Organizing Committee, said of androstenedione, "There's not enough research being done on these drugs. . . . Athletes who take them are guinea pigs."[13] Journalists quite openly raise these concerns. For instance, Angella Issajenko, who took Human Growth Hormone, steroids, and testosterone, was called a "drug guinea pig for the Mazda track group."[14]

Lamenting McGwire's use of androstenedione and creatine, Professor Charles Yesalis, author of *The Steroids Game,* worried about kids rushing out to buy it. As he put it, this is not like taking vitamin C. The impact on others should not go unnoticed. In fact, "since home-run king Mark McGwire admitted to using androstenedione [in the summer of 1998] andro use among kids has soared fivefold."[15]

Unfortunately, few independent studies have been done on androstenedione. It is thought that the side effects would mirror those of testosterone.[16] It is generally regarded that steroids are not benign. In the short term they cause acne, cause the liver to function abnormally, affect cholesterol patterns, affect sperm production, increase aggressiveness, masculinize women and, have potentially long-term effects; such as possible links to liver tumors and potential harm to the endocrine system. It is worse for adolescents; e.g., both males and females could become permanently sterile.[17]

As for creatine: Dr. Jeffrey Diaz, member of the Major League Baseball's health advisory group, said, "No one knows what it is, what it can do, what it can't do. It's often represented as something that has been tested, but it's not been tested and it's not consistent." In July 1998, the FDA warned consumers to consult a doctor before taking creatine, and is investigating whether a link exists between creatine and the development of seizures and brain tumours."[18] EPO has its risks too. As reported in 1997, internationally 18 cyclists have died and there have been several deaths in other sports that may have been caused by EPO,[19] called the Tour de France drug of choice. EPO has also been used in distance running, Nordic skiing, and tennis.

Then there are stimulants such as amphetamines, which are said to provide a rush of energy and are used by sprinters, cyclists, and swimmers. Sixty percent of the US Olympic team in 1994 supposedly had asthma, necessitating the use of asthma medications containing amphetamines.[20] Speaking to the Assembly of the American Academy of Family Physicians on the use of amphetamines in high school students, Dr. Joseph Snyder warned of their possible side effects. These include high blood pressure, heart attacks, and strokes.[21] Human growth hormones also raise concerns; for instance it was noted in the *British Medical Journal* that some growth hormone preparations may be associated with Creutzfeldt-Jakob (alias mad-cow) disease.[22]

In other words, those who use performance-enhancing drugs are basically human subjects at unclear risk. Whatever the potential fame and glory, it is at a cost. As Dr. Snyder affirmed, the use of performance-enhancing drugs is a threat to an athlete's health. IOC president Juan Antonio Samaranch announced plans to set up a special agency to coordinate drug testing. In his view: "As for performance-enhancing drugs, there is not a single one that is not harming the health of the athletes." He estimated that the Olympic movement currently spends $20 million on drug testing.[23]

We cheer the Rocky's of the world who overcome obstacles to achieve greatness. But we expect this success is achieved honestly, without resorting to duplicitous means. Granted Mark McGwire did not attempt to hide his use of performance-enhancing drugs. However, he is said to have accused the Associated Press reporter who wrote of his use of androstenedione of "snooping."[24]

Questions arise: Is there a problem in using any supplement that is solely intended to enhance performance and otherwise has no medical benefit? Is there a problem in using drugs that are not banned in the sport in question but are banned in other fields? Does this damage the athlete's integrity? Are *any* supplements acceptable when the difference between the one in first place and those in second, third, and fourth may be computed in fractions of seconds (as, e.g., in sprinting, swimming, bicycling)? What is the honest athlete to do?

If we permit the addition of drugs and dietary supplements, we fundamentally change the way we look at the sport itself. That's at the heart of the issue here. And this goes beyond health risks. It goes to issues of individual integrity and the moral fabric of our society. Part of the problem with considering certain drugs permissible while others are not is that we find ourselves on a morally slippery slope.

Consider the possible analogy of memory-enhancing drugs. Suppose we said buying a paper from someone is unacceptable, but peering over at a fellow student's paper is not. Suppose I could buy a drug or herbal remedy that allowed me to memorize 20 pages at a time and hold it in my mind for a few hours, or a few days, before it would fade away. We might say the person on memory-enhancing drugs is getting the answers by herself; whereas the one who looks at a neighbor or bought the test and memorized the answers is clearly a cheater. But there's still something disturbing at work here.

One of the issues in assessing integrity is not just looking at short-term gains but long-term consequences. Who would you consider the more learned of these two candidates: Bob, who took a memory-enhancing drug that allows him to memorize chapters and retain it for two hours or two days — (long enough to be tested and answer questions in great detail and get a 95% on the test), or Betty, who didn't use any drugs and got 88% on the test? Who would you rather hire? You might prefer Bob if you planned to enter him in memory competitions; but this might be exploitative, especially if these drugs have negative side effects.

A Utilitarian, or anyone else looking at the short term, might argue for using Bob anyway, so long as they can maximize benefits over risks —especially if Bob was a willing participant. As suggested in an article on ethical issues raised by cognitive-enhancers, "we might want to allow enhanced individuals to benefit personally so that society can obtain the accompanying benefit."[25]

But this points to the consequence for Bob and presumably for athletes who use performance-enhancing drugs. This is that such individuals are being sacrificed—or are sacrificing themselves—for the good of the team, the company, or the society. The big winners here are not those using the various methods of enhancing performance but those who *use* the athletes for their own profit. Even if they compensate them handsomely, they let them go when they no longer function and ready replacements are available. Loyalty and gratitude don't seem to be a factor here. In this regard the winners are not the athletes—but the owners, stockholders, and advertisers who sell products around teams and players. We might, nevertheless, argue that the athletes freely chose what path to take. This brings up the issue of liberty.

There are two major concerns regarding the ethical basis for testing performance drugs according to Don Catlin and Thomas Murray in an article in *JAMA*.[26] One is that efforts to limit their use are paternalistic and an infringement on liberty. The other is that it is impossible to distinguish acceptable versus unacceptable forms of enhancement, which seems more a matter of quality control than ethics.

Let us then look at paternalism versus liberty. Paternalism basically involves making decisions for someone else without their consent, but presumably with their best interests in mind. As a society, we favor liberty and regard risks as something a competent adult can assess and then make up their own minds. Most sports have risks anyway and some are inherently risky (such as downhill skiing, luge, diving, and football). However, decision making doesn't take place in a vacuum. If athletes

discover their competitors are using performance-enhancing drugs, they may feel compelled to do so as well in order to level the playing field.[27]

Commentators struggle to find an analogy to performance-enhancing drugs. One potential analogy is that they are like an athlete entering the Boston Marathon wearing roller skates. The wheels provide such a massive competitive advantage that they alter the meaning of the sport as a foot race.[28] One difference, of course, is that the runner on roller skates is obvious, whereas the sprinter on steroids or the baseball player on creatine and androstenedione, has an advantage not nearly as easy to detect.

Another possible analogy is the use of breast implants, since those were introduced without any testing on human subjects. A closer one might be the case of the Japanese prostitutes who injected their breasts with liquid silicon in World War II because American men liked big breasts— or the breast implant, La Même, that was covered with upholstery foam. Even then, the issue with implants centers on appearance, rather than performance. However, a better analogy to performance-enhancing drugs might be in comparing the human and the cyborg in the movies *Terminator* and *T2: Judgment Day*. There the cyborg moved in human society without being detected except by dogs (who barked at them). The cyborg, alias the Terminator, had vastly superior strength to humans. In fact, the only advantage humans had was their creativity. By their own imagination, they could, hopefully, outsmart the cyborg long enough to terminate HIM.

Unfortunately, quick wits don't usually counter the newfound abilities of those using performance-enhancing drugs. The drug user has a decided advantage. Because of this, an unscrupulous athlete or one who is ethically challenged may be tempted to try performance-enhancing drugs also. This is particularly if the constraints were minimal and the risks minor. Of course, the issue of constraints deserves to be looked at, as well as risks. The most powerful constraints are the following:

- **a sense of honor, or the Authenticity Principle.** By this we have an inherent sense of integrity having its own reward and, thus, we are honest as a matter of duty.

- **a sense of fairness, or the Justice Principle.** By this we have a sense of what is just and unjust in our relations with others and strive to achieve justice and fairness and avoid injustice.

- **a sense of fear of legal repercussions, or the Deterrence Principle.** By this we see the punitive side of the law as a kind of cattle prod, by which we avoid the illegal behavior, regardless of any sense of this being related to doing the right thing.

- **a sense of individual pride and standards, or the Excellence Principle.** By this we are guided by our own individual notion of what the excellent athlete would do, regardless of others falling far from this goal or anyone else either noticing or caring.

- **a sense of community and teamwork, or the Loyalty Principle.** By this we strive to be a good team player, to do what is right so we not let others down and disappoint our community, our team, our buddies.

- **a sense of personal legacy, or the Role Model Principle.** By this we look at our own behavior in terms of its effect on others and particularly upon those, like children, who may look up to us as a model of what to do and what is right.

Any one of these six constraints may be powerful enough to keep an athlete away from performance-enhancing drugs. Of course, we, as a society, provide the groundwork, ethical guidance, and support for individual athletes who face decisions around whether or not to seek shortcuts to success. If we applaud those who refuse to succumb to drug use, we send a clear message. If, however, we celebrate as heroes those who make it by using such tricks of the trade as performance-enhancing drugs, then we give another message.

Ours is a society that elevates athletes to hero status and employs such terms as "superathlete" for those who have earned the recognition and an entry into the big money sweepstakes of sports competitions. If performance-enhancing drugs helped an athlete become a better person or contribute to the well-being of others—as for instance could possibly be the case with cognitive-enhancing drugs—we might not only see them as morally permissible, but as desirable. They could win first place, a medal, money, or fame for themselves or for the team. But little else. And note that the "advantage" disappears if all competitors were similarly drugged.

On the other hand, it may be very hard to draw the line between what is acceptable and what is not. For example, should it be an offense to take androstenedione in football, but not in baseball? Are those who take anabolic steroids or EPO more culpable than those on androstenedione? And are athletes using androstenedione more morally repugnant than those taking creatine?

Supposedly both Mark McGwire and Sammy Sosa took creatine—does that mean they are both morally reprehensible for doing so? Or is McGwire more morally culpable than Sosa since he also took androstenedione? Or should the line be drawn further, so neither is thought guilty of any transgression, since no legal boundary was crossed?

Well, let us try a more Libertine approach. What if we try a variation of what John Robertson calls "procreative liberty"[29] as a justification of surrogate parenting. By this view, procreation, even with the use of third parties, is thought to be constitutionally protected, a kind of privacy right. Maybe it should be argued that athletes also have rights to privacy that allow the use of performance-enhancing drugs. This is the view of Toronto journalist, Peter Worthington, who lamented what he called "the Orwellian ethics people who sit inquisitorially in judgment of others."[30]

At issue is whether athletes have the right of self-determination—so that they are free to decide what they do to their own bodies. Athletes could then be said to have the right of what we will call "performance liberty." It would be a personal decision whether to take performance-enhancing drugs, so long as they voluntarily consent and are properly informed of the risks and benefits.

John Stuart Mill addressed individual liberty. As he put it, "The only purpose for which power can be rightfully exercised over any member of a civilized community, against his will, is to prevent harm to others. His own good, either physical or moral, is not a sufficient warrant. He cannot rightfully be compelled to do or forbear because it will be better for him to do so, because it will make him happier, because, in the opinions of others, to do so would be wise, or even right."[31]

Over oneself, over one's own body and mind, the individual is sovereign, Mill asserts. For Mill, then, if the athlete wants to self-destruct with performance-enhancing drugs, then he or she should have the right to do so, especially if this contributes to the happiness or good of the general public and no one else is harmed. Mill would, therefore, likely agree with IOC president Juan Antonio Samaranch's call for the legalization of performance-enhancing drugs, so long as they don't damage an athlete's health. However, as Mill notes above, liberty is not an absolute. It is bounded by non-maleficence (the duty not to harm others). So when an athlete's behavior harms others, then the society has both the right and the duty to intervene. Our question here is whether others are harmed by those who use performance-enhancing drugs and whether others are harmed when an athlete takes drugs or supplements, whether or not the athlete personally suffers.

Is it a harm to lose the pennant, come in second or third in a sports competition, win the silver and not the gold at the Olympics because the winners are using drugs? Is the society itself harmed by athletes who do drugs, blood doping, or surgical interventions?

It could be said that we are all harmed by any acts of dishonesty that are not justified for some greater good, such as to prevent serious harm to others. Sir Arthur Gold, former head of the British Olympic Association, suggests there are societal harms from any drug use. Gold called Samaranch's remarks unwise. He said, "To use drugs is to cheat whether they damage your health or not."[32]

But surely this is one of the problems. Athletes employing performance-enhancing drugs are not always cognizant of the risks they are taking for the sole potential benefit of sharpening their competitive edge. Moreover, we might wonder whether it is voluntary, when coaches, doctors, and fellow teammates pressure them to use drugs and over-the-counter supplements. All the enablers bear responsibility too. For example, Willy Voet, the physiotherapist of the French Festina cycling team in the Tour de France, was quoted as saying the team doctor, Eric Ryckaert, injected riders with banned drugs.[33]

Another example comes from football: former NFL player Walter Sweeney filed an action in 1999 alleging that he and his teammates were urged to take anabolic steroids in his first year with the San Diego Chargers. Sweeney says that if they didn't take the drugs, they were fined a game check (approximately fifty dollars). Moreover, trainers and coaches made amphetamines available to the players by placing them in lockers and training kits, Sweeney claims. He says that, when he was traded to the Washington Redskins, coach George Allen once told the team, "If it takes amphetamines to win, I will bring it in by the truckload."[34]

Of course there's always the option of turning a blind eye or even legalizing performance-enhancing drugs. One worry, though, is that athletes might be expected to use them for that competitive edge. Plus, either ignoring or legalizing their use would imply that the health risks and moral costs are minimal.

So the circle of moral accountability seems to widen. Athletes aren't the only ones lured by the smell of victory at any cost; it has been recognized that strategies to evade bans and drug-testing programs fuel a growth industry. Writing in the *New Statesman*, Matt Barnard said that the former Soviet states poured money into developing performance-enhancing drugs "using the athlete as guinea pig—the individual as the servant of the collective."[35] He compares athletes to test pilots, who take high risks and sometimes get injured or killed; but without any safety checks. He goes further to suggest that sport sponsors covertly encourage drug use on the part of athletes but abandon and condemn them if they are caught.

There are a number of issues and concerns here. They include questions about the athletes themselves and how we judge them in terms of morality. There are questions about professional sports in general—and what sorts of standards should be set down and upheld. There are questions about physicians and coaches and what sorts of ethical guidelines they should be expected to follow in their handling of athletes. And what we do as a society to encourage or discourage the use of performance-enhancing drugs.

What standards should doctors and coaches be held to? Surely they have a professional obligation and moral duty to do no harm, as set down by the Hippocratic Oath. We might see that there are also moral duties, such as honesty, justice, doing no harm, and acting as a role model for others. There are issues for enablers with all of these duties. As well, the Nuremberg Code can be seen to have relevance here, given the experimental nature of some of the drugs and treatments being used by athletes. The Nuremberg Code not only demands previous animal studies but requires that the benefits to the society must never be put above the risks to the individual human subject.

It could hardly be argued that performance-enhancing drugs are risk-free. Doctors and coaches who participate in or condone their use

should also be held accountable. We need to do more than punish athletes whenever others are involved in the use and access to performance-enhancing drugs by athletes. As a *New York Times* journalist speculated, "We're giving McGwire standing ovations, but I wonder what we're celebrating: the work of a hero or the spectacle of a hero fashioning his own destruction—for our pleasure."[36]

NOTES

1. Josiah D. Rich et al., "Insulin Use by Body-builders," (letter) to the *Journal of the American Medical Association*, Vol. 279 (20), 27 May 1998, p. 1613.

2. See Domhnall MacAuley, "Fortnightly Review: Drugs in Sport," *British Medical Journal*, Vol. 313, 27 July 96, pp. 211.

3. See Michael P. Milton, "Should Drug and Alcohol Addictions Be Compensable Disabilities under the NFL Player Retirement Plan? An Analysis of the Sweeney Case," *Sports Lawyers Journal*, Spring 1998.

4. As noted by Mike Fish, "Women in Sports: Growing Pains," *The Atlanta Journal Constitution*, 23 Sept 98, sec. D, p. 9.

5. See Nick Thorpe, "Olympics Chief's Call to 'Go Soft' on Drugs Attacked," *The Scotsman*, 28 July 98.

6. See John Jeansonne, "My Turn/USOC Makes Waves for Naught," *Newsday*, 1 Nov 98.

7. See Duncan McKay, "Joyner Hopes Autopsy Ends Frenzy on Flo-Jo," *The Irish Times*, 24 Oct 98.

8. See Associated Press, "Plus Cycling: Federation Bans and Fines 3 Riders," *The Lancet*, 1 Oct 98.

9. See Deborah Josefson, "Concern Raised about Performance Enhancing Drugs in the US," *British Medical Journal*, Vol. 317, 12 Sep 98, p. 702.

10. See Janet Goshu and Ann Endo, "To Your Health/Steering Away from Steroids," *The Daily Yomiuri (Tokyo)*, 17 Oct 98.

11. See Mike Dodd, "McGwire's Use of 'Andro' Concerns IOC," *USA Today*, 15 Sep 98.

12. See "The Drug in the Controversy," *The New York Times*, 31 Aug 98, sec. C, p. 4.

13. See Janice Lloyd, "Officials Campaign Against Use of 'Andro'," *USA Today*, 17 Sep 98.

14. See Steve Buffery, "Issajenko Living in Denial Over Effects of Drugs?" *The Toronto Sun*, 2 Oct 98.

15. Sharon Begley and Martha Brant, "The Real Scandal," *Newsweek*, 13 Feb 99, p. 48.

16. See Deborah Josefson, "Concern Raised about Performance Enhancing Drugs in the US," *British Medical Journal*, Vol. 317, 12 Sep 98, p. 702.

17. See Janet Goshu and Ann Endo, "To Your Health/Steering Away from Steroids," *The Daily Yomiuri (Tokyo)*, 17 Oct 98.

18. See Deborah Josefson, "Concern Raised About Performance Enhancing Drugs in the US," *British Medical Journal*, Vol. 317, 12 Sep 98.

19. See Karen Birchard, "Ireland to Pioneer Compulsory Drug Testing for Athletes," *The Lancet*, 26 July 97. See *supra* note 25.

20. As noted by Sharon Begley and Martha Brant, "The Real Scandal," *Newsweek*, 15 Feb 99, p. 48.

21. See E.J. Mundell, "Performance Drugs Problem in Teen Athletes," *Kids Health at the AMA*.

22. Domhnall MacAuley, "Fortnightly Review: Drugs in Sport," *British Medical Journal*, Vol. 313, 27 July 96, p. 213.

23. See "IOC Seeks to Form Anti-Doping Agency: Summer's Drug Scandals Result in Bold Move," *The Montreal Gazette*, 21 Aug 98.

24. See William C. Rhoden, "Baseball's Pandora's Box Cracks Open," *New York Times*, 25 Aug 98.

25. Peter Whitehorse, et al, "Enhancing Cognition in the Intellectually Intact," *The Hastings Center Report*, vol. 27, no. 3 (1997), p. 14.

26. Don H. Catlin and Thomas H. Murray, "Performance-Enhancing Drugs, Fair Competition, and Olympic Sport," *Journal of the American Medical Association*, Vol. 276 (3), 17 July 96, pp. 231–237.

27. Ibid.

28. See Peter Whitehorse et al., "Enhancing Cognition in the Intellectually Intact." See *supra* note 25.

29. For instance, see John A. Robertson, *Children of Choice: Freedom and the New Reproductive Technologies* (Princeton, NJ: Princeton University Press, 1994).

30. Peter Worthington, "When Willing is the Only Thing—Mark McGwire and the Steroid Controversy, Is he a Hero or a Bum?", *The Toronto Star*, 1 Sep 98.

31. From *On Liberty*, as quoted by Thomas A. Mappes and Jane S. Zembaty (eds.), *Biomedical Ethics* 3rd edition, (New York: McGraw-Hill, Inc., 1991), p. 33.

32. See "IOC Head's Drug Comments Draw Angry Reaction," Associated Press, 1 Nov 98—espn.sportszone.com.

33. See "Virenque Accused of Taking Drugs," *The Irish Times*, 24 Sep 98.

34. See Michael P. Milton, "Should Drug and Alcohol Addictions Be Compensable Disabilities Under the NFL Player Retirement Plan? An Analysis of the Sweeney Case," *Sports Lawyers Journal*, Spring 98, p. 206.

35. See Matt Barnard, "Drugs and Darwin Fuel Athletes; Performance-Enhancing Drugs Usage in Sports," *New Statesman*, 25 Sep 98.

36. See William C. Rhoden, "Baseball's Pandora's Box Cracks Open," *New York Times*, 25 Aug 98.

"Decoding" Informed Consent: Insights from Women Regarding Breast Cancer Susceptibility Testing

GAIL GELLER, MISHA STRAUSS, BARBARA A. BERNHARDT, and NEIL A. HOLTZMAN

THE PROLIFERATION OF TESTS for genetic predisposition to common but complex adult-onset diseases such as cancer provides us with an opportunity to reconsider informed consent. . . . Our own research on women's reactions to the availability of genetic susceptibility testing for breast cancer dramatically underscores that informed consent ought to be individualized based on patient beliefs and preferences, and take place in the context of an ongoing relationship with a trusted health care provider. . . . Although our focus is on informed consent for breast cancer susceptibility testing, our analysis has broader applicability. . . . Two essential goals of informed consent include assuring that patients have substantial understanding and assuring that their decisions to accept or reject interventions are substantially voluntary.[1]

How patients understand factual information is contingent upon their background assumptions and personal history. People tend to incorporate information into a framework of pre-existing knowledge and beliefs. . . . To achieve intelligibility, we tend to interpret new information in such a way as to preserve the coherence of our be-

GAIL GELLER is Associate Professor in the Department of Pediatrics, with primary affiliations in Genetics and Public Policy Studies; she has a joint appointment in the Dept of Public Health Policy and Management; Johns Hopkins University.

liefs . . . First, patients may come to an encounter with an idiosyncratic, if not incorrect, understanding of facts, even before the provider has a chance to disclose any new information. . . . This reasoning also highlights the danger in assuming that disclosure of factual information alone ensures understanding. Second, some patients report fatalistic or superstitious beliefs about the likelihood of developing cancer. Such beliefs may reflect the degree to which people feel that they have control over their lives. For example, fatalists believe the diseases that befall them, and the timing and manner of their death, are foreordained. Therefore, the individual has no control over whether he or she will develop cancer.

By contrast, some people believe that their thoughts and behaviors directly influence what happens to them: talking about bad things such as cancer might precipitate their onset.[2] . . . Third, patients receiving risk information will potentially latch on to anecdotes, personal experience, and fears more readily than to general facts and statistics, often causing them to distort their own risk. . . . Furthermore, stories and experiences of other individuals, such as family members, close friends, coworkers, or neighbors, are likely to resonate very deeply with listeners. For example, one woman in our focus groups, whose mother died of breast cancer at an early age, said, "I have breasts, anyone with breasts can get breast cancer, and if I get breast

The Hastings Center Report (March/Apr 1997): 28–33. Reprinted by permission of Gail Geller and The Hastings Center. Copyright, 1997 The Hastings Center.

cancer I will die." This woman is planning to have a prophylactic mastectomy no matter what her genetic test shows. . . .

Because patient decision-making is influenced by one's personal exposure to a disease, providers must be able to distinguish between what they think reflects rational decision-making and that which is material to the patient.[3] . . . Although the participants indicated a preference for recommendations rather than orders from their physician, some wanted to hear a single recommended course of action, while others wanted to hear all the options. Choice is considered important in both cases . . . choice lies in hearing the physician's recommendation and deciding whether to follow it; whereas to others, a choice means hearing all the options and deciding for yourself which of them to follow. Those who only want unambiguous guidance are likely to express frustration with physicians who do not provide any recommendation. Since the physician is perceived as the medical expert, such patients are likely to complain either that the physician is not fulfilling her duty or that the patient is not getting her money's worth.

Often, when this kind of patient wants her physician to play an advisory role, she wants to hear recommendations based on the physician's experience with other patients who have faced similar situations. In addition to the technical knowledge that physicians can provide, patients value their physician's input because the physician presumably has encountered this problem before, can speak from experience about different choices other patients have made, and can describe actual outcomes of different options. . . . Lauritzen says that "to offer your experience as your truth is not to claim that you have the Truth with a capital T. It is a starting point, an invitation to conversation."[4] . . . Providers ought to be genuine patient advocates. Such advocacy can take the form of expressing an interest in the patient's personal life. . . . Providers can potentially abuse patient trust in order to get patients to do what they want them to do. Ideally, the in-

formed consent process should function to check the physician's influence on patient decision-making. However, there is evidence in the research context that patient-subjects are more likely to be influenced by the trust they have in their physicians than by what is disclosed during informed consent.[5]

This suggests that we need to explore carefully how physicians can promote patient trust in a way that ensures rather than "hinder[s] adequate fulfillment of the informed consent process." Development of patient trust does not entitle physicians to assume the role of parents and treat patients like dependent children, as traditional professional notions of trust imply.[6] . . . [T]he evolution of trust challenges providers to engage in the more difficult task of learning to trust themselves to "face up to and acknowledge the . . . limitations of their own professional knowledge; their inability to impart all their insights to patients; and their own personal incapacities . . . to devote themselves fully to their patients' needs." . . .

Despite our agreement with the fundamental importance of the elements of understanding and voluntariness to any adequate model of informed consent, evidence of incongruence between consumer and provider expectations[7] raises the question whether our current conceptualization of these elements is adequate. Can the informed consent process ensure fair and ethical decision-making regarding cancer susceptibility testing in particular and other situations in which benefits do not clearly outweigh risks? The technological capacity to conduct predisposition testing, the decision-making preferences expressed by the women in our focus groups, and the realities of the current health care delivery system challenge the implementation of the informed consent process as we ideally envision it. . . . [I]f decision-making regarding genetic testing for breast cancer risk is to maximize understanding and voluntariness, it must involve an in-depth exploration by providers of patients' affective and cognitive processes.

We also saw the important ways in which a trusting, ongoing relationship with a provider who seeks to meet the patient's expectations would facilitate decision-making. Providers who rely on a discrete or short-term approach to informed consent are unlikely to succeed at understanding fundamental patient beliefs and preferences and thereby have little hope of obtaining truly informed consent. Therefore, two major challenges for the informed consent process during both its disclosure (education) and decision-making (counseling) components, are encouraging providers to learn what patients understand and believe about genetics and risk of disease, and ensuring that they consider patients' wishes with regard to the role they want to play in decision-making. . . .

If one of the primary objectives in the consent process must be an attempt, on the part of providers, to understand patients' concerns, values, and (mis)perceptions, this should include a recognition of the degree to which their own beliefs support or conflict with those of their patients. In addition, our research urges that providers develop a reasonably sophisticated understanding of patient beliefs as well, if they are to fulfill their professional obligations. When confronted with inconsistent beliefs, providers typically do not have enough information about the patient to understand what is motivating those beliefs. Consequently, providers are likely to miss important explanations for the decisions patients make.

For example, the woman who receives a negative test result and still wants a prophylactic mastectomy might seem irrational to a provider. Without background information about her mother's death and its impact on the patient's own sense of mortality, her provider would think that her decision reflects an incorrect understanding of genetic risk information rather than a different perception of risk or a different set of values and priorities. . . . Providers who acknowledge to their patients, and to themselves, that they are interested in information that pa-

tients can provide are likely to engender trust in the patient.

Second, by listening to patients, providers would receive guidance as to how their end of the conversation should proceed. In some cases, providers might attempt to correct patients' misperceptions, such as inflated views of their risk of disease, or misunderstandings about the risk factors or causes of disease. For example, a woman who believes that her sister developed breast cancer because she "resembles her mother's side of the family" might incorrectly conclude that she herself is at low risk for breast cancer because she resembles her father's side. In the case of such misunderstanding, it is morally defensible, indeed obligatory, for providers to correct the false beliefs as long as they do so with sensitivity. Providers who understand the basis for such perceptions are less likely to respond in a condescending fashion and more likely to facilitate an accurate assessment of risk for the patient and her relatives. In the process, patients will become better educated but will be spared from feeling either like receptacles of objective facts that have little or no meaning in their lives, or patronized and misunderstood by their providers. . . .

Concerns about autonomy should be broadened from a sole focus on the voluntariness of the decision itself to include a focus on the voluntariness of the decision-making process. That is, in addition to learning about patients' values and beliefs, providers ought to explore what kind of role expectations the patient has for herself and her provider. . . . We are not recommending that patients relinquish the decision to the doctor. Instead, we are suggesting that patients who are able to play their preferred role in decision-making are, in this way, exercising their autonomy. . . .

In cases where the benefits of genetic susceptibility testing do not clearly outweigh the risks, as is true for breast cancer,[8] providers should be very careful in distinguishing between advice intended to correct factual misunderstanding and advice aimed at modifying patient values that are discordant with those of the provider. The rationale for this caution is the likelihood of discordance between patient's and provider's values, particularly regarding perception of and comfort with risk. When such values differ enough to affect the way each would make a decision, giving advice could prevent patients from making decisions that are consistent with their own values and thereby compromise autonomy. . . .

Consistent with concerns about abandonment, most of the women we studied argued for their provider's assistance with decision-making, as long as they have the right to "veto" the recommendation. They seemed to view the withholding of recommendations as an obstacle to autonomous decision-making, not as a means of promoting it. . . . With such respect, patients are more likely to exercise their right to "veto" the provider's recommendation when it differs from their own preferences. . . .

[T]he informed consent process obliges providers to learn what patients understand, believe, and desire from the encounter, both in terms of content and of decision-making preferences. An attempt should be made to offer education and counseling that solicits patients' beliefs about risk, corrects their misunderstandings, and accounts for the likelihood that patient's views and desires change over time and according to circumstances. . . . The decision-making part of the informed consent process should reflect patients' wishes with regard to the role they want to play at that time, and include the provision of provider recommendations if requested by the patient.

Patients who can exercise some control over the process of decision-making are more likely to feel that they have control over the decision itself.

Whether patients follow their provider's advice or veto it, they will be asserting their freedom to make the decision in a way that is best for them, and trusting that their provider will continue to function in the patient's best interests. . . . The informed consent process must be afforded the time to foster a full appreciation of the dynamic nature of patient preferences, and the unique implications of an individual's values and beliefs for his or her autonomous decision-making.

REFERENCES

1. Ruth R. Faden and Tom L. Beauchamp in collaboration with Nancy M. P. King, *A History and Theory of Informed Consent* (New York: Oxford University Press, 1986), p. 238.

2. Joseph Carrese and Loma A. Rhodes, "Western Bioethics on the Navajo Reservation: Benefit or Harm?" *JAMA* 274 (1995): 826–29.

3. Gail Geller and Nancy E. Kass, "Informed Consent in the Context of Prenatal HIV Screening," in *AIDS, Women and the Next Generation: Toward A Morally Acceptable Public Policy on HIV Screening of Pregnant Women and Newborns,* ed. Ruth R. Faden, Gail Geller, and G. Madison Powers (New York: Oxford University Press, 1991).

4. Paul Lauritzen, "Ethics and Experience: The Case of the Curious Response," *Hastings Center Report* 26, no. 1 (1996): 615, at 6.

5. Nancy E. Kass et al., "Trust: The Fragile Foundation of Contemporary Biomedical Research," *Hastings Center Report* 26, no. 5 (1996): 25–29.

6. Jay Katz, *The Silent World of Doctor and Patient* (New York: The Free Press, 1984), pp. 101–103.

7. Myers et al., "Involving Consumers"; Richard M. Allman, William C. Yoels, and Jeffrey M. Clair, "Reconciling the Agendas of Physicians and Patients," in *Sociomedical Perspectives on Patient Care,* ed. J. M. Clair and R. M. Allman (Lexington, Ky.: University Press of Kentucky, 1993), 29–46, at 33.

8. Francis S. Collins, "BRCA1-Lots of Mutations, Lots of Dilemmas," *NEJM* 334 (1996): 186–88.

The Body as Property

The Body Bazaar:
The Market in Human Organs Is Growing

KAREN WRIGHT

BLOOD, KIDNEYS, EGGS, SPERM—name a body part, there's a price on it. Think of it as a commodities market for the twenty-first century. There's a bank in central Boston that offers its customers a unique investment opportunity. For an initial outlay of $1,500 and yearly fees of $95, investors can realize returns of incalculable value —or, more often, no returns at all. Unlike most business deals, this one involves the extraction of blood. But participants in the Boston scheme give up the blood willingly, because blood is the very substance of their investment.

The institution in question is Viacord, the nation's largest commercial banker of blood from fetal umbilical cords. In recent years cord blood has become something of a hot commodity, as medical research has demonstrated its potential for treating leukemia and certain immune disorders. A few tablespoons of the blood can be drawn quickly and painlessly from a baby's umbilical cord right after delivery and frozen for future use. Because it is rich in the so-called stem cells that give rise to all other blood cells, cord blood can be used to reconstitute immune systems damaged by disease or radiation treatments. Although nonprofit centers have begun banking donated cord blood, private bankers like Viacord can guarantee customers—that is, expectant parents—future access to their own baby's blood, thereby increasing the likelihood of a match should the child or a relative someday need to restore a crippled immune system.

Viacord takes custody of the samples at Hoxworth Blood Center, a part of the University of Cincinnati Medical Center that has been contracted to process and store the cord blood. Small plastic packets of whole blood in containers arrive by courier from hospitals all over the country 24 hours a day, seven days a week. More than 1,400 samples of cord blood are stowed in cylindrical liquid-nitrogen freezers set at −320.8 degrees. The frozen blood could represent roughly $2 million in revenue for Viacord. But no one knows what cord blood will be worth to the families who have paid to keep it. Viacord's president and founder, Cynthia Fisher, calls cord-blood banking a kind of insurance. Critics say that it is an attempt to capitalize on parents' worst fears.

Cord-blood banking is just one of many enterprises that make up the late-twentieth-century trade in body parts and products. Advances in medical technology have created a marketplace for everything from organs and tissues to genes and sex cells. Prices vary: $300 for a pint of plasma (the fluid in which blood cells are suspended), $50 for a sample of sperm, $10,000 for a nine-month lease on a surrogate mother's womb. In this country, organs cannot be sold for transplant, but the charges surrounding a donated organ can turn into tens of thousands of dollars. It costs about $20,000, for example, to remove and transport a donor kidney. This commerce is conspicuous and unapologetic. But other companies—such as those that sell parts of aborted fetuses to medical researchers—prefer to keep the nature of their trade and the size of their profits to themselves.

Blood was the first commodity on the market, and it is still the most commonly sold body product. . . . As blood banks were established across the country, two competing models soon emerged: commercial suppliers, which pay blood donors, and nonprofit collection centers, which depend on volunteers to donate blood. The two ended up splitting the market. Today the vast majority of transfusions are done with donated blood, while commercial centers provide almost all of the blood used by the pharmaceutical industry in developing vaccines, diagnostics, and drugs. International trade in plasma products from paid blood donors—antibodies, clotting factors, and other blood components— is a multimillion-dollar industry in which the United States is a leading exporter.

Paid blood donors typically earn from $50 to $500 per pint; those with rare blood types or components may get more. . . . The League of Red Cross Societies and other international organizations have expressed concern that the financial incentives offered by the blood trade constitute a subtle form of coercion for impoverished or otherwise disadvantaged groups.

But concerns about donor exploitation have not succeeded in halting blood buying and selling in several countries, including the United States. Part of the reason may be that, in legal terms as well as popular perception, blood is more a body "product" than a body "part." The U.S. National Organ Transplant Act (NOTA), which in 1984 banned interstate commerce in organs for transplant, specifically excluded "replenishable tissues such as blood or sperm" from its prohibitions. That blood is a renewable resource seems to set it apart from the more finite entities that the transplant act was designed to regulate. But that may be reading more into the statute than lawmakers intended.

"There's no coherent legal, ethical, or political theory of the body in the United States," says George Annas, . . . "The regulations have come about in a patchwork fashion, because they've come in response to certain things that were perceived as abuses." Historically, says Annas, the states have had authority over the body, and states have proved reluctant to interfere with trade in pieces of their citizens. "There's no uniform act even proposed about body parts." NOTA itself was passed in response to the transplant successes of the late 1970s. From the beginning, organ-transplant programs have been beset by a supply-and-demand crisis. . . .

Before the transplant act, there were cases of would-be donors advertising for potential buyers, and of organ brokers offering to match the two in exchange for a piece of the action. Though kidneys were—and still are—the item living donors were most likely to part with, they could also contribute lungs, eyes, and skin. Sales of less expendable items, such as hearts and livers, were also proposed. The idea was to make the arrangements in advance of death, sort of like life insurance. The extent of these transactions isn't well documented. But the market interest in organ sales made lawmakers queasy—much as does the business interest in cloning today. One of the inciting events in the passage of NOTA, in fact, was a proposed scheme to bring impoverished people to the United States and let them swap organs for money.

Al Gore, then a senator, got wind of this proposal and, horrified, prodded Congress to ban payment for organs. Doctors who tracked the development of transplantation techniques anticipated the organ shortage and took steps to relieve it. In 1968, prompted by the first transplant of a human heart the year before, a committee at Harvard Medical School recommended revising the definition of death so that hearts could be "harvested" from people whose brains had ceased to function but whose breathing was sustained via artificial respirators. Today the concept of brain death has won widespread acceptance. But organs are still in desperately short supply, and thousands of people die each year waiting for transplants. Hence while NOTA has shut down organ brokers here, unregulated and poorly documented markets for organs are believed to flourish elsewhere, mostly in India and Brazil.

Cases have been reported in both India and Egypt of living donors selling kidneys . . . most often just to make money to get by. Some ethicists have argued that body parts constitute a natural asset and that individuals should be free to make contracts regarding their disposal. But most reports about the organ trade concern the exploitation of groups that are anything but free. Several years ago, staffers of a state mental hospital in Argentina were accused of murdering patients to sell their organs. More recently, two Chinese men were arrested in New York for trying to arrange the sale of body parts from prisoners executed in China. And earlier this year, a state representative in Missouri floated the idea of permitting prisoners on death row to donate organs in exchange for a life sentence. Meanwhile, organs and tissues are still being bought

and sold—legally—in this country. While NOTA prohibits traffic in organs for transplantation, it allows such commerce if the body parts in question are to be used in research or product development and testing . . .

"I'm amazed by the scope of the market here, you know, the fact that hospitals with existing tissue banks are getting large financial rewards in joint ventures with biotech companies that want to have access to them," says Lori Andrews, a professor at Chicago-Kent College of Law. "Right now the code of federal regulations says that if there is existing tissue on the shelf, and it is used in an anonymous way in research, you do not have to get informed consent from the individual. But I don't think there's any tissue 'on the shelf' anymore. I see it all in a pipeline to commercialization."

Oddly enough, you and your relatives may have more to say about what happens to your body parts after you're dead than you do premortem. There are laws protecting the inviolability of cadavers but almost none to protect what happens to tissues and organs removed from a patient who's still alive. "The next of kin have a lot more authority over your dead body than you have over your live body," says Annas. One of the most complicated issues in body-shop policy is the traffic in fetal parts, which are gleaned almost exclusively from fetuses that have been selectively aborted (rather than from miscarried or stillborn fetuses, which tend to have defects and are harder to harvest). Fetal tissue—once, like cord blood, a medical waste—has been a prized medical resource ever since research demonstrated its potential for treating Parkinson's disease, diabetes, and Alzheimer's, as well as spinal-cord injuries and hemophilia.

Combined markets for cures of these diseases have been estimated at more than $6 billion. But when a company began in the mid-1980s to develop a treatment involving transplanted fetal cells, right-to-life protests erupted, and in 1988 Congress passed an amendment to NOTA—the only amendment to NOTA—extending the act's restrictions to include fetal organs and tissues. Of course, fetal body parts are still being collected for use in research. A lab at the University of Washington in Seattle can supply "tissue from normal or abnormal embryos and fetuses of desired gestational ages between 40 days and term" by overnight express, and at least a half-dozen brokers of fetal parts harvest tissue from abortion clinics and hospitals across the country. The women who donate the tissue are supposed to sign a consent form, and they cannot legally receive payment for the fetal tissue. The brokers, however, pay a small fee to clinics for collecting the tissue, and charge, in turn, a handling fee of between $50 and $150 per specimen to their customers in the private research community.

The transplantation of fetal cells and tissues into human patients is still allowed, if the procedure is done in the name of approved clinical research. Another segment of the body-parts market prices the goods and services for assisted reproduction. At present, money can buy sperm ($50 to $100), eggs (starting at $2,000), embryos (market value varies), and a place to put them (gestational surrogates start at $10,000, not including brokers' fees). These arrangements have bred some formidable contract disputes, as the courts struggle to spell out what belongs to whom—or more precisely, what exactly is being purchased in such transactions. In one memorable case, contractual parents told their surrogate just two weeks before her due date that they would not accept any male children. When the surrogate delivered a twin brother and sister, the boy was put up for adoption and the couple left the hospital with the girl. The surrogate and her husband then decided to keep the boy and threatened legal action to regain custody of the girl. Though the other couple agreed to give back the girl, it's not clear that they would have been legally compelled to do so.

. . . In cases involving gestational surrogates, who bring to term a genetically unrelated baby created from other people's gametes, the Califor-

nia courts tend to favor the rights of genetic mothers over those of gestational mothers. But when an infertile woman buys someone else's eggs in an attempt to conceive, it is commonly assumed that the egg donor has no legal claim over the resulting embryos or children. That assumption has yet to be tested in court.

Advances in medical industry are stirring up other, more far-reaching questions about ownership. At the heart of the controversy are conflicting perceptions of genetic material. "Genes are an abstract entity to most people," says sociologist Dorothy Nelkin of New York University, who shares a National Science Foundation grant with Lori Andrews to study legal disputes over uses of body tissues in biotechnology. "They're not seen as body parts." Yet, says Nelkin, when it comes to an individual's DNA, genes are perceived . . . as embodying the very essence of a person's identity.

The more than 1,900 claims for patents on human DNA that have so far been registered create an image of genes as commodities, and observers like Nelkin fear that commodification could ultimately infringe on individual rights. A patent on the gene for Huntington's disease may seem abstract, for example, until it turns out to be one of your genes and employers or insurers discriminate against you based on results from a test developed by the patent holder. Researchers and economic analysts also disagree on whether gene patents will speed medical progress or impede it. Proponents of the practice claim that patents provide financial incentive for investment in DNA research, a lure for venture capital, and protection for privately funded scientists who wish to disclose their findings to the public.

John Doll, director of Biotechnology Examination at the U.S. Patent and Trademark Office, has likened the role of DNA and gene patents in the growth of the biomedical industry to the role of patented polymer components in the plastics industry. But other experts insist that the patenting of human DNA will present obstacles to research if too many different owners hold rights to materials and procedures that are necessary for new discoveries. They fear that the simplest experiment could get hung up in a snare of licensing agreements.

The story of cord-blood banking may present an object lesson in commercialization, though the moral of the story is not quite clear. Some ten years ago, when techniques for transplanting cord blood were still being worked out, a number of scientists formed a company called Biocyte to commercialize the technology. Investors put up money for the new venture, and Biocyte developed the clinical procedures, informed consent practices, patient counseling and education, and storage protocols for cord-blood banking. And then, with more than 200 cord-blood samples stored in a freezer in a Pittsburgh blood center, investors decided they could not continue the service. The company is still trying—so far unsuccessfully—to recoup its investment through patents on its cord-blood retrieval and storage procedures.

And Biocyte's 200 patrons can still gain access to their banked blood. But they probably never will. Even now, the only proven use for fetal cord blood is as a substitute for bone-marrow transplants, and at least one expert has predicted that the average person's chance of ever needing to use the blood banked is 1 in 200,000. Nevertheless, the idea of cord-blood banking seems to be taking off. More than a dozen companies, in addition to Viacord, now offer banking services. And people are buying. . . . more than half of Viacord's families have no apparent need for the blood at all. Champions of cord-blood banking maintain that they have turned a medical waste product into a valuable resource. But critics of the trafficking in human anatomy claim that no matter how many lives are saved (or created), any such commerce inevitably violates the sanctity of the human body. . . .

In the United States, animals engineered with human genes and tissues have already been patented. . . . The Thirteenth Amendment to the Constitution, which outlawed slavery, would seem to prohibit the patenting of a human being. But when does a human part, or a part-human, become a full-fledged person? The ever-expanding scope of biomedical commerce is forcing answers to such improbable questions. As the market races forward, issues that were once the province of the very ill or the very thoughtful may soon become everybody's business.

Homo Economicus: Commercialization of Body Tissue in the Age of Biotechnology

DOROTHY NELKIN and LORI ANDREWS

IN RECENT YEARS, biotechnology techniques have transformed a variety of human body tissue into valuable and marketable research materials and clinical products. Blood can serve as the basis for immortalized cell lines for biological studies and the development of pharmaceutical products; the catalogue from the American Tissue Culture Catalogue lists thousands of people's cell lines that are available for sale. Snippets of foreskin are used for the development of artificial skin. Biopsied tissue is used to manufacture therapeutic quantities of genetic material.

Body tissue also has commercial value beyond the medical and research contexts. Placenta is used to enrich shampoos, cosmetics, and skin care products. Katy Mullis, a Nobel Prize-winning geneticist, founded a company called Star Gene that uses gene amplification techniques to make and market jewelry containing DNA cloned from famous rock stars and athletes. The idea, says Mullis, is that "teenagers might pay a little money to get a piece of jewelry containing the actual piece of amplified DNA of somebody like a rock star."[1]

There is also a market for services to collect and store one's tissue outside the body. People can pay to store blood prior to surgery or embryos in the course of in vitro fertilization. A Massachusetts company, BioBank, stores excess tissue removed during cosmetic or other surgical procedures for the patient's future use. New companies such as Safe-T-Child and Child Trail have formed to collect and store tissue samples to identify children who have been kidnapped. And a company called Identigene advertises on taxicabs and billboards (call 1-800-DNA-TYPE) for a service to collect tissue for DNA identification that would establish paternity in child support disputes. There are about fifty private DNA testing centers in the United States, hundreds of university laboratories undertaking DNA research, and over 1,000 biotechnology companies developing commercial products from bodily materials.

These expanding markets have increased the value of human tissue, and institutions with ready access to tissue find they possess a capital resource. Access to stored tissue samples is sometimes included in collaborative agreements between hospitals and biotechnology firms. In a joint venture agreement, Sequana Therapeutics, Inc., a California biotechnology firm, credited the New York City cancer hospital, Memorial-Sloan Kettering, with $5 million in order to obtain access to its bank of cancer tissue biopsies that could be useful as a source of genetic information.[2]

Physicians who treat families with genetic disease are approaching geneticists and offering to "sell you my families"[3]—meaning that they will, for a fee, give the researcher their patients' blood samples. Scientists who isolate certain genes are then patenting them and profiting from their use

DOROTHY NELKIN is a University Professor at New York University in Sociology and in the School of Medicine.
LORI B. ANDREWS is a Professor of Law; Director of the Institute of Science, Law and Technology; and Associate Vice President.

The Hastings Center Report 28, 5 (Sep–Oct 98): 30–39. Reprinted by permission of Dorothy Nelkin, Lori Andrews, and The Hastings Center. Copyright 1998, The Hastings Center.

in genetic tests. Hospitals in Great Britain and Russia sell tissue in order to augment their limited budgets. Between 1976 and 1993 Merieux UK collected 360 tons of placental tissue each year from 282 British hospitals and sent them to France for use in manufacturing drugs.[4] Human tissue has become so valuable that it is sometimes a target for corporate espionage and theft.

In the United States the potential for commercial gain from the body grew as a consequence of legislative measures that were enacted in the 1980s to encourage the commercial development of government-funded research.[5] Legislation allowed universities and nonprofit institutions to apply for patents on federally funded projects and also provided tax incentives to companies investing in academic research. At the same time, changes in patent law turned commercial attention toward research in genetics. A landmark U.S. Supreme Court case in 1980 granted a patent on a life form—a bacterium—setting the stage for the patenting of human genes.[6] In the mid-1980s the U.S. Patent Office began granting patent rights for human genes.[7] It has since received over 5,000 patent applications and has granted more than 1,500, including patents for bone and brain tissue and DNA coding for human proteins.

Today, joint ventures between industry and universities are thriving, and research scientists are increasingly tied to commercial goals. Industry has become a significant source of funding for genetics research. As Francis Collins observed, companies have resources for gene hunting that the academies cannot match: "It's important not to ignore the way things have changed in the last 3 years in human genetics [because of industry]. Gene hunting used to be a purely academic exercise."[8] Nearly every major geneticist is associated with a biotechnology firm; some as directors, others as consultants. And scientists, hospitals, and universities are patenting genes.

The body, of course, has long been exploited as a commercial and marketable entity, as athletes, models, prostitutes, surrogate mothers, and beauty queens are well aware. Yet there is something strange and troubling about the traffic in body tissue, the banking of human cells, the patenting of genes. In the 1984 public hearings concerning anatomical gifts, Albert Gore, then a U.S. Congressman, was troubled by a growing tendency to treat the body as a commodity in a market economy: "It is against our system of values to buy and sell parts of human beings. . . . The notion has perhaps superficial attraction to some because we have learned that the market system will solve lots of problems if we just stand out of the way and let it work. It is very true. This ought to be an exception because you don't want to invest property rights in human beings. . . . It is wrong."[9]

But what *is* troubling about the commodification of the body? What is the problem with the growing interest in human tissue for the manufacturing of pharmaceutical or bioengineered products? Clearly the interest in the body is driven by instrumental and commercial values; but so too, as Gore suggested, are most technological endeavors. Moreover, much of the body tissue useful for biotechnology innovation—hair, blood, sperm—is replenishable. And we normally regard body materials such as umbilical cord blood, foreskin, the tissue discarded after surgery—and, in some cases, even the excess embryos created for in vitro fertilization—as simply refuse, like bloodied bandages and other medical wastes. Why not, then, view the body as a useful and exploitable resource if this can advance scientific research, contribute to progress, or provide lifesaving benefits to others? Why are there demonstrations against the privatization of cord blood, lawsuits against the commercialization of cell lines, protests against the patenting of genes? Why are commercial developments in the removal, storage, and transformation of human tissue controversial?

To answer these questions, we undertook a study of several prominent disputes over the ownership of the body, the collection of human tissue, and its distribution as a resource. These disputes reflect the collision between commercial claims for body tissue and individual interests or cultural values. They reflect a conviction that turning tissue, cell lines, and DNA into commodities violates body integrity, exploits powerless people, intrudes on community values, distorts research agendas, and weakens public trust in scientists and clinicians.

HISTORICAL CONTROVERSIES

Research and clinical uses of body parts have been controversial since the early days of anatomical dissection. The process of cutting and fragmenting the body once evoked images of evil, and Dante-esque visions of Hell.[10] As the Renaissance brought growing interest in anatomy, the use of bodies in medical schools was gradually accepted. Yet dissection remained controversial well into the nineteenth century, mainly due to the exploitative manner of obtaining anatomical specimens and the commercial interests involved. Bodies, in short supply, became, as historian Michael Sappol described them, valuable commodities, "objects of exchange whose value fluctuated according to the law of supply and demand."[11] Anatomy departments paid between $10 and $35 for a body, more than the weekly wage of a skilled worker at that time. Body snatching became a lucrative business as dead bodies were obtained in devious ways—through grave robbing, the bribing of hospital attendants, and even the murder of beggars. Historian Ruth Richardson describes how corpses were "quarried": "Parts extracted were sold to those who could use them, such as dentists and wigmakers, and to those who assisted medical research and study, such as articulators of bones for medical skeletons and medical specimen makers. Profits were to be made at every stage."[12] Despite riots and demonstrations,[13] the practice of body snatching continued in America until anatomy laws, passed in various states throughout the nineteenth century, eased the shortage by allowing medical schools to use the bodies of executed murderers and the unclaimed dead.[14] These laws regularized the practice of

dissection, but throughout the nineteenth century, writes Sappol, people remained sensitive to the dangers of commercialization, insisting that the body remain "outside the capital nexus, outside the exchange of goods, . . . sequestered from the market economy."[15]

Later experiments in organ transplantation were welcomed as "medical milestones," but still evoked worries about market exploitation. As organs became valuable commodities, would physicians hasten deaths? Would valuable organs be harvested for a fee from needy people or from citizens of the Third World?[16]

The historical disputes over dissection and organ transplants reflected several concerns about the effect of commercial interest in the body: the violation of body integrity as corpses were "snatched" for profit and cut into parts; the devaluation of personal characteristics as the body was viewed as an object with replaceable and collectible parts; and conflict between the interests of doctors and scientists and those of patients and their families. These concerns were ultimately assuaged by the passage of the Uniform Anatomical Gift Act (1968) and the National Organ Transplantation Act (1984), which assure the noncommercial, voluntary donation of bodies and their parts for research and transplantation.

Today, old tensions have taken on new dimensions as the commercial potential of human tissue has caught the entrepreneurial imagination. Few laws are in place to address the proper uses of cells, tissues, and genes. Instead, disputes over the ownership, collection, and distribution of human tissue have ended up in the media and in the courts.

THE OWNERSHIP OF BODY TISSUE

John Moore, a patient with hairy cell leukemia, had his spleen removed at the University of California, Los Angeles School of Medicine in 1976. His physician, Dr. David W. Golde, patented certain chemicals in Moore's blood purportedly without his knowledge or consent and set up contracts with a Boston company, negotiating shares worth $3 million. Sandoz, the Swiss pharmaceutical company, paid a reported $15 million for the right to develop the Mo cell line.

Moore began to suspect that his tissue was being used for purposes beyond his personal care when UCLA cancer specialists kept taking samples of blood, bone marrow, skin, and sperm for seven years. When Moore discovered in 1984 that he had become patent number 4,438,032, he sued the doctors for malpractice and property theft.[17] His physicians claimed that Moore had waived his interest in his body parts when he signed a general consent form giving the UCLA pathology department the right to dispose of his removed tissue. But Moore felt that his integrity was violated, his body exploited, and his tissue turned into a product: "My doctors are claiming that my humanity, my genetic essence, is their invention and their property. They view me as a mine from which to extract biological material. I was harvested."[18]

The court held that clinicians must inform patients in advance of surgical procedures that their tissue could be used for research, but it denied Moore's claim that he owned his tissue. Who then should reap the *profits* from parts taken from an individual's body? The court decided that the doctor and biotechnology company rather than the patient should profit. The decision rested on the promise of biotechnology innovation. The court did not want to slow down research by "threaten[ing] with disabling civil liability innocent parties who are engaged in socially useful activities, such as researchers who have no reason to believe that their use of a particular cell sample is against a donor's wishes." The court was concerned that giving Moore a property right to his tissue would "destroy the economic incentive to conduct important medical research."[19]

Justice Stanley Mosk, dissenting, objected to the notion that the body—"the physical and temporal expression of the unique human persona" —could be regarded as a product for commercial exploitation. For, he argued, the spectre of direct abuse, of torture, of involuntary servitude haunts the laboratories and boardrooms of today's biotechnological research industrial complex (p. 515).

The privileging of biotechnology companies encouraged a genetics gold rush. In 1992 Craig Venter, a molecular biologist, left the National Institutes of Health to form The Institute for Genomic Research (TIGR), where he compiled the world's largest human gene data bank containing at least 150,000 fragments of DNA sequences. The Institute for Genomic Research was initially funded by a $70 million grant from a firm, Human Genome Services (HGS). Two months after the agreement, HGS contracted with SmithKline Beecham, which gained an exclusive stake in the database with first rights on patentable discoveries. Geneticist David King described the situation: "You have a corporation trying to monopolize control of a large part of the whole human genome, literally the human heritage. Should this become private property?"[20]

The concerns about commercial exploitation of the body expressed in *Moore* have assumed more complex dimensions in disputes over the collection of human tissue in a global context. Scientists and biotechnology companies are searching the world for disease genes. But critics have viewed the collection of tissue from indigenous populations as a violation of cultural values, and associate these efforts with past forms of exploitation.

COLLECTING TISSUE FROM INDIGENOUS POPULATIONS

Because people from isolated populations may have unique body tissue, western geneticists, biotechnology companies, and researchers from the Human Genome Diversity Project (HGDP) are seeking blood and hair samples from indigenous groups throughout the world. Their goals are to find disease genes by identifying families with a high rate of genetically linked conditions; to develop genetic tests and therapeutic products; and to "immortalize" the DNA from "vanishing populations."[21]

In March 1995 researchers from the National Institutes of Health obtained a virus-infected cell line from a man from the Hagahai tribe in Papua, New Guinea. The cell line, which could be used to develop a diagnostic test, became patent number 5,397,696. Accused of exploitation, the NIH withdrew the patent claim in December 1996. Meanwhile, Sequana Therapeutics, collaborating with the University of Toronto, collected DNA samples from the island of Tristan de Cunha for research on asthma and then sold the rights to develop therapeutic technologies for $70 million to a German company, Boehringer Ingelheim.[22] Western scientists are also negotiating contracts to collect DNA samples from Chinese families with genetic diseases. But China's eugenics policies include efforts to identify families with genetic abnormalities so as to prevent them from reproducing. Thus the DNA samples may also be a valuable resource for Chinese authorities seeking to implement oppressive eugenics laws.

The HGDP has confronted angry opposition. Indigenous groups view the taking of their tissue as exploitation. They have accused the program of violating community values, "biopiracy" or "biocolonialism," one more effort to divide their social world. A representative of an indigenous group opined, "You've taken our land, our language, our culture, and even our children. Are you now saying you want to take part of our bodies as well?"[23] Some objections reflect beliefs, expressed in collective rituals involving blood or body parts, about the social meaning of body tissue—its role in maintaining the integrity of the community and the relationship of the individual to the collective.[24] Others believe that their future might be compromised by the collection of their DNA. Once scientists have what they need from them, there would be no reason to help them stay alive. This pessimistic view was fueled by researchers who promoted the project as a way to "immortalize" the cell lines of groups that will become extinct.

Indigenous groups also question the relevance of the scientific work to their own health needs, which have less to do with genetic disease than with common disorders such as diarrhea. They argue that DNA is collected, often without adequate knowledge or consent, and then used for products relevant only in wealthy nations. And Native Americans suspect that genetic data will be used against them: just as criteria of blood quanta were used to define political entitlements to land and social services, so DNA could be used to override long-standing social relationships. Thus in 1993 the World Council of Indigenous Peoples unanimously voted to "categorically reject and condemn the Human Genome Diversity Project as it applies to our rights, lives, and dignity."[25]

In response to concerns about exploitation of indigenous resources, the United Nations Convention on Biodiversity (1992) had sought to assure that national governments receive just compensation for commercial use of both human and agricultural resources. But the interest in genetic resources suggests that this approach may lead to further exploitation of indigenous groups as they become profit centers for their governments. Moreover, some groups do not want compensation—the very idea of commercializing the body offends them and contradicts their world view. For them, the body has a social meaning tied to colonial history, traditional communal rituals, and concerns about continued exploitation.

THE DISTRIBUTION OF BODY TISSUE

Commercial interests are also involved in the distribution of products derived from the body. The market involvement in the distribution of umbilical cord blood has become controversial as a resource considered communal became privatized. In 1988 a French research team headed by Dr. Eliane Gluckmann developed a way to process umbilical cord blood so that it could be used as an alternative for bone marrow in treating life-threatening diseases. Blood from the umbilical cord is rich in stem cells that produce mature red and white blood cells and platelets. Its use for transplantation has several advantages: it is readily available—at least 10,000 umbilical cords are routinely clamped, cut, and discarded each day in the United States. Cord blood is also less immunoreactive than bone marrow. The researchers envisioned a system of nonprofit cord blood banks where the frozen blood would be stored and available for distribution with minimal delay to those in need of transplantation. It was to be a communal resource.

The likelihood that a newborn infant will ever need his or her umbilical cord blood is less than one in 10,000. However, attracted by potential markets, cord blood companies created private banks and urged prospective parents to store their infant's cord blood privately as "insurance" against future medical needs. In effect, these companies are creating a market and generating a need.[26]

The commercialization of the product led to the use of strong-arm marketing tactics. Cord blood companies employ a direct marketing approach obtaining mailing lists from diaper services and magazine subscriptions to sell the promise of innovation and future progress to vulnerable prospective parents. Cord blood, they say, is a "low cost edge on an uncertain future."[27] In case of emergency it is "immediately available off the shelf." This marketing strategy plays on the risk-aversive sentiments of those who prefer to rely on their own resources rather than on the state, and it exploits parental guilt—the desire to "do right" by one's children.

In 1991 an American company, Biocyte Corporation, sought a patent for its method for cryopreserving newborn blood stem cells to se-cure rights to its storage and distribution. Biocyte obtained European and U.S. patents covering "hemopoietic stem and placenta cells of neonatal and fetal blood, that are cryopreserved, and the therapeutic uses of such cells."[28] These patents gave the company rights over storage of stem cells from cord blood and also over therapeutic services. The European Group on Blood and Marrow Transplantation protested, claiming that patenting would impede further research and discourage the formation of nonprofit banks. The idea of patenting also evoked moral outrage against commodifying a "natural" substance and turning a product of childbirth into a commercial object.[29] Cord blood, once a body substance discarded as useless, became a hot clinical property, and a focus of tension over commercialization of the body and the equitable distribution of body tissue for therapeutic purposes.

THEFT— THE ULTIMATE SYMBOL OF COMMODIFICATION

Products that attain commercial value are inevitably subject to theft, a not uncommon form of redistribution. The traffic in body parts has persisted, spurred as in the nineteenth century, by a shortage of organs and tissue. Body parts have been bought from coroners, stolen from the site of accidents, and sold to meet the demands of industry and medicine.[30] Today, cell lines are a target for international espionage.[31] In a sting operation, agents of the Food and Drug Administration posed as representatives of a tissue bank and ordered tissue from a California dentist who tried to sell them body parts at a discount.[32] In France, a government investigation exposed an embezzlement scheme in which private companies billed local hospitals for synthetic ligament tissue that, it turned out, came from human tissue, which in France cannot legally be bought and sold.[33]

Funeral home personnel and coroners have also engaged in tissue theft. In one case, a morgue employee allegedly stole body parts and sold them nationally—a situation uncovered unexpectedly when the body of a twenty-one-day-old infant was exhumed for other purposes and, found to be missing his heart, lungs, eyes, pituitary gland, aorta, kidneys, spleen, and key brain parts.[34] In Britain seventeen people who contracted Creutzfeld Jacob disease from human growth hormone accused the Medical Research Council and the Department of Health of unlawfully buying, from mortuaries, the pituitary glands from 900,000 bodies to extract the growth hormone. The tissue was taken without the consent of the individuals before death or their families, in violation of British law.[35]

Demands for spare embryos have also led to undercover redistribution in the in vitro fertilization business. At the University of California at Irvine, over 75 couples were affected by theft of eggs and embryos at the university clinic where Dr. Ricardo Asch had apparently been secretly selling some of the eggs extracted from his infertility patients to other patients who were duped into thinking they were from legitimate donors. More than forty civil lawsuits were filed. In July 1997 the university agreed to pay $14 million to seventy-five couples; two dozen lawsuits still remain. Embryo theft was "predictable, almost inevitable," says Boston University health law professor George Annas. "The field [of in vitro fertilization] is so lucrative and so unregulated that someone was just bound to do it."[36]

PROBLEMS WITH THE BUSINESS OF BODIES

References to body parts in the medical and scientific literature increasingly employ a language of commerce—of banking, investment, insurance, compensation, and patenting. Gene sequences are patented; cord blood is a "hot property," the body is a "medical factory." Companies "target" appropriate markets for their products. Pathology organizations lobby the government to allow them to use stored tissue samples without consent, for they view such samples as "treasure troves" or "national resources" for research. Geneticists talk of "prospecting" for genes. The body is a "project"—a system that can be divided and dissected down to the molecular level. In a striking statement in the *Moore* case, the defendant, UCLA, claimed that even if Moore's cells were his property, as a state university it had a right to take the cells under "eminent domain."

The body tissue disputes we have described—over the ownership, collection, and distribution of body tissue—raise questions about the assumptions underlying this language of commerce. Who will profit? Who will lose? How will exploitation be avoided? They reflect conflicting beliefs about the body. Is body tissue to be defined as waste, like the material in a hospital bed pan? Is it refuse that is freely available as raw material for commercial products? Or does body tissue have inherent value as part of a person? Are genes the essence of an individual and a sacred part of the human inheritance? Or are they, as a director of SmithKline Beecham purportedly claimed, "the currency of the future."[37]

Disputes suggest that commodifying human tissue, usually without the person's knowledge or consent, is troubling because it threatens the well-being of individuals and violates social assumptions about the body.[38] And they suggest that commercialization can also have serious implications for science and medical practice.

REFERENCES

1. "Kary Mullis," *Omni Magazine,* April 1992, p. 69.
2. "Cancer Genetics Joint Venture," *Business Wire,* 20 August 1996.
3. David Cox, Stanford University, personal communication.
4. Heather Kirby, "Something Nasty in the Night Cream," *The Times* (London), 3 April 1992.

5. See, for example, Andrew Kimbrell, *The Human Body Shop: The Engineering and Marketing of Life* (San Francisco: Harper San Francisco, 1993); Sheldon Krimsky, *Biotechnics and Society* (New York: Praeger, 1991); and Paul Rabinow, *Making PCR* (Chicago: University of Chicago Press, 1996).

6. Diamond v. Chakabarry, 447 U.S. 303 (1980). Initially, researchers assumed that genes were not patentable since patent law covers "inventions" and prohibits patenting the "products of nature."

7. See, for example, Rebecca S. Eisenberg, "Patenting the Human Genome," *Emory Law Journal* 39 (1990): 721–45.

8. Quoted in Jon Cohen, "The Genomics Gamble," *Science* 275 (1997); 767–72, at 767.

9. House Hearing on H.R. 4080, "National Organ Transplant Act": Hearing Before the Subcommittee on Health and the Environment of the House Committee on Energy and Commerce, 98th Cong., 1984, p. 128.

10. Caroline Bynum, *The Resurrection of the Body* (New York: Columbia University Press, 1995).

11. Michael Sappol, "The Cultural Politics of Anatomy in 19th Century America: Death, Dissection, and Embodied Social Identity." Unpublished doctoral thesis, Columbia University, 1997, pp. 526–28. Forthcoming, Princeton University Press, 1998.

12. Ruth Richardson, "Fearful Symmetry, Corpses for Anatomy: Organs for Transplantation," in *Organ Transplantation: Meanings and Realities,* ed. Stuart J. Youngner, Renée C. Fox, and Lawrence O'Connell (Madison: University of Wisconsin Press, 1999), ch. 5 at 82.

13. Sappol, "Cultural Politics of Anatomy," documents and describes these riots and their goals.

14. The first anatomy law was passed in Massachusetts in 1831.

15. Sappol, "Cultural Politics of Anatomy," p. 196.

16. Kimbrell, *The Human Body Shop.*

17. Moore v. Regents of the University of California, 793 P.2d 479 (Cal. 1990).

18. Quoted in John Vidal and Hohn Carvel, "Lambs to the Gene Market," *The Guardian* (London), 12 November 1994.

19. Moore v. Regents of the University of California, p. 495.

20. Quoted in "Staking Their Claims to Parts of Your Body," *The Independent,* 6 December 1994.

21. The distribution of genes across populations can also help answer intriguing questions about human origins and patterns of migration. L. L. Cavalli-Sforza, A. C. Wilson, C. R. Cantor et al., "Survey of Human Genetic Diversity: A Vanishing Opportunity for the Human Genome Project," *Genomics* 11 1991): 490–91.

22. Global Information Network, 8 December 1995 (Westlaw Data Base); "$2 Million Received for Gene Discovery Program," *Gene Therapy Weekly,* 6 November 1995.

23. Zef Productions Ltd., "The Gene Hunters," documentary film, aired by British Broadcasting, Channel 4, 1995.

24. See, for example, Michael O'Hanlon, *Reading the Skin: Adornment, Display and Society Among the Wahgi* (London: British Museum, 1989).

25. World Council of Indigenous People, "Resolution on the HGDP," Native Net Archive Page http://broco9.uthsca.edu/natnet/archive/nl/hgdp.html.

26. Sugarman et al., "Ethical Issues in Umbilical Cord Blood Banking," *JAMA* 278 (1997): 938–43.

27. Frank Molloy, "Banking Fetal Cells," *Hartford Courant,* 19 August 1995.

28. Declan Butler, "U.S. Company Comes Under Fire on Patent on Umbilical Cord Cells," *Nature* 382 (1996): 99; Susan Kelleher and Kim Christensen, "Fertility Patients Fight over Twins," *Orange County Register,* 18 February 1996.

29. Interview with Helena Paul, Gaia Foundation, 11 April 1997, London.

30. "The Human Body Parts Trade," *World Press Review* 1, no. 4 (1994): 38.

31. Charles M. Sennott, "New Cold War: Spies Target Corporation," *Boston Globe,* 19 January 1997.

32. CBS Evening News, 21 May 1996.

33. Catherine Tastemain, "Oversight for Tissue Transplants," *Nature-Medicine,* 1, no. 5 (1995): 397.

34. Frank J. Murray, "Survivors May Sue Over Theft of Body Parts," *Washington Times,* 6 November 1995.

35. Dominic Kennedy. "Families Challenge Legality of Trade in Pituitary Glands," *The Times* (London), 4 September 1995.

36. Karen Brandon, "Emerging Fertility Scandal Has Californians Rapt," *Chicago Tribune,* 24 March 1996.

37. Global 2000, Communiqué, 1997.

38. Lori Andrews and Dorothy Nelkin, "Whose Body Is It Anyway?" *The Lancet* 351 (1997): 53–57.

A Ray of Light about Frozen Embryos

ELLEN WRIGHT CLAYTON

ABSTRACT. The Tennessee Supreme Court's decision in *Davis v. Davis,* a case that raises the question of how to allocate frozen embryos in the event of divorce, addresses many of the legal issues posed by in vitro fertilization. The decision considers the interests of the progenitors as well as of the children who may result. For example, the court held that gamete providers' discretion regarding the disposition of embryos can be limited only when their decisions would harm the children who might be born. The court also made clear that efforts to seek genetic parenthood are protected only when accompanied by a desire to raise the resulting children, a conclusion that also affects other reproductive technologies. In addition to elaborating an analytic framework, the court set guidelines for resolving disputes when the couples had made no prior agreements, including holding that while the embryos are ex-utero the desire to avoid genetic parenthood almost always trumps the wish to become a parent. The well-reasoned analysis in *Davis v. Davis* should help shape legal and ethical discussion regarding the use of in vitro fertilization for many years to come.

MORE AND MORE people are choosing to cryopreserve (freeze) some embryos that are produced during in vitro fertilization (IVF). This practice permits embryos to be saved for later implantation. But the fact that an extended period of time can elapse between fertilization and

ELLEN WRIGHT CLAYTON is an associate professor of pediatrics at the Vanderbilt University School of Medicine and an associate professor of law at Vanderbilt's School of Law.

the implantation of any resulting embryos has enormous implications.

Couples may choose to proceed with cryopreservation for a host of reasons. They usually want to decrease the need for the woman to undergo repeated hormonal stimulation and egg harvest and to increase the overall chance of a viable pregnancy. They may simply see this as a part of the process of in vitro fertilization. Couples may also be acting out of a respect for the potential represented by the embryos.

However, while couples usually feel that frozen embryos represent hope for the future when they embark on this course, things can change. They may discover later that they do not want to use the embryos themselves. And, not uncommonly, couples come to disagree about what to do with the embryos, especially in the event of divorce.

While the propriety of governments or physicians placing limits on the disposition of "extra" embryos has been an issue since the advent of IVF (*Smith v. Hartigan,* 556 F. Supp. 157 (ND Ill. 1983)), the existence now of thousands of frozen embryos has increased the intensity of the debate, resulting in a flood of scholarly comment (e.g., Andrews 1986; Bonnicksen 1989; Robertson 1990a & b), and presenting new opportunities for legal intervention. Although many countries regulate the practice of in vitro fertilization, sometimes with great specificity (Knoppers and LeBris 1990; Price 1989; Scott 1990), the use of this reproductive technology in the United

Kennedy Institute of Ethics Journal, *2, 4 (1992): 347–359. Copyright 1992. Reprinted with permission of The Johns Hopkins University Press.*

States has developed relatively free of legal over-sight (Bonnicksen 1989). When legislators recently began to turn their attention to IVF, they most often were concerned with issues of access, such as who should or should not have to pay for this procedure (insurance, the state, the progenitors, etc.) and for whom third party payment ought to be available (married couples or other individuals).[1] Very few lawsuits asserted that IVF had gone awry (*Del Zio v. Columbia Presbyterian Medical Center,* No 74-3558 (SDNY, filed 12 April 1978)).

But the growing use of cryopreservation has meant that the hands-off stance of the law in this country toward IVF has begun to change. Legal intervention occurred slowly at first. In a statute that has not been contested, Louisiana required that all extra embryos be donated to another couple, a rule that dramatically decreases the availability of IVF since there are few potential donees (*La. Rev. Stat. Ann.* 1992 (West), sec. 9:130). A federal district court in Virginia ruled that a gamete-providing couple had the right to take the resulting embryo to another clinic over the objections of the clinic that had initially performed the harvest and fertilization (*York v. Jones,* 717 F. Supp. 421 (ED Va. 1989)). These examples, however, seem to have provided little guidance for the rest of the country. Louisiana's statute is not easily generalized because it reflects a stance toward procreative autonomy, as evidenced by that state's uniquely restrictive abortion law, which is among the least permissive in the country. *York*'s impact is limited by the perception that the appropriate resolution in that case was rather clear from the outset.

By contrast, a recent decision by the Tennessee Supreme Court, *Davis v. Davis* (18 Fam. L. Rptr. 2029 (Tenn. 1992)), will likely influence future legal discourse about IVF and other reproductive technologies, both because of the notoriety of the case and the breadth of the court's analysis. *Davis v. Davis* is certainly the sort of "hard case" that lawyers say usually makes "bad law."

The fight between Mary Sue and Junior Davis during their divorce over the disposition of seven frozen embryos can only be described as a tragedy. After several tubal pregnancies and an effort to adopt in which the birth mother changed her mind, the Davises turned to IVF. Ms. Davis underwent six of these procedures, but none resulted in pregnancy. Shortly after the last attempt, Mr. Davis filed for divorce. When asked why he had agreed to pursue IVF when he knew of their marital problems, he said that he had hoped that having a child would make things better between the two of them. On the last round, the couple had agreed to freeze the seven "extra" embryos, setting the stage for the dispute to come.

After the marriage fell apart, Mr. Davis did not want the embryos to be implanted. His fears for the children who might be born were colored by his dramatic personal experience of profound separation from his parents as a young child. Ms. Davis (now Stowe) initially wanted to have the embryos implanted in herself. After she later remarried, she wished to donate them to someone else, in hopes that some child would be born after all she had been through. What makes this case particularly sad is that the Davises were not asked at the time they agreed to cryopreservation to consider what should be done with the embryos should their circumstances change. As a result, they apparently did not anticipate the possibility of divorce, and their later disagreement caught the attention of the national media and was laid out for all the world to see.

In the early stages, this "hard case" resulted in some very bad law. In a lengthy opinion subject to a host of criticisms, the trial court ruled in essence that the embryos were children, over "whom" their "parents" had little say (*Davis v. Davis,* 15 Fam. L. Rptr. 2097 (Tenn. Cir. Ct. 1989)). The judge concluded that the embryos should be implanted in Mary Sue Davis, who was thereby cast in the role of a potentially involuntary, if actually willing, "uterine hostess." At a conference that Judge Young and I addressed a few months after he rendered his decision, he denied that he meant to rule this broadly, but the implications of his decision were clear. The intermediate appellate court overturned the trial court's decision, ruling that embryos are not children and briefly discussing the right not to procreate (*Davis v. Davis*, 16 Fam. L. Rptr. 1535 (Tenn. Ct. App. 1990)). Incredibly enough, however, that court left it up to the Davises to decide what to do with the embryos even though their inability to agree was a major reason why this case was in court at all.

The Tennessee Supreme Court took this mess of complex human experience and shoddy law and, in a thoughtful opinion, set forth an extensive legal analysis, which it then applied to reach a reasonable resolution of the Davises' claims (*Davis* 1992). In the process, the court took several steps that provide specific guidance to those who participate in cryopreservation.

The first, and most central, is that the court made clear that couples' decisions regarding the disposition of the embryos created from their gametes should prevail in almost all circumstances. In reaching this conclusion, the court made important points along the way. It began by discussing an array of bright-line rules that could apply when questions arise regarding the desirability of continuing with IVF. These included (1) a mandate like the one in Louisiana that all embryos be implanted; (2) the adoption of an "implied contract" model in which the decision to embark on IVF is assumed to include a commitment to continue the process to the end; (3) a requirement that all unused embryos be discarded and none frozen; (4) a rule that the embryos simply be divided between the two parties; and (5) a decision to vest total control in the woman, based on the greater burdens usually placed on her by the process of IVF. The court rejected all these possible solutions even though it recognized that such rules would be relatively straightforward to apply and would provide clear guidance for all those concerned. It reasoned that adopting an easy answer was precluded by the constraints of law, science, and ethics.

The justices then discussed these constraints, beginning their analysis with a consideration of the status of the frozen embryos and holding that they are less than fully "persons" in the eyes of the law. Thus, while the court acknowledged a role for respecting embryos as potential life, it implicitly rejected the position advocated by some that embryos ought never be destroyed and that physicians should be permitted only to attempt to create as many embryos as might be used on any particular round so that there would be none left to discard or freeze (Browne and Hynes 1990; Congregation for the Doctrine of Faith 1987). The Tennessee Supreme Court did, however, conclude that the embryos were more than property because of the chance that they could be transferred into a woman's body and brought to term and that some events before or during transfer might cause *harm* to the resulting *children*.

This emphasis on avoiding injury to children illuminates the court's holding that the intermediate status of the embryos justifies some publicly defined limits on gamete donors' discretion. Progenitors' decisions to discard embryos or to keep them cryopreserved could not be overridden because such choices would simply mean that no children would be born who could then be harmed. But what sort of harm would justify vetoing gamete providers' decisions to attempt to bring an embryo to term? Viewed from the perspective of the potential child whose claim would be couched in terms of wrongful life (Wright 1978), the injury would have to be very great indeed since the alternative would be not to be born at all. A child born, for example, to a divorced woman who received the embryo as a gift from the gamete providers could not be heard to complain in court that he would have been better off had he been born into an intact family. From the state's point of view, its interest in avoiding burdens similarly would not suffice to sustain rules forbidding the use of embryos by single women or the implantation of embryos at known risk for having genetic disorders.

Deliberate experimentation with embryos intended for later transfer, however, may be another matter. It is quite likely that a statute that forbade implanting an embryo that had been the object (subject?) of nontherapeutic experimentation or transferring a human embryo to an animal's uterus (perhaps for a brief period of transport) would be upheld under the *Davis* court's avoidance of harm analysis (*Minn. Stat. Ann.* 1991 (West), sec. 145.422; *New Mex Stat. Ann.* 1991, sec. 24-9A-1-6), even if it might fail on other grounds (*Lifchez v. Hartigan,* 735 F. Supp. 1361 (ND Ill.) *aff'd,* 914 F.2d 260 (7th Cir. 1990), *cert. denied sub nom, Scholberg v. Lifchez,* Ill. S.Ct. 787 (1991)). Interestingly, some of the few statutes in other states that already forbid research on and subsequent implantation of embryos do not distinguish between nontherapeutic and therapeutic intervention (*NH Rev. Stat. Ann.* 1991, sec. 168-B:15) even though there is already discussion about the possibility of performing gene therapy on embryos ex utero (Andrews 1987; Robertson 1992). A question that remains then is whether a state could prohibit the latter type of research under the *Davis* court's rule.

Having addressed the status of the embryo, the court next considered the enforceability of contracts between gamete donors regarding the disposition of their embryos. The media coverage of the dispute between Mary Sue and Junior Davis made clear that couples are well-advised to consider such possibilities as divorce or abandonment of the program before they embark on cryopreservation. The Tennessee Supreme Court's opinion, however, put gamete donors on notice that they will be held to the terms of their agreements regarding the disposition of the frozen embryos they create. The court acknowledged that individuals' views on these matters may change as their relationship with one another changes but held that, in order to minimize the risks to the parties, "initial agreements

may later be modified [only] *by agreement*" (p. 2034).

Some commentators agree with this rule (Poole 1990; Robertson 1990a & b) but others support a less stringent approach. The American Medical Association's Board of Trustees, for example, would make such contracts enforceable "unless changed circumstances make enforcement of the agreement unreasonable" (AMA Board of Trustees 1990, p. 2484). While a universal requirement that couples abide by their prior agreements may be desirable because of increased predictability, approaches such as those suggested by the AMA may be more in line with current rules on legal enforcement of intrafamilial relationships. For while the trend is toward increasingly strict enforcement of contractual arrangements between spouses such as antenuptial agreements (*Edwardson v. Edwardson,* 798 S.W.2d 941 (Ky. 1990); *Simeone v. Simeone,* 581 A.2d 162 (Pa. 1990)), courts in general still tend to look particularly closely at the circumstances under which such agreements were entered into and to allow more opportunities for escape than are permitted under general contract law. It is also noteworthy that the court did not address the possibility that clinics may start requiring couples to sign such contracts as a condition for obtaining IVF, a practice that some commentators condemn (AMA Board of Trustees 1990).

But what the *Davis* court ultimately had to confront was not an effort by the state to wrest control of the embryos away from a pair of gamete donors who were united in their desires, nor a squabble over a prior agreement, but rather the facts that Mary Sue and Junior Davis had never agreed about what they would do with the embryos in the event of divorce and that doing nothing effectively gave complete veto power to Mr. Davis.

As the first step toward resolving this dilemma, the court elaborated a right of procreational autonomy under the federal and state constitutions, which incorporated far-reaching, although not unlimited, rights both to procreate and not to procreate. What was particularly striking about the court's analysis was the extent to which these freedoms were based on the implications of becoming a parent. These consequences, in turn, were drawn very broadly to include not only the joys of wanted parenthood, but also the economic and psychological burdens of having a child, whether initially wanted or not, with whom one may have little or no contact.

This focus on the enormity of parenthood led the court to conclude first that there was no state interest evidenced in Tennessee law that would justify removing control outright from the couple because "no one else bears the consequences of these decisions in the way that the gamete-providers do" (p. 2037, fn. om.). It also led the court to create a presumption in favor of the party who did not want the embryos to be implanted that could be overridden only if the party seeking to use the embryos "could not achieve parenthood by any other reasonable means" (p. 2039), including further efforts at IVF with another partner and even adoption if he or she would be "satisfied by the child-rearing aspects of parenthood alone" (p. 2039). Thus, when conflicts arise in the absence of a prior agreement, the desire to avoid genetic parenthood almost always trumps the wish to become a genetic parent.

The court's analysis of who has the right to make decisions about genetic parenthood has legal implications for many of the participants in reproduction, whether by old or new techniques. While it is possible, for example, that some people seek to procreate simply to get their genes into the world, the opinion makes clear that the aspect of reproduction that merits legal protection is the desire to have children to raise, or "genetic + social parenthood." Having a baby simply to ensure that one's genes are passed on to the next generation when unaccompanied by a commitment to rear the resulting child is not what reproduction is all about in the law's eyes.

This refusal to view procreation solely as a means to achieve genetic connection can affect the legal responses to other new reproductive technologies as well. If one were to apply this insistence that genetic parenthood not be viewed in isolation from raising the resulting children, for example, to the case of *Baby M*, one would conclude that the New Jersey Supreme Court was incorrect when it said that Mr. Stern's "right to procreate is very simply the right to have natural [read genetic] children . . ." and then suggested that his interest would be fulfilled from the law's perspective by the birth of Baby M even if Ms. Whitehead had gotten exclusive custody of the child (*In re Baby M.*, 537 A.2d 1227 (1988), p. 1253). One cannot award absolute custody to one gamete donor and assert that the other's right to procreate has nonetheless been vindicated.

This strategy of refusing to view genetic parenthood as separate from all other aspects of parental hopes and responsibilities also begins to respond to some concerns that focusing on genetic connections is bad for children because it undermines not only social parenting, including adoption, but also broader societal norms about responsibility for children in general (Developments in the Law 1990). At least this opinion affirms that having children entails an obligation to care for them. Even if children are somehow harmed or commodified by an emphasis on genetic ties, we need to realize that there never was a halcyon time when genetic connections did not matter, when all children were cared for regardless of where they came from or their characteristics. At most, the new reproductive technologies simply add to an already deeply ingrained social concern with biologic ties.

With regard to fears that enabling individuals to try to have a genetically connected child interferes with the adoption of other children, especially those with special needs, it is difficult to believe that these couples who try so hard to procreate would provide the latter children with permanent homes if only the new technologies were banned. The claims of children individually and in the aggregate are better served by policies that enable families to care for their offspring and that provide direct assistance particularly to those children whose needs are not met within the home, not by what would doubtless be largely futile efforts to shift our focus away from genetics.

The protection of those who seek "genetic + social parenthood" outlined in *Davis* provides less direct guidance regarding claims against third parties. In particular, does this interest mean that gamete providers are entitled to seek help from another woman in the case of classical or gestational surrogacy, or that sperm donors can have any control over whether their partners continue their pregnancies after implantation? After all, the *Davis* court found that Mr. Davis had sufficient interest in avoiding the responsibility of genetic parenthood that he could bar the implantation of frozen embryos over the opposing wishes of his ex-wife, or potentially, of the state. But while interrupting an ongoing pregnancy or asserting a claim for custody of a child who had been brought to term following surrogacy were not at issue, the court's approach suggests that it would not rely solely on the interest in genetic parenthood to resolve these sorts of questions. It is hard to imagine that this court would permit a sperm donor who changed his mind to require that either his wife or a gestational mother obtain an abortion or that it would resolve a gestational surrogacy case on the basis of genetic connections alone while ignoring the experience of pregnancy, as did the California courts in *Anna J. v. Mark C.* (286 Cal. Rptr. 369 (Cal. App. 1991)).

But even if gamete donors may not be able to control or contract to use the bodies of others in order to effectuate their choices about genetic parenthood, one can still ask whether they have a right to financial assistance from their insurers or the state for procedures such as IVF. The abortion funding cases made abundantly clear that the state need not provide the financial resources needed for, nor force others to remove economic barriers to, an individual's exercise of a constitutional right.[2] If the state is not constitutionally required to fund abortion, it does not have to mandate that IVF be paid for either. Many insurers provide such coverage, however, either as a matter of choice or because a few states require them to do so, but usually only to married heterosexual couples (O'Rourke 1992). This practice of limiting resources for procreation on the basis of marital status may also survive scrutiny although it raises a closer constitutional question (*Eisenstadt v. Baird,* 405 U.S. 438 (1972)). But perhaps more important than the issue of its ultimate legality is the fact that this sort of discrimination reinforces a notion of the family as a married couple with children that at present applies to only one-quarter of the households in America (Married With Children 1992).

A more fundamental question than the rights and obligations of all those potentially affected by IVF is how firm the realm of protected procreational autonomy really is. After all, the *Davis* court relied in part on the absence in Tennessee law of any evidence of public policy protecting early embryos. The legislature may have failed to enact such laws in part because of concern that *Roe v. Wade* (410 U.S. 113 (1973)) and its progeny limited the state's power to protect fetal and embryonic life prior to viability (Op. Tenn. Att'y. Gen. 89-28, Feb. 22, 1989). One could always argue that the absence of legislation regarding frozen embryos is telling nonetheless because the state could have asserted that the lack of direct conflict with a woman's bodily integrity meant that it could have protected embryos ex utero without contravening *Roe,* but *Roe's* broad shadow makes this convoluted argument seem less compelling.

The Supreme Court, however, changed the legal landscape when it held in *Planned Parenthood of Southeastern Pennsylvania v. Casey* (112 S.Ct. 2791 (1992), p. 2064) that the state has a "substantial interest in potential life" even prior to viability and that the state is free to assert that interest so long as regulations do not have "the purpose or effect of placing a substantial obstacle in the path of a woman seeking an abortion of a nonviable fetus." This increased power to intervene prior to viability on behalf of the child who might be born, which was presaged in some of the preceding opinions (*Webster v. Reproductive Health Services*, 492 U.S. 490 (1989)), sends a clear invitation to the states. Other states have already passed statutes that evince an interest in life from the moment of conception,[3] and the day could come when Tennessee enacts laws that seek to protect embryos and fetuses from the time of fertilization or shortly thereafter. At that point, the constitutional protection of procreative autonomy would become a much closer issue although the *Davis* court's heavy emphasis on the privacy rights of gamete providers grounded in the state's constitution suggests that a couple would probably still prevail, at least as a matter of state law.

Yet even if the constitutional foundation and consequences of protecting "genetic + social parenthood" are not entirely clear, it probably was appropriate for Junior Davis to "win" in light of the positions of the parties by the time that the case reached them. His concerns that it would be difficult for him to have children who would not be raised in a home with two parents seem much more immediate than Mary Sue Davis Stowe's wish that the embryos be donated to unknown third parties to be gestated and reared. There is, however, a dichotomy here that both is troubling in its own terms and points out an inherent limitation in the decision to focus on the implications of "genetic + social parenthood" for the future. The court was willing to weigh Mr. Davis's experiences of being largely abandoned by his parents during childhood in considering the poignancy of his fears of what could happen to the children who might be born. At the same time, the justices gave virtually no heed to the "sweat equity" that Ms. Davis had invested in the creation of the embryos in the first place. Looked at in personal terms, it seems unjust for his earlier pain to count while hers did not.

This dichotomy also makes clear that in focusing on the disposition of the embryos that were in storage as the central issue, the court chose one

out of an array of potential points on the time line of IVF—a time line that begins when a couple seeks medical help for infertility and continues through a process of harvesting and fertilizing the woman's eggs, ending sometimes in failure and sometimes in giving birth. All that the Davises and particularly Ms. Davis had undergone before the embryos were frozen was essentially ignored. In addition, when it held that the gamete providers were equally situated with regard to making decisions about how the embryos were to be used, the court seemed to have in mind a world in which men and women share equally in the joys and burdens of parenthood. This ideal flies in the face of the reality that in most instances today women perform the overwhelming majority of child care duties (Areen 1992, p. 195).

The court's approach may be laudable to the extent that it encourages men to take parenthood more seriously (Schultz 1990). It is important to acknowledge, however, that the rules adopted in *Davis* run the risk of undervaluing the pain and suffering associated with the earlier stages of IVF and the disproportionate role that women currently play in caring for children. This approach also does little to address fears that pressure to do more and more to have a genetically connected child to raise commodifies women by reinforcing deep-seated views that value women primarily as baby-makers (Baruch, D'Adamo, and Seager 1988; Corea 1985; Rothman 1992; Stanworth 1987). Addressing these concerns, however, will require a radical transformation of the social construction of the new reproductive technologies and of the value placed on child-rearing in the society at large (Rothman 1989). Adopting a rule that gives more weight to the woman's contribution to IVF would go only a small part of the way toward this revolution, and only at the cost of minimizing men's roles in social parenthood, at least in the short term.

That some questions and even some quibbles remain should not detract from the Tennessee Supreme Court's achievement in *Davis v. Davis*. The opinion provides concrete guidance to all the potential participants in IVF and remarkably rich material for further discussion. While other state courts obviously are not bound by this opinion, justices in other jurisdictions will find it difficult to ignore this thoughtful analysis. But no matter how sweeping the import of *Davis* may be on the legal and ethical debate about IVF and other reproductive technologies, perhaps the most desirable outcome of this case would be that all couples recognize and consider the problems that may arise before they decide to embark on cryopreservation.

I would like to thank Jay Clayton for his insightful reading of earlier versions of this paper and Margaret L. Schmucker for her invaluable research assistance.

NOTES

1. *Ark. Stat. Ann.* 1992 (Michie), secs. 23-85-101, 23-85-137, 23-86-101, 23-86-118; *Haw. Rev. Stat* 1991, secs. 431 10A 116.5, 432.1-604; *1991 Ill. Laws* 87-681, sec. 1; *Ky. Rev. Stat. Ann.* 1991 (Michie), sec. 311.715.

2. *Harris v. McRae*, 448 U.S. 297 (1980); *Maher v. Roe*, 432 U.S. 464 (1977); *Poelker v. Doe*, 432 U.S. 519 (1977).

3. *La. Rev. Stat. Ann.* 1992 (West), sec. 14.87; *Mo. Ann. Stat.* 1992 (Vernon), sec. 1.205.1(1); *Utah Code Ann.* 1992, secs. 76-7-301, 301.1.

REFERENCES

Andrews, Lori B. 1986. The Legal Status of the Embryo. *Loyola Law Review* 32: 357–409.

———. 1987. *Medical Genetics: A Legal Frontier.* Chicago: American Bar Foundation.

AMA Board of Trustees. 1990. Frozen Pre-embryos. *Journal of the American Medical Association* 263: 2484–87.

Areen, Judith. 1992. *Family Law—Cases and Materials.* 3rd ed. Westbury, NY: Foundation Press.

Baruch, Elaine Hoffman; D'Adamo, Jr., Amadeo F.; and Seager, Joni, eds. 1988. *New Reproductive Technologies.* New York: Harrington Park Press.

Bonnicksen, Andrea L. 1989. *In Vitro Fertilization: Building Policy from Laboratories to Legislatures.* New York: Columbia University Press.

Browne, Colleen M., and Hynes, Brian H. [Note] 1990. The Legal Status of Frozen Embryos: Analysis and Proposed Guidelines for a Uniform Law. *Journal of Legislation* 17: 97–122.

Congregation for the Doctrine of the Faith. 1987. *Instruction on Respect for Human Life in Its Origin and on the Dignity of Procreation: Replies to Certain Ques-* *tions of the Day.* Boston: St. Paul Editions. Reprinted in Hull, Richard R., ed. 1990. *Ethical Issues in the New Reproductive Technologies,* pp. 21–39. Belmont, CA: Wadsworth Publishing Co.

Corea, Gena. 1985. *The Mother Machine: Reproductive Technologies from Artificial Insemination to Artificial Wombs.* New York: Harper & Row.

Developments in the Law. 1990. Medical Technology and the Law. *Harvard Law Review* 103: 1519–1676.

Knoppers, Bartha M., and LeBris, Sonia. 1991. Recent Advances in Medically Assisted Conception: Legal, Ethical and Social Issues. *American Journal of Law and Medicine* 17: 329–61.

Married with Children: The Waning Icon. 1992. *New York Times* (23 August): 2, sec. 4, col. 1.

O'Rourke, Melissa R. 1992. The Status of Infertility Treatments and Insurance Coverage: Some Hopes and Frustrations. *South Dakota Law Review* 37: 343–87.

Poole, Elisa Kristine. 1990. Allocation of Decision-Making Rights to Frozen Embryos. *American Journal of Family Law* 4: 67–102.

Price, Frances. 1989. Establishing Guidelines: Regulation and the Clinical Management of Infertility. In *Birthrights: Law and Ethics at the Beginnings of Life,* ed. Robert Lee and Derek Morgan, pp. 37–54. New York: Routledge.

Robertson, John A. 1990a. In the Beginning: The Legal Status of Early Embryos. *Virginia Law Review* 76: 437–517.

———. 1990b. Prior Agreements for Disposition of Frozen Embryos. *Ohio State Law Journal* 51: 407–24.

———. 1992. Ethical and Legal Issues in Preimplantation Genetic Screening. *Fertility and Sterility* 57: 1–11.

Rothman, Barbara Katz. 1989. *Recreating Motherhood: Ideology and Technology in a Patriarchal Society.* New York: W. W. Norton.

———. 1992. Not All That Glitters Is Gold. *Hastings Center Report* 22 (4): S11–15.

Schultz, Marjorie Maguire. 1990. Reproductive Technology and Intent-Based Parenthood: An Opportunity for Gender Neutrality. *Wisconsin Law Review* 1990: 297–398.

Scott, Russell. 1990. The Regulation of Artificial Procreation: Law, Ethics, and Other Options. *International Digest of Health Legislation* 41: 173–78.

Stanworth, Michelle, ed. 1987. *Reproductive Technology: Gender, Motherhood, and Medicine.* Minneapolis: University of Minnesota Press.

Wright, Ellen E. [Note] 1978. Father and Mother Know Best: Defining the Liability of Physicians for Inadequate Genetic Counseling. *Yale Law Journal* 87: 1488–1515.

Fetal Experimentation:
The Question of Ownership and Exploitation

WANDA TEAYS

As the "magic bullet,"[1] fetal tissue "is to medicine what superconductivity is to physics."[2] Fetal tissue transplants helped cure nearly 10,000 laboratory animals of diabetes,[3] successfully treated Parkinson's symptoms in monkeys induced with the disease,[4] and directly benefited patients with Parkinson's disease.[5] Fetal tissue is considered less "immunologically reactive," so the potential for rejection is minimal and the success rate promising.[6] In 1986, Robert Gale used fetal liver transplants on Chernobyl victims.[7] Fetal tissue transplants may help Alzheimer's disease, diabetes, Huntington's Chorea, spinal cord injuries, leukemia, blindness, aplastic anemia, stroke, certain kinds of brain damage,[8] and in studying AIDS.[9] A biotech firm, Hana Biologics, estimates a market potential of $8 billion for treating diabetes and $7 billion for supplying fetal neural cells to treat Parkinson's disease.[10] "The fact that demand for fetal organs and tissues greatly exceeds the available supply," observes James Roberts, "makes the fetus even more valuable."[11] The list of potential recipients is staggering—"millions of people."[12]

Against this backdrop of medical promise is the fear of scrupulous women willing to use their own bodies for a cut of the action. John Hillebrecht says if the technology fulfills its promise and competition for fetal tissue grows tight, "billions of dollars in temptation bodes ill for self-restraint on the part of corporate America. It is easy to imagine abortion clinics or indi-

Wanda Teays is Professor of Philosophy and Philosophy Department Chair at Mount St. Mary's College, Los Angeles.

vidual women holding out for a "piece of the action."[13] One specter raised is "the exploitation of women's reproductive capacity" and the subsequent treatment of the aborted fetus as a simple commodity.[14] In the face of such "commercialization of human life"[15] are ethical issues and public policy concerns and that, if we remove the profit incentive, a number of suspicions—such as the unjustified view of women—can be alleviated.

PART ONE: ETHICAL ISSUES AND CONCERNS

In the absence of clearly delineated Constitutional protection, the issues have generally been transferred onto the level of states [for policy considerations] and medical professions and ethics committees [for considerations of consent and use]. As of 1986, twenty-five states had addressed the issue,[16] with the guidelines both diverse and ambiguous. There is little agreement on research guidelines. At least eight states have statutes that prohibit the experimental use of cadaveric fetal tissue from induced abortions.[17] As Nicholas Terry[18] notes, Indiana regulates the transportation of an aborted fetus out of the state for experimentation purposes. Massachusetts prohibits all research on live human fetuses. Tennessee set guidelines for "possession" of any fetus born alive as a result of a voluntary abortion. California regulates the actual storage of fetal remains. Some states prevent the commercial disposition of fetuses; but, unless addressed by state statute, dead fetal tissue can be sold.[19] Nineteen states ban any non-therapeutic research on a live aborted fetus, while Arkansas and Utah permit all types of fetal research on a living aborted fetus.[20] Embryo experimentation has received some attention, with embryo sale and transfer already prohibited or restricted by some states.[21]

In Spring 1997 Arthur Caplan reported that retrieving sperm from dead men is raising issues of informed consent.[22] Embryo research "has taken place in something of a legal vacuum" and some regulatory regimes, such as the Uniform Anatomical Gift Act and Health Department regulations, apply to fetuses but not to embryos.[23] "For the purposes of the criminal law . . . the live embryo *in vitro* lacks any nominate legal protection, fitting within neither 'property' nor 'persons' regimes."[24]

There is also the conflict of rights between woman and fetus: Treating the fetus as if it were outside a woman's body is seen as a "political act."[25] There is considerable ambivalence about pregnancy. "There is a tendency to value the product of pregnancy and childbirth (the foetus, the infant) over the mother herself."[26] The very use of language like "farming fetuses," "organ farms," "harvesting fetuses," "spare embryos," suggests the fetus "has become a new type of property; it is now the sort of thing one can own."[27] Formerly a "vessel of lust"[28] the female body is now a vessel of procreation. Moreover, "Absent some form of constraint, the human body could eventually become a breeding factory for fetal tissue"[29] whereby women will become pregnant "to supply relatives, friends, or themselves with fetal tissue."[30] This concern is raised throughout the literature.[31]

The AMA's Council on Scientific Affairs and its Council of Ethical and Judicial Affairs both assert that, "Safeguards to reduce any motivation, reason or incentive by the woman to have an abortion can be developed to allow the benefits of this procedure to be made available to those who are in need of improved therapies."[32] This "specific benevolence," as James Childress calls it, was addressed by the Panel on Human Fetal Tissue Transplantation Research. They recommended that women donating fetal tissue for federally funded research not be permitted to designate the beneficiary, so they wouldn't treat the fetus as a commodity.[33] The warning is this: "We would not want to live in a society where women become pregnant for the purpose of making money."[34] However, the view that women will seek abortion because of fetal experimentation is more speculation than reality. As stated in the Report of Human Fetal Tissue Transplantation Research Panel, "the more than 30 years of publicized research involving fetal tissue has yielded 'no evidence that [such] research has had a material effect on the reasons for seeking an abortion in the past.'"[35]

There are other concerns as well; e.g., biotechnology firms "have spent millions of dollars in research and development positioning themselves to reap some of the billions of dollars to be made from fetal-cell transplants."[36] With *in vitro* fertilization and embryo transfers, the donation, sale or exchange of embryos is before us. Already cases regarding the custody of embryos have hit the courts; e.g., Junior Davis, a Tennessee man, sued his ex-wife to bar her from using any of their fertilized eggs.[37]

We are told that the "transformation of women into 'fetus factories' subject to the pressures of powerful interests is not as far-fetched as might seem."[38] Restricting the supplier, users and producers can profit and the societal moral conscience be appeased. That is, if the supplier of fetal tissue cannot participate in fetal sales, then we have not committed an indignity on the fetal body. Using fetal tissues in biomedical products can both compensate for that loss to the human community and be medically beneficial to others. The fact that middle men, the biotech corporations, stand to profit gets dismissed.[39] "Without a profit incentive," C. Ann Sheehan argues, "the benefits of such a therapy [using fetal tissue] may never be realized."[40] The fear is that, "If refining the proliferation of technology became a non-profit endeavor, the pace of advancement would slacken."[41]

We need to consider legal and moral authority around fetal experimentation. These five major arguments justify giving decision-making control to researchers, ethics committees, "storage authorities," governmental agents—rather than the woman, who is seen as most morally suspect. Christine Neff claims that, since *Roe v. Wade,* "In adopting for itself the role of defender of fetal rights, the state reveals its latent suspicion that a pregnant woman is untrustworthy, irresponsible, and an adversary to her fetus. Privacy doctrine has permitted the state to exercise increasing control.[42] Let us examine these arguments and counter-arguments below.

1. The Abdication of Maternal Responsibility

A pregnant woman necessarily abdicates her maternal duties by electing to abort. By so choosing, she loses all rights to direct use or disposal of the fetus. James David Roberts asserts that, " A woman's decision to put her personal autonomy ahead of her maternal duties to the fetus implies that she has rejected those maternal duties . . . it therefore operates as a legal abandonment."[43] The aborted fetus, subsequently, becomes the property of the hospital or "storage authority" for purposes of disposal or "donation In other words, an abortion disallows the woman from further control over or interest (legal, moral, or financial) in the fetus. Robert Morison agrees, holding that any fetal research poses "no particular ethical difficulty," since "the experimental subjects would be fetuses whose prospective parents will have specifically renounced the possibility of parenthood."[44] The woman should no more determine the fetus' future than we would allow a murderer to donate his victim's corpse for anatomical study.[45] Andrew Simons declared, "It is, purely and simply, cannibalism."[46]

Counter-Argument

Nicholas Terry says permitting anyone other than the aborting woman to determine such an issue puts an impermissible burden on the abor-

tion decision and he insisted that she decide the fetus' fate.[47]

2. The Argument from Special Moral Status

The fetus or embryo has some, but not all, rights accorded to a person and, thus, deserves protection. This claim takes various forms, according to the way the fetus gets classified. These categories are:

(i) *The Class of Human Beings:* The embryo is seen "as an individual human being, not with the same claims and rights as a newborn baby, but at least an individual deserving some protection."[48]

(ii) *The Class of Morally Distinct Entities:* The fetus is in a distinctive, relatively unique moral category, in which its status is close to but not identical with that of a typical adult and is both different from and superior to that of the 'higher' animals."[49]

(iii) *The Class of Vulnerable Beings:* The fetus is analogous to a newborn infant, an unconscious patient, a dying patient (spontaneous abortion), and to a condemned person (induced abortion)."[50]

(iv) *The Class of Conscious Beings:* Moral obligation arises at the point of fetal brain function and, with that, the couple's rights to control disposal is no longer a given. Embryo research must be subject to strict controls when the embryo has consciousness or some brain function. Before that, the embryo has no more status than an egg or sperm and, so, "there is no moral obligation to preserve the life of the embryo."[51]

Counter-Argument

The strongest case against these four versions of the Special Moral Status argument comes from Mary Anne Warren, who argues that, lacking the criteria of personhood, a fetus has no significant moral status or right.[52] There would be no ethical grounds for opposing fetal experimentation.

We might also consider legal precedent in trying to ascertain the moral status of the fetus. For example, in *Planned Parenthood of Central Missouri v. Danforth, Attorney General of Missouri*,[53] the Supreme Court noted that, the fetus cannot, in English law have any right of its own at least until it is born and has a separate existence from the mother. That permeates the whole of the civil law of this country and is, indeed, the basis of the decisions in those countries where the law is founded on the common law.[54]

A similar decision was reached in *Roe v. Wade*, that "embryos, like foetuses, are not treated as legal persons."[55] For Britain's Warnock Commission, appointed to appraise the new technologies, "the embryo had no legal status per se."[56] However, governmental agencies are not to be in total accord with the Court's perspective. For instance, the Report and Conclusions of the *HEW Support of Research Involving Human In Vitro Fertilization and Embryo Transfer* (4 May 1979), claimed that, "the Board is in agreement that the human embryo is entitled to profound respect, but this respect does not necessarily encompass the full legal and moral rights attributed to persons."[57] The fetus has a special moral status—effectively separating it from a mere thing or possession and, so, the woman has no legal or moral authority over the aborted fetus. Either she has no power over directing its disposal or allocation to medical research or she has consensual power.

3. The Argument from Consent

This argument has three variations, all centering on the question of informed consent and what can or should be assumed.

(i) *The Argument from Consent:* The woman has the right to give consent or proxy consent for use of the fetus in an experiment or for transplant purposes. In the case, for instance, of the Uniform Anatomical Gift Act, there must be consent of one parent in

the absence of resistance from the other.[58] Willingness to give "consent," however, is construed as a relinquishing of any further rights, control, or profit from resulting experimentation. In assenting to fetal experimentation, the woman is thus erased as a figure of any legal force.

Counter-Argument

Childress claims that, "In general, the level of information disclosure that would be expected in informed consent for therapy or research is not required for fetal tissue donation, although *the pregnant woman may request any information* prior to making a decision about donation."[59] Arthur Caplan notes, "the use of foetal tissue derived from abortuses is a practice that is shrouded in secrecy in the United States and most other nations."[60] Also, state laws governing the procurement and distribution of foetal tissues resulting from abortions are poorly understood by health care providers, patients and their next-of-kin.[61] The failure to provide information needed to make an informed consent suggests a desire to withhold it. It is unlikely the woman would be told of commercial possibilities of the fetal tissue, so no "consent" would have been given.

(ii) *The Argument from Permission:* As Annas, Glantz and Katz observe, "Only a small portion of the controversy surrounding fetal research is directly related to the issue of informed consent."[62] Shannon claimed that "consent" is a consistently emphasized and examined concept in discussions of this issue, testifying to the very difficulty of applying the notion to fetal research.[63] The doctrine of informed consent, which arose in *Salgo v. Leland Stanford Jr. Univ. Board of Trustees*,[64] has come to require that "a person or an entity with presumptively superior information as to risks, contents, or consequences take affirmative steps to disclose that information at the time another individual is faced with a decision for which it might prove pertinent."[65] It is now widely used when a substituted judgement is thought necessary. The National Commission for the Protection of Human Subjects of Biomedical and Behavioral Research does not use "proxy consent" or "consent of a legally authorized representative"—instead, the parent or guardian is asked to give "permission."[66]

Counter-Argument

Robert Veatch sees both the woman and the fetus as research subjects. Both actual and proposed experimentation has involved research on the soon-to-be-aborted fetus *in vitro*. In a study of rubella vaccine, for example, women who requested an abortion were asked to take the vaccine and to postpone the abortion procedure for three to four weeks.[67] "By the canons of medical experimentation," Veatch asserts, "the researchers cannot give such proxy consent for the fetuses *as research subjects.*[68] One issue is what should happen if a 24-week old (nonviable) fetus is maintained for a two-week experimentation and, as of 26 weeks, may be viable (and more distinctly human life).[69] For Veatch, we would then face a situation of one moral wrong needed to rectify another.

(iii)   *The Argument from Assumed Consent:* A variation on proxy consent, the argument is that we are a human family and can assume altruism. Mary Mahowald assumes a predisposition to donate organs or otherwise act in a way beneficial to humanity.[70] This predisposition is seen as natural, if not innate; thus permitting use of fetal tissue for therapeutic purposes. Arguing in terms of human need, Mahowald thinks the notion of proxy consent applies here.

Counter-Argument

A great deal is presumed in arguing a predisposition toward humanity. However much we *ought*

to give of ourselves freely to help others, it is not an obligation ordinarily perceived. For example, in *Belchertown School v. Saikewicz,* the Court was asked to approve the removal of a kidney from an incompetent patient for transplant into an ailing family member. The Court ruled that, "Individual choice is determined not by the vote of the majority but by the complexities of the singular situation viewed from the unique perspective of the person called on to make the decision.[71] In other words, "the problems of arriving at an accurate substituted judgment in matters of life and death vary greatly in degree, if not in kind, in different circumstances."[72] Perhaps, with fetal experimentation, the notion is stretched too far and, so, as did the National Commission, switch to "permission."

4. Argument from the Doctor-Patient Relationship

Rosalind Petchesky asserts that there is a "growing tendency of ob-gyn practitioners to view the fetus as their 'patient' independently of the woman who carries it."[73] The result is that the woman's womb has been "deprivatized" and she is no longer the primary patient.[74] Her womb is now a "maternal environment" or a "fetal container."[75] This was the Court's position in *Johnson v. Calvert,* where Crispina Calvert (the genetic mother) was deemed the "real mother"— and Anna Johnson (the gestational mother) was deemed a "foster mother,"[76] and described as a "human incubator."[77] With fetal experimentation, the doctor-*fetal* relationship has become a doctor-*patient* relationship. This elevates the position of the fetus to the status of patient for life-saving and life-enhancement purposes—as, e.g., argued for by Arthur Dyck.[78] Christine Overall observed, "The assumption is that the advocate for the fetus/newborn is, or should be, the doctor, not the pregnant woman/new mother."[79]

This shift would affect the woman's role in *any* medical decisions to be made regarding the fetus (*in utero* or *ex utero*). There have already been lawsuits regarding alleged negligent behavior or drug use of pregnant women, forced Caesarian sections, and sustaining brain-dead pregnant women until a Caesarian section could be performed.

Counter-Argument

Abortion procedures often result in the destruction, crushing, or breaking up of the fetus. Those with the least risk to the woman are the most damaging to the fetus. Should these priorities be switched? Hysterotomies are being performed—right now only on "volunteers." Since *Colautti v. Franklin*[80] disallowed the forced use of a hysterotomy to save the fetus in an abortion, doctors and researchers must rely on the "goodwill" of the pregnant woman. That women ever agreed to unnecessary hysterotomies suggests the potential for controlling both the timing[81] and method of abortions. In *Quinlan* it was ruled that the doctor has no right independent of the patient. "He can act only if the patient explicitly or implicitly, directly or indirectly, gives him the permission [with the rights and duties of the family dependent upon the presumed will of the unconscious patient]."[82] The application to fetuses, *qua patient,* may be inferred. Doctors should see themselves as advocates of both the woman and the fetus.[83] The fetus cannot give permission. Neither the woman nor the doctor here can presume to know what the "presumed will" of the fetus could possibly be.

5. The Argument from Sacrifice for the Public Good

Hans Jonas brings up an argument that could justify fetal research based on a notion of the common good. He says,

> . . . the unknown in our problem is the so-called common or public good and its potentially superior claims, to which the individual good must or might sometimes be sacrificed, in circumstances that in turn must also be counted

among the unknowns of our questions. Note that in putting the matter in this way—that is, in asking about the right of society to individual sacrifice—the consent of the sacrificial subject is no necessary part of the *basic* question.[84]

Counter-Argument

Adherents of individual sacrifice would seem to run afoul with the Thirteenth Amendment which prohibits involuntary servitude. The utilitarian benefits of sacrificing to public good are overshadowed by individual rights, as we saw in *Belchertown School v. Saikewicz,* where the Court was concerned that we not place "a lesser value on [the incompetent patient's] intrinsic worth and vitality."[85] *Saikewicz* may act as a precedent if we assume a special moral status on the part of the fetus. Moreover, *Saikewicz* might be applicable, since fetal transplantation may involve the use of live fetuses; particularly with Parkinson's or Alzheimer's, where live fetal brain grafts or cells must be used.[86]

PART TWO: THE QUESTION OF COMMERCIAL RIGHTS AND EXPLOITATION

> . . . the California Legislature recognized "that medical experimentation on human subjects is vital for the benefit of mankind," but declared that "such experimentation shall be undertaken with due respect to the preciousness of human life and the right of individuals to determine what is done to their own bodies."[87]

The possibility of commercial profits seems imminent. We might ask, "If the biotechnology corporations stand to make millions of dollars off the tissue of one person, does not basic fair play demand some sharing of the wealth?"[88] As Hillbrecht says, "Cell lines developed from unique tissues can prove to be commercial gold mines. Trade in fetal tissue may represent an even richer vein and could dwarf the present indus-try."[89] We are warned, however, against doing anything to deter the development of cell-lines, where only "compelling reasons" could slow down this corporate momentum.[90]

People do not want to talk in terms of "own-ership." George Annas, for instance, rejects this concept, suggesting that frozen embryos be de-stroyed when the purpose for freezing them has been fulfilled or when the gamete donors have both died. Lori Andrews claims that the progen-itors have the right to control disposition of em-bryos, including the right to allow them to ex-pire.[91] The Tennessee judge deciding over the frozen embryos rejected the notion of ownership in place of custody, drawing upon a personhood-upon-conception argument. Ms. Davis' attorney said the embryos "should be labeled preborn children."[92]

People sell blood, men sell sperm, and women are paid to bear another couple's child, and pay-ments to hospitals are made for embryos and fe-tuses. And, as we saw with the California Supreme Court decision in *John Moore v. The Re-gents of the University of California*,[93] ownership and property rights may collide with scientific re-search and biomedical patents. When such a con-flict happens ownership may be limited and property rights circumscribed. The fact that money actually changes hands around sperms, embryos, and fetuses raises some questions of commerce. That hospitals receive processing or administrative fees for each of the hundreds of thousands of fetuses used annually for research purposes means some degree of commodifica-tion has already occurred.

This calls for our participation in decision-making. As Childress observes, "Since she [the aborting woman] is donating for transplantation research, she may also have an interest in know-ing any plans for commercialization."[94] Women have the right to be informed. This is not a view widely held. For example, the British Polking-horne report (1989) recommended the pregnant

woman have "no knowledge of what will actu-ally happen to the fetus or fetal tissue" and not allow her "to make any direction regarding the use of her fetus or fetal tissue."[95] The concern is: "a woman's right to exercise control over her body does not include the right to exploit an aborted fetus."[96]

The Human Fetal Tissue Transplantation Re-search Panel (1988) recognizes the woman's moral authority over the disposal of fetal re-mains. "She still has a special connection with the fetus and she has a legitimate interest in its disposition and use. Furthermore, the dead fetus has no interests that the pregnant woman's dona-tion would violate."[97] The question of her com-mercial or property rights, however, is yet an-other matter. We simply do not envision someone making a windfall profit on our re-mains. The idea that a beneficiary of an organ, the researchers, or others profit from our do-nated remains seems unfathomable. The concern that women will seek to abort[98] or go into the fetus-making business appears to be a serious misunderstanding of (a) the health risks; (b) the moral distaste or revulsion women might feel; (c) the low probability for commercial profit. Nevertheless many commentators wish to pre-vent "the morally unpleasant result of women in-tentionally conceiving human life for the sole purpose of harvesting the fetus for spare parts."[99]

In his dissent in *Moore*, Justice Mosk of the California Supreme Court voiced criticism of the majority's failure to recognize Moore's property rights; arguing that the commercialization of biomedical products that would not have been possible without the patient's contribution; i.e., without his unique genetic contribution.[100] Mosk suggested the idea of joint contributors or co-inventors to recognize the contributions of both the patient and the researcher. The fear that women will somehow abuse their reproductive abilities and turn pregnancy into pregnancy-for-profit ignores the great social and personal costs that would ensue from commercializing procreation. In a footnote the *Moore* Court noted: "We are not called upon, nor are we attempting, to resolve the complex issues relating to the human fetus."[101] Nevertheless, the possible application of *Moore* to fetal experimentation remains to be seen.

Fetal tissues and cells are not in a distinct category separate from the woman's own cells and tissues. It may be abhorrent to think of the aborted fetus as the "property" of the woman who nurtured it, but she may yet have an "interest rightfully obtained" (a quasi-property right) over that fetus. The fetus developed only by means of the use of her body. A miscarriage or abortion may not negate the rights and interests she has accrued. The consent to an abortion is not a consent to give the doctor control over the fetus. "Disposal" is not equivalent to "donation." An agreement to an abortion is not an agreement to commercial exploitation.

We could amend Mark Danis' suggestion that we "construct a 'Chinese wall' between the donor and the recipient"[102] and extend that wall to separate donors and researchers as well. This would prevent the sort of abuses found in the Moore case. There are serious issues facing us as a society around biomedical experimentation and the commercial use of human tissue, body parts, and, in this case, fetuses.[103] As Justice Mosk observed in *Moore,* "Such research tends to treat the human body as a commodity—a means to a profitable end."[104] There are significant concerns that, with fetal experimentation, researchers are also treating the human body as a commodity, as a means to an end.

We ought to disallow the commercial exploitation of aborted fetuses, embryos, and fetal remains. We may be wiser to remove the profit motive from the picture altogether. As Nadine Taub says, "It's a hard one, whether fetuses should be treated as renewable body tissue that can be sold, or as organs that can't be. I don't think fetal tissue should be saleable. And it seems to me that if women can't make money off it,

companies shouldn't be able to make money off it, either."[105]

REFERENCES

1. John M. Hillebrecht, "Regulating the Clinical Uses of Fetal Tissue: A Proposal for Legislation," in *The Journal of Legal Medicine,* Vol. 10, No. 2, 1989 at 269.
2. C. Ann Sheehan, "Fetal Tissue Implants: An Explosive Technology Needs National Action," in *Dickinson Law Review,* Vol. 92, No. 4, Summer 1988 at 897, quoting from Gorman, "A Balancing Act of Life and Death," *Time,* Feb. 1, 1988 at 62. Lieberman later suggested the analogy to the fountain of youth. (cf. 897–8, footnote 25)
3. Hans Sollinger, testimony before National Institutes of Health Human Fetal Tissue Transplantation Research Panel (NIH Panel) Sept. 14–15 1988, Transcript at 90 as quoted by Rachel Benson Gold and Dorothy Lehrman, "Fetal Research Under Fire: The Influence of Abortion Politics," in *Family Planning Perspectives,* vol. 21, no. 1., January/February 1989 at 7.
4. Mahowald, Silver, and Ratcheson, "The Ethical Options in Transplanting Fetal Tissue," *Hastings Ctr. Report,* Feb. 1987 at 10, as quoted by Michael J. Walker, "Fetal Tissue Harvesting: Should Courts be the Final Arbiter?" in *Gonzaga Law Review,* Vol. 23, no. 3, 1987/88 at 622.
5. Thomas H. Maugh II, "Fetal Tissue Eases Symptoms of Parkinson's, Team Finds," *Los Angeles Times,* 2 Feb 1990, A 25, col. 1.
6. Mahowald, Silver, & Ratcheson, at 10, as quoted by Walker, *supra* note 4 at 622.
7. Gold and Lehrman, *supra* note 3 at 7.
8. C. Ann Sheehan, *supra* note 2 at 897.
9. Lindsay Tanner, "Fetal Tissue Use Raises Questions," *Los Angeles Times,* June 26, 1989, col. 3.
10. Hillebrecht, *supra* note 1 at 289–290. He notes that Hana "obviously" now wants to make a great deal of money selling the fetal cell line and these cells will be marketed under the registered trademark "Cytograft." See p. 308.
11. James David Roberts, "The Intentional Creation of Fetal Tissue for Transplants: The Womb as a Fetus Farm?" in *The John Marshall Law Review,* Vol. 21, No. 4, Summer 1988 at 857.
12. Bioethicist Arthur Caplan, as quoted by Hillebrecht at 286. Hillebrecht cites such potential recipients of fetal cell treatment as: 1.5 million people with Parkinson's, 2.5 to 3 million with Alzheimer's disease, 6

million diabetics, 400,000 stroke victims and hundreds of thousands of accident victims. See Hillbrecht pp. 285–86.

13. Hillebrecht, *supra* note 1 at 290.

14. Id. at 287.

15. Walker, *supra* note 4, at 627.

16. Nicholas P. Terry, "Alas! Poor Yorick, I Knew Him *Ex Utero:* The Regulation of Embryo and Fetal Experimentation and Disposal in England and the United States," *Vanderbilt Law Review,* Vol. 39, No. 3: April 1986 at 468.

17. *Report of the Human Fetal Tissue Transplantation Research Panel* 1988, I: 13, as noted in James F. Childress, "Ethics, Public Policy, and Human Fetal Tissue Transplantation," *Kennedy Institute of Ethics Journal,* Vol. 1, No. 2, June 1991, at 113.

18. Terry, *supra* note 16, at 437–439.

19. The National Organ Transplant Act, 42 U.S.C. sec. 274e (Supp. 1984), as noted by Sheehan, *supra* note 2 at 901.

20. Sheehan, *supra* note 2 at 911.

21. Id.

22. Noted by Gina Kolata, "Uncertain Area for Doctors: Saving Sperm of Dead Men," *New York Times,* 30 May 97.

23. Terry, *supra* note 16 at 456.

24. Terry, *supra* note 16 at 458.

25. Rosalind Pollack Petchesky "Foetal Images: The Power of Visual Culture in the Politics of Reproduction," in Michelle Stanworth, ed., *Reproductive Technologies: Gender, Motherhood and Medicine* (Minneapolis: University of Minnesota Press, 1987) at 65.

26. Michelle Stanworth, "Reproductive Technologies and the Deconstruction of Motherhood," in Michelle Stanworth, *supra* note 25 at 26–27.

27. Id. at 50.

28. As noted by Zillah R. Eisenstein, *The Female Body and the Law* (Berkeley: University of California Press, 1988) at 83, referring to Peter Gay's comment of the nineteenth-century view of women.

29. Walker, *supra* note 4 at 627. Clearly the human body to which Walker refers here is a human *female* body.

30. Mark, W. Danis, "Fetal Tissue Transplants: Restricting Recipient Designation," in *The Hastings Law Journal,* Vol. 39, No. 5, July 1988, at 1080. Even Danis, however, admitted that, whereas there have been reports of women desiring to do this, there have been no reported instance of it actually occurring. (Danis at 1080).

31. See, e.g., Jenn Swenson Bregman, "Conceiving to Abort and Donate Fetal Tissue: New Ethical Strains in the Transplantation Field—A Survey of Existing Law and a Proposal for Change," in *UCLA Law Review,* Vol. 36, No. 6, August 1989 at 1194. See also Hillebrecht, *supra* note 1 and Childress, *supra* note 17 at 106.

32. Tanner, *supra* note 9 at col. 3.

33. Childress, *supra* note 17 at 106.

34. Hillebrecht, *supra* note 1 at 290, quoting in agreement Nancy Dubler, director of Montefiore Medical Center.

35. Gold and Lehrman, *supra* note 3 at 11.

36. Hillebrecht, *supra* note 1 at 291. Hillebrecht, himself, does not necessarily approve of this, since he seeks to balance the needs of the sick and dying against the risks of such an industry. In his view legislation is the only way to meet this challenge.

37. See "Custody of Stored Embryos Disputed in Divorce Trial," in *Los Angeles Times,* 8 August 1989.

38. Hillebrecht, *supra* note 1 at 320. Hillebrecht's solution, as most others, is to prohibit the sale of fetal tissue.

39. As we will see in the discussion of the John Moore case in the last section of this article, even the Court is loathe to discourage medical research and biomedical technology by giving any commercial rights to the person from whom cells were taken and used to profitable ends.

40. Sheehan, *supra* note 2 at 907.

41. Hillebrecht, *supra* note 1 at 309.

42. Christine L. Neff, "Woman, Womb, and Bodily Integrity," in *Yale Journal of Law and Feminism,* Vol. 3, No. 2, Spring 1991 at 331.

43. It might be argued that, at least in many cases, a "sale" rather than "donation" transpires, since hospitals often get paid a nominal sum ($75 in 1975) to cover expenses, processing, and so on. See James David Roberts, "The Intentional Creation of Fetal Tissue for Transplants: The Womb as a Fetus Farm," *John Marshall Law Review,* Summer 88, Vol. 21, No. 4, at 854.

44. As quoted by Robert M. Veatch, *Case Studies in Medical Ethics,* (Cambridge, Ma: Harvard Univ. Press, 1977) at 210.

45. Terry, *supra,* note 16 at 469. This, however, disregards the questionable abortion/murder and fetus/person parallels drawn in his analogy.

46. Andrew Simons, "Brave New Harvest," *Christianity Today,* 19 November 1990, at 26.

47. Terry, *supra* note 16 at 469. He cites, as legal support, *Planned Parenthood Ass'n v. Fitzpatrick,* 401 F. Supp. 554 (E.D. Pa. 1975) and *Franklin v. Fitzpatrick,* 428 U.S. 902 (1976).

48. Marcia Wurmbrand, "Frozen Embryos: Moral, Social, and Legal Implications," *So Cal Law Rev.,* Vol. 59: 1986 at 1089.

49. Richard Wasserstrom, "Ethical Issues Involved in Experimentation on the Nonviable Human Fetus," from James M. Humber and Robert F. Almeder, eds., *Biomedical Ethics and the Law* (New York: Plenum Press, 1976) at 287.

50. As noted in Paul Ramsey, "The Limited Role of Informed Consent in Protecting the Unborn," in George J. Annas, Leonard H. Glantz, and Barbara F. Katz, *Informed Consent to Human Experimentation: The Subject's Dilemma* (Cambridge, Ma: Ballinger Pub. Co., 1977), at 198.

51. Id. at 70.

52. Mary Anne Warren, "On the Moral and Legal Status of Abortion," in Robert Baird and Stuart Rosenbaum, eds., *The Ethics of Abortion* (Buffalo, N.Y.: Prometheus Books, 1989). See especially 76–79.

53. [428 U.S. 52(1976)]

54. As noted by R.D. Mackay, "The Relationship Between Abortion and Child Destruction in English Law," *Medicine and Law*, Vol. 7, No. 2, 1988 at 78.

55. Cited in Janet Gallagher, "Eggs, Embryos and Foetuses: Anxiety and the Law," Michelle Stanworth, *supra* note 25 at 142.

56. Warnock, 1985, section 11.16, as noted by Janet Gallagher, *supra* note 55 at 141. She quotes from the Warnock Commission's report in which, generally speaking, the Commission declared that the human embryo "is not under the present law in the UK accorded the same status as a living child or adult, nor do we necessarily wish it to be accorded the same status." (sec. 11.17 Warnock report), as quoted Gallagher, *supra* note 55 at 141.

57. As quoted by Peter Singer and Deane Wells, *Making Babies: The New Science and Ethics of Conception* (New York: Scribners, 1985), at 184.

58. Mary B. Mahowald, "Ethical Aspects of Neural Fetal Tissue Transplantation," public lecture Mount St. Mary's College, 16 March 1989.

59. James F. Childress, *supra* note 17 at 114. My emphasis.

60. Arthur L. Caplan, "Should Foetuses or Infants be Utilized as Organ Donors?" *Bioethics*, Vol. 1, No. 2, 1987 at 124.

61. Id.

62. Annas, Glantz, and Katz, *supra* note 50 at 195.

63. cf., Thomas A. Shannon, *Bioethics*, Third Edition, (NY: Paulist Press, 1976) at 255.

64. 317 P. 2d 170 (Cal 1957).

65. Lynn A. Baker, "I Think I Do: Another Perspective on Consent and the Law," *Law, Medicine and Health Care*, Vol. 16, No. 3–4, Fall/Winter 1988 at 256.

66. As noted by Robert J. Levine, "Clarifying the Concepts of Research Ethics," in Shannon, *supra* note at 63 at 308.

67. From *Research on the Fetus*, "Report and Recommendations of the National Commission for the Protection of Human Subjects of Biomedical and Behavioral Research," as quoted by Annas, Glantz, and Katz, *supra* note 50 at 197.

68. Id. at 212.

69. Id. at 212.

70. Public Lecture, "Ethical Aspects of Neural Fetal Tissue Transplantation," Mount St. Mary's College, 16 March 1989.

71. As quoted by Thomas A. Shannon and Jo Ann Manfra, eds., *Law and Bioethics: Texts With Commentary on Major U.S. Court Decisions* (New York: Paulist Press, 1982) at 182–3.

72. Id. at 183.

73. Rosalind Pollack Petchesky, *Abortion and Woman's Choice: The State, Sexuality, and Reproductive Freedom*, (Boston: Northeastern Univ Press, 1984) at 352.

74. Id. at 353.

75. Attributed to George Annas by Nancy Rhoden, "Cesareans and Samaritans," in George Annas and Nancy Rhoden, eds., *Ethical Issues in Modern Medicine*, 3rd ed. (Mountain View, Ca.: Mayfield Publishing Company, 1989) at 329.

76. No. X63190 (Cal.Super. Ct. Oct. 22, 1990), as noted by Nicole Miller Healy, "Beyond Surrogacy: Gestational Parenting Agreements Under California Law," in *UCLA Women's Law Journal*, Vol. 1:53, 1991 at 90.

77. *Los Angeles Times*, Oct. 23, 1990, at A24, col. 3, as noted in Healy, *supra* note 76, at 115, footnote 113.

78. From "Ethical Issues in Community and Research Medicine," as excerpted by Jay Katz, *Experimentation with Human Beings: The Authority of the Investigator, Subject, Professions, and State in the Human Experimentation Process* (New York: Russell Sage Foundation, 1972) at 505.

79. Christine Overall, *Ethics and Human Reproduction, A Feminist Analysis* (Boston: Allen and Unwin, 1987) at 6.

80. 439 U.S. 379 (1979), as discussed in James J. Nocon, "Physicians and Maternal-Fetal Conflicts: Duties, Rights, and Responsibilities," in 5 *J. Law & Health* (1990–1991) at 20.

81. This warrants our concern, given that "fetal age is an important factor. The best fetus for one purpose may be useless for another . . . While neurosurgical grafts have worked at 13 weeks, some researchers believe that about the ninth week is the best time to retrieve the tissue. For Diabetes, the 20th week seems best." cf. Hillebrecht, *supra* note 1 at 256, footnote 117.

82. Supreme Court statement in the *Quinlan* case, as excerpted in Thomas A. Shannon and Jo Ann Manfra, *supra* note 71 at 155.

83. Or, according to James Nocon, "the obstetrician is the mother's advocate." (See Nocon, *supra* note 80 at 19). Minimally, however, the doctor should not position herself as an adversary to the woman, nor should the pregnant woman and her fetus be treated as adversaries.

84. Hans Jonas, "Philosophical Reflections on Experimenting with Human Subjects," in Shannon, *supra* note 63 at 255.

85. As quoted by Shannon, *supra* note 63 at 183.

86. As raised by Robert J. White, "The Aborted Fetus: A Commercial Prize?" in *America,* Jan. 23, 1988, at 53.

87. Health and Safety. Code, sec. 24172–24175, as noted by *John Moore v. The Regents of University of California,* 202 Cal.App.3d 1230 - Cal. Rptr. - [July 1988] at 1267.

88. Hillebrecht, *supra* note 1 at 309.

89. Id. at 288.

90. Id. at 309.

91. As noted by Janet Gallager, "Eggs, Embryos and Foetuses: Anxiety and the Law," in Michelle Stanworth, *supra* note 25 at 149.

92. "Divorce Case Raises a New Issue: Status of Fertilized Human Eggs," *New York Times,* 9 August 1989.

93. 202 Cal.App.3d 1230.

94. Childress, *supra* note 17 at 114.

95. Childress, *supra* note 17 at 114.

96. Hillebrecht, *supra* note 1 at 319.

97. *Human Fetal Tissue Transplantation Research Panel* 1988 I:6, as quoted by Childress, *supra* note 17 at 112.

98. As Roberts contends this is already a reality, though "physicians have generally refused [approaches by women to conceive and abort] stating that the idea is medically and ethically unsound." See Roberts, *supra* note 18 at 853.

99. Roberts, *supra* note 18 at 853–854.

100. *John Moore v. The Regents of the University of California et al,* No. S006987, Supreme Court of California, 202 Cal App. 3d 1230, - Cal. Rptr. July 1988 at 187.

101. *John Moore,* at 1248.

102. Danis, *supra* note 48 at 1092.

103. Patricia Martin and Martin L. Lagod, "Biotechnology and the Commercial Use of Human Cells: Toward an Organic View of Life and Technology," in *Daily Journal Report,* 25 August, 1989.

104. *John Moore v. The Regents of the University of California, et al,* R 006987, California Supreme Court, at 183.

105. As quoted by C. Ann Sheehan, *supra* note 2 at 907, footnote 105.

The Telltale Heart: Public Policy and the Utilization of Non-Heart-Beating Donors

ARTHUR L. CAPLAN

ABSTRACT. The transplant community has quietly initiated efforts to expand the current pool of cadaver organ donors to include those who are dead by cardiac criteria but cannot be pronounced dead using brain-based criteria. There are many reasons for concern about "policy creep" regarding who is defined as a potential organ donor. These reasons include loss of trust in the transplant community because of confusion over the protocols to be used, blurring the line between life and death, stress on family members, and burdens imposed on health care providers when a long-standing policy regarding who can serve as a cadaver organ donor is unilaterally changed. While these concerns are not sufficient reason for abandoning efforts to broaden existing eligibility standards for cadaver donation, they are sufficient reasons for the transplant community to desist in changing existing standards without widespread professional and public discussion.

IN RECENT YEARS much attention has been paid to the problem of scarcity with respect to organs available for transplant (Caplan et al. 1992). Some centers have relaxed the criteria they use to determine eligibility for donation in order to allow the use of organs from older donors (Alexander, Vaughn, and Carey 1991). Other

ARTHUR CAPLAN is Director, Center for Bioethics and Trustee Professor of Bioethics, University of Pennsylvania, Professor of Molecular and Cellular Engineering and Professor of Philosophy, and Chief, Division of Bioethics, University of Pennsylvania Medical Center.

transplant programs are turning to living donors (Caplan 1992a). A few have begun to pursue strategies wherein the organs of recently deceased persons are preserved inside the body in order to permit requests to be made to next-of-kin about donation. Some transplant centers in the United States such as Pittsburgh, Minnesota, Stanford, Columbia, Loma Linda as well as in many other nations are pursuing research on the feasibility of using animals as sources of organs. And many centers are continuing research into the development of artificial organs including heart, liver, lung, and pancreas.

A few transplant programs including the University of Pittsburgh in collaboration with their regional organ procurement organizations, have decided to pursue a strategy of trying to obtain organs from those who meet the criteria for cardiopulmonary death as a result of the elective removal of life-support technologies and the forgoing of resuscitative efforts. This decision is a response to the recognition that the prospects for obtaining significant increases in the supply of transplantable organs from cadaver sources under existing eligibility criteria are exceedingly poor. The number of persons who die each year in the United States under circumstances which permit the determination of "brain death" is so small that it is unlikely that any change in existing public policy is going to greatly influence the overall availability of cadaver organs for transplantation to those in need. In order to obtain

Kennedy Institute of Ethics Journal 3, 2 (1993): 251–262. Copyright 1993. Permission granted by Arthur L. Caplan and The John Hopkins University Press.

large increases in the supply of organs it will be necessary to do more than change public attitudes or laws. The only way to achieve a significant expansion in the overall number of available organs is to significantly enlarge the number of potential sources or donors.

The number of persons eligible to donate organs who die when heart and lung functions stop is believed to be much larger than the number who are pronounced "brain-dead" while on life-support. There appears to be a sizable number of persons who die while on life-support but who, for various reasons, are not or cannot be pronounced "brain-dead" (Hibberd et al. 1992). This is a number that could be made even larger if terminally ill persons were placed on life-support prior to death solely for the purpose of obtaining organs for transplantation to others. If the families of all persons who die according to cardiac criteria could be approached about the possibility of organ donation, and if methods could be designed to procure viable organs from those who die of irreversible cardiac failure rather than irreversible loss of all brain function, the size of the pool of potential donors could be greatly expanded (Feest et al. 1990; Hibberd et al. 1992).

The strategy of utilizing persons who suffer death as a result of the irreversible loss of cardiac function is, as those in the transplant community who support this approach are eager to point out, not unprecedented. The strategy has been used in the United States and other nations, and unlike the United States, a few countries never abandoned it (DeVita, Snyder, and Grenvik 1993). Before brain-based criteria for death were articulated and the standard was codified into state laws, non-heart-beating cadaver donors (NHBCDs) constituted a significant source of kidneys for what were then experimental attempts to use non-related cadaver kidneys for transplants (Fox and Swazey 1978).

The fact that there are precedents for using NHBCDs provides some moral ballast for those who now suggest pursuing procurement strategies that would allow the use of NHBCDs. So does the constant invocation of shortage and the inability to save lives which always accompany discussions in the professional literature of the merits of using NHBCDs. The fact that current proposals to expand the donor pool using those with irreversible cardiac failure invoke the past or research in other nations is, however, also a sign of just how fraught with potential moral problems the use of NHBCDs is.

The best strategy for gaining support for the expansion of the cadaver pool from those pronounced "brain-dead" to include those who meet some agreed upon standard of cardiac death is to depict the proposed expansion as an incremental transition rather than a drastic break with existing policy. Incremental change is an easier road to travel in terms of changing public policy concerning organ procurement than arguing for a drastic break with existing practice. Moreover, if the general public and legislators can be gradually familiarized with the practice of utilizing NHBCDs by having a few transplant procurement programs retrieve organs from such sources, then what might best be termed 'policy creep' becomes a possibility. Once a few centers have actually retrieved organs and successfully transplanted them to needy recipients it becomes easier to make the case for changing procurement practices.

While incrementalism is already in evidence with respect to the use of NHBCDs as a way to alleviate the frustrating shortage in the supply of organs, the moral problems associated with the use of NHBCDs are of such a magnitude that policy creep may not be possible. If these problems are not adequately and explicitly addressed, there is a very real danger that policy creep with respect to procuring organs from NHBCDs could result in a public relations disaster for the transplant field.

Five areas loom as especially controversial. First, what are the factors really fueling the search for new donor sources on the part of the transplant community? Unspoken or unacknowledged motives could be especially damaging to efforts to gain support for a redefinition of donor eligibility. A second set of ethical issues revolves around problems raised by the handling, management, and treatment of terminally ill or grievously injured patients when organ procurement is an acknowledged goal. A third area of controversy concerns the responsibilities and interest of families who would be involved in procurement from NHBCDs and the impact such a strategy might have upon them. Another set of third parties influenced by a shift in procurement practice are providers not connected directly to the transplant field. What responsibilities and duties would procurement from NHBCDs impose upon them? Finally, to what extent would the lines between life and death and killing and letting die be blurred or, be perceived as being blurred, by allowing procurement from those who have suffered cardiac death or who would be managed so as to allow their death to occur in a manner that would maximize the chance for obtaining organs?

MOTIVES FOR EXPANDING THE DONOR POOL

One of the critical determinants of the general public's reaction to proposed changes in the definition of who can serve as a source or donor of organs is the presumed motives of those seeking change. The dominant theme regarding motive in the literature of organ and tissue procurement in recent years has been the elimination of scarcity. Many suggestions have been made for changing public policy regarding organ transplantation. These include ensuring that requests are made of the families of those pronounced "brain-dead" (Caplan 1988a, 1992b); moving toward a public policy of presumed consent (Matas et al. 1985); reciprocal altruism (Kleinman and Lowy 1992); and use of markets (Peters 1991; Cohen 1991). Other suggestions involve shifting the composition of the donor pool:

living donors (Spital 1991; Caplan 1992a), NHBCDs (Anaise et al. 1989; Rapaport 1991; DeVita, Snyder, and Grenvik 1993), animals (Caplan 1992b, 1992c), prisoners condemned to death (Guttmann 1992), or anencephalic infants (Caplan 1988b; Grenvik 1992). Every one of the rationales given for change is couched exclusively in terms of the need to narrow or eliminate the gap between the supply and need for organs for transplants.

It seems impolite, if not downright paranoid, to wonder about the motives of those who argue for a shift in professional practice or public policy in the procurement of organs when lives are being lost every day for want of organs. Indeed, some have argued (Caplan 1992b) that it is morally incumbent on health care professionals who face situations, such as organ transplantation, in which rationing is necessary, to make every effort to alter the conditions that create scarcity; therefore, those who pursue strategies aimed at securing more organs are doing what is morally required. Those who are made uneasy by efforts to ameliorate scarcity and wonder about what motives lie behind them are often put in the position of appearing to defend abstract sentiments instead of saving lives (Fox and Swazey 1992; Kass 1992).

Scarcity and the deaths which result from it are indisputably real. But, the motive for expanding the supply of donors is not confined to the desire to help those on waiting lists or who might get on waiting lists if there were more organs. These motives must be analyzed and scrutinized since if the public believes that those in the field of transplantation are not being entirely forthcoming about their motives in seeking a wider base for organ procurement this will create enormous resistance to any proposed changes in existing policy.

An important motive for seeking more organs is the desire to see the transplant field grow. Unless significantly more organs become available, continued growth in the number of hospitals that perform transplants, the teams that obtain organs, and the number of surgeons who do these procedures will be impossible. It has become all but impossible to justify additional kidney or heart transplant centers in the United States. Organ procurement organizations are feeling pinched as the ceiling on the supply of organs brings pressure to bear to centralize and streamline their procurement activities. The only way for the field of transplantation to grow is to secure more organ donors.

A related motive for aggressively seeking an expansion in the pool of potential organ donors is money. The companies that manufacture immunosuppressive drugs such as cyclosporine and FK-506 would like to see what are already extremely lucrative markets expand. So would hospital administrators and boards of trustees who see transplantation as a useful marketing tool as well as a source of significant income. Large transplant centers keep many beds and lots of specialists occupied doing evaluations and post-transplant care. The only way to market more immunosuppressive drugs and to keep beds filled at a time of increasing pressures to contain health care costs is to find more organs to transplant.

The perception of motives plays a crucial role in the public's willingness to accept changes in public policy in areas as culturally sensitive as dying and death (Fox and Swazey 1992). Expanding the class of potential donors to include NHBCDs may seem sensible, even obligatory when the sole motive for doing so is saving lives. However, such efforts may appear unseemly, ghoulish, or even immoral if other factors such as professional self-interest, competition, and profit are at work but are swept under the rug.

CARE OF THE DYING

An obvious source of moral difficulty surrounding calls for the expansion of the donor pool to include NHBCDs or to permit the creation of NHBCDs by changes in the management of terminal illness and injury is the implications such

changes would have for public expectations, attitudes, and concerns about medical care. The protocol for the management of terminally ill patients who might become NHBCDs adopted in April of last year by the University of Pittsburgh Medical Center reflects this concern.

The overwhelming majority of the procedures and recommendations outlined in the Pittsburgh policy are aimed at ensuring that there is no conflation of decisions about patient care and the cessation of life-support with the desire for organ procurement. The protocol explicitly mandates that decisions about medical treatment "must be made separately from and prior to discussions of organ donation" (UPMC Policy 1993, p. A-1) and that no intervention may be undertaken "whose primary intention is to shorten the patient's life" (UPMC Policy 1993, p. A-2).

It is not easy to implement policies that try to draw boundaries between the management of the care of dying patients and the identification and management of cadavers for organ procurement. Current practices with respect to organ donation bear this out. Tales abound of hospitals mistakenly referring patients to OPOs as candidates for transplant without any effort having been made to pronounce "brain death," or on the basis of grossly inadequate "brain death" protocols. Every once in a while a story appears in the media about the decision of a procurement team to proceed with harvesting based on a judge's court order only to have relatives arrive after the fact, malpractice lawyers in tow, complaining about the unseemly exploitation of their loved ones. Surgeons and organ procurement organization personnel directly involved in organ retrieval know that once death is imminent, it is hard—if not impossible—not to manage patients as potential donors rather than simply as dying patients when there is reason to think that donation might be a possibility.

The reality is, however, that even if health care professionals are taught and firmly believe that they have a duty to keep the boundaries distinct between patient care and organ retrieval, their efforts to do so will be persuasive to the general public only to the extent that the public trusts the health care system. The level of trust in the American health care system is especially low among certain groups, notably African Americans, Native Americans, and some other minorities, and is weakening in society as a whole as the public begins to wonder about the influence of economic concerns on health care access and practice (Caplan 1992b; Priester 1992). Many Americans will not carry donor cards for fear that they will not receive aggressive care should they require it (Caplan et al. 1992). Given the distrust engendered by inadequate access to the present health care system, it is not likely that policies aimed at expanding the donor pool that are perceived as further fuzzing the line between life and death will elicit a positive response once they become known in the general community.

While there is a great deal of befuddlement expressed in the transplant community about why it is that relatively few Americans carry donor cards or actually give consent to organ donation when a relative dies, a key factor is that there are a large number of Americans who are either skittish about organ procurement for religious or aesthetic reasons or who simply do not trust doctors, nurses, and the health care system. Others believe that they cannot trust their lives to doctors because they lack insurance or are members of a minority group. And still others are extremely wary of organ donation under the circumstances in which it currently exists simply because they do not believe the system is fair with respect to the distribution of the organs that are available for transplant (Novello 1992).

Policy changes aimed at keeping a firm wall between procurement and the management of the dying in order to permit NHBCDs to be eligible for donation are emerging in a climate of growing distrust. It is not likely that those who now refuse to carry a donor card for fear they will be allowed to die or even killed for their parts will find much solace in administrative policies promulgated by committees of physi-

cians at large transplant centers. Assurances that the management of the dying will not be influenced by interest in organ retrieval are likely to fall on ears that are already skeptical about current practices and safeguards.

FAMILIES

Very little is known about the impact of requests concerning organ and tissue donation upon family members and friends. While some studies of families who have consented to donation indicate that the vast majority did not feel troubled or unduly stressed by requests (Batten and Prottas 1987), almost nothing is known about families who refuse requests. Since many more families say "no" than "yes" to requests, there is reason for concern that families may find the topic of organ donation troubling or stressful. Proposals to expand the pool of potential donors by including NHBCDs, or by managing the terminally ill to allow them to become NHBCDs, may increase the burdens of grieving families and friends.

Those who believe that the goal of public policy is to permit individuals maximum autonomy will find concerns about the impact on families irrelevant. Respect for autonomy requires that those who want to be organ donors be allowed to do so. Regardless of changes in public policy and professional practice individuals would decide whether to complete organ donor cards.

The problem with this line of argument is that it is neither persuasive nor realistic. When someone is terminally ill and unable to speak for themselves, or is newly dead, the interests of families inevitably begin to displace that person's interests. And to some extent they should.

Whether we are willing to admit it or not, autonomy yields in the face of death. And it should. Both the family and community have strong interests in the management of the terminally ill who are close to dying and the recently dead. Even if we accord high value to personal autonomy, any practice involving the management of dying—including the setting, the treatment of the corpse, the grief of survivors and the costs—that is seen as disturbing to the family is unlikely to be tolerated by society. If the management of NHBCDs is perceived as improper, disrespectful, callous, or crude then this strategy for increasing the supply of organs will quickly bump up against significant public policy obstacles (Fox and Swazey 1992).

HEALTH CARE PROFESSIONALS

To date, the greatest resistance to the development of protocols permitting donation from NHBCDs has come from nurses and physicians not directly connected to transplantation activities. Professional disquiet seems to center around fears that efforts to include NHBCDs may result in actions that hurry or hasten the death of a dying or terminally ill patient. Health care professionals do not want to be made party to killing in the name of organ procurement.

A different but equally problematic dilemma for health care professionals arose when Loma Linda University attempted to institute a protocol to permit the management of anencephalic babies in order to allow them to serve as organ donors. The protocol permitted the use of life-sustaining treatment with such babies in order to preserve organs until such time as cardiac death could be pronounced. However, interventions aimed at providing organ support had, at least apparently in some cases, the unintended effect of prolonging the dying of these infants. Nurses in particular were greatly troubled by being asked to participate in the administration of protocols which they felt were disrespectful to the infants and their parents. Ultimately the protocol was abandoned due to protests from health care professionals at Loma Linda.

A similar situation could arise with respect to NHBCDs. Technically, anencephalic infants still might fit into such protocols. But, even if they were excluded, it is possible that efforts to manage the terminally ill and dying might lead to the prolongation rather than the shortening of life. Furthermore, there is a real likelihood that efforts to allow persons to have life-support removed should they fall into a permanent vegetative state, locked-in syndrome, or other severely disabling and painful condition could create situations regarding organ donation which health care professionals would find extremely disquieting. In the future, changes in public policy with respect to physician-assisted suicide could elicit even stronger feelings of ambivalence on the part of health care providers asked to participate in organ procurement when a death is planned.

No change in organ donor eligibility can be instituted without the enthusiastic support of health care professionals who care for the terminally ill and dying. If changes in public policy result in changes in the management of death and dying in our society it may be too much to expect health care professionals to absorb additional changes in organ retrieval policy at the same time.

BLURRING THE BOUNDARIES OF LIFE AND DEATH

It is commonly said that the only reason the concept of "brain death" exists is organ donation. Behind such comments are the criticisms or even fear that the boundary between life and death was shifted purely to serve the transplant profession's and society's interest in having more organs available to transplant.

Perhaps the greatest obstacle to public policy change with respect to NHBCDs is the public perception that the transplant community is too willing to draw the boundary between life and death wherever it happens to maximize the chances for organ procurement. Public fears about how and where the line is drawn are likely to be exacerbated by the current emphasis on cost containment and rationing, which now dominate political discussions of health care policy.

While it may be possible to arrive at a social consensus regarding the definition of who is and is not eligible to be a donor, what steps can be taken to facilitate donation, and what criteria should be used to define cardiac death, there should be little doubt that the public will find very little assurance about how these definitions, steps, and criteria have been drawn if the decision-making process is limited to physicians who work at major transplant centers. If anything is clear in American society, it is that the public will not trust groups seen as having vested interests to design, monitor, and regulate matters pertaining to life and death. The definition of death is seen as both a legal and a medical matter, and as such, efforts to institute new standards of practice in the management of NHBCDs require more publicity and accountability than they have received to date (Cole 1993).

None of these areas of concern raises sufficient problems to argue that the idea of using NHBCDs as donors is doomed on ethical grounds. But these problems are of sufficient weight that they should give those who would favor pursing an incremental strategy of policy creep pause about the wisdom of going very far down that road.

REFERENCES

Alexander, J. W.; Vaughn, W. K.; and Carey, M. A. 1991. The Use of Marginal Donors for Organ Transplantation. *Transplantation Proceedings* 23: 905–9.

Anaise, D.; Yland, M. J.; Ishimaru, M.; et al. 1989. Organ Procurement from Non-Heartbeating Cadaver Donors. *Transplantation Proceedings* 21: 1211–14.

Batten, Helen Levine, and Prottas, Jeffrey M. 1987. Kind Strangers: The Families of Organ Donors. *Health Affairs* 6: 35–47.

Caplan, Arthur L. 1988a. Professional Arrogance and Public Misunderstanding: Threats to the Health of Required Request Legislation. *Hastings Center Report* 18 (2): 34–37.

———. 1988b. Ethical Issues in the Use of Anencephalic Infants as a Source of Organs and Tissues for Transplantation. *Transplantation Proceedings* 20: 42–50.

———. 1992a. Living Dangerously: Ethical Issues in Living Donation of Lobes of Liver. *Cambridge Quarterly of Ethics* 1: 311–17.

———. 1992b. If I Were a Rich Man Could I Buy a Pancreas? Bloomington: Indiana University Press.

———. 1992c. Is Xenografting Morally Wrong? *Transplantation Proceedings* 24: 722–27.

———; Siminoff, Laura; Arnold, Robert; and Virnig, Beth. 1992. Increasing Organ and Tissue Donation: What Are the Obstacles, What Are Our Options? In *Surgeon General's Workshop on Increasing Organ Donation*, ed. Antonia C. Novello, pp. 199–232. Washington, DC: DHSS.

Cohen, Lloyd. 1991. A Market for Increasing the Supply of Cadaveric Organs. *Clinical Transplantation* 5: 462–70.

Cole, David. 1993. Statutory Definitions of Death and the Management of Terminally Ill Patients Who May Become Organ Donors after Death. *Kennedy Institute of Ethics Journal* 3: 145–55.

DeVita, Michael A.; Snyder, James V.; and Grenvik, Ake. 1993. History of Organ Donation by Patients with Cardiac Death. *Kennedy Institute of Ethics Journal* 3: 113–29.

Feest, T. G.; Riad, H. N.; Collins, C. H.; et al. 1990. Protocol for Increasing Organ Donation after Cerebrovascular Deaths in a District General Hospital. *Lancet* 335: 1133–35.

Fox, Renée C., and Swazey, Judith P. 1978. *The Courage to Fail.* 2nd ed. Chicago: University of Chicago Press.

———. 1992. *Spare Parts.* New York: Oxford University Press.

Grenvik, Ake. 1992. Brain Death and Organ Transplantation, A 40 Year Review. *Opmear* 37: 33–40.

Guttmann, Ronald D. 1992. On the Use of Organs from Executed Prisoners. *Transplantation Reviews* 6: 189–93.

Hibberd, A. D.; Pearson, I. Y.; McCosker, C. J.; et al. 1992. Potential for Cadaveric Organ Retrieval in New South Wales. *British Medical Journal* 304: 1339–43.

Kass, Leon. 1992. Organs for Sale? Propriety, Property, and the Price of Progress. *The Public Interest* 107: 65–86.

Kleinman, Irwin, and Lowy, Frederick H. 1992. Ethical Considerations in Living Organ Donation and a New Approach. *Archives of Internal Medicine* 152: 1484–88.

Matas, Arthur J.; Arras, John; Muyskens, James; et al. 1985. A Proposal for Cadaver Organ Procurement: Routine Removal with Right of Informed Refusal. *Journal of Health Politics, Policy and Law* 10: 231–44.

Novello, Antonia C., ed. 1992. *Surgeon General's Workshop on Increasing Organ Donation.* Washington, DC: DHSS.

Peters, Thomas G. 1991. Life or Death: The Issue of Payment in Cadaveric Organ Donation. *Journal of the American Medical Association* 265: 1302–5.

Priester, Reinhard. 1992. A Values Framework for Health System Reform. *Health Affairs* 11: 84–107.

Rapaport, F. T. 1991. Progress in Organ Procurement: The Non-Heart Beating Cadaver Donor and Other Issues in Transplantation. *Transplantation Proceedings* 23: 2699–701.

Spital, Aaron. 1991. Living Organ Donation: Shifting Responsibility. *Archives of Internal Medicine* 151: 234–35.

UPMC Policy. 1993. UPMC Policy for the Management of Terminally Ill Patients Who May Become Organ Donors after Death. University of Pittsburgh Medical Center, 18 May 1992. Reprinted in *Kennedy Institute of Ethics Journal* 3: A-1–A-15.

The Case for Allowing Kidney Sales

JANET RADCLIFFE-RICHARDS et al.*

WHEN THE PRACTICE of buying kidneys from live vendors first came to light some years ago, it aroused such horror that all professional associations denounced it[1,2] and nearly all countries have now made it illegal.[3] Such political and professional unanimity may seem to leave no room for further debate, but we nevertheless think it important to reopen the discussion.

The well-known shortage of kidneys for transplantation causes much suffering and death. Dialysis is a wretched experience for most patients, and is anyway rationed in most places and simply unavailable to the majority of patients in most developing countries.[5] Since most potential kidney vendors will never become unpaid donors, either during life or posthumously, the prohibition of sales must be presumed to exclude kidneys that would otherwise be available. It is therefore essential to make sure that there is adequate justification for the resulting harm.

Most people will recognize in themselves the feelings of outrage and disgust that led to an outright ban on kidney sales, and such feelings typically have a force that seems to their possessors to need no further justification. Nevertheless, if we are to deny treatment to the suffering and dying we need better reasons than our own feelings of disgust.

In this paper we outline our reasons for thinking that the arguments commonly offered for prohibiting organ sales do not work, and therefore that the debate should be reopened.[6,7] Here we consider only the selling of kidneys by

*J. Radcliffe-Richards, A. S. Daar, R. D. Guttmann, R. Hoffenberg, I. Kennedy, M. Lock, R. A. Sells, and N. Tilney

JANET RADCLIFFE RICHARDS is a lecturer in Philosophy at Open University.

living vendors, but our arguments have wider implications.

The commonest objection to kidney selling is expressed on behalf of the vendors: the exploited poor, who need to be protected against the greedy rich. However, the vendors are themselves anxious to sell,[8] and see this practice as the best option open to them. The worse we think the selling of a kidney, therefore, the worse should seem the position of the vendors when that option is removed. Unless this appearance is illusory, the prohibition of sales does even more harm than first seemed, in harming vendors as well as recipients. To this argument it is replied that the vendors' apparent choice is not genuine. It is said that they are likely to be too uneducated to understand the risks, and that this precludes informed consent. It is also claimed that, since they are coerced by their economic circumstances, their consent cannot count as genuine.[9]

Although both these arguments appeal to the importance of autonomous choice, they are quite different. The first claim is that the vendors are not competent to make a genuine choice within a given range of options. The second, by contrast, is that poverty has so restricted the range of options that organ selling has become the best, and therefore, in effect, that the range is too small. Once this distinction is drawn, it can be seen that neither argument works as a justification of prohibition.[7]

If our ground for concern is that the range of choices is too small, we cannot improve matters by removing the best option that poverty has left, and making the range smaller still. To do so is to make subsequent choices, by this criterion, even less autonomous. The only way to improve matters is to lessen the poverty until organ selling no longer seems the best option; and if that could be achieved, prohibition would be irrelevant because nobody would want to sell.

The other line of argument may seem more promising, since ignorance does preclude informed consent. However, the likely ignorance of the subjects is not a reason for banning altogether a procedure for which consent is required. In other contexts, the value we place on autonomy leads us to insist on information and counselling, and that is what it should suggest in the case of organ selling as well. It may be said that this approach is impracticable, because the educational level of potential vendors is too limited to make explanation feasible, or because no system could reliably counteract the misinformation of nefarious middlemen and profiteering clinics. But even if we accepted that no possible vendor could be competent to consent, that would justify only putting the decision in the hands of competent guardians. To justify total prohibition it would also be necessary to show that organ selling must always be against the interests of potential vendors, and it is most unlikely that this would be done.

The risk involved in nephrectomy is not in itself high, and most people regard it as acceptable for living related donors.[10] Since the procedure is, in principle, the same for vendors as for unpaid donors, any systematic difference between the worthwhileness of the risk for vendors and donors presumably lies on the other side of the calculation, in the expected benefit. Nevertheless the exchange of money cannot in itself turn an acceptable risk into an unacceptable one from the vendor's point of view. It depends entirely on what the money is wanted for.

In general, furthermore, the poorer a potential vendor, the more likely it is that the sale of a kidney will be worth whatever risk there is. If the rich are free to engage in dangerous sports for pleasure, or dangerous jobs for high pay, it is difficult to see why the poor who take the lesser risk of kidney selling for greater rewards—perhaps saving relatives' lives,[11] or extricating themselves from poverty and debt—should be thought so misguided as to need saving from themselves.

It will be said that this does not take account of the reality of the vendors' circumstances: that risks are likely to be greater than for unpaid donors because poverty is detrimental to health, and vendors are often not given proper care. They may also be underpaid or cheated, or may waste their money through inexperience. However, once again, these arguments apply far more strongly to many other activities by which the poor try to earn money, and which we do not forbid. The best way to address such problems would be by regulation and perhaps a central purchasing system, to provide screening, counselling, reliable payment, insurance, and financial advice.[12]

To this it will be replied that no system of screening and control could be complete, and that both vendors and recipients would always be at risk of exploitation and poor treatment. But all the evidence we have shows that there is much more scope for exploitation and abuse when a supply of desperately wanted goods is made illegal. It is, furthermore, not clear why it should be thought harder to police a legal trade than the present complete ban.

Furthermore, even if vendors and recipients would always be at risk of exploitation, that does not alter the fact that if they choose this option, all alternatives must seem worse to them. Trying to end exploitation by prohibition is rather like ending slum dwelling by bulldozing slums: it ends the evil in that form, but only by making things worse for the victims. If we want to protect the exploited, we can do it only by removing the poverty that makes them vulnerable, or, failing that, by controlling the trade.

Another familiar objection is that it is unfair for the rich to have privileges not available to the poor. This argument, however, is irrelevant to the issue of organ selling as such. If organ selling is wrong for this reason, so are all benefits available to the rich, including all private medicine, and, for that matter, all public provision of medicine in rich countries (including transplantation of donated organs) that is unavailable in poor ones. Furthermore, all purchasing could be done by a central organization responsible for fair distribution.[12]

It is frequently asserted that organ donation must be altruistic to be acceptable,[13] and that this rules out payment. However, there are two problems with this claim. First, altruism does not distinguish donors from vendors. If a father who saves his daughter's life by giving her a kidney is altruistic, it is difficult to see why his selling a kidney to pay for some other operation to save her life would be thought less so. Second, nobody believes in general that unless some useful action is altruistic it is better to forbid it altogether.

It is said that the practice would undermine confidence in the medical profession, because of the association of doctors with money-making practices. That, however, would be a reason for objecting to all private practice; and in this case the objection could easily be met by the separation of purchasing and treatment. There could, for instance, be independent trusts[12] to fix charges and handle accounts, as well as to ensure fair play and high standards. It is alleged that allowing the trade would lessen the supply of donated cadaveric kidneys.[14] But although some possible donors might decide to sell instead, their organs would be available, so there would be no loss in the total. And in the meantime, many people will agree to sell who would not otherwise donate.

It is said that in parts of the world where women and children are essentially chattels there would be a danger of their being coerced into becoming vendors. This argument, however, would work as strongly against unpaid living kidney donation, and even more strongly against many far more harmful practices which do not attract calls for their prohibition. Again, regulation would provide the most reliable means of protection.

It is said that selling kidneys would set us on a slippery slope to selling vital organs such as hearts. But that argument would apply equally to the case of the unpaid kidney donation, and nobody is afraid that that will result in the donation of hearts. It is entirely feasible to have laws and professional practices that allow the giving or selling only of non-vital organs. Another objection is that allowing organ sales is impossible because it would outrage public opinion. But this claim is about western public opinion: in many potential vendor communities, organ selling is more acceptable than cadaveric donation, and this argument amounts to a claim that other people should follow western cultural preferences rather than their own. There is, anyway, evidence that the western public is far less opposed to the idea, than are medical and political professionals.[15]

It must be stressed that we are not arguing for the positive conclusion that organ sales must always be acceptable, let alone that there should be an unfettered market. Our claim is only that none of the familiar arguments against organ selling works, and this allows for the possibility that better arguments may yet be found.

Nevertheless, we claim that the burden of proof remains against the defenders of prohibition, and that until good arguments appear, the presumption must be that the trade should be regulated rather than banned altogether. Furthermore, even when there are good objections at particular times or in particular places, that should be regarded as a reason for trying to remove the objections, rather than as an excuse for permanent prohibition.

The weakness of the familiar arguments suggests that they are attempts to justify the deep feelings of repugnance which are the real driving force of prohibition, and feelings of repugnance among the rich and healthy, no matter how strongly felt, cannot justify removing the only hope of the destitute and dying. This is why we conclude that the issue should be considered again, and with scrupulous impartiality.

REFERENCES

1. British Transplantation Society Working Party. Guidelines on living organ donation. *BMJ* 1986; 293: 257–58.

2. The Council of the Transplantation Society. Organ sales. *Lancet* 1985; 2: 715–16.

3. World Health Organization. A report on developments under the auspices of WHO (1987–1991). WHO 1992 Geneva. 12–28.

4. Hauptman PJ, O'Connor KJ. Procurement and allocation of solid organs for transplantation. *N Engl J Med* 1997; 336: 422–31.

5. Barsoum RS. Ethical problems in dialysis and transplantation: Africa. In: Kjellstrand CM, Dossetor JB, eds. *Ethical problems in dialysis and transplantation*. Kluwer Academic Publishers, Netherlands. 1992: 169–82.

6. Radcliffe-Richards J. Nephrarious goings on: kidney sales and moral arguments. *J Med Philosph*. Netherlands: Kluwer Academic Publishers, 1996; 21: 375–416.

7. Radcliffe-Richards J. From him that hath not. In: Kjellstrand CM, Dossetor JB, eds. *Ethical problems in dialysis and transplantation*. Netherlands: Kluwer Academic Publishers, 1992: 53–60.

8. Mani MK. The argument against the unrelated live donor. In: Kjellstrand CM, Dossetor JB, eds. *Ethical problems in dialysis and transplantation*. Netherlands: Kluwer Academic Publishers, 1992: 164.

9. Sells RA. The case against buying organs and a futures market in transplants. *Trans Proc* 1992; 24: 2198–202.

10. Daar AD, Land W, Yahya TM, Schneewind K, Gutmann T, Jakobsen A. Living-donor renal transplantation: evidence-based justification for an ethical option. *Trans Reviews* (in press) 1997.

11. Dossetor JB, Manickavel V. Commercialisation: the buying and selling of kidneys. In: Kjellstrand CM, Dossetor JB, eds. *Ethical problems in dialysis and transplantation*. Netherlands: Kluwer Academic Publishers, 1992: 61–71.

12. Sells RA. Some ethical issues in organ retrieval 1982–1992. *Trans Proc* 1992; 24: 2401–03.

13. Sheil R. Policy statement from the ethics committee of the Transplantation Society. *Trans Soc Bull* 1995; 3: 3.

14. Altshuler JS, Evanisko MJ. *JAMA* 1992; 267: 2037.

15. Guttmann RD, Guttmann A. Organ transplantation: duty reconsidered. *Trans Proc* 1992; 24: 2179–80.

Transplantation through a Glass Darkly

JAMES LINDEMANN NELSON

BIOETHICAL PROBLEMS TAKE many different forms, and fascinate many different kinds of people. Physicians and philosophers, lawyers and theologians, policy analysts and talk show hosts are all drawn by the blend of practical urgency and moral complexity that characterize these issues.

But there seem to be only two kinds of bioethical problems that typically pull into their orbits not only theorists and practitioners, but pickets and protesters as well. When it comes to the treatment of fetuses and animals, people take to the streets. On the same day that demonstrators on both sides of the abortion issue lamented the Supreme Court's decision in *Casey,* representatives of PETA (People for the Ethical Treatment of Animals) gathered at the University of Pittsburgh to protest the implantation of a baboon's liver in a thirty-five-year-old man—the father of two children—whose own liver had been destroyed by hepatitis B virus.

There is, of course, a big difference in the way the disputes are perceived: abortion's bona fides as a central ethical issue are well established, but despite an upsurge of interest among ethicists over the past decade and a half, concern about animals still seems a bit quirky, too exclusively the domain of zealots who maintain the moral equality of all species, and thereby mark themselves as fundamentally out of sympathy with our basic ethical traditions. Here I try to pull

JAMES LINDEMANN NELSON is a Professor at the Center for Applied and Professional Ethics, University of Tennessee at Knoxville.

moral consideration of nonhumans closer to the ethical center, arguing that thinking about the fate of nonhumans at our hands shares with abortion—indeed, with many of our culture's most difficult moral issues—a fundamental problem: we don't really know what we are talking about. More concretely, we're at a loss to say what it is about baboons that makes their livers fair game, when we wouldn't dare take vital organs from those of our own species whose abilities to live rich, full lives are no greater than those of the nonhumans we seem so willing to prey upon. Unless we're able to isolate and defend the relevant moral distinction, we should reject the seductive image of solving the problem of organ shortage by maintaining colonies of animals at the ready for transplantation on demand.

MORAL OUTLIERS

Public protest about abortion is not galvanized by concern about the quality of informed consent, or its impact on the doctor-patient relationship. What *does* lie at the center of the dispute is an absolutely crucial kind of ignorance. As a society, we don't know what fetuses are, and, in an important sense, we don't know what pregnant women are either. Are fetuses babies or tissue? Are pregnant women mothers bound by special duties to their unborn children, or independent adults exercising their right to make important self-regarding decisions under the protection of a mantle of privacy? Because we don't know these things, and

Hastings Center Report 22, 5 (Sept–Oct 1992): 6–8. Reprinted by permission of James Lindemann Nelson and The Hastings Center. Copyright 1992, The Hastings Center.

they matter so much, we have a hard time imagining what responsible compromise might really be like.

And what gets people out into the streets in response to a daring attempt to rescue from certain death a young father of two? What, for that matter, causes medical research advocacy organizations to spend large amounts of money, not on research, but on full-page ads in the *New York Times* defending what scientists do? Is it concerns about justice in the allocation of medical resources? Doubts about the "courage to fail" ethos? Misgivings centered around the independence of IRB review? Surely not. The ground of protest and counter-protest is a similar kind of ignorance about the fundamental terms of the relevant moral discourse: we don't know what animals are, either. We treat them as if they were morally protean; we mold them into anything from much-loved companions and symbols of virtue to mere machines for making food and instruments for scientific research.

Our ignorance as a society about these dark corners of our moral commitments, our lack of consensus about where outliers really fit, is extremely divisive when coupled with individual assurance that there is in fact available knowledge about these matters, that the answers are of surpassing importance, and that there is something suspicious, if not downright evil, about the people who don't get it. While such conclusions cripple civility, and should of course be resisted, our history should be making us nervous. We have so often gotten matters of who counts morally just flatly wrong, and have exacted horrible prices from those shuffled unjustly to the margins of our moral concern.

What fetuses are has at least received a thorough airing in the bioethics literature. Gravid women we still find quite puzzling apparently, as witness current concerns about "forced cesareans" and "maternal-fetal conflict," but at least there is an awareness that getting clear about the moral character of pregnancy is a key to understanding the morality of pregnancy terminations.

But despite their ubiquity in medical research and practice, determining what animals are is not thought of as a paradigmatic bioethics issue. Yet seeing animals clearly is likely to be at least as difficult as the analogous tasks for fetuses and pregnant women. After all, we have a strong stake in the presumption that nonhumans are things whose moral status is at our discretion: the looser we can keep the moral constraints, the freer we are to do as we like with these extremely useful creatures. Further, there is a sense in which animals really are protean. Human beings are animals; so are protozoa. Drawing some moral distinctions is inescapable when facing such a range, and if there's to be a bright line between entities that really matter and those that don't, the human species may very well seem a reasonable place to draw it.

Choosing this line may appear suspiciously self-serving. Yet, at least at first glance, it looks as though there really could be something ethically serious to be said for us. We don't have to rely on the brute fact that we've got all the power, this is a comfort, as "might makes right" has a dubious history as a basis for moral distinctions. Nor do we have to resort to the bare fact of our common species membership—again, all to the good, as such purely biological bases for moral categorization also have a simply horrifying pedigree. Further, we can avoid invoking the soul as a sort of special moral talisman whose possession elevates us above all others: purely metaphysical entities aren't much use when we're trying to do ethics with an eye to public policy in a pluralistic society. Besides, imagine what we would do if someone were to argue that the subjugation of women was justified on the grounds that all and only men possess "schmouls," an empirically undetectable entity that inexplicably gives them extra moral worth.

The distinction we wish to draw between humans and the rest of creation seems much more respectable than distinctions based on might, on species, or on sectarian metaphysics. One could say that the appeal to such things as the range and power of the human intellect, the complexity and depth of our interpersonal relationships, our passions, both personal and aesthetic, our sense of morality, and of tragedy makes good sense. If these abilities and vulnerabilities don't matter morally, it's hard to imagine what would.

But if these are the characteristics that matter morally, it is not only baboons who lack them; not all of us humans have them either. Many humans have lost, or will never have, powerful intellects, deep relationships, rich passions, or the intimations of mortality. Think of the profoundly mentally ill, the comatose, and those who have sustained severe brain injuries. While such humans are themselves instances of tragedy, they have no sense of what tragedy is.

Despite this sad fact, our convictions about the importance of simply being human are so strong that we hesitate to use organs from newborns with anencephaly, a condition incompatible with either sensation or life. Given this hesitation, one can imagine the response if a leading transplant surgeon were to call for the maintenance of colonies of mentally handicapped orphans, to be well cared for until needed, but whose organs would then be "humanely" harvested for use in dying but otherwise "normal" people—infants with hypoplastic left heart syndrome, young fathers with HVB. Yet this scenario—with baboons and other primates substituting for handicapped orphans—is precisely what some transplant surgeons have been advocating since at least the 1960s, and is quite explicitly part of the agenda underlying the recent effort in Pittsburgh. If we are morally repulsed by a call to use handicapped orphans, but are eager to see whether colonies of baboons mightn't become a solution to our endemic lack of transplantable organs, it surely behooves us to have a good answer to the question, "What's so different about the two kinds of creature?"

Perhaps there is a good answer to that question—a difference, or set of overlapping differences, that will end up ethically supporting our practice. Perhaps we could, without arbitrary prejudice, keep all mentally handicapped humans, no matter how damaged or how alone in the world they might be, in the ethical family, so to speak. Perhaps it's appropriate to see all nonhumans, no matter how intelligent or complex their lives might be, as largely discretionary items, to be cast into the outer darkness if anything approaching a serious purpose seems to demand it. Or perhaps the real moral of the story here is that it is not baboons we should respect more, but humans who are their emotional and intellectual peers we should respect less; consider the research and therapeutic bonanza *that* would yield! But defending either of these conclusions would take a powerful argument, and there's very little evidence that any of the people most enthusiastically thumping the tub for more and better xenotransplantation have come up with reasons of the kind that are needed. Typically, their strategy is simply to point to the human cost of not pushing the xenograft agenda—the "three people who die every day waiting for a necessary organ" argument—without any serious attempt to balance that cost against the debit incurred to the victims of those grafts. Nor do we see much effort to set the xenograft strategy against the costs and benefits incurred by trying to enforce the required request laws that are already on the books, or to enact "presumed consent" or "routine retrieval" policies for organ procurement.

DISCERNMENT IN THE DARK

This, of course, returns us to our original problem: we don't even know how to begin that balancing act, and it seems that we aren't very keen on learning. A simple reliance on our moral intuitions isn't enough. As the history of medical research in the nineteenth and even twentieth century reveals, we have been more than willing to subject those who were "clearly less valuable" to the rigors of research—only then, the ones who were obviously less valuable were Jewish, or people of color. Our gut instincts simply aren't good enough as reliable moral guides when we're dealing with those whom we've pushed to the margin of moral discourse. The question is not whether we're generally able to move deftly within our ordinary understanding of morality, but whether, when it comes to the moral outliers, that ordinary understanding itself is adequate.

Cross-species transplantation crystallizes a certain kind of moral conflict between humans and other animals—perhaps too sharply. Pitting the life of the father of two against that of a baboon is sure to strike most of us as no contest. The glare of the contrast distracts us from such realities as the fact that, at the point of decision-making, the animal's death buys only a chance, not a guarantee, or that the outcome of acting is not always better than the outcome of refraining, even when death is inevitable if we stay our hand. If we reflect about our moral duties and liberties more broadly, it may strike us that we are apparently quite comfortable allowing many tragic deaths to occur daily, when what it would take to stop them is not the life of an intelligent animal, but merely the cost of drinks after work.

On the other hand, if we do refuse to take the baboon's life in an effort to save the human's out of a sense that the moral parity between baboons and mentally handicapped humans leaves us no other option, then we need to ask what else that sense of parity implies. The animal who provided the liver in the Pittsburgh case was at least killed in an effort to save the life of an identifiable person. But most of what we do with the lives of animals is—at best—only distantly related to the lives and health of people in general. If it is wrong to kill a baboon to try to save a man's life, is it wrong to kill a pig because sausages taste so good? To kill a kid to make elegant gloves? Crit-

ics of xenograft whose main concern is with the "sacrificed" animal may find it relatively easy to adopt vegan diets and eschew wearing leather. But do they really advocate that ill people begin a wholesale boycott of a medical system in which the training and research leading up to its quite standard offerings are, as it were, drenched in the blood of nonhumans?

The implications of all this for the development of xenograft and the creation of "donor" colonies are comparatively clear. There are numerous ways in which we might strive to save and enhance lives, including many that are more efficient than killing animals who resemble us in no small degree—ways that do not burden us by reinforcing our commitment to moral positions we do not fully understand, and may not be able to maintain. If we feel morally constrained to continue organ transplantation as an important way of saving and enhancing human lives, we ought not to try to respond to that moral challenge with the technological fix of a better anti-rejection drug that will allow us to use non-humans as organ sources, but rather by figuring out better ways to engage the altruism of the human community, until at last it strikes us all as mighty peculiar that anyone would want to hang on to her organs after death, when she has no conceivable use for them.

We ought to drop xenograft research and therapy, investing the resources of human effort, ingenuity, and money it consumes elsewhere. We don't now know what the judgment of history regarding our relationship with nonhumans will be, but there's no reason to be sanguine about it. What this uncertainty says for our overall relationship with animals may still be a matter for debate, but there's no compelling need to make matters any worse.

Societal and Environmental Issues

Executive Summary and Guide to Final Report

ADVISORY COMMITTEE ON HUMAN RADIATION EXPERIMENTS

THE CREATION OF THE ADVISORY COMMITTEE

On January 15, 1994, President Clinton appointed the Advisory Committee on Human Radiation Experiments. The president created the Committee to investigate reports of possibly unethical experiments funded by the government decades ago.

The members of the Advisory Committee were fourteen private citizens from around the country: a representative of the general public and thirteen experts in bioethics, radiation oncology and biology, nuclear medicine, epidemiology and biostatistics, public health, history of science and medicine, and law.

President Clinton asked us to deliver our recommendations to a Cabinet-level group, the Human Radiation Interagency Working Group, whose members are the Secretaries of Defense, Energy, Health and Human Services, and Veterans Affairs; the Attorney General; the Administrator of the National Aeronautics and Space Ad-

ministration; the Director of Central Intelligence; and the Director of the Office of Management and Budget. Some of the experiments the committee was asked to investigate, and particularly a series that included the injection of plutonium into unsuspecting hospital patients, were of special concern to Secretary of Energy Hazel O'Leary. Her department had its origins in the federal agencies that had sponsored the plutonium experiments. These agencies were responsible for the development of nuclear weapons and during the Cold War their activities had been shrouded in secrecy. But now the Cold War was over.

The controversy surrounding the plutonium experiments and others like them brought basic questions to the fore: How many experiments were conducted or sponsored by the government, and why? How many were secret? Was anyone harmed? What was disclosed to those subjected to risk, and what opportunity did they have for consent? By what rules should the past be judged? What remedies are due those who

U.S. Government Printing Office.

were wronged or harmed by the government in the past? How well do federal rules that today govern human experimentation work? What lessons can be learned for application to the future? Our Final Report provides the details of the Committee's answers to these questions. This Executive Summary presents an overview of the work done by the Committee, our findings and recommendations, and the contents of the Final Report.

THE PRESIDENT'S CHARGE

The President directed the Advisory Committee to uncover the history of human radiation experiments during the period 1944 through 1974. It was in 1944 that the first known human radiation experiment of interest was planned, and in 1974 that the Department of Health, Education and Welfare adopted regulations governing the conduct of human research, a watershed event in the history of federal protections for human subjects.

In addition to asking us to investigate human radiation experiments, the President directed us to examine cases in which the government had intentionally released radiation into the environment for research purposes. He further charged us with identifying the ethical and scientific standards for evaluating these events, and with making recommendations to ensure that whatever wrongdoing may have occurred in the past cannot be repeated.

We were asked to address human experiments and intentional releases that involved radiation. The ethical issues we addressed and the moral framework we developed are, however, applicable to all research involving human subjects.

The breadth of the Committee's charge was remarkable. We were called on to review government programs that spanned administrations from Franklin Roosevelt to Gerald Ford. As an independent advisory committee, we were free to pursue our charge as we saw fit. The decisions we reached regarding the course of our inquiry and the nature of our findings and recommendations were entirely our own.

THE COMMITTEE'S APPROACH

At our first meeting, we immediately realized that we were embarking on an intense and challenging investigation of an important aspect of our nation's past and present, a task that required new insights and difficult judgments about ethical questions that persist even today.

Between April 1994 and July 1995, the Advisory Committee held sixteen public meetings, most in Washington, D.C. In addition, subsets of Committee members presided over public forums in cities throughout the country. The Committee heard from more than 200 witnesses and interviewed dozens of professionals who were familiar with experiments involving radiation. A special effort, called the Ethics Oral History Project, was undertaken to learn from eminent physicians about how research with human subjects was conducted in the 1940s and 1950s.

We were granted unprecedented access to government documents. The President directed all the federal agencies involved to make available to the Committee any documents that might further our inquiry, wherever they might be located and whether or not they were still secret.

As we began our search into the past, we quickly discovered that it was going to be extremely difficult to piece together a coherent picture. Many critical documents had long since been forgotten and were stored in obscure locations throughout the country. Often they were buried in collections that bore no obvious connection to human radiation experiments. There was no easy way to identify how many experiments had been conducted, where they took place, and which government agencies had sponsored them. Nor was there a quick way to learn what rules applied to these experiments for the period prior to the mid-1960s. With the assistance of hundreds of federal officials and agency staff, the Committee retrieved and reviewed hundreds of thousands of government documents. Some of the most important documents were secret and were declassified at our request. Even after this extraordinary effort, the historical record remains incomplete. Some potentially important collections could not be located and were evidently lost or destroyed years ago.

Nevertheless, the documents that were recovered enabled us to identify nearly 4,000 human radiation experiments sponsored by the federal government between 1944 and 1974. In the great majority of cases, only fragmentary data was locatable; the identity of subjects and the specific radiation exposures involved were typically unavailable. Given the constraints of information, even more so than time, it was impossible for the Committee to review all these experiments, nor could we evaluate the experiences of countless individual subjects. We thus decided to focus our investigation on representative case studies reflecting eight different categories of experiments that together addressed our charge and priorities. These case studies included:

- experiments with plutonium and other atomic bomb materials
- the Atomic Energy Commission's program of radioisotope distribution
- nontherapeutic research on children
- total body irradiation
- research on prisoners
- human experimentation in connection with nuclear weapons testing
- intentional environmental releases of radiation

- observational research involving uranium miners and residents of the Marshall Islands

In addition to assessing the ethics of human radiation experiments conducted decades ago, it was also important to explore the current conduct of human radiation research. Insofar as wrongdoing may have occurred in the past, we needed to examine the likelihood that such things could happen today. We therefore undertook three projects:

- A review of how each agency of the federal government that currently conducts or funds research involving human subjects regulates this activity and oversees it.

- An examination of the documents and consent forms of research projects that are today sponsored by the federal government in order to develop insight into the current status of protections for the rights and interests of human subjects.

- Interviews of nearly 1,900 patients receiving out-patient medical care in private hospitals and federal facilities throughout the country. We asked them whether they were currently, or had been, subjects of research, and why they had agreed to participate in research or had refused.

THE HISTORICAL CONTEXT

Since its discovery 100 years ago, radioactivity has been a basic tool of medical research and diagnosis. In addition to the many uses of the x ray, it was soon discovered that radiation could be used to treat cancer and that the introduction of "tracer" amounts of radioisotopes into the human body could help to diagnose disease and understand bodily processes. At the same time, the perils of overexposure to radiation were becoming apparent.

During World War II the new field of radiation science was at the center of one of the most ambitious and secret research efforts the world has known—the Manhattan Project. Human radiation experiments were undertaken in secret to help understand radiation risks to workers engaged in the development of the atomic bomb.

Following the war, the new Atomic Energy Commission used facilities built to make the atomic bomb to produce radioisotopes for medical research and other peacetime uses. This highly publicized program provided the radioisotopes that were used in thousands of human experiments conducted in research facilities throughout the country and the world. This research, in turn, was part of a larger postwar transformation of biomedical research through the infusion of substantial government monies and technical support.

The intersection of government and biomedical research brought with it new roles and new ethical questions for medical researchers. Many of these researchers were also physicians who operated within a tradition of medical ethics that enjoined them to put the interests of their patients first. When the doctor also was a researcher, however, the potential for conflict emerged between the advancement of science and the advancement of the patient's well-being.

Other ethical issues were posed as medical researchers were called on by government officials to play new roles in the development and testing of nuclear weapons. For example, as advisers they were asked to provide human research data that could reassure officials about the effects of radiation, but as scientists they were not always convinced that human research could provide scientifically useful data. Similarly, as scientists, they came from a tradition in which research results were freely debated. In their capacity as advisers to and officials of the government, however, these researchers found that the openness of science now needed to be constrained.

None of these tensions were unique to radiation research. Radiation represents just one of several examples of the exploration of the weapons potential of new scientific discoveries during and after World War II. Similarly, the tensions between clinical research and the treatment of patients were emerging throughout medical science, and were not found only in research involving radiation. Not only were these issues not unique to radiation, but they were not unique to the 1940s and 1950s. Today society still struggles with conflicts between the openness of science and the preservation of national security, as well as with conflicts between the advancement of medical science and the rights and interests of patients.

KEY FINDINGS

Human Radiation Experiments

- Between 1944 and 1974 the federal government sponsored several thousand human radiation experiments. In the great majority of cases, the experiments were conducted to advance biomedical science; some experiments were conducted to advance national interests in defense or space exploration; and some experiments served both biomedical and defense or space exploration purposes. As noted, in the great majority of cases only fragmentary data are available.

- The majority of human radiation experiments identified by the Advisory Committee involved radioactive tracers administered in amounts that are likely to be similar to those used in research today. Most of these tracer studies involved adult subjects and are unlikely to have caused physical harm. However, in some nontherapeutic tracer studies involving children, radioisotope exposures were associated with increases in the potential lifetime risk for developing thyroid cancer that would be considered unacceptable today. The Advisory Committee also identified several studies in which patients died soon after receiving external radiation or radioisotope doses in the therapeutic range that were associated with acute radiation effects.

- Although the AEC, the Defense Department and the National Institutes of Health recognized at an early date that research should proceed only with the consent of the human subject, there is little evidence of rules or practices of consent except in research with healthy subjects. It was commonplace during the 1940s and 1950s for physicians to use patients as subjects of research without their awareness or consent. By contrast, the government and its researchers focused with substantial success on the minimization of risk in the conduct of experiments, particularly with respect to research involving radioisotopes. But little attention was paid during this period to issues of fairness in the selection of subjects.

- Government officials and investigators are blameworthy for not having had policies and practices in place to protect the rights and interests of human subjects who were used in research from which the subjects could not possibly derive direct medical benefit. To the extent that there was reason to believe that research might provide a direct medical benefit to subjects, government officials and biomedical professionals are less blameworthy for not having had such protections and practices in place.

Intentional Releases

- During the 1944–1974 period, the government conducted several hundred intentional releases of radiation into the environment for research purposes. Gener-

ally, these releases were not conducted for the purpose of studying the effects of radiation on humans. Instead they were usually conducted to test the operation of weapons, the safety of equipment, or the dispersal of radiation into the environment.

- For those intentional releases where dose reconstructions have been undertaken, it is unlikely that members of the public were directly harmed solely as a consequence of these tests. However, these releases were conducted in secret and despite continued requests from the public that stretch back well over a decade, some information about them was made public only during the life of the Advisory Committee.

Uranium Miners

- As a consequence of exposure to radon and its daughter products in underground uranium mines, at least several hundred miners died of lung cancer and surviving miners remain at elevated risk. These men, who were the subject of government study as they mined uranium for use in weapons manufacturing, were subject to radon exposures well in excess of levels known to be hazardous. The government failed to act to require the reduction of the hazard by ventilating the mines, and it failed to adequately warn the miners of the hazard to which they were being exposed.

Secrecy and the Public Trust

- The greatest harm from past experiments and intentional releases may be the legacy of distrust they created. Hundreds of intentional releases took place in secret, and remained secret for decades. Important discussion of the policies to govern human experimentation also took place in secret. Information about human experiments was kept secret out of concern for embarrassment to the government, potential legal liability, and worry that public misunderstanding would jeopardize government programs.

- In a few instances, people used as experimental subjects and their families were denied the opportunity to pursue redress for possible wrongdoing because of actions taken by the government to keep the truth from them. Where programs were legitimately kept secret for national security reasons, the government often did not create or maintain adequate records, thereby preventing the public, and those most at risk, from learning the facts in a timely and complete fashion.

Contemporary Human Subjects Research

- Human research involving radioisotopes is currently subjected to more safeguards and levels of review than most other areas of research involving human subjects. There are no apparent differences between the treatment of human subjects of radiation research and human subjects of other biomedical research.

- Based on the Advisory Committee's review, it appears that much of human subjects research poses only minimal risk of harm to subjects. In our review of research documents that bear on human subjects issues, we found no problems or only minor problems in most of the minimal-risk studies we examined.

- Our review of documents identified examples of complicated, higher-risk studies in which human subjects issues were carefully and adequately addressed and that included excellent consent forms. In our interview project, there was little evidence that patient-subjects felt coerced or pres-

sured by investigators to participate in research. We interviewed patients who had declined offers to become research subjects, reinforcing the impression that there are often contexts in which potential research subjects have a genuine choice.

- At the same time, however, we also found evidence suggesting serious deficiencies in aspects of the current system for the protection of the rights and interests of human subjects. For example, consent forms do not always provide adequate information and may be misleading about the impact of research participation on people's lives. Some patients with serious illnesses appear to have unrealistic expectations about the benefits of being subjects in research.

Current Regulations on Secrecy in Human Research and Environmental Releases

- Human research can still be conducted in secret today, and under some conditions informed consent in secret research can be waived.

- Events that raise the same concerns as the intentional releases in the Committee's charter could take place in secret today under current environmental laws.

. . . .

KEY RECOMMENDATIONS

Apologies and Compensation

The government should deliver a personal, individualized apology and provide financial compensation to those subjects of human radiation experiments, or their next of kin, in cases where:

- efforts were made by the government to keep information secret from these individuals or their families, or the public, for the purpose of avoiding embarrassment or potential legal liability, and where this secrecy had the effect of denying individuals the opportunity to pursue potential grievances.

- there was no prospect of direct medical benefit to the subjects, or interventions considered controversial at the time were presented as standard practice, and physical injury attributable to the experiment resulted.

Uranium Miners

- The Interagency Working Group, together with Congress, should give serious consideration to amending the provisions of the Radiation Exposure Compensation Act of 1990 relating to uranium miners in order to provide compensation to *all* miners who develop lung cancer after some minimal duration of employment underground (such as one year), without requiring a specific level of exposure. The act should also be reviewed to determine whether the documentation standards for compensation should be liberalized.

Improved Protection for Human Subjects

- The Committee found no differences between human radiation research and other areas of research with respect to human subjects issues, either in the past or the present. In comparison to the practices and policies of the 1940s and 1950s, there have been significant advances in the federal government's system for the protection of the rights and interests of human subjects. But deficiencies remain. Efforts should be undertaken on a national scale to

ensure the centrality of ethics in the conduct of scientists whose research involves human subjects.

- One problem in need of immediate attention by the government and the biomedical research community is unrealistic expectations among some patients with serious illnesses about the prospect of direct medical benefit from participating in research. Also, among the consent forms we reviewed, some appear to be overly optimistic in portraying the likely benefits of research, to inadequately explain the impact of research procedures on quality of life and personal finances, and to be incomprehensible to lay people.

- A mechanism should be established to provide for continuing interpretation and application in an open and public forum of ethics rules and principles for the conduct of human subjects research. Three examples of policy issues in need of public resolution that the Advisory Committee confronted in our work are: (1) Clarification of the meaning of minimal risk in research with healthy children; (2) regulations to cover the conduct of research with institutionalized children; and (3) guidelines for research with adults of questionable competence, particularly for research in which subjects are placed at more than minimal risk but are offered no prospect of direct medical benefit.

Secrecy: Balancing National Security and the Public Trust

Current policies do not adequately safeguard against the recurrence of the kinds of events we studied that fostered distrust. The Advisory Committee concludes that there may be special circumstances in which it may be necessary to conduct human research or intentional releases in secret. However, to the extent that the government conducts such activities with elements of secrecy, special protections of the rights and interests of individuals and the public are needed.

Research Involving Human Subjects

The Advisory Committee recommends the adoption of federal policies requiring:

- the informed consent of all human subjects of classified research. This requirement should not be subject to exemption or waiver.
- that classified research involving human subjects be permitted only after the review and approval of an independent panel of appropriate nongovernmental experts and citizen representatives, all with the necessary security clearances.

Environmental Releases

There must be independent review to assure that the action is needed, that risk is minimized, and that records will be kept to assure a proper accounting to the public at the earliest date consistent with legitimate national security concerns. Specifically, the Committee recommends that:

- Secret environmental releases of hazardous substances should be permitted only after the review and approval of an independent panel. This panel should consist of appropriate, nongovernmental experts and citizen representatives, all with the necessary security clearances.
- An appropriate government agency, such as the Environmental Protection Agency, should maintain a program directed at the oversight of classified programs, with suitably cleared personnel.

. . . .

"The Only Feasible Means": The Pentagon's Ambivalent Relationship with the Nuremberg Code

JONATHAN D. MORENO

IN THE EARLY YEARS of the 1950s, advisory committees in the United States Department of

JONATHAN D. MORENO is a Professor and Director of the Center for Biomedical Ethics at the Virginia School of Medicine.

Defense (DOD) engaged in highly classified discussions about the permissible use of human subjects in military research. In spite of grave reservations expressed by many military officers

Hastings Center Report 26, 5 (1996): 11–19. Reprinted by permission of Jonathan D. Moreno and The Hastings Center. Copyright 1996, The Hastings Center.

and physician consultants, Pentagon officials not only adopted a formal set of rules to govern these activities, they settled upon the Nuremberg Code *verbatim,* making it even more rigorous with the addition of a requirement for written subject consent. Subsequently, however, the Pentagon policy was accorded limited influence not only in the defense establishment, but also among physician-investigators who were DOD contract researchers.

This strange and rich story has been largely unknown to medical historians and philosophers. A few commentators have alluded to the Pentagon policy in the bioethics literature,[1] but only recently has it become possible to place the document in historical context. Precious work on this subject has been limited by the classified status of many of the background documents and the complexity of the story in which they are imbedded.

But on 15 January 1994 President Clinton created the Advisory Committee on Human Radiation Experiments. The committee was charged with uncovering the history of these experiments and of the intentional releases of radiation, identifying the ethical and scientific standards for judging them, and recommending ways to ensure that any wrongdoing could not be repeated. Along with the executive order that created the committee, the president also ordered a massive declassification process throughout the federal bureaucracy of any material that would shed light on this story.

As a member of the committee staff, I was charged with poring over thousands of once secret documents that might help tell the story of the evolution of federal standards in relation to the use of human subjects.[2] Especially critical was the tense decade following World War II, characterized by the early cold war, the Korean War, and McCarthyism. How did government advisors and policymakers weigh considerations of national security and human rights in this extraordinary time?

MOTIVATIONS FOR POLICY CREATION AFTER WORLD WAR II

Following the end of World War II there was a perceived need at the highest levels of the defense establishment for information from human experiments. This perception stemmed from two sources. First, it was believed that the Soviet Union was engaged in an intensive research and development program not only in conventional weapons but also in atomic, biological, and chemical warfare. Since Pentagon defense planners in the late 1940s and early 1950s assumed that the United States and the Soviet Union were on a collision course to armed conflict, this was a threat that had to be answered in kind. Second, many argued that the lessons that could be gleaned from animal research were inherently limited, a view often employed to explain the value of human experimentation. In the specific realm of radiation, by the late 1940s scientists had begun to learn from human "experiments of opportunity." These included several radiation accidents among Manhattan Project laboratory workers, the mass exposures at Hiroshima and Nagasaki, and the frustrating clean-up effort following the underwater detonation at Operation Crossroads in 1947. In particular, the Crossroads experience impressed war planners with the insidious nature of radiation hazards, hazards that are invisible and therefore hard for military commanders to manage. Panic reactions among both civilian populations and armed forces personnel were considered perhaps the greatest single threat posed by atomic warfare, and they could be studied only with human subjects. A desire began to emerge for more controlled experiments to explore such matters.[3]

Also in this period, radiation safety concerns shifted from laboratory workers to military personnel. Along with the widespread assumption that World War III was soon to be fought was

Agencies Created after the End of World War II

Armed Forces Medical Policy Council (AFMPC)

The AFMPC, established by the secretary of defense in 1951, was formerly the Office of Medical Services. Its members included a civilian physician as chairman, other civilians from medicine or related fields, and the surgeons general of the three services. It developed basic medical and health policies for DOD and reviewed the medical and health aspects of the policies, plans, and programs of other DOD agencies. The AFMPC was succeeded by the Assistant Secretary of Defense for Health and Medicine in late 1953.

Atomic Energy Commission (AEC)

The AEC was established by the 1946 McMahon Act. It was headed by five civilian commissioners. The AEC assumed responsibility for the Manhattan Project's activities and contracts, including nuclear weapons development and the production and distribution of radioisotopes for civilian use. It was succeeded in 1974 by two agencies: the Nuclear Regulatory Commission and the Energy Research and Development Agency, which was in turn succeeded in 1977 by the current Department of Energy.

Committee on Medical Sciences
Committee on Chemical Warfare

These were both committees of the DOD's Research and Development Board, which reviewed, evaluated, and directed all research and development conducted by or for DOD. These functions were transferred to the Assistant Secretary of Defense for Research and Development and the Assistant Secretary of Defense for Research and Engineering in late 1953.

Nuclear Energy Propulsion for Aircraft Medical Advisory Committee (NEPA)

The NEPA program had its origins in 1946 as a venture that included the Manhattan Project's Oak Ridge site, the military, and private aircraft manufacturers. Later it became a joint project of the AEC and the DOD. Members of the NEPA Medical Advisory Committee were civilian health physicists who had a critical role in the debate about using human subjects.

United States Department of Defense (DOD)

Under the 1947 National Security Act the armed services were put under the authority of the newly created National Military Establishment (NME), to be headed by the secretary of defense. In 1949 the National Security Act was amended, and the NME was transformed into an executive department: the Department of Defense.

---

the notion that it would take place on an atomic battlefield. Therefore it was important not only to prepare combatants for the experience of nuclear warfare, but also to understand how best to protect them from radiation effects so that they could be maximally effective as fighters in such an environment, and how to treat them for the ill-effects of exposures. Another major concern was how to protect and care for noncombatants who were at high risk of exposure in an era of "total war." Radiobiologists had long accepted the view that there is a threshold of acceptable exposure; defense planners needed to know what that threshold was and how field medicine could best respond if that exposure was exceeded. Some planners explicitly expressed less concern about long-term effects of radiation, which, of course, would not hinder troop battlefield performance. Several surveys of health physicists and others expert in radiation biology at that time produced wildly disparate estimates of permissible dose, a matter of considerable frustration to military officials. . . .

Similar issues were raised by biochemical warfare research. In December 1951, for example, the secretary of defense expressed concern in a DOD directive about "our lack of readiness in chemical and biological warfare," and ordered the three services to increase their activities in these areas.[4] Similarly, a joint meeting of representatives of all three service branches on 11 February 1952 was held to discuss "increased emphasis on CW and BW" (chemical and biological warfare). The minutes of that meeting include the summary statement: "That we have a serious need for increased testing of these weapons, in particular, experiments involving humans."[5] Reporting on these meetings to the secretary of defense on 25 April 1952, the assistant for special security programs emphasized the problem by stating: "if the signal to retaliate were given tomorrow, or even within the next year, the United States could make little more than a token effort."[6] To concerns about what might be called the "biochem gap" were gradually added similar worries about radiation preparedness, and by sometime in 1952 all three areas were routinely considered together as "ABC warfare research."

Therefore, a union of national security, scientific, and medical concerns emerged in this period, along with the view of many national security officials that human experiments were necessary. Yet defense planners also appreciated that human experimentation had unsavory associations in the public mind. The revelations of Nazi crimes and the Nuremberg doctors' trial did nothing to assuage such suspicions, and in their deliberations Pentagon medical advisory committees evidenced some awareness of the importance of these events for policymaking. At the same time, it was also widely believed that there was no moral similarity between what the Americans were contemplating and the Nazis' exploitation of concentration camp inmates. Nuremberg appears to have exercised both moral and public relations constraints on Pentagon officials and advisors; the question that divided many, especially between 1950 and 1952, was what the appropriate response should be to these constraints.

To be sure, there were also legal concerns about human experimentation in the DOD at mid-century. Fear of suit by aggrieved service personnel was probably not the primary motivation for these concerns, since that kind of action was significantly less likely even to be seriously considered than is the case today. Rather, difficult insurance questions arose concerning indemnification of civilian volunteers in case of injury related to an experiment. Military personnel were automatically covered for injuries incurred during service, and at this time the armed forces did not require that experiment volunteers from the ranks give up their rights to be compensated.[7]

Finally, DOD administrators were engaged in an extensive reorganization process in the early 1950s. During that process it became evident that the Pentagon lacked the technical authority to conduct human experiments according to its own operating policies, experiments that many defense planners thought highly desirable. This is not to suggest that the defense department was not conducting medical experiments involving human subjects during this period, but that the controversial nature of the new experiments that were proposed impelled the department to develop a more formal policy. In a memo dated 5 February 1953, the director of the executive office of the secretary of defense wrote of proposed atomic, biological, and chemical warfare experiments. "There is no DOD policy on the books which permits this type of research."[8] Thus the lack of a rule on human experiments became another important impetus to introduce some kind of formal policy. More difficult was just what kind of policy to introduce.

THE ROBERT S. STONE CONTROVERSY

A paper by Robert S. Stone, M.D., dated 31 January 1950 apparently formed the basis of a discussion within the office of the secretary of defense about conducting human experiments that would make it possible to predict the biological effects of radiation exposure.[9] This discussion is a window into the themes and tensions that suffused this question. Stone was professor of radiology at the University of California at San Francisco and a member of the Nuclear Energy Propulsion for Aircraft (NEPA) Medical Advisory Committee. His nine-page paper is a systematic and scholarly defense of the proposition that human radiation testing is needed and that it is ethical. Not only the nuclear powered aircraft then being researched, but also the prospect that soldiers and sailors would be exposed to radiation from weapons as a result of international hostilities, formed the strategic basis of the need argument. From a scientific standpoint, Stone noted the wide disagreement among radiologists about doses that would produce "specific effects" in humans. Thus Stone recommended that some people be exposed to 25 r (roentgens) and observed. If there were no "significant" changes then the dosage would be doubled, and then repeated a week later. If there were again no significant changes the amount should be at least doubled. Based on experience with sick patients at these levels, Stone writes, "it seems unlikely that any particular person would realize that any damage had been done to him by such exposure." Stone argued that the small risks of "undetectable genetic effect" on the life span or possibly on the blood must be weighed against the advantages of actual human exposure, such as reassuring pilots who would carry out a particular mission.

Stone noted that the use of human subjects in medical experiments was not new, citing Jenner's development of a smallpox vaccine, Walter Reed's yellow fever work, the use of federal prisoners by the Public Health Service, and armed forces research on malaria with Illinois state prisoners. In a section entitled "The Ethics of Human Experimentation," Stone cited Dr. Andrew Ivy's well-known article published in *Science* on 2 July 1948. Dr. Ivy was a medical ethics advisor to the Nuremberg judges, and in his article he states that the most important ethical requirement is that subjects be volunteers who are under no "undue pressure" to participate. Stone also cited the American Medical Association's code of ethics, and the analysis of a committee appointed by Governor Dwight H. Green of Illinois (chaired by Dr. Ivy) concerning the use of prisoners as experimental subjects, published in *JAMA* on 14 February 1948.

Stone concluded that the proposed radiation experiments met all ethical criteria, and he recommended that a subject population be identified that could be followed years after exposure: "Life prisoners are the one group of people that are likely to remain in one place where they can be observed for a great many years." To obtain "short term results," other types of subjects might be used. "Patients with incurable cancer such as those having multiple metastases might volunteer . . . Certain scientists might be willing to volunteer for specific doses," as well as some in the "general population," but again they might be hard to follow. Those under twenty-one should be ruled out because they cannot legally volunteer, and "those below the menopause (unless they have incurable cancer) probably should not be used because of psychological factors." The advantages and disadvantages of these two populations for research purposes would be revisited time and again in secret discussions.

Stone's paper generated considerable reaction in the DOD and in the Atomic Energy Commission (AEC) during the following months. For example, at the Pentagon's Committee on Medical Sciences meeting on 31 January–1 February 1950, the members were deeply split on the question of human experiments. Some appeared to support the view that there was a need for human experiments under "safe" conditions using "volunteers," and others were clearly opposed to any such studies. The following exchanges are representative not only of the division within the committee on this issue, but also of the breadth of the subjects covered and the uncertainty among many members about the right approach to take.

Dr. Fenn [Dr. Wallace O. Fenn, University of Rochester]:[10] Mr. Chairman, I'd like to say a word about human experimentation because I have a feeling that is a very dangerous route to get started on and that we shouldn't sanction human experimentation without careful consideration . . . I think we will get the information that is required from animals, animal experimentation and accidental exposure and shouldn't approve routine experimentation on volunteers. I'd like to hear some discussion about it.

Gen. Armstrong [Maj. Gen. Harry C. Armstrong, U.S. Air Force Medical Corps]: I don't believe we can adopt that stand because if we do it for that we should do it for all areas of research, and certainly, many of our valuable findings in the past have been based on volunteer human experimentation. I think that the actual research should be evaluated in each individual case and certainly given every possible safeguard but if we go on record as being opposed to human research experimentation in this field we should apply it, I believe, to all fields.

Dr. Fenn: I wouldn't make it quite as broad as that. I'd qualify that a little.

Gen. Armstrong: I don't see there is any great difference in principle in undertaking a hazardous procedure. It seems to me it doesn't make much difference whether it's an atomic energy or using an ejection seat at 530 miles an hour. They are both likely to kill you, and I don't see any particular reason why we should include any area, or if you include one you must include them all. I don't see where you should make any distinction.

Dr. Blake [Dr. Francis G. Blake, Chairman]: In individual cases it comes down to assessment of risk, doesn't it?

Gen. Armstrong: That's right. I certainly don't think we should advocate widespread and superficial plunging into this thing by any means, but I don't think we can solve that by simply saying we are not in favor of any human experimentation.[11]

Contrasting with the ambivalence within the DOD was the reaction of the advisory committee of the AEC's Division of Biology and Medicine in their meeting of 8 and 9 September 1950. The committee recorded its opposition to human experiments "at the present time," noting also "serious repercussions from a public relations standpoint if undertaken by an agency that has to do a portion of its work in secret . . ."[12]

The Pentagon's Committee on Medical Sciences met again on 23 May 1950. This time they considered a proposal to use "long-term prisoners" as subjects for the radiation research. There was agreement that, if this were to be done, the studies would have to be in conformity with the research principles adopted by the AMA in December 1946. The author of these rules, Dr. Andrew Ivy, was also the AMA's advisor on the Nuremberg prosecution of medical war criminals and an expert witness at the trial. The Nuremberg tribunal evidently used his memorandum to the AMA as the basis for much of the language contained in the Nuremberg Code. Although published in small print in *JAMA* in 1946 as part of other association business,[13] the AMA's formal position was well known enough to be part of a Pentagon committee's conversation.

A fascinating debate ensued in the Committee on Medical Sciences that day about whether long-term prisoners or cancer patients being treated with radiation therapy would be more appropriate subjects considering the questions at issue.

Admiral Greaves [Rear Adm. F C. Greaves, Medical Corps, U.S. Navy]: I agree with Colonel

Stone in that there certainly is a need for this type of information, particularly in view of the fact that we are going to be confronted with the problem of protecting personnel, not only in airplanes, but also in submarines, of this type of thing . . . But this is a long-range think [sic], and people who have types of diseases in which it is necessary to give them x-ray therapy may not be with us long enough to make the information we get valid.

Col. Stone [This is a different person from Dr. Robert S. Stone, mentioned above.]: Admiral Greaves, I'd like to point out that from the Army's viewpoint, at least, the levels that we are particularly interested in are those of relatively short duration. In other words, a man may develop a cancer twenty years later but if he is in the middle of combat we don't think that would actually deter from actually something [sic], so that what we are interested in is what level is going to make this man sick or noneffective within a period of thirty days, in all probability. Now we are very much interested in long-term effects, but when you start thinking militarily of this, if men are going out on these missions anyway, a high percentage is not coming back, the fact that you may get cancer twenty years later is just of no significance to us.

Dr. Coggeshall [Dr. Lowell T. Coggeshall]: What about the other way around? Do you believe you can get answers from people subjected to radiation therapy usually by reason of neoplastic disorders?

Col. Stone: I think it would have to be a selective study. For instance, take any of our big centers where we have quite a lot of cases of carcinomas (you can't pick lymphomas, but carcinomous types of metastasis); a number of those individuals will live in varied states of health from a period of six to eight months and x-ray therapy was indicated in epilating measures [doses sufficient to cause hair loss], and I think when we study our material on the population in Japan, plus our combined animal work, then we might logically draw up a series of bracketing experiments in which you probably get thirty to fifty such cases in a hospital like Memorial Hospital, for instance, in New York, or certain hospitals in other cities, by carefully selecting the cases and getting the amount of radiation from that bracket we might be able to get a very satisfactory answer.

Adm. Greaves: I agree with that absolutely. We could use information from whatever source, but I am wondering if we are not being a little too skiddish [sic] about this. We have a problem on our hands and I think we should consider it very seriously, but whether it is enough of a problem to go ahead and take a chance . . .

Col. Stone: Well, we think it is a problem, all right, and certainly willing [sic] to take a chance on this thing. It is a question about whether you are going to get the best information in the most scientific manner. . . .

. . . .

Col. DeCoursey [Col. Elbert DeCoursey, Medical Corps, U.S. Army]: . . . I must say that in my own mind I realize that all of these things are important to know and we must know them, but it is difficult for me to come to a decision of whether or not you should go into human experimentation on this because of the world opinion on the experimentation in Germany. That bothers me.

Adm. Greaves: I find it very difficult, too.

. . . .

Dr. Fenn: . . . I question, myself, whether the end is going to justify the means. We certainly ought to do every other method until we are absolutely certain it can't give us any information. I think the important thing is whether you take the decision to go down this road of human experimentation and work on prisoners, even though they are volunteers, and start the idea that as long as they are prisoners it really doesn't matter very much what you do to them, and it is no great loss to society, which I think it isn't, but it is a bad decision.

Dr. Coggeshall: I'd say, in comment on this, they are already down this road. There is quite a bit of human utilization of prisoners, of one type or another. It seems to me it differs only in the type of work they propose to do, not in the opinions of the thing. That doesn't make it right, necessarily, but . . . [ellipses in transcript].

Adm. Greaves: I think the reasoning behind the proposal to use prisoners was that they are long-term prisoners and that they would be available for observation and study. I don't think the reason for the proposal to use prisoners is because they were prisoners to society, or little use to society. The reason was that they would be there and you can put your finger on them and observe them for a long period of time. That isn't true of volunteers from the rest of the world, either Armed Forces or otherwise. They are here maybe this year and gone next. You lose track of them. This is a long-term thing.[14]

The proposal was referred to the Armed Forces Medical Policy Council (AFMPC) on 30 June 1951, a body that subsequently played an important role in the promulgation of the draft human experiments policy. The issue of experimentation on human subjects was not confined to radiation studies, but also had implications for research on biological and chemical warfare. On 17 December 1951 the AFMPC endorsed the principle that "final realistic evaluation of biological warfare must await appropriate field trials in which human subjects are used."[15] Sympathy for the view that human experimentation was unavoidable was growing. At its 8 September 1952 meeting the AFMPC heard a presentation from the chief of preventive medicine of the army surgeon general's office concerning the medical services' role in the development of defensive measures and devices. "Following detailed discussion, it was unanimously agreed that the use of human volunteers in this type of research be approved."[16] Interestingly, the proposition that human subjects were needed prevailed in the immediate context of biological and chemical rather than radiation experiments. What the debate did not provide (an explicit policy on human radia-

tion experiments) would become available as an indirect result of worries about the future of biological and chemical weapons development.

ADOPTING THE NUREMBERG CODE

Now that human experimentation was accepted in principle, the problem of exactly what kind of rules should govern it remained. In October 1952 the AFMPC decided to adopt the ten rules of the Nuremberg Code, based on the advice of its legal counsel, Stephen S. Jackson, the Pentagon's assistant general counsel for manpower and personnel. Jackson also advised that there should be no exception for physicians who used themselves as subjects, and that an eleventh rule should be added that explicitly prohibited experiments with prisoners of war.[17]

It is hard to escape the conclusion that the decision to adopt the code was driven by legal reasons such as concern about insurance coverage in the event of injury to subjects, and that these kinds of concerns finally forced the issue, quite apart from the internal Pentagon debate that had been going on for several years. An extraordinary sentence from a letter written on 2 March 1953, the day it was learned that Eisenhower's new secretary of defense, Charles E. Wilson, had signed the memo, vividly documents Jackson's central role in crafting the DOD policy based on the Nuremberg Code:

> It was on Mr. Jackson's insistence that the "Nuremberg Principles" were used in toto in the document [the Wilson memo], since he stated, these *already had international juridical sanction,* and to modify them would open us to severe criticism along the line—"see they use only that which suits them."[18] [emphasis added]

The italicized passage in the above quotation is remarkable: a senior administration official in 1953 seems to have cited the 1947 ruling by the judges at the Nuremberg doctors' trial as setting international legal precedent to which American researchers should be held.

Jackson's superior, Anna M. Rosenberg, Assistant Secretary for Manpower and Personnel, was another important participant in drafting the ultimate proposal. Rosenberg was a nationally recognized authority on labor relations and had been an influential New Dealer. The highest-ranking woman to serve in the defense establishment up to that time, Rosenberg insisted that a further rule be added to the proposed policy, that "consent be expressed in writing before at least one witness."[19]

Several Pentagon medical advisory committees were then asked to comment on the draft proposal and gave it at best a cool reception. The Committee on Medical Sciences opposed any policy at all, on the grounds that it "would probably do the cause more harm than good; for such a statement would have to be 'watered down' to suit the capabilities of the average investigator. Thus, it would be restrictive to the exceptional research worker."[20] The committee also expressed the view that "human experimentation within the field of medical sciences has, in years past, and is at present governed by an unwritten code of ethics," which is "administered informally" and "considered to be satisfactory . . . To commit to writing a policy on human experimentation would focus unnecessary attention on the legal aspects of the subject."

At least one other DOD committee was engaged in the discussion and ultimately advanced an alternative recommendation. The Committee on Chemical Warfare, in its 10 November 1952 meeting, was read a draft of the Nuremberg Code-based proposal. After the reading one member remarked to general laughter, "If they can get any volunteers after that I'm all in favor of it."[21] The committee advanced an alternative proposal that a British-style system of rewards for volunteers should be employed. A consent form could then "be subject to the interpretation that uniformed volunteers could be assigned to

temporary duty at the experimental installation for the purpose of engaging in the program as test subjects."[22]

In spite of the reservations of these advisory committees, the AFMPC proposal had already been endorsed by the general counsel and an assistant secretary. That top officials were committed to the eventual adoption of the Nuremberg Code-based draft is dramatically evidenced by a handwritten note from George V. Underwood, director of the executive office of the secretary of defense, to Deputy Secretary Foster dated 4 January 1953:

I believe Mr. Lovett [secretary of defense under President Truman] has a considerable awareness of this proposed policy. It has been under development for some time. Because of the importance and controversial character of the policy, I strongly recommend advance clearance with Service Sec'ys [sic] thru joint Sec'y's [sic] group. If you agree, we'd like to recapture the case so that copies can be made available to Service Sec'ys [sic].

Since consequences of this policy will fall upon Mr. Wilson, it might be wise to pass to him as a unanimous recommendation from the "alumni."[23]

A new administration was about to take power in Washington, and the top echelon of the Pentagon wanted to make sure that an important but controversial matter was placed before the new secretary of defense with all the support needed to make it easier for him to approve the proposed policy. To maximize support, the plan was to mobilize heavy artillery in the form of the service secretaries. But Underwood's plan failed. On 8 January 1953 Foster and the three service secretaries were briefed on the policy. The secretaries did not object but also were not enthusiastically favorable. One reason for this result might have been the absence of Secretary Lovett, who was testifying before Congress that day. It was decided only to refer the matter to Secretary Wilson because it was controversial and, in any case, would be up to him to implement it if it were approved.

THE WILSON MEMORANDUM

In spite of the cool reception by other groups within the DOD, on 13 January 1953 the AFMPC's memo to the secretary of defense "strongly recommended that a policy be established for the use of human volunteers (military and civilian employees) in experimental research at Armed Forces facilities," and that such use "shall be subject to the principles and conditions laid down as a result of the Nuremberg Trials."[24]

Finally, on 26 February 1953 the new secretary did sign off on the proposed policy. His memorandum began with the following paragraph:

> Based upon a recommendation of the Armed Forces Medical Policy Council, that human subjects be employed, under recognized safeguards, as the only feasible means for realistic evaluation and/or development of effective preventive measures of defense against atomic, biologic or chemical agents, that policy set forth below will govern the use of human volunteers by the Department of Defense in experimental research in the fields of atomic, biological and/or chemical warfare.[25]

In the hustle and bustle of a new administration it is unlikely that defense secretary Wilson had very much time to consider the implications of the new policy on the use of human subjects, but probably took it on faith that the AFMPC and the previous administration had done its homework. The memorandum was given the number TS-01188, "TS" standing for top secret.[26]

As the Pentagon's Committee on Medical Sciences began its meeting the next day, 27 February, they did not know about the new secretary's action. During a discussion of the potential harms of hepatitis studies, when it was mentioned that there had been three deaths in the Pentagon's program of prison studies, another remarkable debate about the use of human subjects took place:

Col. Wood [Col. John R. Wood, Medical Corps., U.S. Army, Army Chemical Center, Maryland]: I think if we have men volunteer who are satisfied that they are taking a full risk and they fully understand what this risk is, then we are justified in going ahead on the basis of absolute necessity and there being no alternative whatsoever. So I have mixed feelings about this thing. I would not be willing to be a volunteer. However, on the other hand, there is no other way to do this work.

Capt. Shilling [Capt. Shilling, M.D., Medical Corps, U.S. Navy]: In connection with the human volunteer problem in general, I think we have all discussed this for the last six months at all levels in the Department of Defense. There is one thing that disturbs me a great deal, and that is at the DOD level and at the Medical Policy Council Level [sic] there is a strong urge to try and set up an over-all policy for the conduct of human experimentation. They even go back to the Buchenwald trials, and they are trying to work ought [sic] an over-all pattern that will, if you meet this pattern — To me, this is utterly fantastic as a method of approach.

As far as the Navy is concerned, I have cleared this with policy, and we want to strongly urge that human research be conducted as it is now outlined from a policy standpoint; namely, that the field or the individual or the groups who want to do the research prepare a complete experimental design, showing exactly what they want to do, what the safeguards are going to be, what the program is, why it has to be human rather than animal, and so forth, and then come in and be evaluated by the Surgeons General involved in the Army, Navy, and Air Force, and then that it go up to the Secretary informed for final permission. This is the way we do it now and I think we are going to get into a horrible mess if we try to set up an over-all standard for every type of research. What happens is that you put so many safeguards on that we cannot do the multitude of things we are trying to do.

Moments later, the chair interrupted:

The Chairman: We have here a document which was just brought in which is signed by Mr.

Wilson, dated February 26th. With your permission, I would like to release this information. However, in order to do so, it will be necessary for any member of the audience to excuse himself if he does not have a top secret clearance.[27]

After the letter was read to the committee there was an off-the-record discussion of the new policy. Obviously, any further general objections to the policy were now academic.

The Wilson memo appears to represent a very high ethical standard in the spirit of the Nuremberg Code. But the standard is more limited than might at first be apparent. It is unclear, for example, how the policy was to apply to civilian contractors, or to those who are not normal volunteers (the population to which the Nuremberg Code seems limited), but individuals with active medical problems. These ambiguities were to be vexing in the future.

In the shorter term, the fact that the memorandum was at first top secret and only gradually downgraded prevented the new policy from being implemented as efficiently as it might have been, as we shall see. Some explanation for the top secret classification of the Wilson memo may be gleaned from the spirit of a 3 September 1952 memorandum from the secretary of the joint chiefs of staff to the joint chiefs; it also raises other questions about the determination the military's interest in medical research conducted out of the public eye:

> 2. The Joint Chiefs of Staff further consider that responsible agencies should: . . . d. Insure, insofar as practicable, that all published articles stemming from the BW or CW research and development programs are disassociated from anything which might connect them with U.S. military endeavors.[28]

WHY THE WILSON MEMO?

At least two interesting conclusions can be drawn about the process leading up to the Wilson memorandum. First, the idea to use the Nuremberg Code as the basis of a policy was received without enthusiasm among relevant advisory groups in the defense department. Second, apart from that reception, the question of what sort of policy the Pentagon should adopt concerning human experiments, and if they were needed at all, was a matter of vigorous debate even before the Wilson memo was presented in draft in 1952. This debate was further fueled when the draft policy was circulated.

Yet the debate that began at least as early as 1950 in the Pentagon was flawed. The protagonists spent most of their time staking out abstract philosophical positions for and against human experimentation in general. The real question, however, was not whether human experiments would take place (for human subjects were being used in medical research at that time, both inside and outside the military), but rather how human subjects may be used. There seems to have been little or no discussion of some basic questions: What is the meaning of "volunteering" once one is in the military? What are the limits of possible harm to which military personnel may acceptably be exposed? How can it be assured that no more individuals will be used in an experiment than are absolutely necessary?

Nor is there evidence, as yet, that those who promulgated the Nuremberg Code as the basis of a policy understood its implications. Had this been the case, difficult questions would surely have been raised in anticipation of efforts to apply the code.

The "controversy" about the use of human subjects and about the draft proposal that came out of the AFMPC thus largely missed the point. Interestingly, in spite of its lukewarm reception, the controversy behind it, and its potentially far-reaching consequences, the Nuremberg-like policy went from proposal to policy in a matter of months. Reading the documents, one has the sense that the poorly understood proposal had a momentum that was independent of the debate surrounding it, and was certainly independent of the substance of the proposed policy. Indeed, the most reasonable explanation of its eventual formal success, and its ultimate practical limitations, is precisely that the Wilson memo grew out of the decisionmaking of a few top officials of the Lovett defense department, especially the general counsel's office and Assistant Secretary Rosenberg, rather than out of the advisory process of internal experts on military medical research.[29]

It was the defense department's legal counsel and labor relations expert, not its physicians or defense planners, who seem to have originated and promoted the idea of using the Nuremberg Code and adding to it signed and witnessed consent, as well as an explicit bar to the use of prisoners of war. And it was high officials in the office of the secretary of defense who carried it forward into the new administration. Members of the DOD upper echelon thus crafted a document that was state-of-the-art for the day, but not one that would enjoy the widespread allegiance of those who would have to implement it —or perhaps even the full understanding of those who promulgated it.

In a sense, the motivation of top officials to create a policy was straightforward: following the 1950 Department of Defense Reorganization Act there was a perceived need for such a policy to cover the use of military personnel in experiments having to do with atomic, biological, and chemical warfare, experiments that were in turn regarded as imperative in the confrontation with the Soviet Union. Human experiments involving "unconventional" forms of warfare, and especially radiation, were likely to be highly sensitive with the American public. Thus, the experiments being contemplated seemed to planners to fall into a different category, as compared with more familiar kinds of military exercises or clinically based medical experiments.

This also explains why the comment process by Pentagon committees turned out to be largely a formality. For as the documents show, the office of the secretary of defense wanted to have some sort of policy on the books as soon as possible. The legal and personnel management impetus behind the draft proposal had its own *raison d'etre*. But while the theory behind the Wilson memo triumphed in a formal sense, it did not settle the doubts among the officers and researchers who would have to live according to its rules. The military-medical bureaucracy's failure to embrace the memorandum's spirit was not a matter of insubordination, which would have been clear and relatively easy to manage; it was, rather, a matter of cultural resistance, and therefore far more subtle and difficult to control. It was perhaps for this reason, more than any other, that the policy's consent requirements were at best sporadically applied in the two decades that followed.

Indeed, not only the military establishment but American society as a whole only began to come to terms with the issues embodied in this debate nearly twenty-five years later in the mid-1970s, and then only after some highly publicized abuses of human subjects. In retrospect, it might be said that high Pentagon advisors and officials could hardly have been expected to resolve issues that continue to generate new and difficult questions following decades of further experience and reflection.

ACKNOWLEDGMENTS

The author worked on the staff of the Advisory Committee on Human Radiation Experiments. The enclosed views are those of the author and do not represent the views of the Advisory Committee. The findings, recommendations, and analysis of the Advisory Committee are expressed in the "Final Report of the Advisory Committee on Human Radiation Experiments," available from Oxford University Press under the title *The Human Radiation Experiments* (1996).

I want to thank the many committee members and staff who helped me understand the significance of the materials presented in this paper and influenced my thinking about them: Jim David, Ruth Faden, Patrick Fitzgerald, Dan Guttman, Jon Harkness, Greg Herken, Jay Katz, Jeff Kahn, Pat King, Sue Lederer, Ruth Macklin,

Phil Russell, and Gil Whittemore. Special thanks to my research associate, Valerie Hurt. This was an extraordinarily talented and dedicated group with whom I will always feel privileged to have worked.

REFERENCES

1. George J. Annas and Michael A. Grodin, eds., *The Nazi Doctors and the Nuremberg Code: Human Rights in Human Experimentation* (New York: Oxford University Press, 1992), pp. 343–45.

2. Like some other committee and staff members, I was granted a "top secret" security clearance so that I could inspect other potentially relevant documents and, as needed, recommend that they be put on a "fast track" for declassification.

3. Advisory Committee on Human Radiation Experiments, *The Human Radiation Experiments* (New York: Oxford University Press, 1996), pp. 5–13.

4. Secretary of Defense Directive, 21 December 1951. This and all subsequently referenced documents gathered by the Advisory Committee are on deposit in Record Group 220 (Presidential Committees, Commissions, and Boards) at the National Archives and Records Administration, Washington, D.C. Whenever possible, I have provided specific record identifiers from the ACHRE document collection system. Unfortunately, many of the documents cited were processed and assigned "ACHRE numbers" after I worked with them. It is my hope that future scholars will be able to retrieve the relevant documents based upon the information I am able to provide in the citations.

5. Minutes of a meeting of Department of Defense service representatives, 11 February 1952.

6. Memorandum from the Assistant Secretary for Special Security Programs to the Secretary of Defense, 25 April 1952.

7. Advisory Committee, *The Human Radiation Experiments*, pp. 55–56.

8. George V. Underwood, Director, Executive Office, Office of the Secretary of Defense to Mr. Keys, Deputy Secretary of Defense. 5 February 1953, ("Use of Human Volunteers in Experimental Research") (ACHRE No. DOD-062194-A).

9. Robert S. Stone, 31 January 1950, paper presented to Department of Defense, NEPA Medical Advisory Committee ("Irradiation of Human Subjects as a Medical Experiment") (ACHRE No. NARA 070794-A). It is evident that the navy and the Joint Panel on Medical Aspects of Atomic Warfare (which included AEC and DOD representatives) favored the use of human subjects at this time, while the army and the Committee on Medical Sciences of the Pentagon's Research and Development Board did not. This episode is also covered in Gilbert Whittemore, "A Crystal Ball in the Shadows of Nuremberg and Hiroshima: The Ethical Debate over Human Experimentation to Develop a Nuclear Powered Bomber, 1946–1951," in *Science, Technology and the Military*, ed. Everett Mendelsohn, Merritt Roe Smith, and Peter Weingart (Dordrecht: Kluwer Academic Publishers, 1988), pp. 431–62. A propos the present paper, Whittemore observes: "ethical arguments may be much more common [in high level national security debates] than one would judge from published material alone" (p. 432).

10. Identifications are based on information provided in the documents themselves; further information is not always available.

11. Transcript of the Meeting of the Committee on Medical Sciences of the Research and Development Board, Department of Defense, 31 January–1 February 1950, pp. 61–66.

12. Minutes of the Advisory Committee for Biology and Medicine, Atomic Energy Commission, 8–9 September 1950.

13. "Supplementary Report of the Judicial Council," Proceedings of the House of Delegates Annual Meeting, 9–11 December 1946, *JAMA* 132 (1946): 1090.

14. Transcript of the Meeting of the Committee on Medical Sciences of the Research and Development Board, Department of Defense, 23 May 1950.

15. Annual Report of the Armed Forces Medical Policy Council, Department of Defense, to the Secretary of Defense, 30 June 1951.

16. Melvin Casberg, Chairman, AFMPC, to the Secretary of Defense, DOD, 24 December 1952 ("Human Volunteers in Experimental Research") (ACHRE No. NARA -101294-A).

17. Stephen S. Jackson, Assistant General Counsel in the Office of the Secretary of Defense and Counsel for the Armed Forces Medical Policy Council, DOD, to Melvin A. Casberg, Chairman of the Armed Forces Medical Policy Council, 13 October 1952 (ACHRE No. NARA-101294-A).

18. Adam J. Rapalski, Administrator, Armed Forces Epidemiological Board, DOD, to Colin MacLeod, President, Armed Forces Epidemiological Board, DOD, 2 March 1953 ("The attached letter I believe is self-explanatory") (ACHRE No. NARA-012395-A-5).

19. Stephen S. Jackson, Assistant General Counsel in the Office of the Secretary of Defense and counsel for the Armed Forces Medical Policy Council, DOD, to Melvin A. Casberg, Chairman of the Armed Forces

Medical Policy Council, 22 October 1952 (ACHRE No. NARA-101294-A).

20. F. Lloyd Mussells, Executive Director, Committee on Medical Sciences, RDB, DOD, to Floyd L. Miller, Vice Chairman, Research and Development Board, DOD, 12 November 1952 ("Human Experimentation") (ACHRE No. NARA-071194-A-2).

21. Transcript of the Meeting of the Committee on Chemical Warfare, RDB, DOD, 10 November 1952, p. 128 (ACHRE No. NARA-1025).

22. H. N. Worthley, Executive Director, Committee on Chemical Warfare, RDB, DOD, to the Director of Administration, Office of the Secretary of Defense, 9 December 1952 ("Use of Volunteers in Experimental Research") (ACHRE No. NARA-101294-A).

23. Underwood, 5 February 1953, ACHRE No. DOD-062194-A.

24. Melvin A. Casberg, Chairman of the Armed Forces Medical Policy Council, DOD, to the Secretary of Defense, 13 January 1953 ("Digest: Use of Human Volunteers in Experimental Research") (ACHRE No. DOD-042595-A).

25. Secretary of Defense to the Secretary of the Army, Secretary of the Navy, Secretary of the Air Force, 26 February 1953 ("Use of Human Volunteers in Experimental Research") (ACHRE No. DOD-082394-A).

26. Secretary of Defense to the Secretary of the Army, Secretary of the Navy, Secretary of the Air Force, 26 February 1953 ("Use of Human Volunteers in Experimental Research") (ACHRE No. DOD-082394-A).

27. Transcripts of the Meeting of the Committee on Medical Sciences, RDB, DOD, 27 February 1953.

28. W. G. Lalor, Secretary, Joint Chiefs of Staff to Chief of Staff, U.S. Army, Chief of Naval Operations, Chief of Staff, U.S. Air Force, 3 September 1952 ("Security Measures on Chemical Warfare and Biological Warfare") (ACHRE No. NARA-012495-A) .

29. This point was forcefully made by Jay Katz in our discussions during my work for the Advisory Committee.

The Prospects for Consensus and Convergence in the Animal Rights Debate

GARY E. VARNER

CONTROVERSIES OVER THE USE of non-human animals (henceforth animals) for science, nutrition, and recreation are often presented as clear-cut standoffs, with little or no common ground between opposing factions and, consequently, with little or no possibility for consensus-formation. As a philosopher studying these controversies, my sense is that the apparent

GARY E. VARNER is an associate professor in the department of philosophy at Texas A&M University, College Station, Tex.

intransigence of opposing parties is more a function of political posturing than theoretical necessity, and that continuing to paint the situation as a clear-cut standoff serves the interests of neither side. A critical look at the philosophical bases of the animal rights movement reveals surprising potential for *convergence* (agreement at the level of policy despite disagreement at the level of moral theory) and, in some cases, *consensus* (agreement at both levels).[1] Recognizing this should make defenders of animal research take

Hastings Center Report 24, 1 (Jan–Feb 1994): 24–28. Permission granted by Gary E. Varner and The Hastings Center. Copyright 1994, The Hastings Center.

animal rights views more seriously and could re-focus the animal rights debate in a constructive way.

In response to the growth of the animal rights movement, animal researchers have begun to distinguish between animal rights views and animal welfare views, but they have not drawn the distinction the way a philosopher would. Researchers typically stress two differences between animal welfarists and animal rightists. First, welfarists argue for reforms in research involving animals, whereas rightists argue for the total abolition of such research. Second, welfarists work within the system, whereas rightists advocate using theft, sabotage, or even violence to achieve their ends. A more philosophical account of the animal rights/animal welfare distinction cuts the pie very differently, revealing that many researchers agree with some animal rights advocates at the level of moral theory, and that, even where they differ dramatically at the level of moral theory, there is some potential for convergence at the level of policy.

ANIMAL WELFARE: THE PROSPECTS FOR *CONSENSUS*

Peter Singer's *Animal Liberation* is the acknowledged Bible of the animal rights movement. Literally millions of people have been moved to vegetarianism or animal activism as a result of reading this book. PETA (People for the Ethical Treatment of Animals) distributed the first edition of the book as a membership premium, and the number of copies in print has been cited as a measure of growth in the animal rights movement. However, Singer wrote *Animal Liberation* for popular consumption, and in it he intentionally avoided discussion of complex philosophical issues.[2] In particular, he avoided analyzing the concepts of 'rights' and 'harm,' and these concepts are crucial to drawing the animal rights/animal welfare distinction in philosophical terms.

In *Animal Liberation,* Singer spoke loosely of animals having moral "rights," but all that he intended by this was that animals (at least some of them) have some basic moral standing and that there are right and wrong ways of treating them. In later, more philosophically rigorous work— summarized in his *Practical Ethics,* a second edition of which has just been issued[3]—he explicitly eschews the term *rights,* noting that, as a thoroughgoing utilitarian, he must decry not only that animals have moral rights, but also that human beings do.

When moral philosophers speak of an individual "having moral rights," they mean something much more specific than that the individual has some basic moral standing and that there are right and wrong ways of treating him or her. Although there is much controversy as to the specifics, there is general agreement on this: to attribute moral rights to an individual is to assert that the individual has some kind of special moral dignity, the cash value of which is that certain things cannot justifiably be done to him or her (or it) for the sake of benefit to others. For this reason, moral rights have been characterized as "trump cards" against utilitarian arguments. Utilitarian arguments are based on aggregate benefits and aggregate harms. Specifically, utilitarianism is the view that right actions maximize aggregate happiness. In principle, nothing is inherently or intrinsically wrong, according to a utilitarian; any action could be justified under some possible circumstances. One way of characterizing rights views in ethics, by contrast, is that there are some things which, regardless of the consequences, it is simply wrong to do to individuals, and that moral rights single out these things.

Although a technical and stipulative definition of 'rights,' this philosophical usage reflects a familiar concept. In day-to-day discussions, appeals to individuals' rights are used to assert, in effect, that there is a limit to what individuals can be forced to do, or to the harm that may be inflicted upon them, for the benefit of others. So the philosophical usage of rights talk reflects the common-sense view that there are limits to what we can justifiably do to an individual for the benefit of society.

To defend the moral rights of animals would be to claim that certain ways of treating animals cannot be justified on utilitarian grounds. But in *Practical Ethics* Peter Singer explicitly adopts a utilitarian stance for dealing with our treatment of nonhuman animals. So the author of "the Bible of the animal rights movement" is not an animal *rights* theorist at all, and the self-proclaimed advocates of animal welfare are appealing to precisely the same tradition in ethics as is Singer. Both believe that it is permissible to sacrifice (even involuntarily) the life of one individual for the benefit of others, where the aggregated benefits to others clearly outweigh the costs to that individual. (At least they agree on this as far as animals are concerned. Singer is a thoroughgoing utilitarian, whereas my sense is that most animal researchers are utilitarians when it comes to animals, but rights theorists when it comes to humans.)

Many researchers also conceive of harm to animals very similarly to Singer, at least where non-mammalian animals are concerned. In *Animal Liberation,* Singer employs a strongly hedonistic conception of harm. He admits that the morality of killing is more complicated than that of inflicting pain (p. 17) and that although pain is pain wherever it occurs, this "does not imply that all lives are of equal worth" (p. 20). This should be stressed, because researchers commonly say that according to animal rights philosophies, of which Singer's is their paradigm, all animals' lives are of equal value. No fair reading of Singer's *Animal Liberation* would yield this conclusion, let alone any fair reading of *Practical Ethics,* where he devotes four chapters to the question of killing.

The morality of killing is complicated by competing conceptions of harm. In *Animal Liberation,* Singer leaves the question of killing in the background and uses a strongly hedonistic conception of animal welfare. He argues that the

conclusions reached in the book, including the duty to refrain from eating animals, "flow from the principle of minimizing suffering alone" (p. 21). To conceive of harm hedonistically is to say that harm consists in felt pain or lost opportunities for pleasure. For a utilitarian employing a hedonistic conception of harm, individuals are replaceable in the following sense. If an individual lives a pleasant life, dies a painless death, and is replaced by an individual leading a similarly pleasant life, there is no loss of value in the world. Agriculturalists appear to be thinking like hedonistic utilitarians when they defend humane slaughter in similar terms. Researchers employ a similarly hedonistic conception of harm when they argue that if all pain is eliminated from an experimental protocol then, ethically speaking, there is nothing left to be concerned about.

Singer conceives of harm to "lower" animals in hedonistic terms and thus agrees with these researchers and agriculturalists. He even acknowledges that the replaceability thesis could be used to defend some forms of animal agriculture, although not intensive poultry systems, where the birds hardly live happy lives or die painless deaths. However, Singer argues that it is implausible to conceive of harm in hedonistic terms when it comes to "self-conscious individuals, leading their own lives and wanting to go on living" (p. 125), and he argues that all mammals are self-conscious in this sense.

Singer equates being self-conscious with having forward-looking desires, especially the desire to go on living. He argues that such self-conscious individuals are not replaceable, because when an individual with forward-looking desires dies, those desires go unsatisfied even if another individual is born and has similar desires satisfied. With regard to self-conscious individuals, Singer is still a utilitarian, but he is a *preference* utilitarian rather than a *hedonistic* utilitarian. Singer cites evidence to demonstrate that the great apes are self-conscious in his sense (pp. 11–16) and states, without saying what specific research leads him to this conclusion, that neither fish nor chickens are (pp. 95, 133), but that "a case can be made, though with varying degrees of confidence," that all mammals are self-conscious (p. 132).

It is easy to disagree with Singer about the range of self-consciousness, as he conceives of it, in the animal kingdom.[4] Probably most mammals have forward-looking desires, but the future to which they look is doubtless a very near one. Cats probably think about what to do in the next moment to achieve a desired result, but I doubt that they have projects (long-term, complicated desires) of the kind suggested by saying that they are "leading their own lives and wanting to go on living."

However, even if we grant Singer the claim that all mammals have projects, so long as we remain utilitarians this just means that research on mammals carries a higher burden of justification than does research on "lower" animals like reptiles or insects, a point many researchers would readily grant. A preference utilitarian is still a utilitarian, and in at least some cases, a utilitarian must agree that experimentation is justified.

In the following passage from *Practical Ethics*, Singer stresses just this point:

> In the past, argument about animal experimentation has often . . . been put in absolutist terms: would the opponent of experimentation be prepared to let thousands die from a terrible disease that could be cured by experimenting on one animal? This is a purely hypothetical question, since experiments do not have such dramatic results, but as long as its hypothetical nature is clear, I think the question should be answered affirmatively—in other words, if one, or even a dozen animals had to suffer experiments in order to save thousands, I would think it right and in accordance with equal consideration of interests that they should do so. This, at any rate, is the answer a utilitarian must give. (p. 67)

Singer doubts that most experiments are justified, not because he believes experimentation is wrong *simpliciter*, but because he doubts that the benefits to humans significantly outweigh the costs to the animals. In the pages preceding the passage just quoted, Singer cites examples of experiments he thinks cannot plausibly be said "to serve vital medical purposes": testing of new shampoos and food colorings, armed forces experiments on the effects of radiation on combat performance, and H. F Harlow's maternal deprivation experiments. "In these cases, and many others like them," he says, "the benefits to humans are either nonexistent or uncertain, while the losses to members of other species are certain and real" (p. 66).

So the disagreement between Singer and the research establishment is largely empirical, about how likely various kinds of research are to lead to important human benefits. Researchers often argue that we cannot be expected to know ahead of time which lines of research will yield dramatic benefits. Critics respond that these same scientists serve on grant review boards, whose function is to permit funding agencies to make such decisions all the time. Here I want only to emphasize that this is an empirical dispute that cannot be settled *a priori* or as a matter of moral theory. One of the limitations of utilitarianism is that its application requires very detailed knowledge about the effects of various actions or policies. When it comes to utilitarian justifications for animal research, the probability—and Singer is correct that it is never a certainty—that various lines of research will save or significantly improve human lives must be known or estimated before anything meaningful can be said. Singer is convinced that most research will not meet this burden of proof; most researchers are convinced of just the opposite.

ANIMAL RIGHTS: THE PROSPECTS FOR *CONVERGENCE*

Most animal researchers agree to a surprising extent with the Moses of the animal rights movement. Their basic ethical principles are the same (at least where nonhuman animals are concerned), and they apply to all animals the same conception of harm which Singer applies to all animals except mammals. Where they disagree with Singer is at the level of policy; they see the same ethical theory implying different things in practice. Dramatic disagreement at the level of moral theory emerges only when we turn to the views of Tom Regan, whose ethical principles and conception of harm are dramatically different from Singer's and the researchers'.

Regan's *The Case for Animal Rights*[5] is a lengthy and rigorous defense of a true animal rights position. It is impossible to do justice to the argument of a 400-page book in a few paragraphs, so here I will simply state the basic destination Regan reaches, in order to examine its implications for animal research.

For Regan, there is basically one moral right: the right not to be harmed on the grounds that doing so benefits others, and all individuals who can be harmed in the relevant way have this basic right. Regan conceives of harm as a diminution in the capacity to form and satisfy desires, and he argues that all animals who are capable of having desires have this basic moral right not to be harmed. On Regan's construal, losing an arm is more of a harm than stubbing one's toe (because it frustrates more of one's desires), but death is always the worst harm an individual can suffer because it completely destroys one's capacity to form and satisfy desires. As to which animals have desires, Regan explicitly defends only the claim that all mentally normal mammals of a year or more have desires, but he says that he does this to avoid the controversy over "line drawing," that is, saying precisely how far down the phylogenetic scale one must go to find animals that are incapable of having desires. Regan is confident that at least all mammals and birds have desires, but acknowledges that the analogical evidence for possession of desires becomes progressively weaker as we turn to herpetofauna (reptiles and amphibians), fish, and then invertebrates.[6]

Regan defends two principles to use in deciding whom to harm where it is impossible not to harm someone who has moral rights: the miniride and worse-off principles. *The worse-off principle* applies where *noncomparable* harms are involved, and it requires us to avoid harming the worse-off individual. Regan's discussion of this principle makes it clear that for him, harm is measured in absolute, rather than relative terms. If harm were measured relative to the individual's original capacity to form and satisfy desires, rather than in absolute terms, then death would be uniformly catastrophic wherever it occurs. But Regan reasons that although death is always the greatest harm which any individual can suffer (because it forecloses all of that individual's opportunities for desire formation and satisfaction), death to a normal human being is noncomparably worse than death to any nonhuman animal, because a normal human being's capacity to form and satisfy desires is so much greater. To illustrate the use of the worse-off principle, Regan imagines that five individuals, four humans, and a dog are in a lifeboat that can support only four of them. Since death to any of the human beings would be noncomparably worse than death to the dog, the worse-off principle applies, and it requires us to avoid harming the human beings, who stand to lose the most.

The *miniride principle* applies to cases where *comparable* harms are involved, and it requires us to harm the few rather than the many. Regan admits that, where it applies, this principle yields the same conclusions as the principle of utility, but he emphasizes that the reasoning is nonutilitarian. The focus, he says, is on individuals rather than the aggregate. What the miniride principle instructs us to do is minimize the overriding of individuals' rights, rather than to maximize aggregate happiness. To illustrate the miniride principle's application, Regan imagines that a runaway mine train must be sent down one of two shafts, and that fifty miners would be killed by sending it down the first shaft but only one by sending it down the second. Since the harms that the various individuals in the example would suffer are comparable (only humans are involved, and all are faced with death), the miniride principle applies, and we are obligated to send the runaway train down the second shaft.

Regan argues that the rights view (as he labels his position) calls for the total abolition of animal research. In terms of the basic contrast drawn above between rights views and utilitarianism, it is easy to see why one would think this. The fundamental tenet of rights views is opposition to utilitarian justifications for harming individuals, and as we saw above, researchers' justification for animal research is utilitarian. They argue that by causing a relatively small number of individuals to suffer and die, a relatively large number of individuals can live or have their lives significantly improved.

However, Regan's worse-off principle, coupled with his conception of harm, would seem to imply that at least *some* research is not only permissible but required, even on a true animal rights view. For as we just saw, Regan believes that death for a normal human is noncomparably worse than death for any nonhuman animal. So if we knew that by performing fatal research on a given number of nonhuman animals we could save even one human life, the worse-off principle would apply, and it would require us to perform the research. In the lifeboat case referred to above, Regan emphasizes that where the worse-off principle applies, the numbers do not matter. He says:

> Let the number of dogs be as large as one likes; suppose they number a million; and suppose the lifeboat will support only four survivors. Then the rights view still implies that, special considerations apart, the million dogs should be thrown overboard and the four humans saved. To attempt to reach a contrary judgment will inevitably involve one in aggregative [i.e., utilitarian] considerations. (p. 325)

The same reasoning, in a hypothetical case like that described by Singer (where we *know*, with absolute certainty, that one experiment will save human lives) would imply that the experiment should be performed.

One complication is that the empirical dispute over the likelihood of significant human benefits emerging from various lines of research, which makes utilitarian justifications of experimentation so complex, will reappear here. Having admitted that some research is justified, animal rights advocates would doubtless continue to disagree with researchers over which research this is. Nevertheless, the foregoing discussion illustrates how the implications of a true animal rights view can converge with those of researchers' animal welfare philosophy. Even someone who attributes moral rights in the philosophical sense to animals, and whose ethical theory thus differs dramatically from most animal researchers', could think that some medical research is justified. This warrants stressing, because researchers commonly say things like, "According to animal rightists, 'a rat is a pig is a dog is a boy,'" and, "Animal rightists want to do away with all uses of animals, including life-saving medical research." However, no fair reading of either Singer or Regan would yield the conclusion that they believe that a rat's or a pig's life is equal to a normal human's. And, consequently, it is possible for someone thinking with Singer's or Regan's principles to accept research that actually saves human lives.

It is *possible,* but Regan himself continues to oppose all animal research to benefit humans. His basis is not the worse-off principle, but that the principle applies, "special considerations apart." One of those considerations is that "risks are not morally transferrable to those who do not voluntarily choose to take them," and this, he claims, blocks application of the worse-off principle to the case of medical experimentation (p. 377). For example, subjects used to screen a new vaccine run higher risks of contracting the disease when researchers intentionally expose them to it. Humans can voluntarily accept these risks, but animals cannot. Consequently, the only kind of research on "higher" animals (roughly, vertebrates) that Regan will accept is that which tests a potential cure for a currently incurable disease on animals that have already acquired the disease of their own accord.

However, most people believe that in at least some cases, we can justifiably transfer risks without first securing the agreement of those to whom the risks are transferred. For instance, modifying price supports can redistribute the financial risks involved in farming, and changing draft board policies in time of war can redistribute the risk of being killed in defense of one's country. Yet most people believe such transfers are justifiable even if involuntary. In these cases, however, the individuals among whom risks are redistributed are all members of a *polis* through which, arguably, they give implicit consent to the policies in question. Still, in some cases there cannot plausibly be said to be even implicit consent. When we go to war, for instance, we impose dramatic risks on thousands or even millions of people who have no political influence in our country. But if the war is justified, so too, presumably, are the involuntarily imposed risks.

THE PROSPECTS
FOR CONVERSATION

It has not been my purpose in this paper to decide which particular forms of experimentation are morally justifiable, so I will not further pursue a response to Regan's abolitionist argument. My goal has been to refocus the animal rights debate by emphasizing its philosophical complexity. The question is far more complicated than is suggested by simplistic portrayals by many researchers and in the popular media.

According to the common stereotype, an animal rights advocate wants to eliminate all animal research and is a vegetarian who even avoids wearing leather. But the first "serious attempt . . . to assess the accuracy of" this stereotype, a survey of about 600 animal activists attending the June 1990 "March for Animal Rights" in Wash-

ington, D.C., found that: nearly half of all activists believe the animal rights movement should not focus on animal research as its top priority; over a third eat red meat, poultry, or seafood; and 40 percent wear leather.[7] I have often heard agriculturalists and scientists say that it is hypocritical for an animal rights advocate to eat any kind of meat, wear leather, or use medicines that have been developed using animal models. But it would only be hypocritical if there were a single, monolithic animal rights philosophy that unambiguously ruled them all out.

In this essay, I have stressed the philosophical diversity underlying the animal rights movement. The "animal rights philosophies" of which many researchers are so contemptuous run the philosophical gamut from a utilitarianism very similar to their own to a true animal rights view that is quite different from their own. On some of these views, certain kinds of animal agriculture are permissible, but even on a true animal rights view like Regan's, it is possible to endorse some uses of animals, including experimentation that is meaningfully tied to saving human lives.

Continuing to paint all advocates of animal rights as unreasoning, anti-science lunatics will not make that movement go away, any more than painting all scientists who use animal models as Nazis bent on torturing the innocent will make animal research go away. Animal protection movements have surfaced and then disappeared in the past, but today's animal rights movement is squarely grounded in two major traditions in moral philosophy and, amid the stable affluence of a modern, industrialized nation like the United States, cannot be expected to go away. By the same token, twentieth-century medical research has dramatically proven its capacity to save lives and to improve the quality of human life, and it cannot be expected to go away either. So the reality is going to involve some level of some uses of animals, including some kinds of medical research.

A more philosophical understanding of the animal welfare/animal rights distinction can help replace the current politics of confrontation with a genuine conversation. Researchers who understand the philosophical bases of the animal rights movement will recognize similarities with their own views and can rest assured that genuinely important research will not be opposed by most advocates of animal rights. In the last analysis, what animal rights views do is increase the burden of proof the defenders of research must meet, and this is as it should be. Too often, pain and suffering have been understood to be "necessary" whenever a desired benefit could not be achieved without them, without regard to how important the benefit in question was.[8]

When it comes to research on animals, "academic freedom" cannot mean freedom to pursue any line of research one pleases, even in the arena of medical research. In most areas of research, someone who spends her career doing trivial work wastes only the taxpayers' money. But a scientist who spends his career doing trivial experiments on animals can waste the lives of hundreds or even thousands of sentient creatures. There will be increasing public oversight of laboratory research on animals, because major traditions in Western ethical theory support at least basic moral consideration for all sentient creatures. Researchers who react by adopting a siege mentality, refusing to disclose information on research and refusing to talk to advocates of animal rights, only reinforce the impression that they have something to hide.

REFERENCES

1. I owe this account of the consensus/convergence distinction to Bryan G. Norton, *Toward Unity among Environmentalists* (New York: Oxford University Press, 1991), pp. 237–43.
2. Peter Singer, *Animal Liberation,* 2nd ed. (Avon Books: 1990), pp. x–xi.
3. Peter Singer, *Practical Ethics,* 2nd ed. (New York: Cambridge University Press, 1993).
4. In any case, as Raymond Frey has pointed out, it is not clear that having forward-looking desires is a necessary condition for being self-conscious. R G. Frey, *Rights, Killing, and Suffering: Moral Vegetarianism and Applied Ethics* (Oxford: Basil Blackwell, 1983), p. 163.
5. Tom Regan, *The Case for Animal Rights* (Berkeley and Los Angeles: University of California Press, 1983).
6. This evidence is reviewed in my *In Nature's Interests? Interests, Animal Rights, and Environmental Ethics,* in manuscript.
7. S. Plous, "An Attitude Survey of Animal Rights Activists," *Psychological Science* 2 (May 1991): 194–96.
8. Susan Finsen, "On Moderation," in *Interpretation and Explanation in the Study of Animal Behavior,* ed. Marc Bekoff and Dale Jamieson, vol. 2 (Boulder: Westview Press, 1990), pp. 394–419.

Case Study Exercises

1. Share your thoughts on the radiation studies and the Gulf Vet studies, in light of the Nuremberg Code and/or the Helsinki Declaration. To what extent would you say these codes were followed?

2. In Fall 1995 an AIDS patient, Jeff Getty, underwent a highly risky experimental treatment that resulted in considerable controversy and debate: Baboon bone marrow cells were transplanted into Getty in hopes of slowing down or stopping the progress of Getty's advanced AIDS. The experiment involved killing the baboon, which angered animal rights activists, who contend that it is immoral to harvest or exploit other species to benefit humans. The experiment also involved radiation and drug therapy before the transplantation. A major goal of the experiment was to determine the safety of the radiation and drug therapy used to prepare a patient for a cross-species transplant. Some scientists opposed the experiment because it could potentially introduce new viruses and diseases into humans along the lines of the HIV virus, for which there is no known cure. (See Lawrence K. Altman, "Baboon Cells Fail to Thrive, But AIDS Patient Improves," *New York Times,* 9 February 1996.)

   a. Should cross-species experiments be permitted? Discuss the case from the standpoint of societal interests and global risks.

    b. Should there be any limits to such experiments? Discuss this case from the standpoint of animal rights concerns.

    c. Is it right to create what may be false hopes for seriously ill patients? Discuss this case from the standpoint of the patient.

    d. Is it right for scientists to conduct such medical experiments without any direct benefit to the patient? Discuss this case from the standpoint of the researchers and medical profession.

3. How do you think we should respond to concerns about xenotransplants running the risk of transmitting a virus, such as HIV, to humans? Not only has this issue been raised about the use of pig livers, but, as the following demonstrates, it also comes up with the use of baboons as a source for organs:

> A man who received a baboon liver in an experimental transplant became infected with a virus from the animal, revealing another obstacle in the way of animal-to-human transplants, researchers said. . . . The man, a 35-year-old HIV patient, died of his liver disease just over two months after the transplant, which took place in 1992 amid great publicity. But tests of his tissues in later years show he became infected with a virus from the baboon whose organ he received, Marian Michaels of the University of Pittsburgh said. . . . The patient was suffering from liver damage caused by the hepatitis B virus and had had his spleen removed after a car accident a few years before, so he was very ill. He received the baboon liver in an experimental procedure. He was given a full load of antibiotics, plus the antiviral drug ganciclovir. He and the baboon were infected with a herpes virus known as cytomegalovirus (CMV). Baboons are known to carry CMV—about 98 percent of all animals in the wild and in the laboratory are infected. It does them no harm. But CMV, which also infects many humans, was believed to be species-specific. That is, the strain that infects one species, such as baboons, was not believed to be able to infect humans. "I think it is quite concerning that an animal virus thought to be species-specific could be transmitted," Michaels said. . . . She said the finding strikes a blow to the idea that primates could be used for animal-to-human transplants . . . Michaels said it would be possible to raise animals in totally sterile conditions for use in transplants, but doing so with primates would raise ethical issues. (See "Baboon Liver Passes virus to Man," *Reuters,* 30 September 1999.)

4. Discuss the ethical implications of the creation of "transgenic" organisms. Consider, for example, the case of a biotech firm, Nextran, that is putting human DNA into pigs in hopes of decreasing the chance of the rejection of pig livers transplanted into humans.

> Today, despite fears that pig-to-human transplants could unleash a deadly new virus, the dream is closer than ever to reality. In August, a long-awaited safety study conducted by Nextran's chief competitor, Imutran Ltd., of Cambridge, England, found no evidence of active infection in 160 people who had been treated with pig tissue for a variety of conditions. The findings come as the companies are laying the groundwork to begin testing transplanted organs in people. Sometime within the next few years, and possibly as soon as the end of next year, either the British or the Americans will grab the brass ring: approval from a regulatory agency, either the United States Food and Drug Administration or its equivalent in Britain, to perform the world's first animal-to-human transplant using a heart or a kidney from a genetically engineered pig.
>
> Nobody expects cross-species transplants to be successful overnight. But with time, xenotransplantation could solve the most pressing crisis in medicine—the organ shortage. It could also make the companies very rich. Unlike human organs, which are donated, pig organs will be sold, and in a climate in which demand far outstrips supply, the seller will

name the price. By greatly expanding the donor pool, pigs could make transplants possible for tens of thousands of people who, because of the current rationing system, never even make the list, not to mention those in some Asian nations, where taking organs from the dead is culturally taboo. Imagine a therapy as revolutionary as penicillin and as lucrative as Viagra rolled into one. (See Sheryl Gay Stolberg, "Could This Pig Save Your Life?," *The New York Times,* 3 October 1999.)

5. Do you think it is necessarily wrong to trade, purchase, or barter organs, like kidneys, that are needed for transplants? Discuss whether or not you agree with the position set out in the following:

   . . . Congress had very good reason to want to ban transactions involving organs even if they were not "for profit." Creating contractual arrangements involving organs is inherently problematic, as even recent headlines suggest. Richard McNutt, suffering from kidney failure, allegedly romanced Dorothy Zauhar solely to get her to convince one of her relatives to donate a kidney to him. After her brother did in fact make such a donation, McNutt broke off their engagement. Zauhar and her brother sued McNutt, claiming he swindled the brother out of an organ by breaking his promise to marry Zauhar. Whatever else one things of this set of circumstances, this is not a "for profit" transaction. Zauhar's brother—like the donors in the kidney swap—was acting solely to benefit his relative. Yet the spectacle of people using the courts to fight about alleged promises concerning an organ is unseemly, at best, and may diminish respect and confidence for the organ donation system. The judge in the Zauhar-McNutt case properly ended up dismissing Ms. Zauhar's claims, pointing out that the alleged contract would have been illegal, given state and federal laws that criminalize the purchase and sale of organs. (See Jerry Menikoff, "Organ Swapping," *The Hastings Center Report,* Nov/Dec 1999.)

6. Should pesticide companies be allowed to experiment on humans? Manufacturers test pesticides on human subjects to obtain results that are used by the Environmental Protection Agency to set limits on the use of chemicals on crops, in the home, and elsewhere. Share your thoughts on the excerpt below:

   Because regulators cannot be sure that the highly toxic chemicals affect people in the same way they do animals, they first use the animal tests to estimate safe doses and then use an extra margin of safety, called an uncertainty factor, to make the legal limits 10 times safer. To avoid the uncertainty factor, industry officials have told the E.P.A., the companies are increasingly likely to use humans or tests for some chemicals. (See John H. Cushman Jr., "Group Wants Pesticide Companies to End Testing on Humans," *New York Times,* 28 July 1998.)

7. There are other issues, when it comes to pesticides. For instance, occasionally officials undertake the aerial spraying of pesticides (such as malathion to combat white flies on oranges and other crops), even in urban, heavily populated areas. Under what conditions, if any, do you think such aerial spraying should be permitted?

8. In June 2000 the Clinton administration decided to reject the use of human experiments in setting regulatory limits for pesticides (raised in exercise 6, above). The Environmental Protection Agency (EPA) will adopt a policy of officially ignoring any studies using human subjects in establishing legal limits for pesticides in food and water. Physician David Wallinga, who contended that such tests were analogous to lining up soldiers in front of nuclear blasts to see what would happen, remarked that "Studies that dose people intentionally with pesticides are scientifically and morally bankrupt." (See "U.S. to Reject

Human Testing for Pesticides," *Los Angeles Times,* 7 June 2000.) Do you think there is more than "officially ignoring" such studies that the government ought to do when it comes to using human subjects to test pesticides?

9. To what degree should we consider cosmetic surgery medical experimentation? Should we require long-term studies before allowing a drug or procedure to be marketed? Draw up a list of ethical issues and concerns that should be considered regarding cosmetic surgery.

10. Soldiers during the Gulf War were given experimental drugs and vaccines intended to protect them from chemical and biological weapons. In addition to the potential risks of combining the vaccines, soldiers testifying before Congress charged that these drugs and vaccines were administered to them without getting their informed consent.

   Approximately 20,000 of the troops who served in the Persian Gulf war have reported debilitating symptoms like fatigue, skin rashes, muscle and joint pain, headaches, memory loss, shortness of breath, and gastrointestinal problems. Troops were exposed to smoke from oil well fires, diesel fumes, toxic paints, pesticides, and depleted uranium used in munitions and armor. They were also given at least three drugs under special circumstances in which the military and FDA waived the usual informed consent procedures. These drugs included pyridostigmine bromide, an unapproved vaccine to combat botulism, and a licensed vaccine to protect against anthrax. (See Marlene Cimons, "Stricken Veterans Blame the Military for Health Hazards," *Los Angeles Times,* 7 May 1994.)

   a. Under what conditions, if any, should the military and the FDA be permitted to waive the usual informed-consent guidelines?
   b. If you were a member of Congress hearing the testimony of the Gulf War veterans, what would you recommend?

11. Arthur Caplan studied 273 infertility centers and found that sperm had been removed from 25 dead men at 14 centers in 11 states between 1980 and 1995. Most requests are from family members. (See Gina Kolata , "Uncertain Area for Doctors: Saving Sperm of Dead Men," *New York Times,* 30 May 1997.) Here are some of the moral dilemmas: Does a man have the right to his gametes, and therefore should his written permission be necessary before anyone could take his sperm? Does a wife have the right to assume her (dead) husband would consent to fathering a child with her? What sort of policy makes sense here?

12. Should a competent adult be allowed to donate both of his kidneys? Were medical ethicists justified in opposing a kidney donation by a 38 year-old prisoner, David Patterson, whose daughter had undergone two kidney transplants? The most recent transplant used Patterson's first kidney, which was being rejected, possibly because the girl was negligent in taking antirejection medication. Certain ethical issues arise from allowing anyone to donate an organ when the donor will incur harm in doing so. (See Evelyn Nieve, "Girl Awaits Father's 2d Kidney, and Decision by Medical Ethicists," *New York Times,* 5 December 1998.) In looking at the case, it may be helpful to consider:
   1. The fact that the father is competent.
   2. The fact that approximately 3,100 people are waiting for kidneys in the state of California, with an average wait of three to four years.
   3. The fact that the girl had been on dialysis three times a week for seven years, unable to go to school, and had been abandoned by her father when she was a baby (he has been in prison nine years thus far).

13. Do you think we ought to have a federal policy regarding the stock of viruses, like smallpox, that are no longer considered health threats (except possibly as biowarfare agents)?

14. Reported in the June 2, 1999, *Journal of the American Medical Association,* the drug androstenedione (used by baseball player Mark McGwire, among others) did not build muscle. Rather, it increases the risk of heart disease, pancreatic cancer, and breast enlargement. The study provided the first scientific evidence on the safety of the drug. Researchers found no difference in added strength, muscle mass, or testosterone levels in those using the drug and those taking a placebo. (See Holcomb B. Noble, "Study Shows Drug Does Not Build Muscle," *New York Times,* 2 June 1999.)

    1. Given these results, do you think the FDA should prohibit the sale of supplements and performance-enhancing drugs until sufficient research has been done to attest to their safety?
    2. What sorts of risks should consumers be allowed to take with substances that have no clear health benefits?

15. Among material released by the President's Advisory Committee on Human Radiation Experiments were documents from the Atomic Energy Commission detailing attempts in the 1950's to collect bone and tissue from cadavers without obtaining the family's consent. Evidently, the federal government established a worldwide network to collect tissue in order to secretly monitor the effects of radioactive fallout (in particular strontium-90) from nuclear weapons tests. (Ironically, the enterprise was termed "Project Sunshine.") More than 1,500 samples were gathered and 500 were analyzed, according to the report. (See Warren E. Leary, "U.S. Collected Human Tissue to Monitor Fallout," *New York Times,* 21 June 1995.)

    a. Discuss what this information tells about the federal government's presumptions about what is allowable in the name of national security.
    b. Do you think such studies ought to be morally permissible? If not, how can we prohibit them?

16. Do you think hand transplants raise significantly different ethical concerns from those that organ transplants raise? Can you think of any good reason we ought to prohibit hand transplants? Discuss whether or not you find them morally acceptable. What about foot and leg transplants?

17. The results of the first American trial of a Russian technique for fetal transplantation to help diabetics are in: Transplanted fetal pancreatic cells have resulted in increased insulin production and improved control of blood sugar levels, with virtually all of the experimental subjects benefiting from the transplant. (See Thomas H. Maugh II, "Transplants of Cells Aided Diabetics, Doctors Say," *Los Angeles Times,* 12 April 1995.) Proponents of the use of fetuses in transplantation feel that these optimistic results give further evidence that we should condone such experimentation. Opponents, however, remain unmoved, arguing that using fetal cells is morally wrong, because (a) most come from aborted fetuses and (b) the sanctity of human life demands that we respect dead fetuses by not exploiting them even for medical purposes. How might we resolve the debate as to whether the use of fetal transplantation is justified?

18. On May 10, 2000, the FDA decided to permit McGhan Medical Corporation and Mentor Corporation, the two largest makers of breast implants, to continue marketing the devices. This decision was made in spite of new scientific evidence that they pose a significant risk of infection, tissue hardening, and breast pain as well as the need for repeat surgeries. Five studies of over 9,000 women indicated "relatively high rates of complications and rupture." (See *N.Y. Times News Service,* "Breast Implants Ok'd Despite Risks," *The Bakersfield Californian,* 11 May 2000.)

    a. In light of this latest evidence that breast implants do pose significant risks, do you think the FDA requirement that companies inform women of the risks is sufficient?

    b. In light of the risks, should breast implants only be permitted for reconstructive surgery (e.g., after a mastectomy), rather than for cosmetic surgery?

    c. In light of the risks, should breast implants be disallowed altogether?

19. To what degree should we factor in an animal's species in deciding whether or not to proceed with a particular experiment? A British poll found that many people felt lines need to be drawn in animal experimentation:

> The survey found that attitudes to animal experimentation vary dramatically with the purpose of the experiment, the animal species, and the degree of pain suffered. While 65% were prepared for mice to suffer in experiments to develop a drug to cure leukemia, only 52% would let monkeys be used in the same experiments. In the case of an AIDS vaccine, the figures fell to 56% and 44% respectively. When asked about less emotive treatments, such as new painkilling drugs, the percentages dropped to 47% and 35%. Fundamental research, such as studying the sense of hearing, was opposed by 61% and 75% respectively if the animals suffered in any way. (See Richard Woodman, "Explanations Shift Attitudes to Animal Experiments," *British Medical Journal,* 29 May 1999.)

Set out your recommendations on restricting the use of primates in experiments, taking into account the issue of the purpose of the experiment.

20. According to reports, the U.S. government has quietly been releasing "lightly contaminated" radioactive scrap metal from the nation's defense arsenal and selling it to demolition contractors, scrap dealers, and recyclers for use in such things as jewelry, automobiles, silverware, leg braces, and hip replacements. Environmental groups are concerned that repeated exposure to small doses of radiation over many years is a potential hazard. (See Frank Clifford, "Widespread Use of Radioactive Scrap Assailed," *Los Angeles Times,* 12 June 2000.) How might consumers and environmental groups effectively bring this into the public eye as a safety concern? Share your ideas on this issue.

21. To what degree do you think religious leaders should take a public stand on such issues as the traffic in organs and body parts? Set out your recommendations after reading the following:

> The organs trade is extensive, lucrative, explicitly illegal in most countries, and unethical according to every governing body of medical professional life. It is therefore covert. In some sites the organs trade links the upper strata of biomedical practice to the lowest reaches of the criminal world. The transactions can involve police, mortuary workers, pathologists, civil servants, ambulance drivers, emergency room workers, eye bank and blood bank managers, and transplant coordinators.
>
>   The rapid transfer of organ transplant technologies to countries in the East (China, Taiwan, and India) and the South (especially Argentina, Chile, and Brazil) created a global scarcity of viable organs that has initiated a movement of sick bodies in one direction and of healthy organs—transported by commercial airlines in ordinary Styrofoam picnic coolers conveniently stored in overhead luggage compartments—often in the reverse direction, creating a kind of "kula ring" of bodies and body parts. . . . No modern pope (beginning with Pius XII) has raised any moral objection to the requirements of transplant surgery. The Catholic Church decided over 30 years ago that the definition of death—unlike the

definition of life—should be left up to the doctors, paving the way for the acceptance of brainstem death. (See Nancy Scheper-Hughes, Joseph S. Alter, Steffan I. Ayora-Diaz, Thomas J. Csordas et al., "The Global Traffic in Human Organs," *Current Anthropology,* vol. 41, no. 2, April 2000.)

22. The commodification of organs has brought with it another twist, namely collateral in dowry. Discuss the human rights issues this raises, after considering the excerpt below:

Lawrence Cohen, who has worked in rural towns in various regions of India over the past decade, notes that in a very brief period the idea of trading a kidney for a dowry has caught on and become one strategy for poor parents desperate to arrange a comfortable marriage for an "extra" daughter. . . . in 1998 Cohen encountered friends in Benares who were considering selling a kidney to raise money for a younger sister's dowry. In this instance, he notes, "women flow in one direction and kidneys in the other." And the appearance of a new biomedical technology has reinforced a traditional practice, the dowry, that had been waning. With the emergence of new sources of capital, the dowry system is expanding, along with kidney sales, into areas where it had not traditionally been practiced." (See Nancy Scheper-Hughes, Joseph S. Alter, Steffan I. Ayora-Diaz, Thomas J. Csordas et al. "The Global Traffic in Human Organs," *Current Anthropology,* vol. 41, no. 2, April 2000.)

InfoTrac College Edition

1. Sheila Mclean, "Human Tissue: Ethical and Legal Issues: The Report from the Nuffield Council on Bioethics Provides a Coherent Legal and Ethical Approach"
2. R. D. Start, W. Brown, R. J. Bryant, M. W. Reed, S. S. Cross, and G. Kent, "Ownership and Uses of Human Tissue: Does the Nuffield Bioethics Report Accord with the Opinion of Surgical Inpatients?"
3. Eliot Marshall, "Panel Faults Research Consent Process"
4. Owen Dyer, "Working Party Speaks Out on Use of Human Tissue"
5. Trevor Harrison, "Globalization and the Trade in Human Body Parts"
6. James V. Delong, "Organ Grinders [Laws on Procurement and Distribution of Human Organs]"
7. Carl Kovac, "'Tissue Trade in Hungary Is Investigated"
8. Gloria J. Banks, "Legal & Ethical Safeguards: Protection of Society's Most Vulnerable Participants in a Commercialized Organ Transplantation System"
9. *Diabetes Forecast,* "Kidney Policies Hurt Black Americans [Adapted from the AMA]"
10. *Alcoholism & Drug Abuse Week,* "Change in Transplant Priorities Spells Bad News for Addicts"
11. David J. Rothman, "Body Shop [Use of Executed Prisoners' Organs in China]"
12. Domhnall Macauley, "Drugs in Sports"
13. Philip Hersh, " Tidal Wave [Drugs and Chinese Swim Teams]"
14. Rebecca Johnson, "Mariel in Balance [Interview with Mariel Hemingway on Breast Implants]"
15. Michelle Kohlmeier, "Malpractice & Negligence: Negligent Undertaking Liability for Silicone Testing—*Dow Chemical Co. v. Mahlum*"
16. *Cancer Weekly Plus,* "U.S. Government Sued for Wrongful Human Radiological Experiments [Hanford Nuclear Reservation Release of Ionizing Radiation into Air]"

17. George J. Annas, "Protecting Soldiers from Friendly Fire: The Consent Requirement for Using Investigational Drugs and Vaccines in Combat [Law, Medicine, and Socially Responsible Research]"
18. L. Christine Oliver and Bruce W. Shackleton, "The Indoor Air We Breathe: A Public Health Problem of the 90's"
19. Richard E. Lehrfeld and Barbara A. Najman, "The Nabobs of Negativism Are Wrong: EPA Should Redirect Some Research on Toxic Airborne Particles"

Web Connections

For links to Medical Experimentation: Historical Considerations Web sites, articles, cases, and more exercises go to our Medical Experimentation page at philosophy.wadsworth.com/teays.purdy/experimentation

Chapter 5

Death and Dying

IT IS HARD for most of us to think about our loved ones dying and the fact that we, too, will one day die. A lot of thought has gone into attempts to make the end of our lives more dignified and less dehumanizing. Most desirable would be the end of our days to have a maximum of satisfying moments and a minimum of suffering.

One issue that arises when we look at death and dying is how and where we will die. Will we die in a hospital, alone or with a caring nurse, doctor, member of the clergy, or loved one near our side? Will we die alone, hooked to a machine in some nursing home, convalescent hospital, or retirement facility? Will we end up in a hospice, letting our lives take their course? Or will we seek to control that end, say by suicide or physician-assisted death? Some of us get to choose; others don't. Some can draw up a living will and, hopefully, others make sure it is carried out. Some die, say in an accident or an act of violence, without ever getting to see their plans for how they die carried out.

Unfortunately, even when we try to draw up a plan for our own ideal way to die we are not always able to see it put into motion. Nevertheless, that fact does not stop people from trying. And so we make our Living Wills and share our values about end-of-life medical treatment with our friends and family in hopes that our wishes will be honored.

Diseases or disabling conditions may make life difficult even when they do not immediately kill; modern treatments and technology can prolong life still further. So although questions about care toward the end of life are by no means new, they are nevertheless pressing because our ability to prolong life still leaves ethical issues unresolved. Social refusal or inability to provide comprehensive, universal health care, especially good palliative care and more effective pain control, complicates the debate still further.

Many religious and moral traditions place a high value on life. Such value is often equated with a prohibition on killing. We might reasonably expect such prohibitions to be absolute, thus excluding capital punishment or killing in war. However, that is not usually the case. Some qualification intended to distinguish between permissible and prohibited killing is usually introduced, such as "guilt" and "innocence." Strictures about when "innocent" life can be ended are common, and taking steps such as physician-assisted suicide that are intended to end life may be morally permissible or even morally required.

Assumptions about the sanctity of life are widespread and deeply felt. As a result, the terms and images used to describe possible courses of action are often highly charged. For example, suicide may be seen as sinful or shameful, physician-assisted suicide as frightful or macabre, and euthanasia as associated with Nazi death camps. On the other hand, there are those who see suicide as an acceptable act of self-determination, physician-assisted suicide as a humane gesture on the part of one's physician, and euthanasia as an act of mercy to relieve the terminally ill of extended suffering.

THE PHILOSOPHICAL DEBATE

Within the philosophical debate on death and dying, we find considerable interest in the growing pressure in our society to take a closer look at how we treat those in insufferable pain (terminally ill or not) and those facing their own deaths. When we examine this issue, we need to consider both acts of omission and acts of commission, such as:

- Heroic acts versus suicide

- Failing to start treatment versus withdrawing treatment

- Refusing treatment versus ending life directly

- Treatment aimed at pain control versus treatment aimed at causing death

- Ending your own life versus asking another to end it

- Ending life to avoid suffering versus ending it for some other reason

- Acts or omissions taken with consent versus those taken without it

The moral relevance of such distinctions is particularly important here because of the prominence of so-called "slippery slope" arguments in debates about the end of life. Such arguments contend that although a specific act is itself morally permissible, allowing it will inevitably lead to a different type of act that is not morally permissible. Therefore, acts of the first type must be prohibited.

A common slippery slope argument about euthanasia is that although it is right to help end the lives of terminally ill individuals who want to die, a public policy permitting such help will inevitably lead to the murder of individuals perceived as burdensome. Additional slippery slope arguments could be found for most of the dichotomies listed above.

Evaluating slippery slope arguments requires us to see if there is a causal connection between an initial action and a purported series of consequences; namely that if we allow one moral action it will invariably lead to another, less desirable one. Such investigations demand conceptual and moral analysis. We may also need to search for elusive empirical clues about potential human behavior. Merely pointing out the possibility of a slippery slope, as some authors do, is not sufficient grounds for prohibiting anything. It is impossible to judge which changes will be problematic without scrutiny of the evidence.

Conceptual analysis and moral judgment are therefore closely related. Consider "suicide." The paradigm case of suicide is one in which somebody ends her life to avoid mental or physical suffering. But are you suicidal if you risk your life for the benefit of others? Are you suicidal if you continue to smoke knowing the evidence of its health risks? Are you suicidal if you choose to forgo painful treatment for some life-threatening medical condition? An issue here is whether a person can be competent and elect to behave suicidally, or whether suicidal behavior is invariably linked to a disturbed state of mind, such as depression.

It seems important to distinguish between foreseen and intended acts, as well as between the goodness or badness of the consequences. Generally, heroes, smokers, alcoholics, and those fearful of medical treatment are not choosing to die; death is merely a more or less probable consequence of a course of action. This distinction between foreseen and intended does not relieve us of responsibility for our actions, but it emphasizes the importance of the ends that are sought.

Judgments about the value of those ends are at the center of the suicide debate. Some people are skeptical about whether reason can show that some ends are better than others. Another view is that autonomous judgments should have priority over other, competing values, and that society does not always have an overriding interest in prolonging life. This position holds that autonomy entails individual judgments about what constitutes unbearable life.

The difficulty with this autonomy-based position is the fact that many suicides are a result of depression temporarily distorting judgment. Such deaths are tragic and should be prevented wherever possible, for the sake both of those who would die and those who would be left behind. However, some people believe suicide can be a rational response to unbearable suffering or a life no longer thought to hold value. Therefore, we need to consider whether an institution should be put in place that fights to save those in danger of making a dreadful mistake but that also recognizes the need for some sort of policy when suicide seems a reasonable course of action. This is a problematic, but significant, issue facing us.

There are those who think that suicide can never be a rational response to the conditions of life, that killing oneself is intrinsically wrong, or that society's interest in life always overrides even an autonomous desire to die. One prerequisite for moral thinking is empathetic understanding of such issues. We need not only to consider if suicide, an action some view as intrinsically wrong, might be justified, we need also to consider whether we have a social interest in continued life for all individuals as well as for its consistency with other social arrangements that affect life and death.

Physician-Assisted Suicide

Entertaining the possibility of a policy permitting physician-assisted suicide requires showing that objections to it can be refuted and that some version of the arguments for it can be defended. In addition, the involvement of physicians must be justifiable. Many people are wary of allowing physicians to be involved in patients' decisions to commit suicide. Traditional objections to this policy are the Hippocratic oath, the possible erosion of trust in physicians, the claim that their proper goal is preserving life and health, and slippery slope arguments that it will inevitably be abused. Daniel Callahan raises such concerns in one of the articles in this chapter. Proponents of physician-assisted suicide question the relevance of the Hippocratic oath, point out the limited role proposed for physicians, and wonder whether this additional authority necessarily erodes trust. Some believe that assistance with suicide could or should be provided by a different member of the health care team. Some, like Timothy Quill, as we see in his article, believe the physician has an important role to play in assisted suicide.

Assisted suicide is a hotly debated issue unlikely to go away in the near future. One reason for this is that as we face the reality of our own death, significant numbers of people will continue to want sufficient control over their deaths to avoid unnecessary suffering. Another reason is that the opposing positions of the issue reflect sharply differing world views.

Measures that would legalize physician-assisted suicide are now appearing on state ballots, and some states, like Oregon, have made it public policy. With the *Glucksberg* decision, the Supreme Court has rejected the argument that there is a constitutional right to assisted suicide. It does not necessarily follow, however, that asserting a right to assisted suicide will be found unconstitutional.

Euthanasia

"Euthanasia" is now being used to cover a variety of situations in which a physician is more directly involved in a decision about the end of life than is the case with physician-assisted suicide. Traditionally, euthanasia has been divided into four moral categories: passive voluntary, active voluntary, passive nonvoluntary, and active nonvoluntary. These categories are the result of applying different combinations of two distinctions:

- Active versus passive

- Voluntary versus nonvoluntary

Active euthanasia involves the intentional termination of a patient's life in order to alleviate suffering from an underlying medical condition. In contrast, passive euthanasia occurs when treatment intended to sustain or prolong life is intentionally withheld or withdrawn. In the latter case (but not the former), it is claimed that the disease, not human action, killed the patient. This is seen as a morally relevant difference. This distinction has come into ever sharper relief as the capacity of health care to prolong dying has increased. A common reaction to the increased potential for such technologically supported dying has been to rely on a variety of principles that justify failing to start care or withdrawing care (such as the Doctrine of Double Effect, boundaries of extraordinary versus ordinary care, and labeling unwanted treatment as legal assault), without justifying direct and intended killing. Many people thus accept passive euthanasia on these grounds, but reject active euthanasia. Whether these principles can bear this weight remains to be shown. However, Consequentialists contend that they cannot. And given that some suffering cannot be relieved, some argue that a humanly engineered quick death may be morally superior to letting nature take its course.

If the differences between passive and active euthanasia are not morally relevant, it would still remain to be shown whether the pair should be rejected or embraced. There is no doubt that many deaths would be worse if every potentially life-prolonging treatment were morally mandatory. Holland has decriminalized certain forms of active euthanasia, but it is as yet far from clear that we ought to follow its example.

Proponents of such a policy contend that it could, if carefully regulated, prevent much suffering without leading to the kinds of consequences feared by opponents. This is an empirical matter that can be tested only by experience. If a state or country legalizes assisted suicide, that will provide some relevant evidence, although opponents would likely find this experience unacceptable. One step the state of Oregon took was to make physician-assisted *suicide* within a patient's reach, but to prohibit a physician from using a lethal injection to take the patient's life.

Voluntary euthanasia is euthanasia requested by a patient. Nonvoluntary euthanasia would take place without the consent of the patient. Although clear in principle, this distinction can be difficult to apply in practice. The simpler case is where a competent patient consistently requests death. But what if a patient is only periodically competent? What if the patient is incompetent, but has a health care proxy, or a living will? And so forth. At the other end of the spectrum, a dying patient may be clear about his or her desire to live as long as possible. Killing such a patient may then be murder. It is less obvious whether such a patient has a right to all the health care resources necessary to prolong life. And what about patients about whom we have no information? The current assumption is that because life is such a fundamental good, society should generally assume that the patient would wish to live as long as possible, and act accordingly. Scarce resources now put this assumption in question; this issue is likely to become increasingly pressing as the large generation of baby boomers ages, straining health care resources.

Scarce resources raise additional questions about euthanasia. Will dying patients be pressured to accept euthanasia because of society's inability or unwillingness to allocate sufficient resources for care? Could there be a duty to die? Even if there were, will there be differential pressure to die on those traditionally perceived to be less valuable members of society? Conversely, does the failure to craft a morally desirable euthanasia policy weigh more heavily on certain groups over others, such as the elderly, those without families, women, the disabled? These questions are not intended to end debate, but rather to make sure that it is set within a realistic context that takes account of how policy affects every member of society.

One of the concerns raised in the *Vacco v. Quill* case, addressed in the second section of readings, is that some disabled people fear that the momentum for physician-assisted suicide may prove a danger to them; that there is the potential for abuse here. As suggested in the Amici Curiae brief, a society that is willing to dispense with the terminally ill may come also to want to eliminate those, like the disabled, sometimes viewed as having less social worth than the so-called normal members of society. For that reason, they urge that we think twice before allowing active euthanasia to become a fixture of our lives.

This chapter's readings fall into three sections. The first looks at euthanasia and physician-assisted death.

1. Arguing for the patient's right to seek physician-assisted suicide, Timothy E. Quill focuses on the case of his patient "Diane," who had advanced leukemia when she sought his assistance in killing herself.

2. In his discussion of the role of physicians in active euthanasia cases, Daniel Callahan argues against the involvement of the medical profession in taking another person's life. He questions arguments based on self-determination and sets out the reasons why he thinks physician-assisted suicide is a mistake.

3. Dena S. Davis looks at euthanasia from a feminist perspective, bringing in issues of personal autonomy and employing a comparison with contraception.

4. H. Tristram Engelhardt, Jr., looks at euthanasia and children. He contrasts it with adult euthanasia, looks at children's moral status and parents' rights, and offers some recommendations about when it would be justified.

5. With respect to hospices, Tracy Albee offers a personal narrative detailing the sorts of fears hospice patients exhibit regarding the alleviation of pain (as a disguised form of euthanasia).

The second section of readings focuses upon ethical and legal guidelines, including ones arising from court decisions.

1. Troyen A. Brennan examines what ought to be done regarding DNR (do-not-resuscitate) orders for incompetent patients when there is no consent on the part of the family.

2. Susan M. Wolf et al. examine the Patient Self-Determination Act of 1990, noting the goals and raising a variety of reservations.

3. In opposition to legalizing physician-assisted suicide, activists for the disabled (Not Dead Yet) submitted an Amici Curiae (friend of the court) brief in the *Vacco v. Quill case* — a case of physician-assisted suicide. We present an excerpt from the brief.

4. Marcia Angell examines the case of Helga Wanglie, who wanted to be kept on a respirator despite the wishes of her husband and children — and contrasts it with "right to die" cases like *Quinlan, Brophy,* and *Cruzan.*

5. We present an example of a Living Will.

In the last section, we look at personal narratives about death and dying.

1. Elisabeth Hansot's letter describes the death of her mother in an intensive care unit of a large hospital and the struggle she had in order to have her advance directives recognized.

2. David S. Pisetsky writes about the death of his father and explains why he was grateful that his father died at home, rather than in a clinical or hospital setting.

Euthanasia and Physician-Assisted Death

Death and Dignity:
A Case of Individualized Decision Making

TIMOTHY E. QUILL

DIANE WAS FEELING TIRED and had a rash. A common scenario, though there was something subliminally worrisome that prompted me to check her blood count. Her hematocrit was 22, and the white-cell count was 4.3 with some metamyelocytes and unusual white cells. I wanted it to be viral, trying to deny what was staring me in the face. Perhaps in a repeated count it would disappear. I called Diane and told her it might be more serious than I had initially thought—that the test needed to be repeated and that if she felt worse, we might have to move quickly. When she pressed for the possibilities, I reluctantly opened the door to leukemia. Hearing the word seemed to make it exist. "Oh, shit!" she said. "Don't tell me that." Oh, shit! I thought, I wish I didn't have to.

Diane was no ordinary person (although no one I have ever come to know has been really or-

TIMOTHY E. QUILL is an Associate Chief of Medicine at Genesee Hospital and a Professor of Medicine and Psychiatry at the Rochester University School of Medicine and Dentistry.

dinary). She was raised in an alcoholic family and had felt alone for much of her life. She had vaginal cancer as a young woman. Through much of her adult life, she had struggled with depression and her own alcoholism. I had come to know, respect, and admire her over the previous eight years as she confronted these problems and gradually overcame them. She was an incredibly clear, at times brutally honest, thinker and communicator. As she took control of her life, she developed a strong sense of independence and confidence. In the previous three-and-one-half years, her hard work had paid off. She was completely abstinent from alcohol, she had established much deeper connections with her husband, college-age son, and several friends, and her business and her artistic work were blossoming. She felt she was really living fully for the first time.

Not surprisingly, the repeated blood count was abnormal, and detailed examination of the peripheral blood smear showed myelocytes. I advised her to come into the hospital, explaining that we needed to do a bone marrow biopsy and make some decisions relatively rapidly. She came

New England Journal of Medicine 324, 10 (March 7, 1991): 691–694. Copyright 1991. Permission granted by the Massachusetts Medical Society. All rights reserved.

to the hospital knowing what we would find. She was terrified, angry, and sad. Although we knew the odds, we both clung to the thread of possibility that it might be something else.

The bone marrow confirmed the worst: acute myelomonocytic leukemia. In the face of this tragedy, we looked for signs of hope. This is an area of medicine in which technological intervention has been successful, with cures 25 percent of the time—long-term cures. As I probed the costs of these cures, I heard about induction chemotherapy (three weeks in the hospital, prolonged neutropenia, probable infectious complications, and hair loss; 75 percent of patients respond, 25 percent do not). For the survivors, this is followed by consolidation chemotherapy (with similar side effects; another 25 percent die, for a net survival of 50 percent). Those still alive, to have a reasonable chance of long-term survival, then need bone marrow transplantation (hospitalization for two months and whole-body irradiation, with complete killing of the bone marrow, infectious complications, and the possibility for graft-versus-host disease—with a survival of approximately 50 percent, or 25 percent of the original group). Though hematologists may argue over the exact percentages, they don't argue about the outcome of no treatment—certain death in days, weeks, or at most a few months.

Believing that delay was dangerous, our oncologist broke the news to Diane and began making plans to insert a Hickman catheter and begin induction chemotherapy that afternoon. When I saw her shortly thereafter, she was enraged at his presumption that she would want treatment, and devastated by the finality of the diagnosis. All she wanted to do was go home and be with her family. She had no further questions about treatment and in fact had decided that she wanted none. Together we lamented her tragedy and the unfairness of life. Before she left, I felt the need to be sure that she and her husband understood that there was some risk in delay, that the problem was not going to go away, and that we needed to keep considering the options over

the next several days. We agreed to meet in two days.

She returned in two days with her husband and son. They had talked extensively about the problem and the options. She remained very clear about her wish not to undergo chemotherapy and to live whatever time she had left outside the hospital. As we explored her thinking further, it became clear that she was convinced she would die during the period of treatment and would suffer unspeakably in the process (from hospitalization, from lack of control over her body, from the side effects of chemotherapy, and from pain and anguish). Although I could offer support and my best effort to minimize her suffering if she chose treatment, there was no way I could say any of this would not occur. In fact, the last four patients with acute leukemia at our hospital had died very painful deaths in the hospital during various stages of treatment (a fact I did not share with her). Her family wished she would choose treatment but sadly accepted her decision. She articulated very clearly that it was she who would be experiencing all the side effects of treatment and that odds of 25 percent were not good enough for her to undergo so toxic a course of therapy, given her expectations of chemotherapy and hospitalization and the absence of a closely matched bone marrow donor. I had her repeat her understanding of the treatment, the odds, and what to expect if there were no treatment. I clarified a few misunderstandings, but she had a remarkable grasp of the options and implications.

I have been a longtime advocate of active, informed patient choice of treatment or nontreatment, and of a patient's right to die with as much control and dignity as possible. Yet there was something about her giving up a 25 percent chance of long-term survival in favor of almost certain death that disturbed me. I had seen Diane fight and use her considerable inner resources to overcome alcoholism and depression, and I half expected her to change her mind over the next week. Since the window of time in which effective treatment can be initiated is rather narrow, we met several times that week. We obtained a second hematology consultation and talked at length about the meaning and implications of treatment and nontreatment. She talked to a psychologist she had seen in the past. I gradually understood the decision from her perspective and became convinced that it was the right decision for her. We arranged for home hospice care (although at that time Diane felt reasonably well, was active, and looked healthy), left the door open for her to change her mind, and tried to anticipate how to keep her comfortable in the time she had left.

Just as I was adjusting to her decision, she opened up another area that would stretch me profoundly. It was extraordinarily important to Diane to maintain control of herself and her own dignity during the time remaining to her. When this was no longer possible, she clearly wanted to die. As a former director of a hospice program, I know how to use pain medicines to keep patients comfortable and lessen suffering. I explained the philosophy of comfort care, which I strongly believe in. Although Diane understood and appreciated this, she had known of people lingering in what was called relative comfort, and she wanted no part of it. When the time came, she wanted to take her life in the least painful way possible. Knowing of her desire for independence and her decision to stay in control, I thought this request made perfect sense. I acknowledged and explored this wish but also thought that it was out of the realm of currently accepted medical practice and that it was more than I could offer or promise. In our discussion, it became clear that preoccupation with her fear of a lingering death would interfere with Diane's getting the most out of the time she had left until she found a safe way to ensure her death. I feared the effects of a violent death on her family, the consequences of an ineffective suicide that would leave her lingering in precisely the state she dreaded so much, and the possibility that a family member would be forced to assist her, with all the legal and personal repercussions that would follow. She discussed this at length with her family. They believed that they should respect her choice. With this in mind, I told Diane that information was available from the Hemlock Society that might be helpful to her.

A week later she phoned me with a request for barbiturates for sleep. Since I knew that this was an essential ingredient in a Hemlock Society suicide, I asked her to come to the office to talk things over. She was more than willing to protect me by participating in a superficial conversation about her insomnia, but it was important to me to know how she planned to use the drugs and to be sure that she was not in despair or overwhelmed in a way that might color her judgment. In our discussion, it was apparent that she was having trouble sleeping, but it was also evident that the security of having enough barbiturates available to commit suicide when and if the time came would leave her secure enough to live fully and concentrate on the present. It was clear that she was not despondent and that in fact she was making deep, personal connections with her family and close friends. I made sure that she knew how to use the barbiturates for sleep, and also that she knew the amount needed to commit suicide. We agreed to meet regularly, and she promised to meet with me before taking her life, to ensure that all other avenues had been exhausted. I wrote the prescription with an uneasy feeling about the boundaries I was exploring—spiritual, legal, professional, and personal. Yet I also felt strongly that I was setting her free to get the most out of the time she had left, and to maintain dignity and control on her own terms until her death.

The next several months were very intense and important for Diane. Her son stayed home from college, and they were able to be with one another and say much that had not been said earlier. Her husband did his work at home so that he and Diane could spend more time together. She spent time with her closest friends. I had her come into the hospital for a conference with our residents, at which she illustrated in a most profound and personal way the importance of informed decision making, the right to refuse treatment, and the extraordinarily personal effects of illness and interaction with the medical system. There were emotional and physical hardships as well. She had periods of intense sadness and anger. Several times she became very weak, but she received transfusions as an outpatient and responded with marked improvement of symptoms. She had two serious infections that responded surprisingly well to empirical courses of oral antibiotics. After three tumultuous months, there were two weeks of relative calm and well-being, and fantasies of a miracle began to surface.

Unfortunately, we had no miracle. Bone pain, weakness, fatigue, and fevers began to dominate her life. Although the hospice workers, family members, and I tried our best to minimize the suffering and promote comfort, it was clear that the end was approaching. Diane's immediate future held what she feared the most—increasing discomfort, dependence, and hard choices between pain and sedation. She called up her closest friends and asked them to come over to say goodbye, telling them that she would be leaving soon. As we had agreed, she let me know as well. When we met, it was clear that she knew what she was doing, that she was sad and frightened to be leaving, but that she would be even more terrified to stay and suffer. In our tearful goodbye, she promised a reunion in the future at her favorite spot on the edge of Lake Geneva, with dragons swimming in the sunset.

Two days later her husband called to say that Diane had died. She had said her final goodbyes to her husband and son that morning, and asked them to leave her alone for an hour. After an hour, which must have seemed an eternity, they found her on the couch, lying very still and covered by her favorite shawl. There was no sign of struggle. She seemed to be at peace. They called me for advice about how to proceed. When I arrived at their house, Diane indeed seemed peaceful. Her husband and son were quiet. We talked about what a remarkable person she had been. They seemed to have no doubts about the course she had chosen or about their cooperation, although the unfairness of her illness and the finality of her death were overwhelming to us all.

I called the medical examiner to inform him that a hospice patient had died. When asked about the cause of death, I said, "acute leukemia." He said that was fine and that we should call a funeral director. Although acute leukemia was the truth, it was not the whole story. Yet any mention of suicide would have given rise to a police investigation and probably brought the arrival of an ambulance crew for resuscitation. Diane would have become a "coroner's case," and the decision to perform an autopsy would have been made at the discretion of the medical examiner. The family or I could have been subject to criminal prosecution, and I to professional review, for our roles in support of Diane's choices. Although I truly believe that the family and I gave her the best care possible, allowing her to define her limits and directions as much as possible, I am not sure the law, society, or the medical profession would agree. So I said "acute leukemia" to protect all of us, to protect Diane from an invasion into her past and her body, and to continue to shield society from the knowledge of the degree of suffering that people often undergo in the process of dying. Suffering can be lessened to some extent, but in no way eliminated or made benign, by the careful intervention of a competent, caring physician, given current social constraints.

Diane taught me about the range of help I can provide if I know people well and if I allow them to say what they really want. She taught me about life, death, and honesty and about taking charge and facing tragedy squarely when it strikes. She taught me that I can take small risks for people that I really know and care about. Although I did not assist in her suicide directly, I helped indirectly to make it possible, successful, and relatively painless. Although I know we have measures to help control pain and lessen suffering, to think that people do not suffer in the process of dying is an illusion. Prolonged dying can occasionally be peaceful, but more often the role of the physician and family is limited to lessening but not eliminating severe suffering.

I wonder how many families and physicians secretly help patients over the edge into death in the face of such severe suffering. I wonder how many severely ill or dying patients secretly take their lives, dying alone in despair. I wonder whether the image of Diane's final aloneness will persist in the minds of her family, or if they will remember more the intense, meaningful months they had together before she died. I wonder whether Diane struggled in that last hour, and whether the Hemlock Society's way of death by suicide is the most benign. I wonder why Diane, who gave so much to so many of us, had to be alone for the last hour of her life. I wonder whether I will see Diane again, on the shore of Lake Geneva at sunset, with dragons swimming on the horizon.

When Self-Determination Runs Amok

DANIEL CALLAHAN

THE EUTHANASIA DEBATE is not just another moral debate, one in a long list of arguments in our pluralistic society. It is profoundly emblematic of three important turning points in Western thought. The first is that of the legitimate conditions under which one person can kill another. The acceptance of voluntary active euthanasia would morally sanction what can only be called "consenting adult killing." By that term I mean the killing of one person by another in the name of their mutual right to be killer and killed if they freely agree to play those roles. This turn flies in the face of a long-standing effort to limit the circumstances under which one person can take the life of another, from efforts to control the free flow of guns and arms, to abolish capital punishment, and to more tightly control warfare. Euthanasia would add a whole new category of killing to a society that already has too many excuses to indulge itself in that way.

The second turning point lies in the meaning and limits of self-determination. The acceptance of euthanasia would sanction a view of autonomy holding that individuals may, in the name of their own private, idiosyncratic view of the good life, call upon others, including such institutions as medicine, to help them pursue that life, even at the risk of harm to the common good. This works against the idea that the meaning and scope of our own right to lead our own lives must be conditioned by, and be compatible

DANIEL CALLAHAN is the Director of International Programs for the Hastings Center. He is an honorary professor at the Charles University School of Medicine, Prague, the Czech Republic.

The Hastings Center Report *22, 2 (March–April 1992): 52–55. Reprinted by permission of Daniel Callahan and The Hastings Center. Copyright 1992, The Hastings Center.*

with, the good of the community, which is more than an aggregate of self-directing individuals.

The third turning point is to be found in the claim being made upon medicine: it should be prepared to make its skills available to individuals to help them achieve their private vision of the good life. This puts medicine in the business of promoting the individualistic pursuit of general human happiness and well-being. It would overturn the traditional belief that medicine should limit its domain to promoting and preserving human health, redirecting it instead to the relief of that suffering which stems from life itself, not merely from a sick body.

I believe that, at each of these three turning points, proponents of euthanasia push us in the wrong direction. Arguments in favor of euthanasia fall into four general categories, which I will take up in turn: (1) the moral claim of individual self-determination and well-being; (2) the moral irrelevance of the difference between killing and allowing to die; (3) the supposed paucity of evidence to show likely harmful consequences of legalized euthanasia; and (4) the compatibility of euthanasia and medical practice.

SELF-DETERMINATION

Central to most arguments for euthanasia is the principle of self-determination. People are presumed to have an interest in deciding for themselves, according to their own beliefs about what makes life good, how they will conduct their lives. That is an important value, but the question in the euthanasia context is, What does it mean and how far should it extend? If it were a question of suicide, where a person takes her own life without assistance from another, that principle might be pertinent, at least for debate. But euthanasia is not that limited a matter. The self-determination in that case can only be effected by the moral and physical assistance of another. Euthanasia is thus no longer a matter only of self-determination, but of a mutual, social decision between two people, the one to be killed and the other to do the killing.

How are we to make the moral move from my right of self-determination to some doctor's right to kill me—from *my* right to *his* right? Where does the doctor's moral warrant to kill come from? Ought doctors to be able to kill anyone they want as long as permission is given by competent persons? Is our right to life just like a piece of property, to be given away or alienated if the price (happiness, relief of suffering) is right? And then to be destroyed with our permission once alienated?

In answer to all those questions, I will say this: I have yet to hear a plausible argument why it should be permissible for us to put this kind of power in the hands of another, whether a doctor or anyone else. The idea that we can waive our right to life, and then give to another the power to take that life, requires a justification yet to be provided by anyone.

Slavery was long ago outlawed on the ground that one person should not have the right to own another, even with the other's permission. Why? Because it is a fundamental moral wrong for one person to give over his life and fate to another, whatever the good consequences, and no less a wrong for another person to have that kind of total, final power. Like slavery, dueling was long ago banned on similar grounds: even free, competent individuals should not have the power to kill each other, whatever their motives, whatever the circumstances. Consenting adult killing, like consenting adult slavery or degradation, is a strange route to human dignity.

There is another problem as well. If doctors, once sanctioned to carry out euthanasia, are to be themselves responsible moral agents—not simply hired hands with lethal injections at the ready—then they must have their own *independent* moral grounds to kill those who request such services. What do I mean? As those who favor euthanasia are quick to point out, some people want it because their life has become so burdensome it no longer seems worth living.

The doctor will have a difficulty at this point. The degree and intensity to which people suffer from their diseases and their dying, and whether they find life more of a burden than a benefit, has very little directly to do with the nature or extent of their actual physical condition. Three people can have the same condition, but only one will find the suffering unbearable. People suffer, but suffering is as much a function of the values of individuals as it is of the physical causes of that suffering. Inevitably in that circumstance, the doctor will in effect be treating the patient's values. To be responsible, the doctor would have to share those values. The doctor would have to decide, on her own, whether the patient's life was "no longer worth living."

But how could a doctor possibly know that or make such a judgment? Just because the patient said so? I raise this question because, while in Holland at the euthanasia conference reported by Maurice de Wachter elsewhere in this issue, the doctors present agreed that there is no objective way of measuring or judging the claims of patients that their suffering is unbearable. And if it is difficult to measure suffering, how much more difficult to determine the value of a patient's statement that her life is not worth living?

However one might want to answer such questions, the very need to ask them, to inquire into the physician's responsibility and grounds for medical and moral judgment, points out the social nature of the decision. Euthanasia is not a private matter of self-determination. It is an act that requires two people to make it possible, and a complicit society to make it acceptable.

KILLING AND ALLOWING TO DIE

Against common opinion, the argument is sometimes made that there is no moral difference between stopping life-sustaining treatment and more active forms of killing, such as lethal injection. Instead I would contend that the no-

tion that there is no morally significant difference between omission and commission is just wrong. Consider in its broad implications what the eradication of the distinction implies: that death from disease has been banished, leaving only the actions of physicians in terminating treatment as the cause of death. Biology, which used to bring about death, has apparently been displaced by human agency. Doctors have finally, I suppose, thus genuinely become gods, now doing what nature and the deities once did.

What is the mistake here? It lies in confusing causality and culpability, and in failing to note the way in which human societies have overlaid natural causes with moral rules and interpretations. Causality (by which I mean the direct physical causes of death) and culpability (by which I mean our attribution of moral responsibility to human actions) are confused under three circumstances.

They are confused, first, when the action of a physician in stopping treatment of a patient with an underlying lethal disease is construed as *causing* death. On the contrary, the physician's omission can only bring about death on the condition that the patient's disease will kill him in the absence of treatment. We may hold the physician morally responsible for the death, if we have morally judged such actions wrongful omissions. But it confuses reality and moral judgment to see an omitted action as having the same causal status as one that directly kills. A lethal injection will kill both a healthy person and a sick person. A physician's omitted treatment will have no effect on a healthy person. Turn off the machine on me, a healthy person, and nothing will happen. It will only, in contrast, bring the life of a sick person to an end because of an underlying fatal disease.

Causality and culpability are confused, second, when we fail to note that judgments of moral responsibility and culpability are human constructs. By that I mean that we human beings, after moral reflection, have decided to call some actions right or wrong, and to devise moral rules to deal with them. When physicians could do nothing to stop death, they were not held responsible for it. When, with medical progress, they began to have some power over death—but only its timing and circumstances, not its ultimate inevitability—moral rules were devised to set forth their obligations. Natural causes of death were not thereby banished. They were, instead, overlaid with a medical ethics designed to determine moral culpability in deploying medical power.

To confuse the judgments of this ethics with the physical causes of death—which is the connotation of the word *kill*—is to confuse nature and human action. People will, one way or another, die of some disease; death will have dominion over all of us. To say that a doctor "kills" a patient by allowing this to happen should only be understood as a moral judgment about the licitness of his omission, nothing more. We can, as a fashion of speech only, talk about a doctor *killing* a patient by omitting treatment he should have provided. It is a fashion of speech precisely because it is the underlying disease that brings death when treatment is omitted; that is its cause, not the physician's omission. It is a misuse of the word *killing* to use it when a doctor stops a treatment he believes will no longer benefit the patient—when, that is, he steps aside to allow an eventually inevitable death to occur now rather then later. The only deaths that human beings invented are those that come from direct killing—when, with a lethal injection, we both cause death and are morally responsible for it. In the case of omissions, we do not cause death even if we may be judged morally responsible for it.

This difference between causality and culpability also helps us see why a doctor who has omitted a treatment he should have provided has "killed" that patient while another doctor—performing precisely the same act of omission on another patient in different circumstances—does not kill her, but only allows her to die. The difference is that we have come, by moral convention and conviction, to classify unauthorized or illegitimate omissions as acts of "killing." We call them "killing" in the expanded sense of the term: a culpable action that permits the real cause of death, the underlying disease, to proceed to its lethal conclusion. By contrast, the doctor who, at the patient's request, omits or terminates unwanted treatment does not kill at all. Her underlying disease, not his action, is the physical cause of death; and we have agreed to consider actions of that kind to be morally licit. He thus can truly be said to have "allowed" her to die.

If we fail to maintain the distinction between killing and allowing to die, moreover, there are some disturbing possibilities. The first would be to confirm many physicians in their already too-powerful belief that, when patients die or when physicians stop treatment because of the futility of continuing it, they are somehow both morally and physically responsible for the deaths that follow. That notion needs to be abolished, not strengthened. It needlessly and wrongly burdens the physician, to whom should not be attributed the powers of the gods. The second possibility would be that, in every case where a doctor judges medical treatment no longer effective in prolonging life, a quick and direct killing of the patient would be seen as the next, most reasonable step, on grounds of both humaneness and economics. I do not see how that logic could easily be rejected.

CALCULATING THE CONSEQUENCES

When concerns about the adverse social consequences of permitting euthanasia are raised, its advocates tend to dismiss them as unfounded and overly speculative. On the contrary, recent data about the Dutch experience suggests that such concerns are right on target. From my own discussions in Holland, and from the articles on that subject in this issue and elsewhere, I believe we can now fully see most of the *likely* consequences of legal euthanasia.

Three consequences seem almost certain, in this or any other country: the inevitability of some abuse of the law; the difficulty of precisely writing, and then enforcing, the law; and the inherent slipperiness of the moral reasons for legalizing euthanasia in the first place.

Why is abuse inevitable? One reason is that almost all laws on delicate, controversial matters are to some extent abused. This happens because not everyone will agree with the law as written and will bend it, or ignore it, if they can get away with it. From explicit admissions to me by Dutch proponents of euthanasia, and from the corroborating information provided by the Remmelink Report and the outside studies of Carlos Gomez and John Keown, I am convinced that in the Netherlands there are a substantial number of cases of nonvoluntary euthanasia, that is, euthanasia undertaken without the explicit permission of the person being killed. The other reason abuse is inevitable is that the law is likely to have a low enforcement priority in the criminal justice system. Like other laws of similar status, unless there is an unrelenting and harsh willingness to pursue abuse, violations will ordinarily be tolerated. The worst thing to me about my experience in Holland was the casual, seemingly indifferent attitude toward abuse. I think that would happen everywhere.

Why would it be hard to precisely write, and then enforce, the law? The Dutch speak about the requirement of "unbearable" suffering, but admit that such a term is just about indefinable, a highly subjective matter admitting of no objective standards. A requirement for outside opinion is nice, but it is easy to find complaisant colleagues. A requirement that a medical condition be "terminal" will run aground on the notorious difficulties of knowing when an illness is actually terminal.

Apart from those technical problems there is a more profound worry. I see no way, even in principle, to write or enforce a meaningful law that can guarantee effective procedural safeguards. The reason is obvious yet almost always overlooked. The euthanasia transaction will ordinarily take place within the boundaries of the private and confidential doctor-patient relationship. No one can possibly know what takes place in that context unless the doctor chooses to reveal it. In Holland, less than 10 percent of the physicians report their acts of euthanasia and do so with almost complete legal impunity. There is no reason why the situation should be any better elsewhere. Doctors will have their own reasons for keeping euthanasia secret, and some patients will have no less a motive for wanting it concealed.

I would mention, finally, that the moral logic of the motives for euthanasia contain within them the ingredients of abuse. The two standard motives for euthanasia and assisted suicide are said to be our right of self-determination, and our claim upon the mercy of others, especially doctors, to relieve our suffering. These two motives are typically spliced together and presented as a single justification. Yet if they are considered independently—and there is no inherent reason why they must be linked—they reveal serious problems. It is said that a competent, adult person should have a right to euthanasia for the relief of suffering. But why must the person be suffering? Does not that stipulation already compromise the principle of self-determination? How can self-determination have any limits? Whatever the person's motives may be, why are they not sufficient?

Consider next the person who is suffering but not competent, who is perhaps demented or mentally retarded. The standard argument would deny euthanasia to that person. But why? If a person is suffering but not competent, then it would seem grossly unfair to deny relief solely on the grounds of incompetence. Are the incompetent less entitled to relief from suffering than the competent? Will it only be affluent, middle-class people, mentally fit and savvy about working the medical system, who can qualify? Do the incompetent suffer less because of their incompetence?

Considered from these angles, there are no good moral reasons to limit euthanasia once the principle of taking life for that purpose has been legitimated. If we really believe in self-determination, then any competent person should have a right to be killed by a doctor for any reason that suits him. If we believe in the relief of suffering, then it seems cruel and capricious to deny it to the incompetent. There is, in short, no reasonable or logical stopping point once the turn has been made down the road to euthanasia, which could soon turn into a convenient and commodious expressway.

EUTHANASIA AND MEDICAL PRACTICE

A fourth kind of argument one often hears both in the Netherlands and in this country is that euthanasia and assisted suicide are perfectly compatible with the aims of medicine. I would note at the very outset that a physician who participates in another person's suicide already abuses medicine. Apart from depression (the main statistical cause of suicide), people commit suicide because they find life empty, oppressive, or meaningless. Their judgment is a judgment about the value of continued life, not only about health (even if they are sick). Are doctors now to be given the right to make judgments about the kinds of life worth living and to give their blessing to suicide for those they judge wanting? What conceivable competence, technical or moral, could doctors claim to play such a role? Are we to medicalize suicide, turning judgments about its worth and value into one more clinical issue? Yes, those are rhetorical questions.

Yet they bring us to the core of the problem of euthanasia and medicine. The great temptation of modern medicine, not always resisted, is to move beyond the promotion and preservation of health into the boundless realm of general human happiness and well-being. The root problem of illness and mortality is both medical and philosophical or religious. "Why must I die?" can be asked as a technical, biological question or

as a question about the meaning of life. When medicine tries to respond to the latter, which it is always under pressure to do, it moves beyond its proper role.

It is not medicine's place to lift from us the burden of that suffering which turns on the meaning we assign to the decay of the body and its eventual death. It is not medicine's place to determine when lives are not worth living or when the burden of life is too great to be borne. Doctors have no conceivable way of evaluating such claims on the part of patients, and they should have no right to act in response to them. Medicine should try to relieve human suffering, but only that suffering which is brought on by illness and dying as biological phenomena, not that suffering which comes from anguish or despair at the human condition.

Doctors ought to relieve those forms of suffering that medically accompany serious illness and the threat of death. They should relieve pain, do what they can to allay anxiety and uncertainty, and be a comforting presence. As sensitive human beings, doctors should be prepared to respond to patients who ask why they must die, or die in pain. But here the doctor and the patient are at the same level. The doctor may have no better an answer to those old questions than anyone else; and certainly no special insight from his training as a physician. It would be terrible for physicians to forget this, and to think that in a swift, lethal injection, medicine has found its own answer to the riddle of life. It would be a false answer, given by the wrong people. It would be no less a false answer for patients. They should neither ask medicine to put its own vocation at risk to serve their private interests, nor think that the answer to suffering is to be killed by another. The problem is precisely that, too often in human history, killing has seemed the quick, efficient way to put aside that which burdens us. It rarely helps, and too often simply adds to one evil still another. That is what I believe euthanasia would accomplish. It is self-determination run amok.

Why Suicide Is Like Contraception:
A Woman-Centered View

DENA S. DAVIS

DESPITE THE FLOOD OF WRITING on assisted suicide in the last few years, relatively little has been written about suicide itself.[1] There are certainly important reasons to distinguish these two subjects. One could, for example, argue that suicide can be a good decision in some situations, but still acknowledge powerful reasons why *medical* people should not blur their mission by taking on this task. However, it is important, before tackling the issue of physician-assisted suicide, to think about suicide *simpliciter*. If one believes that suicide is sometimes a rational, even an admirable, decision, one is at least more sympathetic to the notion of assistance. Whereas someone who believes that virtually all suicides are really "cries for help," responses to social situations that could be ameliorated, or the product of clinical depression is likely to be much more suspicious of any steps society might take to make it easier. In the following pages, let me offer one feminist view of rational suicide.

Women live in a critique relationship with our bodies. Sometimes that is a negative thing, as when we judge ourselves by the "norm" of the tall, skinny model on the cover of *Vogue* and find ourselves wanting, or when we buy into male myths about how women ought to make love and experience orgasm. But it is also a positive thing. Women (at least in the West) learn in adolescence that we must take control of our fertility.

DENA S. DAVIS is an Associate Professor of Law at the Cleveland Marshall School of Law.

We need to view that fertility as *contingent* rather than *given;* we need to evaluate our capacity for procreation with a critical eye, asking how and when that capacity fits into our plans for our lives. To use contraception is to say, *"Despite the fact that my body retains its capacity to be fertile from, say, age eleven to fifty-one, that capacity is not (now) a good for my life but rather a threat to my goals and plans; therefore, I will choose to limit my fertility."* To choose sterilization is to say, *"My fertility has permanently outrun its usefulness for my life and is now a danger, and, therefore, I will exert control by bringing my body's physical capacities into line with my plans for the rest of my life."*

Thus, an important piece of the feminist project has been to argue that biology is not destiny. To decide how to deal with one's fertility—whether by celibacy, pregnancy, contraception, or sterilization—is to exercise choice and will over against the passive acceptance of what would otherwise happen to one's life because of one's bodily proclivities.[2] Sometimes, of course, these are very tragic choices, as when a woman longs for another child but knows that pregnancy will risk her health or the well-being of children already born.[3]

To choose suicide, when one is facing a diagnosis of dementia or the last stages of a terminal illness, is to say, *"My body's continued capacity to pump blood and oxygen is no longer a good for my life but rather a threat to my values and interests in how the final chapter of my life is written; therefore, I will exert control by committing suicide."* These interests might include preserving my

From Physician Assisted Suicide. *Margaret P. Battin, Rosamond Rhodes, and Anita Silvers, eds.*
© *1998. Reproduced by permission of Routledge, Inc.*

387

assets to use in ways consonant with my values (for example, to endow a scholarship or pay for my children's education); sparing family members the experience of coping with protracted dementia and death; preserving friends' and family's memories of me as a vital and competent person; ending my life with a final chapter that is a fitting capstone to the narrative as a whole.

Some religious ethicists, and those with natural law fidelities, will argue that it is arrogant and delusional, "autonomy run amok" as the current phrase has it, to imagine that one can control the course of one's life. In an article tellingly entitled, "Embracing Mystery, Losing Control," William F. May speaks of "a purposeful willing and waiting in the course of letting be and letting go."[4] David Novak mocks autonomy arguments for suicide when he says this:

> We want to die just as we have lived — autonomously. Since we have believed in life that our dignity is to be self-sufficient, we now believe that we must die with that same dignity. Death is no longer the ultimate horizon that teaches us that our essence in this world is not to be in control but to make our peace with an order greater than anything of our own making.[5]

Certainly, there is much that one simply has to accept — such as having terminal cancer or Alzheimer's Disease in the first place. Thus, the decision whether or not to commit suicide is often made in the context of tragedy; one would hugely prefer not to have gotten cancer, or not to live in a society where a nursing home stay will destroy one's assets, or not to be at the mercy of a medical system in which half of dying patients report severe or moderate pain at the end-of-life.[6]

Embracing the idea of suicide as one possible choice among others aligns us on the feminist side of two important divides that are present in the debate over contraception as well: *passive versus active,* and *natural (or "given") versus chosen.*[7]

PASSIVE VERSUS ACTIVE

Not to use contraception, or rather not to include contraception as an active possibility in one's life, is to be passive, to be at the mercy of one's body. Indeed, one of the reasons "moralists" pushed for laws against contraceptives was that they "encouraged" immorality by allowing people to "escape" the consequences of their acts. To be fertile and sexually active without employing contraceptives (or abortion) is to be governed by the vicissitudes of fertility and fate. Given the impact of childbearing and motherhood on women's lives, the consequences for one's health, economic status, and career are enormous.

Conservatives opposed to contraception, especially Christian conservatives, would speak of "openness" rather than passivity, as in this illuminating quote from a woman pro-life activist interviewed by sociologist Kristin Luker:

> Because most pro-life people have a deep faith in God, they also believe in the rightness of His plan for the world. They are therefore skeptical about the ability of individual humans to understand, much less control, events that unfold according to a divine, rather than human, blueprint. From their point of view, human attempts at control are simply arrogance, an unwillingness to admit that larger forces than human will determine human fate. One woman made the point clearly: "God is the Creator of life, and I think all sexual activity should be open to that [creation]. That does not mean that you have to have a certain number of children or anything, but it should be open to Him and His will. The contraceptive mentality denies his will. "It's my will, not your will." And here again, the selfishness comes in.[8]

The idea of life as a "gift" also is common to those who argue for openness and against control. Sydney Callahan, for example, a pro-life feminist who also argues against assisted suicide, says that, "Having received the gift of life and social identity, one has a moral obligation to pre-serve and respect each human life and refrain from suppressing, killing, or destroying self or others."[9] This notion of the self as the receiver of a gift that one is then stuck with, and yet does not own, casts the self as receptive and passive.

By the same token, to allow oneself to be taken over by Alzheimer's Disease or cancer, past the point of possible cure or treatment, is to be passive. With regard to dementia, it is to be the object of others' concern, to be led by the hand, to be unable to drive a car or control one's fi-nances — in short, to return to the infantilized notion of women that prevailed in the West in earlier times (and that still reigns in cultures such as Saudi Arabia). On the other hand, to seize control of one's destiny, perhaps especially under circumstances of great tragedy and limits, is to be active and dominant.

U.S. District Court Judge Barbara J. Roth-stein and the Ninth Circuit Court of Appeals ex-pressed the same point when they relied heavily on the U.S. Supreme Court's abortion decisions to ground the right of terminally ill persons to receive physician assistance in determining the time and manner of their deaths (an argument the Supreme Court ultimately rejected).[10] In *Compassion in Dying,* the Ninth Circuit quoted *Planned Parenthood v. Casey,* a 1992 decision up-holding women's rights to abortion, as saying that:

> At the heart of liberty is the right to define one's own concept of existence, of meaning, of the universe, and of the mystery of human life.[11]

Commenting on the string of contraception and abortion cases that began with *Griswold v. Con-necticut* in 1965, the Ninth Circuit noted that:

> A common thread running through these cases is that they involve decisions that are highly per-sonal and intimate, as well as of great impor-tance to the individual. Certainly, few decisions are more personal, intimate, or important than the decision to end one's life, especially when

the reason for doing so is to avoid excessive and protracted pain.[12]

Most (not all) feminists have long argued that, in the context of abortion, their right to control over their bodies and over the shape of their future lives is supreme. Although the deci-sion whether or not to have an abortion is fraught with moral issues, most feminists have consistently resisted mandatory counseling, waiting periods, spousal notification, and other state interference. If we insist that we can and must be trusted with the power to decide whether or not to destroy a potential human life, how can we not insist on the right to be trusted with the decision whether or not to end our own?

NATURAL VERSUS CHOSEN

One of the principal ways in which women have been oppressed in our society is the identifica-tion of women with that which is "natural," and the demand that women simply accept rather than control their fertility. "Biology is destiny." Women are "made" for childbearing and child-rearing. Birth control is "unnatural" (and will lead to immorality to boot!) Thus, Pope Pius XI, in the 1930 encyclical *Casti Connubii,* wrote:

> It is a divinely appointed law that whatsoever things are constituted by God, the author of nature, these we find the most useful and salu-tary, the more they remain in their natural state, unimpaired and unchanged, inasmuch as God, the Creator of all things, intimately knows what is suited to the constitution and the preserva-tion of each, and by his will and mind has so ordained all things that each may duly achieve its purpose. . . .
>
> The conjugal act is of its very nature designed for the procreation of offspring; and therefore those who in performing it deliber-ately deprive it of its natural power and efficacy, act against nature and do something which is shameful and intrinsically immoral.

Other arguments that rely on a divinely constructed world order are equally pernicious to women, as in the notion of male-female "complementarity" which is so often used to support a "separate but equal" argument against women's full participation in public life.[13] Natural order arguments are also frequently associated with what Charles Curran terms a "negative dualism," in which women are identified with the bodily, the emotional, and the material, while men are identified with spirit and rationality. In this tradition, men are the "head" of the family and women are the "heart."[14]

Until the advent of reasonably dependable birth control in the middle of this century, most women faced the unenviable choice of uncontrolled fertility (often associated with poverty and ill health) or some form of celibacy. For too many poor and Third World women, that description still applies. Today, most feminists believe that access to contraception and sterilization is the *sine qua non* of women's self-determination. And, while long-acting contraceptives (such as Norplant) and the shameful history of forced sterilization of poor and minority women remind us of the problems associated with contraception when it is *forced* upon women, the potential for abuse does not tempt us to give up our support for the principle of contraception itself and women's control over their own fertility.[15] This feminist commitment to a "non-natural," *controlled* approach to our fertility suggests what ought to be our approach to end-of-life decisions as well. To quote Mary Rose Barrington, past chair of EXIT, the London-based Society for the Right to Die with Dignity:

> Very little is "natural" about our present-day existence, and least natural of all is the prolonged period of dying that is suffered by so many incurable patients solicitously kept alive to be killed by their disease. . . . If I seem to be suggesting that in a civilized society suicide ought to be considered a quite proper way for a well-brought-up person to end his life (unless he has the good luck to die suddenly and without warning), that is indeed the tenor of my

argument; if it is received with astonishment and incredulity, the reader is referred to the reception of recommendations made earlier in the century that birth control should be practiced and encouraged. The idea is no more extraordinary and would be equally calculated to diminish the sum total of suffering among humankind.[16]

PHYSICIAN-ASSISTED SUICIDE

It is tempting to carry my analogy to the next step and to argue that, just as medical assistance is the *sine qua non* of access to birth control and the "right" to contraception would be empty without it, the "right" to suicide is empty without the specialized assistance of a healthcare professional to prescribe the drugs and, preferably, to be present to smooth the way and ensure success.[17] Although I am a proponent of rational suicide, I am less convinced that the legalization of physician assistance is a good policy. The many concerns expressed about the effect on the medical profession, and the move to HMOs, with their tendency to look to the cheapest solution to any problem, give me pause. I am also influenced by Joanne Lynn's point about the "routinization" of medical procedures (for example, the routine use of ultrasound and amniocentesis during pregnancy, and the difficulty many pregnant women experience in resisting that expectation).[18] One can imagine that, rather than being an option people have to ask for, even fight for a little, physician-assisted suicide becomes one more track onto which certain patients are shunted.

Thus, we may have to settle for a compromise in which certain compassionate physicians continue to break the law. A better approach would be to look for creative solutions that do not involve the medical profession, for example, lay support groups, end-of-life "midwives," and so on. But this approach assumes a robust and public debate that can shake off the taboo of suicide in the same fashion that we are shaking off the taboo of contraception. Now that the Supreme

Court has declined to find a constitutionally protected liberty interest in assisted suicide and left this question up to the political process in the several states, the time for such debate has certainly begun.[19] However, it is worth noting that, although there is widespread debate at the level of public policy and legislative action, the taboo against discussing suicide still holds in many other areas, including much of medical discourse. For example, when suicide as a response to a probable diagnosis of Huntington or Alzheimer's Disease is mentioned in the medical literature, it is characterized as an "adverse reaction,"[20] or as a "catastrophe."[21] Suicide is always described negatively as a "risk," rather than as a "response" or an "option."[22] Thus, discussions of the usefulness of certain kinds of genetic tests are truncated by the refusal to speak openly about the possibility that some people might use genetic testing to make a rational choice to commit suicide.

To date, the distinctly feminist voices in the debate have been opposed to assisted suicide. Sydney Callahan is one example; Susan M. Wolf is another. Wolf, in common with Callahan, is concerned that women will be particularly threatened by the legitimation of physician-assisted suicide.[23] Together, they note that women are more likely to live long lives, to outlive their spouses, to be poor and underinsured, and to be undermedicated for pain. The historic power inequality between (male) doctors and (female) patients makes it doubly difficult for women to assert themselves to get the medical care they need. Wolf notes that men are statistically more likely to complete acts of suicide, but women are more likely to attempt them. She hypothesizes that women may be more likely to use suicide attempts to effect changes in their environment; but, if a request for assistance in suicide becomes something to which a doctor can easily answer, "Yes," many women might commit suicide who really did not want to.[24] Both Callahan and Wolf find it significant that the majority of Kevorkian's clients have been women (including many who faced diseases, such as Alzheimer's

or multiple sclerosis, that made them increasingly dependent, but not close to death).

Wolf's essay has a number of objectives and arguments. The argument I want to take issue with here is her concern that women's decisions to commit suicide, and society's acceptance of those decisions as appropriate, may be skewed by "a long history of cultural images revering women's sacrifice and self-sacrifice."[25] She worries, in other words, that women are asking (and receiving) suicide assistance for the "wrong" reasons, based on historical and cultural roles that feminists now reject.

Of course, Wolf is correct that self-sacrifice and womanhood have all too easily been considered a natural configuration. But I want to suggest a different way of looking at the content of self-sacrifice. My point is not to denigrate Wolf's picture of the historical and cultural assumptions about women that may play into suicide, but to show that these are actually multifaceted and cut in more than one direction.

Self-sacrifice can be seen, culturally speaking, along a number of different axes. The axis Wolf contemplates is that of resource use. On one end of this axis is the stereotypical mother who doesn't want resources used on her. On the other end is the person who is comfortable having time, money, and resources spent on her, even out of a limited family pool. Wolf argues that women have historically been consigned to the self-sacrificial end. Because women were traditionally expected to fulfill themselves through their families while their husbands pursued success in more public ways, women could all too easily be expected—and expect themselves—to put everyone else's needs first. But there is another sense in which, perhaps unwittingly, the opponents of rational suicide fall into another understanding of self-sacrifice. Here, the self-sacrifice expected is to undergo long periods of pain and disability, perhaps even dementia, rather than to do something as dramatic and unconventional as to put an end to one's life. The ill or dying person is being asked to forgo acting on her own interests in order to (1) avoid making her relatives look like selfish, uncaring brutes in the eyes of the more conventional world; (2) refrain from challenging the comfortable belief that life is always worth living; and (3) avoid giving society at large a push down the slippery slope in the direction of callousness toward those sick and disabled persons who do *not* wish to end their lives. Thus, one could argue that those who oppose rational suicide are asking women to shoulder yet another traditional female burden: the preservation of society's moral and religious values. The stereotypical virtues assigned to Victorian women of "piety, purity, submissiveness, and domesticity," which rightly disturb Wolf, can as easily be harnessed by traditionalists to argue against suicide as for it.[26]

Here again, we see a parallel with enforced motherhood. As Beverly Harrison points out, "We live in a world in which many, perhaps most, of the voluntary sacrifices on behalf of human well-being are made by women, but the assumption of a special obligation to self-giving or sacrifice is male-generated ideology."[27] It is, of course, often a valid argument that the interests of the individual must give way to the good of society as a whole. Although I am not yet persuaded by these arguments, we should certainly consider the concerns of, for example, the New York State Task Force on Life and the Law, which concluded that the probability of "mistake and abuse" was too high to countenance the legalization of physician-assisted suicide,[28] an argument the Supreme Court took very seriously when deciding that assistance in suicide was not a constitutionally protected liberty interest.[29] (We should also consider the accounts of observers in Oregon that the possibility of physician-assisted suicide has actually been *better* for patients, as doctors interpreted Measure 16 as a "wake-up call for medicine" and have been motivated to step up efforts in pain control and hospice care.)[30] But, if we are to make this sort of argument, then let us be honest about it: People are being required to forgo their own interests (and individual values) for the good of society as

a whole. Women, who historically have suffered the brunt of that sort of reasoning, and who have special reasons for avoiding the indignity and dependence of being demented, pain-wracked, and bedridden, may decide that it is not worth the price.

CONCLUSION

There are many different ways in which women's experience can illuminate the complex debate over rational suicide. Some facets of this experience rightly suggest great caution, as women reflect on their greater vulnerability due to age, poverty, and historic oppression. My goal in this essay, by drawing an analogy between contraception and rational suicide, is to highlight one area in which women's experience can argue in favor of support for rational suicide.

NOTES

1. One exception is M. Pabst Battin, *Ethical Issues in Suicide* (Englewood Cliffs, NJ: Prentice-Hall, 1982).

2. Of course, it would be highly preferable for men to take an equal interest in controlling *their* fertility, but women have far more to lose from unplanned pregnancy than do men and, therefore, a much greater interest in contraception.

3. *Infertility* can also challenge women to make very difficult choices. Feminists are divided about whether innovative reproductive technologies give women more choice or less. See, for example, Janice G. Raymond, *Women as Wombs: Reproductive Technologies and the Battle Over Women's Freedom* (San Francisco: Harper, 1993).

4. William F. May, "Embracing Mystery. Losing Control," *The Park Ridge Center Bulletin* 1: 15 (1997).

5. David Novak, "Suicide Is Not a Private Choice," *First Things* 75: 31–34 (1997).

6. The SUPPORT Principal Investigators, "A Controlled Trial to Improve Care for Seriously Ill Hospitalized Patients: The Study to Understand Prognoses and Preferences for Outcomes and Risks of

Treatments (SUPPORT)," *Journal of the American Medical Association* 274: 1591–98 (1996); Joan Stephenson, "Experts Say AIDS Pain 'Dramatically Undertreated,'" *Journal of the American Medical Association* 276: 1369–1370 (1996).

7. I am keenly aware that there is tremendous diversity and controversy in feminist philosophy, and to speak of "the" feminist side is a kind of arrogance. Many feminist philosophers, e.g., Rosemarie Tong, have done a superb job of delineating the many different types of feminist thought and their implications for issues in bioethics. For me, being a feminist means always asking "the woman question," always being alert, as it were, for the impact upon women of a particular policy or perspective. As a liberal feminist, I take equality, justice, and respect for individual autonomy as crucial principles which I seek to extend to women (and to other historically oppressed groups) equally with men. While I agree that equal attention to women's experience will change our notions of how those principles are applied (the abortion issue is an obvious example of this point), I reject the "relational" or "difference" feminism of Carol Gilligan, Robin West, and others.

8. Kristin Luker, *Abortion and the Politics of Motherhood* (Berkeley: University of California Press, 1984), p. 186.

9. Sydney Callahan, "A Feminist Case Against Euthanasia," Health Progress, November–December 1996, pp. 21–29, at p. 23.

10. For an argument against the assertion that the constitutionally protected interest in abortion and treatment refusal embraces a parallel interest in assisted suicide, see Susan M. Wolf, "Physician-Assisted Suicide, Abortion, and Treatment Refusal: Using Gender to Analyze the Difference," in Robert F. Weir, ed., Physician-Assisted Suicide (Bloomington: Indiana University Press, 1997), pp. 167–201.

11. *Compassion in Dying v. State of Washington,* 79 F. 3d (9th Cir. 1996), p. 813.

12. Ibid.

13. Margaret A. Farley, "Feminist Theology and Bioethics," in Lois K. Daly, ed., *Feminist Theological Ethics: A Reader* (Louisville, KY: Westminster John Knox Press, 1994), p. 198.

14. Charles Curran, "Sexual Ethics in the Roman Catholic Tradition," in Ronald M. Green, ed., *Religion and Sexual Health: Ethical, Theological and Clinical Perspectives* (Dordrecht: Kluwer Academic Publishers, 1992), pp. 17–36. See also Margaret Farley, "Feminist Theology and Bioethics," in Lois K. Daly, ed., *Feminist Theological Ethics: A Reader* (Louisville, KY: Westminster John Knox Press, 1994), pp. 192–212.

15. Ellen Moscowitz and Bruce Jennings, eds., *Coerced Contraception? Moral and Policy Challenges of Long-Acting Birth Control* (Washington, DC: Georgetown University Press, 1996).

16. Mary Rose Barrington, "Apologia for Suicide," in M. Pabst Battin and David J. Mayo, eds., *Suicide, The Philosophical Issues* (New York: St. Martin's Press, 1980), pp. 90–103.

17. It is interesting to note that the Supreme Court cases dealing with contraception are not directly about the right of persons to use contraception, but about the criminalization of physicians' and pharmacists' prescription and distribution of contraceptives.

18. Joanne Lynn, "What You Can Do for Your Dying Patient," Presentation at the Cleveland Clinic Foundation, October 10, 1996.

19. *Washington v. Glucksberg,* 117 S. Ct. 2258, 2274 (1997).

20. Medical and Scientific Advisory Committee, Alzheimer's Disease International, "Consensus Statement on Predictive Testing for Alzheimer's Disease," *Alzheimer's Disease and Associated Disorders* 9 (4) (1995): 182–87.

21. Sandi Wiggins, et al., "The Psychological Consequences of Predictive Testing for Huntington's Disease," *New England Journal of Medicine* 327 (20): 1401–1405 (Nov. 12, 1992).

22. Miriam Schoenfeld, et al., "Increased rate of suicide among patients with Huntington's disease," *Journal of Neurology, Neurosurgery, and Psychiatry* 47: 1283–87 (1984).

23. Susan M. Wolf, "Gender, Feminism, and Death: Physician-Assisted Suicide and Euthanasia," in Susan M. Wolf, ed., *Feminism and Bioethics: Beyond Reproduction* (New York: Oxford University Press, 1996).

24. On the other hand, if assisted suicide became open and legal, perhaps women who otherwise would use a suicide attempt as a "cry for help," will be forced to confront and articulate their real needs. To continue to play a societal game in which women "attempt" suicides they don't really intend, perpetuates a situation in which women are rewarded for communicating one thing and meaning another. This makes it more difficult for women to command respect for their real beliefs and wishes, as documented by Steven H. Miles and Allison August in "Courts, Gender and the '"Right to Die,'" *Law, Medicine and Health Care* 18:85–95 (1990). I make a similar argument with respect to Jehovah's Witnesses and refusal of life-saving treatment in "Does 'No' Mean 'Yes'? The Continuing Problem of Jehovah's Witnesses and Refusal of Blood Products," *Second Opinion* 19: 35–43 (1994). (I am indebted for this point to Paul Finkelman.)

25. Ibid., p. 283.

26. Ibid., p. 298.

27. Beverly Wildung Harrison, *Our Right to Choose: Toward a New Ethic of Abortion,* quoted in Janice Raymond, "Reproductive Gifts and Gift-Giving: The Altruistic Woman," in Lois K. Daly, ed., *Feminist Theological Ethics, A Reader* (Louisville, KY: Westminster John Knox Press, 1994), p. 236.

28. The New York State Task Force on Life and the Law, *When Death Is Sought: Assisted Suicide and Euthanasia in the Medical Context* (New York: The New York State Task Force on Life and the Law, 1994).

29. *Washington v. Glucksberg,* 117 Sup. Ct. 2258, 2272–73 (1997).

30. Susan W. Tolle, "How Oregon's Physician-Assisted Suicide Law Spurs Improvements in End-of-Life Care," *Issues and Resources on Dying* (New York: Grantmakers Concerned with Care at the End of Life, 1977), pp. 3–4.

Ethical Issues in Aiding the Death of Young Children

H. TRISTRAM ENGELHARDT, JR.

EUTHANASIA IN THE PEDIATRIC AGE GROUP involves a constellation of issues that are materially different from those of adult euthanasia. The difference lies in the somewhat obvious fact that infants and young children are not able to decide about their own futures and thus are not persons in the same sense that normal adults are. While adults usually decide their own fate, others decide on behalf of young children. Although one can argue that euthanasia is or should be a personal right, the sense of such an argument is obscure with respect to children.

H. TRISTRAM ENGELHARDT, JR., is Professor in the Department of Medicine, as well as in the Departments of Community Medicine, and Obstetrics and Gynecology, Baylor College of Medicine. In addition, he is Professor in the Department of Philosophy, Rice University, Adjunct Research Fellow, Institute of Religion, Houston, Texas, and Member of the Center for Medical Ethics and Health Policy.

Young children do not have any personal rights, at least none that they can exercise on their own behalf with regard to the manner of their life and death. As a result, euthanasia of young children raises special questions concerning the standing of the rights of children, the status of parental rights, the obligations of adults to prevent the suffering of children, and the possible effects on society of allowing or expediting the death of seriously defective infants.

What I will refer to as the euthanasia of infants and young children might be termed by others infanticide, while some cases might be termed the withholding of extraordinary life-prolonging treatment. One needs a term that will encompass both death that results from active intervention and death that ensues when one simply ceases further therapy. In using such a term, one must recognize that death is often not

From Beneficent Euthanasia. *Marvin Kohl, ed. (Amherst, NY: Prometheus Books), 130–135. Copyright 1975. Reprinted by permission of the publisher.*

directly but only obliquely intended. That is, one often intends only to treat no further, not actually to have death follow, even though one knows death will follow.

Finally, one must realize that deaths as the result of withholding treatment constitute a significant proportion of neonatal deaths. For example, as high as 14 percent of children in one hospital have been identified as dying after a decision was made not to treat further, the presumption being that the children would have lived longer had treatment been offered.

Even popular magazines have presented accounts of parental decisions not to pursue treatment. These decisions often involve a choice between expensive treatment with little chance of achieving a full, normal life for the child and "letting nature take its course," with the child dying as a result of its defects. As this suggests, many of these problems are products of medical progress. Such children in the past would have died. The quandaries are in a sense an embarrassment of riches; now that one *can* treat such defective children, *must* one treat them? And, if one need not treat such defective children, may one expedite their death?

I will here briefly examine some of these issues. First, I will review differences that contrast the euthanasia of adults to euthanasia of children. Second, I will review the issue of the rights of parents and the status of children. Third, I will suggest a new notion, the concept of the "injury of continued existence," and draw out some of its implications with respect to a duty to prevent suffering. Finally, I will outline some important questions that remain unanswered even if the foregoing issues can be settled. In all, I hope more to display the issues involved in a difficult question than to advance a particular set of answers to particular dilemmas.

For the purpose of this paper, I will presume that adult euthanasia can be justified by an appeal to freedom. In the face of imminent death, one is usually choosing between a more painful and more protracted dying and a less painful or

less protracted dying, in circumstances where either choice makes little difference with regard to the discharge of social duties and responsibilities. In the case of suicide, we might argue that, in general, social duties (for example, the duty to support one's family) restrain one from taking one's own life. But in the face of imminent death and in the presence of the pain and deterioration of a fatal disease, such duties are usually impossible to discharge and are thus rendered moot. One can, for example, picture an extreme case of an adult with a widely disseminated carcinoma, including metastases to the brain, who because of severe pain and debilitation is no longer capable of discharging any social duties. In these and similar circumstances, euthanasia becomes the issue of the right to control one's own body, even to the point of seeking assistance in suicide. Euthanasia is, as such, the issue of assisted suicide, the universalization of a maxim that all persons should be free, *in extremis,* to decide with regard to the circumstances of their death.

Further, the choice of positive euthanasia could be defended as the more rational choice: the choice of a less painful death and the affirmation of the value of a rational life. In so choosing, one would be acting to set limits to one's life in order not to live when pain and physical and mental deterioration make further rational life impossible. The choice to end one's life can be understood as a non-contradictory willing of a smaller set of states of existence for oneself, a set that would not include a painful death. As such, it would not involve a desire to destroy oneself. That is, adult euthanasia can be construed as an affirmation of the rationality and autonomy of the self.

The remarks above focus on the active or positive euthanasia of adults. But they hold as well concerning what is often called passive or negative euthanasia, the refusal of life-prolonging therapy. In such cases, the patient's refusal of life-prolonging therapy is seen to be a right that derives from personal freedom, or at least from a zone of privacy into which there are no good grounds for social intervention.

Again, none of these considerations apply directly to the euthanasia of young children, because they cannot participate in such decisions. Whatever else pediatric, in particular neonatal, euthanasia involves, it surely involves issues different from those of adult euthanasia. Since infants and small children cannot commit suicide, their right to assisted suicide is difficult to pose. The difference between the euthanasia of young children and that of adults resides in the difference between children and adults. The difference, in fact, raises the troublesome question of whether young children are persons, or at least whether they are persons in the sense in which adults are. Answering that question will resolve in part at least the right of others to decide whether a young child should live or die and whether he should receive life-prolonging treatment.

THE STATUS OF CHILDREN

Adults belong to themselves in the sense that they are rational and free and therefore responsible for their actions. Adults are *sui juris.* Young children, though, are neither self-possessed nor responsible. While adults exist in and for themselves, as self-directive and self-conscious beings, young children, especially newborn infants, exist for their families and those who love them. They are not, nor can they in any sense be, responsible for themselves. If being a person is to be a responsible agent, a bearer of rights and duties, children are not persons in a strict sense. They are, rather, persons in a social sense: others must act on their behalf and bear responsibility for them. They are, as it were, entities defined by their place in social roles (for example, mother-child, family-child) rather than beings that define themselves as persons, that is, in and through themselves. Young children live as persons in and through the care of those who are responsible for them, and those responsible for them exercise the children's rights on their behalf. In this sense children belong to families in ways that most

adults do not. They exist in and through their family and society.

Treating young children with respect has, then, a sense different from treating adults with respect. One can respect neither a newborn infant's or very young child's wishes nor its freedom. In fact, a newborn infant or young child is more an entity that is valued highly because it will grow to be a person and because it plays a social role as if it were a person. That is, a small child is treated as if it were a person in social roles such as mother-child and family-child relationships, though strictly speaking the child is in no way capable of claiming or being responsible for the rights imputed to it. All the rights and duties of the child are exercised and "held in trust" by others for a future time and for a person yet to develop.

Medical decisions to treat or not to treat a neonate or small child often turn on the probability and cost of achieving that future status—a developed personal life. The usual practice of letting anencephalic children (who congenitally lack all or most of the brain) die can be understood as a decision based on the absence of the possibility of achieving a personal life. The practice of refusing treatment to at least some children born with meningomyelocele can be justified through a similar, but more utilitarian, calculus. In the case of anencephalic children one might argue that care for them as persons is futile since they will never be persons. In the case of a child with meningomyelocele, one might argue that when the cost of cure would likely be very high and the probable lifestyle open to attainment very truncated, there is not a positive duty to make a large investment of money and suffering. One should note that the cost here must include not only financial costs but also the anxiety and suffering that prolonged and uncertain treatment of the child would cause the parents.

This further raises the issue of the scope of positive duties not only when there is no person present in a strict sense, but when the likelihood of a full human life is also very uncertain. Clinical and parental judgment may and should be guided by the expected lifestyle and the cost (in parental and societal pain and money) of its attainment. The decision about treatment, however, belongs properly to the parents because the child belongs to them in a sense that it does not belong to anyone else, even to itself. The care and raising of the child falls to the parents, and when considerable cost and little prospect of reasonable success are present, the parents may properly decide against life-prolonging treatment.

The physician's role is to present sufficient information in a usable form to the parents to aid them in making a decision. The accent is on the absence of a positive duty to treat in the presence of severe inconvenience (costs) to the parents; treatment that is very costly is not obligatory. What is suggested here is a general notion that there is never a duty to engage in extraordinary treatment and that "extraordinary" can be defined in terms of costs. This argument concerns children (1) whose future quality of life is likely to be seriously compromised and (2) whose present treatment would be very costly. The issue is that of the circumstances under which parents would not be obliged to take on severe burdens on behalf of their children or those circumstances under which society would not be so obliged. The argument should hold as well for those cases where the expected future life would surely be of normal quality, though its attainment would be extremely costly. The fact of little likelihood of success in attaining a normal life for the child makes decisions to do without treatment more plausible because the hope of success is even more remote and therefore the burden borne by parents or society becomes in that sense more extraordinary. But very high costs themselves could be a sufficient criterion, though in actual cases judgments in that regard would be very difficult when a normal life could be expected.

The decisions in these matters correctly lie in the hands of the parents, because it is primarily in terms of the family that children exist and develop—until children become persons strictly, they are persons in virtue of their social roles. As long as parents do not unjustifiably neglect the humans in those roles so that the value and purpose of that role (that is, child) stands to be eroded (thus endangering other children), society need not intervene. In short, parents may decide for or against the treatment of their severely deformed children.

However, society has a right to intervene and protect children for whom parents refuse care (including treatment) when such care does not constitute a severe burden and when it is likely that the child could be brought to a good quality of life. Obviously, "severe burden" and "good quality of life" will be difficult to define and their meanings will vary, just as it is always difficult to say when grains of sand dropped on a table constitute a heap. At most, though, society need only intervene when the grains clearly do not constitute a heap, that is, when it is clear that the burden is light and the chance of a good quality of life for the child is high. A small child's dependence on his parents is so essential that society need intervene only when the absence of intervention would lead to the role "child" being undermined. Society must value mother-child and family-child relationships and should intervene only in cases where (1) neglect is unreasonable and therefore would undermine respect and care for children, or (2) where societal intervention would prevent children from suffering unnecessary pain.

THE INJURY OF CONTINUED EXISTENCE

But there is another viewpoint that must be considered: that of the child or even the person that the child might become. It might be argued that the child has a right not to have its life prolonged. The idea that forcing existence on a child could be wrong is a difficult notion, which, if true, would serve to amplify the foregoing argument. Such an argument would allow the construal of the issue in terms of the perspective of the child, that is, in terms of a duty not to treat in circumstances where treatment would only prolong suffering. In particular, it would at least give a framework for a decision to stop treatment in cases where, though the costs of treatment are not high, the child's existence would be characterized by severe pain and deprivation.

A basis for speaking of continuing existence as an injury to the child is suggested by the proposed legal concept of "wrongful life." A number of suits have been initiated in the United States and in other countries on the grounds that life or existence itself is, under certain circumstances, a tort or injury to the living person. Although thus far all such suits have ultimately failed, some have succeeded in their initial stages. Two examples may be instructive. In each case the ability to receive recompense for the injury (the tort) presupposed the existence of the individual, whose existence was itself the injury. In one case a suit was initiated on behalf of a child against his father alleging that his father's siring him out of wedlock was an injury to the child. In another case a suit on behalf of a child born of an inmate of a state mental hospital impregnated by rape in that institution was brought against the state of New York. The suit was brought on the grounds that being born with such historical antecedents was itself an injury for which recovery was due. Both cases presupposed that nonexistence would have been preferable to the conditions under which the person born was forced to live.

The suits for tort for wrongful life raise the issue not only of when it would be preferable not to have been born but also of when it would be *wrong* to cause a person to be born. This implies that someone should have judged that it would have been preferable for the child never to have had existence, never to have been in the position to judge that the particular circumstances of life were intolerable. Further, it implies that the person's existence under those circumstances should have been prevented and that, not having been prevented, life was not a gift but an injury. The concept of tort for wrongful life raises an issue concerning the responsibility for giving another

person existence, namely the notion that giving life is not always necessarily a good and justifiable action. Instead, in certain circumstances, so it has been argued, one may have a duty *not* to give existence to another person. This concept involves the claim that certain qualities of life have a negative value, making life an injury, not a gift; it involves, in short, a concept of human accountability and responsibility for human life. It contrasts with the notion that life is a gift of God and thus similar to other "acts of God" (that is, events for which no man is accountable). The concept thus signals the fact that humans can now control reproduction and that where rational control is possible humans are accountable. That is, the expansion of human capabilities has resulted in an expansion of human responsibilities such that one must now decide when and under what circumstances persons will come into existence.

The concept of tort for wrongful life is transferable in part to the painfully compromised existence of children who can only have their life prolonged for a short, painful, and marginal existence. The concept suggests that allowing life to be prolonged under such circumstances would itself be an injury of the person whose painful and severely compromised existence would be made to continue. In fact, it suggests that there is a duty not to prolong life if it can be determined to have a substantial negative value for the person involved. Such issues are moot in the case of adults, who can and should decide for themselves. But small children cannot make such a choice. For them it is an issue of justifying prolonging life under circumstances of painful and compromised existence. Or, put differently, such cases indicate the need to develop social canons to allow a decent death for children for whom the only possibility is protracted, painful suffering.

I do not mean to imply that one should develop a new basis for civil damages. In the field of medicine, the need is to recognize an ethical category, a concept of wrongful continuance of existence, not a new legal right. The concept of injury for continuance of existence, the proposed analogue of the concept of tort for wrongful life, presupposes that life can be of a negative value such that the medical maxim *primum non nocere* ("first do no harm") would require not sustaining life.

The idea of responsibility for acts that sustain or prolong life is cardinal to the notion that one should not under certain circumstances further prolong the life of a child. Unlike adults, children cannot decide with regard to euthanasia (positive or negative), and if more than a utilitarian justification is sought, it must be sought in a duty not to inflict life on another person in circumstances where that life would be painful and futile. This position must rest on the facts that (1) medicine now can cause the prolongation of the life of seriously deformed children who in the past would have died young and that (2) it is not clear that life so prolonged is a good for the child. Further, the choice is made not on the basis of costs to the parents or to society but on the basis of the child's suffering and compromised existence.

The difficulty lies in determining what makes life not worth living for a child. Answers could never be clear. It seems reasonable, however, that the life of children with diseases that involve pain and no hope of survival should not be prolonged. In the case of Tay-Sachs disease (a disease marked by a progressive increase in spasticity and dementia usually leading to death at age three or four), one can hardly imagine that the terminal stages of spastic reaction to stimuli and great difficulty in swallowing are at all pleasant to the child (even insofar as it can only minimally perceive its circumstances). If such a child develops aspiration pneumonia and is treated, it can reasonably be said that to prolong its life is to inflict suffering. Other diseases give fairly clear portraits of lives not worth living: for example, Lesch-Nyhan disease, which is marked by mental retardation and compulsive self-mutilation.

The issues are more difficult in the case of children with diseases for whom the prospects for normal intelligence and a fair lifestyle do exist, but where these chances are remote and

their realization expensive. Children born with meningomyelocele present this dilemma. Imagine, for example, a child that falls within Lorber's fifth category (an IQ of sixty or less, sometimes blind, subject to fits, and always incontinent). Such a child has little prospect of anything approaching a normal life, and there is a good chance of its dying even with treatment. But such judgments are statistical. And if one does not treat such children, some will still survive and, as John Freeman indicates, be worse off if not treated. In such cases one is in a dilemma. If one always treats, one must justify extending the life of those who will ultimately die anyway and in the process subjecting them to the morbidity of multiple surgical procedures. How remote does the prospect of a good life have to be in order not to be worth great pain and expense? It is probably best to decide, in the absence of a positive duty to treat, on the basis of the cost and suffering to parents and society. But, as Freeman argues, the prospect of prolonged or even increased suffering raises the issue of active euthanasia.

If the child is not a person strictly, and if death is inevitable and expediting it would diminish the child's pain prior to death, then it would seem to follow that, all else being equal, a decision for active euthanasia would be permissible, even obligatory. The difficulty lies with "all else being equal," for it is doubtful that active euthanasia could be established as a practice without eroding and endangering children generally, since, as John Lorber has pointed out, children cannot speak in their own behalf. Thus although there is no argument in principle against the active euthanasia of small children, there could be an argument against such practices based on questions of prudence. To put it another way, even though one might have a duty to hasten the death of a particular child, one's duty to protect children in general could override that first duty. The issue of active euthanasia turns in the end on whether it would have social consequences that refraining would not, on whether (1) it is possible to establish procedural safeguards for limited active euthanasia and (2) whether such practices would have a significant adverse effect on the treatment of small children in general. But since these are procedural issues dependent on sociological facts, they are not open to an answer within the confines of this article. In any event, the concept of the injury of continued existence provides a basis for the justification of the passive euthanasia of small children—a practice already widespread and somewhat established in our society—beyond the mere absence of a positive duty to treat.

CONCLUSION

Though the lack of certainty concerning questions such as the prognosis of particular patients and the social consequence of active euthanasia of children prevents a clear answer to all the issues raised by the euthanasia of infants, it would seem that this much can be maintained: (1) Since children are not persons strictly but exist in and through their families, parents are the appropriate ones to decide whether or not to treat a deformed child when (a) there is not only little likelihood of full human life but also great likelihood of suffering if the life is prolonged, or (b) when the cost of prolonging life is very great. Such decisions must be made in consort with a physician who can accurately give estimates of cost and prognosis and who will be able to help the parents with the consequences of their decision. (2) It is reasonable to speak of a duty not to treat a small child when such treatment will only prolong a painful life or would in any event lead to a painful death. Though this does not by any means answer all the questions, it does point out an important fact—that medicine's duty is not always to prolong life doggedly but sometimes is quite the contrary.

Are There Ethical Questions in Hospice?

TRACY ALBEE, R.N.

AFTER TEN YEARS of working as a Registered Nurse in the arena of home health, I felt I

TRACY ALBEE holds a B.S. in Nursing and has been practicing as a RN since 1987. She has spent the majority of her career in the field of home health and has now transitioned into hospice. She is the President and owner of MediLegal, LLC, a legal nurse consulting firm. She is frequently called upon to speak out as an expert on the issues of standards of care in nursing as well as on the future health care needs and costs of the catastrophically injured.

was quite prepared to move on to a new environment. It wasn't so much that I was leaving the home environment, but rather I was leaving the curative environment.

I had spent my career thus far healing the sick. I had spent my days treating illnesses. I used my time looking for new aggressive methods to assist patients and their families to cope with an acute disease process. The disease was usually short-term and therefore I would watch happily

Reprinted by permission of the author.

as the condition improved and the patient was eventually cured of the ailment.

That's not to say that I never dealt with terminal illnesses in home health. I certainly saw my share of diagnoses such as Cancer, Congestive Heart Failure, and Chronic Obstructive Pulmonary Disease. My plan of care at that time included the administration of active medical care to get them through the most recent exacerbation or crisis. Within a couple of weeks after treatment began, a home-health-based decision would be made. If the patient was improving, we were progressing towards discharge from home health and a happy ending, at least for awhile. If no improvement was seen in that few weeks, then the patient would be discharged for a "lack of progress." The ending wasn't so happy in this case and so to make ourselves feel better, we would give a referral to hospice so the patient could get "the care they really need."

Well, now I am the one who gives the patient "the care they really need." I entered the world of hospice and then the once unanswered (at least for me) ethical questions began.

Should we tell him that he is dying? Should we really let him die at home? Is it right to withhold a feeding tube? Will the pain medicine you are giving him kill him? These are the daily questions that I quickly had to learn to answer.

The first three questions were really not so hard to deal with. Each response can be based on the condition of the person with the terminal illness. What have they previously put forth as their wishes? How is the family coping with the impending loss of their loved one? What are each family member's individual goals as they travel down this path that is so unfamiliar to them? It is not difficult to answer their questions with a question and in that way assist them to find their own answers.

"Will the pain medicine you are giving him kill him?" Now this is the question I dread! What is the right answer? Medical research tells us that the use of narcotics in frequent and large doses will decrease the heart rate and the respiration rate. Does this scenario equal death?

The answer is an unequivocal NO. But in this age of "Kevorkianism" and with the increased media coverage of physician-assisted suicide, it is not easy to convince my patients and their families that the morphine I am holding won't be the means to an end.

It might not be so hard to explain the concept of pain management to the average person on the street. While the use of pain medications do indeed decrease our pulse and breathing as the drug relaxes us, the medications do not cause a cessation of our vital signs. Plain and simple!

In hospice though, we are not educating average people. We are working with terminally ill patients who have recently been told that they are going to die and that this death, their death, will be very soon. We are working with people who love these same terminally ill patients and are not yet ready to let them go. While they all agree on the goal of "comfort," they are not sure it's worth the cost of giving up even one extra day on this earth.

As a hospice nurse, I have learned that it is imperative to sit down with my patients and their significant others to explain the process of dying. I educate them to the meaning of hospice. A hospice program provides palliative and supportive care for terminally ill patients and their families. The concept of hospice is that of a caring community of professional and nonprofessional people, supplemented by volunteer services. The emphasis is on dealing with emotional and spiritual issues as well as the medical problems and their symptoms. Hospice is not and has never been in place for the purpose of hastening death or aiding in euthanasia. The purpose is to allow death to take its course while preserving comfort and dignity along the way.

In the end, it is the disease or its complications that bring us to meet Our Maker. Pain medications are given so that the body may be relieved of the suffering that accompanies the dying process. It is imperative that each individual and their loved ones have a clear vision of this perspective from the moment that the first prescription is written.

So now I am spending my career comforting the sick. I spend my days, and more often, my nights, treating symptoms. I use my time looking for new palliative methods to assist my patients and their families to cope with the disease process until the very end of life, and then even longer for the families. I now watch in relief as each of them comes to terms with the events that cannot be sped up nor slowed down.

Yes, it is true; life for a nurse in the hospice world is a little different. Please understand that I am not a murderer when I come forth with my narcotics in hand. For how can I, as a hospice nurse, deliver effective terminal care if those around me are suspicious of my motives? The answer to this question is the easiest one of all: I can't.

Ethical and Legal Guidelines

Do-Not-Resuscitate Orders for the Incompetent Patient in the Absence of Family Consent

TROYEN A. BRENNAN, M.D., J.D., M.P.H.

ADVANCES IN MEDICAL TECHNOLOGY have a habit of raising new, and usually unexpected, ethical and legal questions. Such questions arise when patients or physicians, for a variety of reasons, defer cardiopulmonary resuscitation (CPR) or other treatment with so-called no-code or do-not-resuscitate (DNR) orders. When all parties to the DNR order, including physicians, patient, and family, agree that it is appropriate in a given case, there is rarely controversy. However, when one party dissents from a no-code status, most commentators agree, grave moral, social, and legal questions are raised.[1]

The most troublesome issues concerning DNR orders arise when physicians and family disagree about the appropriateness of such an order in the case of a mentally incompetent patient. These episodes not only raise complex legal issues but also go to the heart of, and challenge, modern medical ethics and the relationship of

TROYEN A. BRENNAN is Professor of Medicine, Professor of Law and Public Health in the Faculty of Public Health, Harvard School of Public Health.

doctor to patient.[2] The physician faced with a family's demands that medical care be limited is forced to examine his or her relationship with both the patient and the family, and also to consider the role of legal constraints in the decision-making process.[3]

The converse situation, when the physician believes a DNR order is appropriate for a mentally incompetent patient whose family wishes "everything done," perhaps raises even more acute legal and ethical questions. Physicians who conclude that further invasive or extraordinary care, including cardiopulmonary resuscitation, is useless given certain clinical criteria[4] may yet feel forced into useless heroic procedures by the family's wishes on behalf of the patient. The family's demands for treatment call upon the physician's traditional obligation to do whatever is possible for the patient, but these demands can challenge the moral sense of a physician who believes such care would only amount to further torture.[5] Most physicians are as unsure about the ethical as about the legal effect of contradicting or deferring to the family's wishes.

Law, Medicine & Health Care 14, 1(1986): 13–19. Copyright 1986. Reprinted with the permission of Troyen A. Brennan and the American Society of Law, Medicine, and Ethics. All rights reserved.

Reviews and discussions of DNR orders in the medical literature shed little light on the physician's duties when the family requests that "everything be done." Almost ten years ago several lawyers wrote that "[f]ailure to obtain and record family approval of orders Not to Resuscitate may expose those involved to charges of negligence or unlawful conduct."[6] Several years later, another commentator stated that "it appears advisable not to give a 'no code' order without the consent of the incompetent patient's immediate family."[7] Nonetheless, a respected bioethicist and his physician collaborator have argued that "even if the patient is incompetent, the wishes of the next of kin have legal force only in three states. The common practice of obtaining prior consent from the next of kin of an incompetent patient has no legal basis."[8] At least one major medical center, however, has adopted a policy of not writing a DNR order if the family disagrees.[9] Other centers have opted for consultation with hospital ethics committees, allowing the input of uninvolved health care and other professionals.[10] The responsibilities of such committees, as well as their power, is, unfortunately, unclear.[11] Indeed, they tend to be directed at "above all, maximizing support for the responsible physician who makes the medical decision to intensify, maintain or limit effort at reversing the illness."[12]

I and other doctors on the staff of the Massachusetts General Hospital in Boston were recently faced with a situation involving a hopelessly ill patient whose family requested he be afforded full care, including CPR and intubation if necessary. Our experience with this case, and its eventual outcome—as well as the confused and contradictory state of the available medical literature—prompted the following review of the ethics of DNR orders issued in contradiction to family wishes.

CASE REPORT

The patient was a fifty-eight-year-old white male with a thirty-year history of alcohol abuse. He had been in relatively good health until two months prior to admission, when he noted a decreasing appetite and increasing problems with balance, including several episodes of falling to the ground. He continued to drink four or five mixed drinks every day. On the day of admission, the patient had fallen down the steps of his home and then walked to the emergency ward. He denied any history of withdrawal syndrome or seizures; any changes in stool patterns or abdominal girth; and any recent fever, chills, or abdominal pain. He also denied any recent rectal bleeding or vomiting of blood, but a hospital record did show that he had undergone endoscopy for evaluation of bleeding in the upper gastrointestinal tract five years prior to this admission. This information raised suspicion that the patient may have had alcoholic liver disease, and thus a predisposition to gastrointestinal bleeding, for some time. The patient listed a female acquaintance as next of kin but also gave the addresses of his sister and brother.

On physical examination, patient was noticeably jaundiced but in no acute distress. His rectal temperature was 100° F. His skin bore spider angiomas, signs of chronic alcoholic liver disease. The liver was enlarged, and its edge was firm and nodular, suggesting end-stage cirrhosis. The presence of gross acites or fluid in the peritoneal cavity also indicated the severity of his liver failure. A rectal examination revealed blood in the stool. All of these findings were consistent with chronic and end-stage alcoholic liver disease.

Laboratory analyses indicated that the patient's blood would not clot properly, a frequent complication of liver disease. His blood chemistries were equally perturbed, his liver function extremely poor, and his renal function minimal. His chest X ray was normal, and a right-upper-quadrant ultrasound test did not reveal any gallstones.

Thus, on initial evaluation, the patient's clinical picture suggested that he had long-standing liver disease that had now reached its final stages. Moreover, he suffered from critical abnormalities in his blood-clotting system, secondary to his poor liver function. This complication, given the patient's predisposition to bleed in the gastrointestinal tract, created the potential for imminent and massive bleeding. Finally, the patient's renal failure undoubtedly represented hepatorenal syndrome, a poorly understood and usually irreversible decline in renal function caused by advanced hepatic failure.

Thus, although the patient had managed to walk into the hospital, it was clear that he would soon die of the complications of liver failure. We could not, however, predict the exact timing of that death, nor the number of days we could prolong his life by providing unlimited care. Moreover, the patient was unable to tell us if he wanted his life prolonged. His sensorium was clouded by the encephalopathy that results from liver disease. While at times he could answer simple questions, he was usually somnolent and was never able to engage in complex or intellectual discussions.

The initial assessment by the house staff team and the gastroenterology consultants, then, concluded that the patient's prognosis was poor. Nonetheless, attempts were made to treat any causes of the decompensation. The patient was given vitamin K, dextrose, thiamine, folate, and lactulose, all of which supplement the liver's normal functions, as well as potent antibiotics to combat the possibility of spontaneous bacterial peritonitis, a life-threatening condition. Antacids were administered as prophylaxis against a gastrointestinal bleed, and intravenous fluids were given to ameliorate renal function. The visiting physician agreed with these steps, noting that the staff team should "address his problems one by one and hope to find some reversible elements, but overall his prognosis is terrible."

On his second hospital day, the patient remained stable. Nonetheless, the house staff felt his problems required constant surveillance, and he was moved to the intensive-care unit. The patient's sister, who had not seen him in three years, visited and was informed of his grave prognosis. She stated firmly that the family wanted everything done for the patient, including CPR and intubation if necessary. The GI

consultant noted that "if this is indeed end-stage alcoholic hepatitis, he has a poor prognosis (as high as 75 percent)." On the third hospital day, the patient's mental status began to deteriorate further. He began to suffer from delirium tremens, an agitated psychosis associated with alcohol withdrawal. His renal function decreased, and a renal consultant described the prognosis as quite poor.

On the fourth hospital day, the patient continued to be tremulous and experienced intermittent hallucinations. Paraldehyde, a sedative, was administered rectally with good effect. Since the tests for infection that had been taken when the patient was first admitted had come out negative, the prophylactic antibiotic therapy was discontinued. Given the lack of response to our therapeutic efforts, however, all observers agreed that death within one week was probable, but we could not exclude a recovery.

On the fifth hospital day, both the renal and the gastrointestinal consultants agreed that the patient was stable. He was visited by his brother and sister, and again they emphasized that he was to receive all possible care. On the sixth hospital day, the team noted a slight improvement in the patient's mental status. The Optimum Care Committee (Massachusetts General's formal ethics committee) evaluated the patient, noting the consultants' opinion that given his blood-clotting problems, the patient's chances of survival following cardiopulmonary resuscitation were extremely small. Therefore, the committee felt that it would be a breach of medical ethics to initiate resuscitation unless requested by the patient. Tests indicated that the patient's renal and hepatic function was minimal.

On his seventh hospital day, the patient's mental status had cleared to the point that he was oriented to person and place. No hallucinations were noted, and he had not received paraldehyde in two days. Intravenous nutrition was begun. However, the patient began to show new signs of infection, and his blood-clotting abnormalities worsened. Thus he was at grave risk of suffering a massive gastrointestinal hemorrhage.

We on the team caring for the patient concluded that we were loath to intubate him in the event of a massive gastrointestinal hemorrhage. Resuscitation and orotracheal intubation, we reasoned, would only complicate the patient's other medical problems. Given the severity of his liver and renal disease, we could be certain that only one or two out of a hundred patients in a similar situation would survive for more than two or three days following CPR and intubation. Again, however, the statistical evidence supporting our estimations did not guarantee that this patient would not survive.

On the patient's eighth hospital day, the Optimum Care Committee gave its final evaluation. The committee noted that recovery was not possible and that decompensation of the heart and lungs would mean sudden death. Since interference, including CPR, in any major decompensation would only guarantee hemorrhage, infection, suffering, and indignity, such measures were contraindicated. The committee concluded that to proceed in such a course would be an ethical violation. Since the patient was not competent to render a judgment, the committee agreed that it ought to be assumed that he, like most other people in such a situation, would "opt out." The psychiatrist associated with the committee expressed the opinion that some family pathology was producing feelings of guilt in the patient's sister and preventing her from seeing reality. She was free to engage a lawyer, the committee noted, but the hospital was willing to pursue a court order to get DNR status for the patient. The psychiatric problems of one individual did not justify mistreatment of another, the committee concluded.

A do-not-resuscitate order was accordingly written by the visiting physician, and the patient was moved out of the intensive-care unit to a general medical floor. Tests showed worsening renal dysfunction and blood-clotting abnormalities. In light of the Optimum Care Committee's determination, we did not re-initiate antibiotic therapy. The patient's family was informed that his liver, not his lungs or heart, was the main problem, and that CPR could not help his liver. The patient remained confused but was oriented to place and person.

On his ninth hospital day, the patient's urine output decreased and he became markedly more confused. No laboratory values were checked. Over the course of the day, the patient became unconscious, and in the early morning of his tenth hospital day he was found pulseless and apneic. He died before his family could arrive. His brother was quite upset, and claimed that the patient had not received full care because he was not wealthy.

DISCUSSION

This case presented many difficult medical and ethical problems. Above all, there was little doubt that the patient was gravely ill, with all the prognostic signs—including increased bilirubin and prothrombin time, and decreased albumin—that indicate increased mortality in alcoholic hepatitis.[13] Even when all these prognostic signs are present, however, one can expect the disease to stabilize over weeks to months if the patient stops consuming alcohol.[14] But once renal failure and severe abnormalities in the clotting system set in, there can be little expectation of recovery. A tiny fraction of cirrhotics with the severity of liver disease present in our patient could survive, but the overwhelming majority would follow the unrelenting course we witnessed. Treating one complication of the disease only allows others to develop. Once a decision is made to pull back from treatment, renal function is no longer followed closely, and sources of infection are not sought, the patient usually dies rapidly. Thus, this case illustrates well the fact that the DNR decision often affects not only the performance of cardiopulmonary resuscitation but also the level of care a physician will offer to a hopelessly ill patient.

This case also illustrates that physicians must act in the absence of complete certainty that a given patient would not recover if offered optimal therapy. Our patient had an extremely small chance of survival, but it was impossible to say definitely that he would die in one day or even one week. It is partly this lack of certainty that inhibits doctors from talking to patients and families about DNR status. Although he was at times oriented to person and place, the patient never demonstrated any ability to think rationally. Thus, he was never asked if he would want to be resuscitated. Nor was the family fully informed about the Optimum Care Committee's opinion or the patient's no-code status. Bedell and Delbanco have found such lack of communication to be common, both with house staff and private physicians.[15] As illustrated above, much of the physician's resistance to discuss DNR status stems from the inability to predict the timing of death, and from the difficulty of determining when a patient is hopelessly ill.

Most importantly, this case squarely raises the question of whether physicians can or should issue DNR orders when a family disagrees. The Optimum Care Committee clearly thought that further intervention, given the limited hopes for success, was very unethical. The committee's reasoning appears sound in light of the medical principle of beneficence: the physician should cause no harm. In this case, then, the ethical act was to let this critically, probably hopelessly, ill patient die. Further attempts to treat him would most likely prove fruitless and would, in the committee's opinion, have amounted to little more than torture. Thus, the decision not to resuscitate this patient, above and beyond any analysis of the family's psychological problems, was defensible.

Unfortunately, reliance on medical ethics for justification of medical moral decisions is rarely straightforward. The concept of "*a* medical ethics" is inaccurate. As Veatch has pointed out: "To be realistic about it, 'theories of medical ethics' is too pretentious. What we really have

before us is a series of unsystematic, unreflective ethical stances or traditions."[16] An enormous variety of codes, of essays by physicians, theologians, and philosophers, and of ethical and moral assumptions are termed "medical ethics." Moreover, different theories of morality can give rise to relatively different prescriptions for ethical activity or ethical behavior.[17] Thus, to assume or mandate that an action is ethical is to assume or mandate the kind of consensus that tends not to exist in a pluralistic society.

For the sake of argument, however, we can assume that a general concept of medical ethics held by many practitioners would be the covenant-fidelity model proposed by Paul Ramsey. As he puts it, "in the language of philosophy, a deontological dimension or test holds chief place in medical ethics, besides logical considerations."[18] Ramsey's characterization of medical ethics as "deontological" means that the moral probity of the doctor–patient relationship is determined by what transpires within the relationship itself, not by the ends that the relationship might produce. The goodness of the relationship cannot be explained by its outcome, but only in the interaction of doctor and patient.

Ramsey develops his theory by emphasizing the loyalty and fidelity between doctor and patient. Unlike the blind trust that professionals purportedly demand of clients, Ramsey states, there is reciprocal trust between doctors and patients. Their relationship is a cooperative agreement: "Faithfulness among men—the faithfulness that is formative for all covenants on moral bonds of life with life—gains specification for the primary relations peculiar to medical practice."[19] This kind of mutual trust between people allows the healing relationship to occur. "[M]en's capacity to become joint adventurers in a common cause makes possible a consent to enter the relation of patient to physician, or of subject to investigator. This means that partnership is a better term than contract in conceptualizing the relation between patient and physician or between subject and investigator."[20] The unification of personalities noted earlier becomes, in this context, a free choice by two people rather than a necessity forced by the physician's much greater knowledge. The physician's authority is generated by the patient's free choice and by the mutual trust and faithfulness of their relationship.

Mutual trust and fidelity, in turn, generate reciprocal duties. The physician is obliged to care for the patient and to ignore issues that would interfere with this care. As Hans Jonas has so beautifully expressed it:

> In the course of treatment, the physician is obligated to the patient and no one else. He is not the agent of society, nor of the interests of medical science, nor of the patient's family, nor of his co-sufferers or future sufferers from the same disease. The patient alone counts when he is under the physician's care. By the simple law of bilateral contract . . . the physician is bound to not let any other interest interfere with that of the patient in being cured. But manifestly more sublime norms than contractual ones are involved. We may speak of a sacred trust; strictly by its terms, the doctor is, as it were, alone with his patient and God.[21]

Again, there is a sense that the doctor's duty and the trust between patient and physician supersedes the need for other sanctions. Jonsen and Hellegers point out that this theory of virtue and duty dominates both Catholic and Jewish medical ethics.[22]

The essential values of duty, commitment, and trust can be expressed in any number of other ways. Fried argues that physicians are special-purpose friends, whose faithfulness and fidelity to the special morality of the doctor-patient relationship takes precedence over other claims.[23] This sentiment is discussed by Jonsen and Jameton, who note that "even radical and reforming physicians who urge the strongest social and political responsibilities are loath to suggest that physicians should neglect patients for higher causes."[24] Twiss calls the special responsibilities of the doctor-patient relationship "role responsibilities," explaining that they pertain "mainly to

the fulfillment of duties designed to further the welfare of others, albeit a defined class of others."[25] These duties, he notes,

> are strongly other-regarding in the sense that they aim to further the welfare of others. . . . [T]hese duties are often nonpre-emptive in character [i.e., not claimed as rights] because they enjoin the kinds of actions that are not performed out of loyalty, devotion and respect. . . . [T]hese duties represent moral requirements that fall under a general concept of concern, concern for another's welfare.[26]

APPLICATION

What light, if any, does such a duty-based ethics cast on the proper care for the patient we came to know over the course of seven days in the intensive-care unit? Did our special responsibility to the patient include doing everything to save his life, no matter what the chances for recovery and with the possibility of unmitigated pain for the patient? Certainly, the ancient roots of medical ethics offer no basis for a duty to prolong life.[27] Nor does that duty logically follow from a duty to put the patient's welfare above all else. Indeed, the partnership between patient and physician, and the physician's fidelity, may at times require the physician to resist the natural but perhaps futile desire to push on, and to face the fact that further intervention is inappropriate. In this situation, the physician must turn away from the professional role as active utilizer of knowledge and technology, and re-emphasize the human commitment of the doctor-patient relationship.

Nonetheless, it is not clear that medical ethics can accept such an interpretation of the physician's duty. As Jonas notes, "the physician is bound to not let any other interest interfere with that of the patient in being *cured*."[28] The emphasis on "cure" provides a clear and undiluted focus on the doctor's duties. The transition from "cure" to "letting die" perhaps undermines the framework of medical ethics. This is what has led Clouser to argue that while a physician has a duty to cure, that duty dissolves when treatment grows more and more fruitless and begins to amount to pointless torture. The physician must at that point act as an ethical person would.[29] Thus, the doctor's role is limited by the limits of humane treatment. Again, however, such prescriptions do little to guide those of us who cared for an encephalopathic man. At what point do a doctor's role-specific duties recede? Is this point medically or ethically determined?

As Trammel notes, attempts to arrive at consistent actions in situations calling for decisions to allow death raise epistemological problems whose solution may be beyond our grasp.[30] Our medical expertise and technology have advanced reality beyond notions of "natural death."[31] Every situation presents specific and unique circumstances. With this in mind, Ramsey, for one, rejects a policy-oriented approach and encourages physicians to rely on the first principles of duty and fidelity. Less radical — or more in the mainstream of philosophers' views on systematic prescriptions for physicians faced with patients like the one discussed above — is the relationship based in special trust that goes beyond contract, as outlined by Jonas.

Many physicians welcome this responsibility and see such decisions as within the domain of medical decision-making.[32] Many others, as did we, feel burdened by such responsibility. Our decision to contradict the family's wishes, at least in some ways, was rather inchoately informed by a sense of fidelity and duty. We hardly came to know the patient before he became encephalopathic, and so we were allowed little time to build the emotional roots for a Kantian mutuality of ends. Thus, our special responsibilities dissolved into what we thought was a humane paternalism. Such paternalism (on behalf of competent patients) has been questioned by insightful observers.[33] Our decision was also undoubtedly, if less than consciously, reinforced by

consideration of limited resources. While some have argued that it is appropriate to consider such factors in deciding whether to treat or not treat,[34] they do conflict with the fidelity model of medical ethics.

In summary, then, medical ethics would appear to abhor policy-based decisions in cases as complicated as ours. The ethicist can offer only limited help to the physician looking for concrete answers and filled with trepidation by a family's desire for full treatment for a hopelessly ill patient. The role of moral philosophy is to provide contexts for analysis and broad guidelines for action. It is up to the physician to integrate these prescriptions into medical decisions. Unfortunately, physicians have little experience with the task of bringing moral and social norms to bear on particular disputes or situations. In turn, ethicists and jurists are not familiar with the medical and emotional nuances associated with the care of acutely ill and dying patients. It is only through honest discussion and careful analysis of difficult cases like the one discussed herein that we can learn to deal with DNR decisions regarding incompetent patients.

The author is indebted to Dr. George Thibault of the Massachusetts General Hospital and to Ms. Wendy Warring, Esq., of Hill and Barlow for their careful reading and thoughtful suggestions.

REFERENCES

1. *President's Commission for the Study of Ethical Problems in Medicine and Biomedical and Behavioral Research, Deciding to Forego Life-Sustaining Treatments* (U.S. Government Printing Office, Washington, D.C., 1983); J.A. Robertson, *The Rights of the Critically Ill* (Ballinger, Boston, 1983); Note, A Structural Analysis of the Physician–Patient Relationship in No-Code Decisionmaking, *Yale Law Journal* 93(2): 362 (December 1983).

2. R.H. McCormick, To Save or Let Die: The Dilemma of Modern Medicine, *JAMA* 229(2): 172 (July 8, 1974).

3. See A.S. Relman, The *Saickewicz* Decision: Judges as Physicians, *New England Journal of Medicine* 298(9): 508 (March 2, 1978); C.H. Baron, Medical Paternalism and the Rule of Law: A Reply to Dr. Relman, *American Journal of Law & Medicine* 4(4): 367 (Winter 1979).

4. N.H. Cassem, Being Honest When Technology Fails, *American Medical School Alumni Bulletin* 53: 23 (1978).

5. K.D. Clouser, Allowing or Causing: Another Look, *Annals of Internal Medicine* 87(5): 622 (November 1977).

6. M.T. Rabkin, G. Gillerman, N.R. Rice, Orders Not to Resuscitate, *New England Journal of Medicine* 295(7): 364 (Aug. 12, 1976).

7. R.B. Schram et al., "No Code Orders": Clarification in the Aftermath of *Saickewicz, New England Journal of Medicine* 299(16): 875, 876 (Oct. 19, 1978).

8. B. Lo, A. Jonsen, Clinical Decision to Limit Treatment, *Annals of Internal Medicine* 93(5): 764 (November 1980).

9. S.H. Miles, R. Cranford, A.L. Schultz, The Do Not Resuscitate Order in a Teaching Hospital, *Annals of Internal Medicine* 96(5): 660 (May 1982).

10. J.A. Robertson, Ethics Committees in Hospitals: Alternative Structures and Responsibilities, *Quality Review Bulletin* 10(1): 6 (January 1984).

11. See R.H. McCormick, Ethics Committees: Promise or Peril?, *Law, Medicine & Health Care* 12(4): 150 (September 1984).

12. Clinical Care Committee of the Massachusetts General Hospital, Optimum Care for Hopelessly Ill Patients, *New England Journal of Medicine* 295(7): 362 (Aug. 12, 1976).

13. C.S. Davidson, R.A. McDonald, Recovery from Active Hepatic Disease of the Alcoholic, *Archives of Internal Medicine* 110: 592 (November 1962); A.A. Mihas, W.G. Doos, J.G. Spenny, Alcoholic Hepatitis—A Clinical and Pathological Study of 142 Cases, *Journal of Chronic Diseases* 31(6/7): 461 (1978).

14. R.A. Helman et al., Alcoholic Hepatitis: Natural History and Evaluation of Prednisolone Therapy, *Annals of Internal Medicine* 74(3): 311 (March 1971).

15. S.E. Bedell, T.L. Delbanco, Choices about Cardiopulmonary Resuscitation in the Hospital, *New England Journal of Medicine* 310(17): 1089 (1984).

16. R.M. Veatch, *A Theory of Medical Ethics* (Basic Books, New York, 1981), at 5.

17. T. Beauchamp, J. Childress, *Principles of Biomedical Ethics,* 2d ed. (Oxford University Press, New York, 1983), at 2, 3.

18. P. Ramsey, *The Patient as Person: Exploration in Medical Ethics* (Yale University Press, New Haven, 1970), at 5.

19. *Id.*

20. *Id.*

21. H. Jonas, Philosophical Reflections on Experimenting with Human Subjects, in *Contemporary Issues in Bioethics* (ed. Walters and Beauchamp) (Wadsworth, Belmont, Cal., 1978), at 417.

22. A. Jonsen, A. Hellegers, Conceptual Foundations for and Ethics of Medical Care, in *Ethics and Health Policy* (ed. Veatch and Bransor) (Ballinger, Boston, 1976), at 23.

23. C. Fried, The Lawyer as Friend: The Moral Foundations of the Lawyer–Client Relation, *Yale Law Journal* 85(8): 1060 (July 1976).

24. A. Jonsen, R. Jameton, Social and Political Responsibilities of Physicians, *Journal of Medicine And Philosophy* 2(4): 376, 388 (December 1977).

25. S. Twiss, The Problem of Moral Responsibility in Medicine, *Journal of Medicine and Philosophy* 2(4): 330 (December 1977).

26. *Id.,* at 339.

27. D.K. Amundsen, The Physician's Obligation to Prolong Life: A Medical Duty Without Classical Roots, *Hastings Center Report* 8(4): 23 (August 1978).

28. Jonas, *supra* note 21, at 416.

29. Clouser, *supra* note 5.

30. R.L. Trammel, The Presumption Against Taking Life, *Journal of Medicine and Philosophy* 3(1): 53 (March 1978).

31. D.M. High, Is Natural Death an Illusion?, *Hastings Center Report* 8(4): 37 (August 1978).

32. Relman, *supra* note 3.

33. Barron, *supra* note 3.

34. Lo and Jonsen, *supra* note 8.

Sources of Concern
about the Patient Self-Determination Act

SUSAN M. WOLF et al.

ON DECEMBER 1, 1991, the Patient Self-Determination Act of 1990 (PSDA)[1] went into effect. This is the first federal statute to focus on advance directives and the rights of adults to refuse life-sustaining treatment. The law applies to all health care institutions receiving Medicare or Medicaid funds, including hospitals, skilled-nursing facilities, hospices, home health and personal care agencies, and health maintenance organizations (HMOs).

The statute requires that the institution provide written information to each adult patient on admission (in the case of hospitals or skilled-nursing facilities), enrollment (HMOs), first receipt of care (hospices), or before the patient comes under an agency's care (home health or personal care agencies). The information provided must describe the person's legal rights in that state to make decisions concerning medical care, to refuse treatment, and to formulate advance directives, plus the relevant written policies of the institution. In addition, the institution must document advance directives in the person's medical record, ensure compliance with state law regarding advance directives, and avoid making care conditional on whether or not patients have directives or otherwise discriminating against

SUSAN M. WOLF, Professor of Law and Medicine, University of Minnesota Law School and Center for Bioethics; Director, Joint Degree Program in Law, Health & the Life Sciences.

them on that basis. Finally, institutions must maintain pertinent written policies and procedures and must provide staff and community education on advance directives. The states must help by preparing descriptions of the relevant law, and the Secretary of Health and Human Services must assist with the development of materials and conduct a public-education campaign. The Health Care Financing Administration has authority to issue regulations.

A goal of the statute is to encourage but not require adults to fill out advance directives—treatment directives (documents such as a living will stating the person's treatment preferences in the event of future incompetence), proxy appointments (documents such as a durable power of attorney appointing a proxy decision maker), or both. There is widespread agreement that directives can have many benefits.[2-5] These include improved communication between doctor and patient, increased clarity about the patient's wishes, and ultimately greater assurance that treatment accords with the patient's values and preferences. Yet few Americans have executed advance directives. Estimates range from 4 to 24 percent[6-8] (and Knox RA: personal communication).

A second goal of the PSDA is to prompt health professionals and institutions to honor advance directives. The U.S. Supreme Court's *Cruzan* decision suggests that advance directives are protected by the federal constitution.[9] The

New England Journal of Medicine *325, 23 (December 5, 1991): 1666–1671. Copyright 1991. Reprinted by permission of the Massachusetts Medical Society. All rights reserved.*

great majority of states and the District of Columbia also have specific statutes or judicial decisions recognizing treatment directives.[10] In addition, all states have general durable-power-of-attorney statutes, and most states further specify how this or another formal can be used to appoint a proxy for health care decisions.[10] Patients thus have a right to use directives that are based in constitutional, statutory, and common law, and others must honor the recorded choices.[11] There is evidence, however, that advance directives are ignored or overridden one fourth of the time.[12]

Efforts to educate patients about directives and to educate health care professionals about their obligation to honor them thus seem warranted. But the PSDA has caused concern.[6,13,14] Implementation may result in drowning patients in written materials on admission, insensitive and ill-timed inquiry into patients' preferences, and untrained bureaucrats attempting a job that should be performed by physicians. Indeed, one can favor directives yet oppose the PSDA because of these dangers. The question is how to accomplish the statute's positive underlying goals while minimizing the potential adverse effects.

The key to avoiding an insensitive and bureaucratic process is to ensure that physicians integrate discussions of directives into their ongoing dialogue with patients about current health status and future care. Many have urged that doctors do this.[4,6,15] Yet the literature shows that physicians still have reservations about advance directives,[6,12,13,16,19] and some remain reluctant to initiate discussion.[7,15,20,21] Only by forthrightly addressing these reservations can we successfully make directives part of practice, realize the potential benefits for all involved, and avoid implementing the PSDA in a destructive way.

Our multidisciplinary group—including physicians, a nurse, philosophers, and lawyers—convened to address those reservations in order to dispell doubts when appropriate and delineate continuing controversy where it exists.

RESERVATIONS ABOUT TREATMENT DIRECTIVES

Patients do not really want to discuss future incompetence and death, and so would rather not discuss advance directives. Future incompetence, serious illness, and death are not easy topics to discuss for either patients or physicians. Yet studies indicate that most patients want to discuss their preferences for future treatment[4,7,18,22] and that such discussion usually evokes positive reactions and an enhanced sense of control.[18,23]

Misconceptions nonetheless remain and may produce anxiety in some patients. Some people wrongly assume that treatment directives are used only to refuse treatments and thus shorten life.[24] But people use directives to request treatments as well.[4,25] Such a demand for treatment can raise important ethical problems later if the physician becomes concerned that the treatment may be medically inappropriate or futile for that patient. These problems are currently being debated.[26-29] Yet they are not peculiar to advance directives: they can arise whenever a patient or surrogate demands arguably inappropriate treatment. The point is that treatment directives are a way to express the patient's preferences for treatment, whatever they may be.

There are substantial advantages to both patients and doctors in discussing and formulating treatment directives. A discussion of future medical scenarios can reduce the uncertainty of patients and physicians, strengthen rapport and facilitate decision making in the future.[16,23,30] Beyond their clinical advantages, directives are one way to fulfill the legal requirement in some states that there be "clear and convincing evidence" of the patient's wishes before life-sustaining treatment is withdrawn.[31,32] The state statutes on treatment directives also generally give physicians a guarantee of civil and criminal immunity when they withhold or withdraw life-sustaining treatment relying in good faith on a patient's directive.

Some debate remains, however, about when directives should first be discussed and with which patients.[4,21,33] The PSDA requires giving information to all adults when they first enter a relevant institution or receive care. This will involve some healthy patients and patients who are expected to return to good health after treatment for a reversible problem. Yet even healthy persons and young people wish to engage in advance planning with their physicians.[4]

Concern nonetheless persists about whether the time of admission or initial receipt of treatment is an appropriate moment to broach the topic of directives. Ideally, initial discussion should take place in the outpatient setting, before the patient experiences the dislocation that often attends inpatient admission. Many patients, however, will reach admission without the benefit of such discussion. If the discussion on admission is handled sensitively and as the first of many opportunities to discuss these matters with the physician and other care givers, admission is an acceptable time to begin the process. For patients who already have directives, admission is a logical time to check the directives in the light of their changed medical circumstances.

Discussion of advance directives takes too much time and requires special training and competence. The discussion of advance directives is an important part of the dialogue between doctor and patient about the patient's condition, prognosis, and future options. But the physician need not discharge this function alone. Others in the health care institution may play an important part in answering questions, providing information, or assisting with documents. The PSDA helpfully makes health care institutions and organizations responsible for the necessary staff education. However, because patients considering treatment directives need to understand their health status and treatment options, physicians have a central role.

Physicians may nonetheless harbor understandable concern about the amount of time that will be required to counsel each patient. An initial discussion of directives structured by a document describing alternative medical scenarios can be accomplished in 15 minutes,[4] but some will undoubtedly find that the initial discussion takes longer, and further discussion is also necessary in any case. Institutions may want to acquire brochures, videotapes, and other materials to help educate patients, and may enlist other personnel in coordinated efforts to assist patients. In addition, the PSDA requires institutions and organizations to engage in community education, which may reach patients before they are admitted. All these efforts promise to facilitate the discussion between doctor and patient.

Treatment directives are not useful, because patients cannot really anticipate what their preferences will be in a future medical situation and because patients know too little about life-support systems and other treatment options. The first part of this objection challenges the very idea of making decisions about medical situations that have not yet developed. Patients who make such decisions will indeed often be making decisions that are less fully informed than those of patients facing a current health problem.[6] Yet the decisions recorded in directives, even if imperfect, give at least an indication of what the patient would want. If the goal is to guide later treatment decisions by the patient's preferences, some indication is better than none.

The question, then, is not whether the decisions embodied in directives are just as informed as those made contemporaneously by a competent patient. It is instead whether the recorded decisions accurately indicate the patient's preferences as best he or she could know them when competent. The answer to that question depends largely on how skillful physicians are in explaining possible medical scenarios and the attendant treatment options. There are many spheres in which we ask people to anticipate the future and state their wishes—wills governing property and most contracts are examples. But in each case the quality of their decisions depends a good deal on the quality of the counseling they receive. It is incumbent on physicians to develop their skills in this regard. Several instruments have been described in the literature to help them communicate successfully with patients.[19,34,35] In addition, the patient's designation of a proxy can provide a person to work with the physician as the medical situation unfolds.

Good counseling by physicians is the best remedy for patients' ignorance about life-support systems, too. Patients need to understand these treatments in order to judge whether the expected burdens will outweigh the benefits in future medical circumstances. Yet a patient choosing in advance will usually have a less detailed understanding than a patient facing an immediate and specific decision, who may even try the treatment for a time to gain more information.[3] This too supports the wisdom of designating a proxy to work with the medical team.

Treatment-directive forms are too vague and open to divergent interpretations to be useful guides to treatment decisions later. Some forms do contain outmoded language. Terms such as "extraordinary" treatment and "heroic" care have been widely discredited as being overly vague.[3,36] (even though "extraordinary" is used in some state laws[37]), and patients should be discouraged from using such generalities. Instead, patients who wish to use treatment directives should be encouraged to specify which treatments they wish to request or refuse, and the medical circumstances under which they want those wishes to go into effect. Although such specification has been challenged,[17] it is a more effective way for patients to communicate their wishes than a general refusal of life-sustaining treatment. The desire for a particular treatment may well vary according to diagnosis and prognosis[4,38]—for instance, artificial nutrition may be desired if the patient is conscious and has a reversible condition, but unwanted if the patient is in a persistent vegetative state. Another way to communicate wishes is for patients to state their preferred goals of treatment, depending on diagnosis[39]—for example, in case of terminal illness, provide comfort care only.

It is nonetheless almost impossible to write a directive that leaves no room for interpretation. Whatever language the patient uses, the goal is to try to determine the patient's intent. Often family members or other intimates can help. Even a vague directive will usually provide some guidance. Some patients will choose to avoid problems of interpretation and application by appointing a proxy and writing no treatment directive. The proxy can then work with the physician as circumstances unfold. Yet the proxy must still strive to choose as the patient would. If the patient has left a treatment directive or other statement of preferences, it will fall to the proxy to determine what the patient intended.

The incompetent patient's best interests should take precedence over even the most thoughtful choices of a patient while competent. Some people argue that the choices stated in a directive are sometimes less relevant than the current experience of the now incompetent patient.[40,41] In the vast majority of cases, this problem does not arise, because the patient's earlier decisions do not conflict with his or her best interests when incompetent. Yet some demented patients, in particular, may seem to derive continued enjoyment from life, although they have a directive refusing life-sustaining treatment. The argument for discounting the directive is that these patients are now such different people that they should not be bound by the choices of their earlier selves, they may no longer hold the values embodied in the directive, and they may appear to accept a quality of life they formerly deemed unacceptable.

Our group did not reach agreement on this argument for overriding some directives. Members who rejected it argued that it is essential that competent patients who record their wishes know those wishes will be followed later, a person's values and choices should govern even after loss of competence because he or she remains essentially the same person, and to recognize the proposed exception would invite widespread disregard of treatment directives. Although we did not resolve this controversy, we did agree on certain procedural safeguards. A treatment directive should not be overridden lightly. In cases in which this controversy arises, only the patient's appointed proxy, a court, or a court-appointed decision maker should be able to consider overriding the directive. Finally, physicians should specifically discuss with patients what the patients' preferences are in the event of dementia.

Even if a directive is valid in all other respects, it is not a reliable guide to treatment because patients may change their minds. Patients may indeed change their minds as their circumstances change. Physicians should therefore reexamine directives periodically with their patients. Data suggest, however, that there is considerable stability in patients' preferences concerning life-sustaining treatment.[16,42–44] In one study of hospitalized patients, 65 to 85 percent of choices did not change during a one-month period, the percentage depending on the illness scenario presented (kappa = 0.35 to 0.70, where 0 represents random and 1 perfect agreement).[42] In another study there was 58 and 81 percent stability in patients' decisions over a six-month period when they were presented with two scenarios (kappa = 0.23 and 0.31).[43] Further research is necessary, but in any case, patients are always free to change or revoke earlier directives. Once a patient has lost competence and the physician can no longer check with the patient about treatment preferences, a directive becomes the most reliable guide to what the patient would want. Physicians cannot justifiably disregard directives because the patient might hypothetically have changed his or her mind.

RESERVATIONS ABOUT PROXY APPOINTMENTS

Patients may appoint a proxy to make treatment decisions in the event of incompetence, using a durable power of attorney or other document. Some patients both appoint a proxy and execute a treatment directive. Proxy appointments raise some different sources of concern than treatment directives.

The appointed proxy may later seem to be the wrong surrogate decision maker. This concern may arise for one of several reasons. The proxy may have had no involvement in the patient's health planning and may not even realize that the patient has chosen him or her as proxy. To avoid this problem the physician should encourage the patient both to secure the proxy's acceptance of the appointment and to consider involving the proxy in the process of making decisions about future care. The proxy will then be prepared to discharge the function and will have some knowledge of the patient's wishes. The physician should also encourage the patient to tell family members and other intimates who the chosen proxy is, especially since some patients will prefer to designate a proxy from outside their families. This will reduce the chance of surprise and disagreement later.

Physicians may nonetheless encounter appointed proxies with little previous involvement in the patient's planning process and daily life. Yet a patient's designation of a proxy is an exercise in self-determination. The physician is bound to contact that person if the patient loses competence and the appointment goes into effect, rather than ignore the appointment and simply turn to someone else. There may be no further problems, because everyone may agree anyway on what course of treatment the patient would wish. But uncertainty or disagreement about the right choice of treatment may force the resolution of questions about who the most appropriate proxy is. If the medical team or the patient's relatives or other intimates have serious doubts about whether the designated proxy can fulfill the required functions, it is their responsibility to address these doubts through discussion. If the problem cannot be resolved in this way, they may need to seek judicial resolution and the appointment of an alternate.

Sometimes the designated proxy seems inappropriate not because the person is too remote but because the person is so involved that his or her own wishes and interests seem to govern, rather than the patient's. Family members and other intimates almost always have to deal with their own emotional and financial issues in serving as a proxy decision maker, and the mere existence of such issues does not disqualify them. Physicians and other members of the medical team have a responsibility to work with proxies, helping them to identify their own matters of concern, to separate those from the patient's, and to focus on the patient's wishes and interests in making decisions about treatment. Occasionally, the medical team will encounter a proxy who simply cannot do this. If efforts among the involved parties to remedy the problem fail, then care givers may have to seek judicial scrutiny and the appointment of another proxy.

Even a diligent proxy cannot tell what the patient wanted without an explicit treatment directive, so a proxy's choice should carry no particular weight. Family members, other intimates, and physicians often fail to select the same treatment the patient chooses when asked.[45–49] In one study there was 59 to 88 percent agreement, depending on the illness scenario the researchers posed (kappa ≤ 0.3 in all cases)[45]; in another study, agreement was 52 to 90 percent (kappa ≤ 0.4 in all cases).[49] Advising the proxy to choose as the patient would, rather than simply asking for a recommendation, seems to act as a partial corrective.[46]

These data should come as no surprise. Even a person's relatives and other intimates are not clairvoyant and may not share identical values. Moreover, proxies are not always adequately informed that their choices for the patient must be based on the patient's wishes and interests, even when those do not accord with the proxy's. Yet there is often no one better informed about the patient's past values and preferences than the proxy, and the patient in any case has manifested trust by appointing that person. Physicians should encourage patients not only to appoint a proxy, but also to provide instructions to guide the proxy. Physicians should also explicitly clarify for the proxy the primacy of the patient's wishes and interests.

The proxy may make a treatment choice contrary to the patient's treatment directive, claiming that the proxy appointment takes precedence over the directive. Some patients will appoint a proxy and leave no treatment directive or other instructions to limit the proxy's authority. Others will guide their proxy by writing a treatment directive or other record of preferences.[5] Problems may then arise if the proxy tries to override the preferences. The law in individual states often directly addresses the relation between proxy appointments and treatment directives.[50–53] In general, the proxy is ethically and legally bound to effectuate the patient's treatment choices. When the patient has failed to make explicit treatment choices, either in a treatment directive or orally, the proxy is bound to extrapolate from what is known of the patient's values and preferences to determine as best he or she can what the patient would want; this is typically labeled an exercise in "substituted judgment." If not enough is known of the patient's values and preferences to ground such a judgment, the proxy is bound to decide in the patient's best interests. A proxy's authority is thus governed by certain decision-making standards, and the proxy is obligated to honor the patient's wishes, whether stated in a treatment directive or elsewhere. One caveat has been noted: there is some disagreement over whether a proxy can override a treatment directive that seriously threatens an incompetent but conscious patient's best interests.

The proxy may make a decision with which the physician or institution disagrees. This is not a problem peculiar to appointed proxies or advance directives. Disagreement surfaces with some frequency between physicians and patients, families, other intimates, and proxies. As always, it is crucial for the physician to discuss the disagreement with the relevant decision maker, attempting to understand the source and resolve the matter. If resolution is elusive, others within the institution can sometimes assist. Judicial resolution is available if all else fails.

One source of disagreement deserves special mention. The proxy (or for that matter, the treatment directive itself) may state a treatment choice that the individual physician believes he or she cannot carry out as a matter of conscience or that violates the commitments and mission of the institution. There has been scholarly discussion[54,55] and some adjudication[56] of the circumstances under which institutions and physicians or other care givers can exempt themselves from carrying out treatment choices. Care givers and institutions are not free to impose unwanted treatment. The PSDA recognizes, however, that a number of states (such as New York) allow providers to assert objections of conscience.[57] Before a patient is admitted, institutions should give notice of any limitation on their willingness to implement treatment choices. Similarly, an individual physician should give as much notice as possible and should assist in the orderly transfer of the patient to a physician who can carry out those choices.

CONCLUSION

Advance directives have provoked a number of reservations. As the PSDA goes into effect, requiring discussion and implementation of directives, it will be essential to address physicians' further reservations as they arise.

Yet that necessary step will not be sufficient to ensure that the PSDA produces more benefit than harm. There is a risk that written advance directives may wrongly come to be viewed as the only way to make treatment decisions for the future. Physicians and other care givers may improperly begin to require an advance directive before treatment may be forgone for incompetent patients. To avoid this, staff education must include discussion of the various ways to decide about life-sustaining treatment and plan future care. Even under the PSDA, not all patients will use advance directives.

There is a further risk of confusion about the procedures and materials to use in implementing the PSDA. All personnel in the relevant institutions will need clarification of the step-by-step process to be followed with patients, the written materials to use, and how to resolve specific questions. The information conveyed to patients must be understandable, accurate in summarizing the patients' rights, and sensitively communicated. All staff members who are involved must be trained. Institutions must design appropriate protocols.

Finally, there is a risk that the PSDA will reduce the discussion of treatment options and directives to a bureaucratic process dominated by brochures and forms. To avoid this, the discussion of advance directives must be part of an ongoing dialogue between physician and patient about the patient's health status and future. Doctors must accept responsibility for initiating these discussions and conducting them skillfully. Such discussions should begin early in the patient's relationship with the doctor, and the content of directives should be reviewed periodically. Institutions and organizations should set up complementary systems to support this effort. The PSDA's requirements must become not a ceiling but a floor—a catalyst for broader innovation to integrate directives into good patient care.

Susan M. Wolf, J.D.
Philip Boyle, Ph.D.
Daniel Callahan, Ph.D.
Joseph J. Fins, M.D.
Bruce Jennings, M.A.

James Lindemann Nelson, Ph.D.

Jeremiah A. Barondess, M.D.

Dan W. Brock, Ph.D.

Rebecca Dresser, J.D.

Linda Emanuel, M.D., Ph.D.

Sandra Johnson, J.D.

John Lantos, M.D.

DaCosta R. Mason, J.D.

Mathy Mezey, Ed.D., R.N.

David Orentlicher, M.D., J.D.

Fenella Rouse, J.D.

REFERENCES

1. Omnibus Budget Reconciliation Act of 1990. Pub. L. No. 101–508 §§ 4206, 4751 (codified in scattered sections of 42 U.S.C., especially § 1395cc, 1396a (West Supp. 1991)).

2. President's Commission for the Study of Ethical Problems in Medicine and Biomedical and Behavioral Research. Making health care decisions: the ethical and legal implications of informed consent in the patient-practitioner relationship. Vol. 1. Report. Washington, D.C.: Government Printing Office, 1982.

3. Guidelines on the termination of life-sustaining treatment and the care of the dying. Bloomington, Ind.: Indiana University Press and the Hastings Center, 1987.

4. Emanuel LL, Barry MJ, Stoeckle JD, Ettelson LM, Emanuel EJ. Advance directives for medical care —a case for greater use. *N Engl J Med* 1991;324: 889–95.

5. Annas GJ. The health care proxy and the living will. *N Engl J Med* 1991:324:1210–3.

6. La Puma J, Orentlicher D, Moss RJ. Advance directives on admission: clinical implications and analysis of the Patient Self-Determination Act of 1990. *JAMA* 1991;266:402–5.

7. Gamble ER, McDonald PJ, Lichstein PR. Knowledge, attitudes, and behavior of elderly persons regarding living wills. *Arch Intern Med* 1991;151: 277–80.

8. Knox RA. Poll: Americans favor mercy killing. *Boston Globe,* November 3, 1991:1, 22.

9. *Cruzan v. Director,* Mo. Dept of Health, 110 S. Ct. 2841 (1990).

10. Society for the Right to Die. Refusal of treatment legislation: a state by state compilation of enacted and model statutes. New York: Society for the Right to Die, 1991.

11. Meisel A. *The right to die.* New York: John Wiley, 1989.

12. Danis M, Southerland LI, Garrett JM, et al. A prospective study of advance directives for life-sustaining care. *N Engl J Med* 1991;324:882–8.

13. White ML, Fletcher JC. The Patient Self-Determination Act: on balance, more help than hindrance. *JAMA* 1991:266:410–2.

14. Greco PJ, Schulman KA, Lavizzo-Mourey R, Hansen-Flaschen J. The Patient Self-Determination Act and the future of advance directives. *Ann Intern Med* 1991;115:639–43.

15. Teno J, Fleishman J, Brock DW, Mor V. The use of formal prior directives among patients with HIV-related diseases. *J Gen Intern Med* 1990;5:490–4.

16. Davidson KW, Hackler C, Caradine DR, McCord RS. Physicians' attitudes on advance directives. *JAMA* 1989;262:2415–9.

17. Brett AS. Limitations of listing specific medical interventions, in advance directives. *JAMA* 1991;266: 825–8.

18. Lo B, McLeod GA, Saika G. Patient attitudes to discussing life-sustaining treatment. *Arch Intern Med* 1986;146:1613–5.

19. Emanuel LL, Emanuel EJ. The medical directive: a new comprehensive advance care document. *JAMA* 1989;261:3288–93.

20. Kohn M, Menon G. Life prolongation: views of elderly outpatients and health care professionals. *J Am Geriatr Soc* 1988;36:840–4.

21. McCrary SV, Botkin JR. Hospital policy on advance directives: do institutions ask patients about living wills? *JAMA* 1989;262:2411–4.

22. Shmerling RH, Bedell SE, Lilienfeld A, Delbanco TL. Discussing cardiopulmonary resuscitation: a study of elderly outpatients. *J Gen Intern Med* 1988;3: 317–21.

23. Finucane TE, Shumway JM, Powers, RL, D'Alessandri RM. Planning with elderly outpatients for contingencies of severe illness: a survey and clinical trial. *J Gen Intern Med* 1988;3:322–5.

24. Ackerman F. Not everybody wants to sign a living will. *New York Times,* October 13, 1989:A32.

25. Molloy DW, Guyatt GH. A comprehensive health care directive in a home for the aged. *Can Med Assoc J* 1991;145:307–11.

26. Callahan D. Medical futility, medical necessity: the-problem-without-a-name. *Hastings Cent Rep* 1991;21(4):30–5.

27. Youngner SJ. Futility in context. *JAMA* 1990: 264:1295–6.

28. *Idem.* Who defines futility? *JAMA* 1988;260: 2094–5.

29. Lantos JD, Singer PA, Walker RM, et al. The illusion of futility in clinical practice. *Am J Med* 1989;87:81–4.

30. Emanuel LL. Does the DNR order need life-sustaining intervention? Time for comprehensive advance directives. *Am J Med* 1989;86:87–90.

31. Orentlicher D. The right to die after *Cruzan*. *JAMA* 1990;264:2444–6.

32. Weir RF. Gostin L. Decisions to abate life-sustaining treatment for non-autonomous patients: ethical standards and legal liability for physicians after *Cruzan. JAMA* 1990;264:1846–53.

33. Hardin SB, Welch HG, Fisher ES. Should advance directives be obtained in the hospital? A review of patient competence during hospitalizations prior to death. *Clin Res* 1991;39:626A, abstract.

34. Doukas DJ, McCullough LB. The values history: the evaluation of the patient's values and advance directives. *J Fam Pract* 1991;32:145–53.

35. Gibson JM. National values history project. *Generations* 1990;14:Suppl:51–64.

36. Eisendrath SJ, Jonsen AR. The living will: help or hindrance? *JAMA* 1983;249:2054–8.

37. North Carolina Gen. Stat. § 90–321(a)(2) (1991).

38. Forrow L, Gogel E, Thomas E. Advance directives for medical care. *N Engl J Med* 1991;325:1255.

39. Emanuel L. The health care directive: learning how to draft advance care documents. *J Am Geriatr Soc* 1991;39:1221–8.

40. Dresser RS. Advance directives, self-determination, and personal identity. In: Hackler C, Moseley R, Vawter DE. eds. *Advance directives in medicine*. New York: Praeger Publishers, 1989:155–70.

41. Buchanan AE, Brock DW. *Deciding for others: the ethics of surrogate decision making*. New York: Cambridge University Press. 1989:152–89.

42. Everhart MA, Pearlman RA. Stability of patient preferences regarding life-sustaining treatments. *Chest* 1990;97:159–64.

43. Silverstein MD, Stocking CB, Antel JP, Beckwith J, Roos RP, Siegler M. Amyotrophic lateral sclerosis and life-sustaining therapy: patients' desires for information, participation in decision making, and life-sustaining therapy. *May Clin Proc* 1991;66:906–13.

44. Emanuel LL, Barry MJ, Stoeckle JD, Emanuel EJ. A detailed advance care directive: practicality and durability. *Clin Res* 1990;38:738A, abstract.

45. Seckler AB, Meier DE, Mulvihill M, Paris BEC. Substituted judgement: how accurate are proxy predictions? *Ann Intern Med* 1991;115:92–8.

46. Tomlinson T, Howe K, Notman M, Rossmiller D. An empirical study of proxy consent for elderly persons. *Gerontologist* 1990;30:54–64.

47. Zweibel NR, Cassel CK. Treatment choices at the end of life: a comparison of decisions by older patients and their physician-selected proxies. *Gerontologist* 1989;29:615–21.

48. Ouslander JG, Tymchuk AJ, Rahbar B. Health care decisions among elderly long-term care residents and their potential proxies. *Arch Intern Med* 1989; 149:1367–72.

49. Uhlmann RF, Pearlman RA, Cain KC. Physicians' and spouses' predictions of elderly patients' resuscitation preferences. *J Gerontol* 1988;43:M115–M121.

50. Kansas Stat. Ann. § 58–629 (Supp. 1990).

51. Vermont Stat. Ann. tit. 14. §§ 3453, 3463 (Supp. 1991).

52. West Virginia Code § 16–30A–4 (Supp. 1991).

53. Wisconsin Stat. Ann. § 155.20 (1989–90).

54. Annas GJ. Transferring the ethical hot potato. *Hastings Cent Rep* 1987:17(1):20–1.

55. Miles SH, Singer PA, Siegler M. Conflicts between patients' wishes to forgo treatment and the policies of health care facilities. *N Engl J Med* 1989;321:48–50.

56. In re Jobes, 529 A.2d 434 (N.J. 1987).

57. New York Pub. Health Law § 2984 (McKinney Supp. 1991).

Amici Curiae Brief of Not Dead Yet . . . [for *Vacco v. Quill*][1]

INTERESTS OF AMICI CURIAE

Amici are two national organizations composed primarily of persons with disabilities, including persons with spina bifida, cerebral palsy, muscular dystrophy, spinal cord injuries, multiple sclerosis, quadriplegia, paraplegia, head and brain injuries, polio, amyotrophic lateral sclerosis, as well as many other disabilities. Most of these persons use assistive devices, including motorized and manual wheelchairs, ventilators, and personal assistance services for meeting their personal hygiene needs, transferring from bed to wheelchair and preparing food.

Not Dead Yet is a national organization of people with severe disabilities who oppose the legalization of assisted suicide because it singles out people with significant health impairments for assistance to die, denying them the equal protection of laws and medical practice standards automatically applied to healthy individuals who are suicidal. . . .

SUMMARY OF ARGUMENT

Discrimination against people with severe disabilities pervades our society. Assisted suicide is the most lethal form of such discrimination. Applied only to people with significant health impairments, assisted suicide is the ultimate expression of society's fear and revulsion regarding disability. . . . Given the pervasive prejudice against and social devaluation of people with severe disabilities and the absence of adequate health care and appropriate supportive services, safeguards cannot be established to prevent abuses resulting in the wrongful death of numerous disabled persons, old and young. If, however, this Court were to uphold a constitutional right to assisted suicide or authorize its legalization by states, such provisions should apply to everyone—regardless of health status or disability—on a nondiscriminatory basis.

ARGUMENT

I. The Creation Of A Right To Assisted Suicide For A Class Of Individuals Based On Health Status Or Disability Is A Lethal Form Of Discrimination Which Violates The ADA.

A. People With Disabilities, With Either Terminal Or Nonterminal Health Impairments, Are The Class Of People Affected By The Proposed Right To Assisted Suicide.

The outcome of this case potentially threatens the lives and well-being of a significant number of the 23,588,000 noninstitutionalized people in the United States who have severe disabilities.[2] They comprise 12.1 percent of the total population, 15 years old and over in the United States. The outcome will also affect the only minority group, people with disabilities, that is open to all regardless of race, gender, nationality, sexual orientation, income, place of residency, political affiliation, or any other characteristic, and the only minority group, from a statistical viewpoint, which only 9 percent of its members join at birth. There are five primary bases for asserting that people with severe disabilities, including nonterminal disabilities, are the actual and potential victims of a right to assisted suicide:

1. Courts in numerous jurisdictions have ruled that people with severe but nonterminal disabilities may legally be denied suicide prevention that nondisabled people routinely receive, but are to be treated like terminally ill people, with respect to the withholding and withdrawal of life sustaining medical treatment.[3]

2. The diagnosis and prognosis of terminal illness is inherently uncertain, as respondents themselves admit.[4] In addition, many doctors conclude that lives of people with severe disabilities are not worth saving, solely because of their disabilities. The potential for error and abuse against people with severe disabilities is too great.

3. Over three quarters of Jack Kevorkian's assisted suicides involved people who were clearly not terminally ill under accepted medical definitions, but were only severely disabled.[5]

4. In the Netherlands, a country in which assisted suicide has been widely accepted and practiced for many years and the country often referred to as "the model" for the United States, a governmental report demonstrates that many people with nonterminal disabilities have been killed, and thousands have been killed involuntarily.[6]

5. Well-known proponents of assisted suicide have written that it should be applied to people with nonterminal disabilities. . . . Many cases in which state courts have expanded the right to refuse treatment demonstrate that prejudice, stereotypes and devaluation of people with disabilities have already had a substantial adverse impact on members of this minority group. Flagrant prejudice against people with disabilities pervades each decision.

Elizabeth Bouvia wanted medical support while starving herself to death. . . . She had a series of emotional blows, including a miscarriage, the death of her brother, serious financial distress, withdrawal from graduate school because of discrimination, and separation from her new husband.[7] A nondisabled person with this history, who refused nutrition and requested physician assistance to commit suicide, would have been diagnosed as suicidal and provided suicide intervention and treatment. But because Ms. Bouvia also had cerebral palsy, a lifelong, nonterminal disability, it was concluded that her decision to die was reasonable and not deserving of intervention.[8] However, only following two years of lengthy court proceedings did Ms. Bouvia decide not to exercise her newly won right. . . .

You're looked upon as a second-rate citizen. People say, 'you're using my taxes. You don't deserve to be here. You should hurry up and leave.' You reach a point where you just can't take it anymore.[9] These five cases are examples of discrimination against and devaluation of people with disabilities. These decisions occurred because the general public, including judges and physicians, share common societal reactions to people with severe disabilities:

1. nondisabled persons fear that they will become disabled themselves and assume that having a severe disability is worse than death itself;

2. nondisabled persons often view people with severe disabilities as lacking in "quality of life," and such people are to be pitied instead of being granted civil rights or equal legal protections; and

3. to many nondisabled persons, disability falsely implies entrapment, loss of control, and loss of dignity.

As a consequence of these reactions, persons with severe disabilities are segregated, put out of sight in institutions, or neglected, abandoned, abused, and increasingly assisted to die. These public misconceptions, however, are refuted by research studies on disabled people's quality of life.[10] Each of these cases dismissed the state interest in protecting the lives of these disabled individuals and found a "right to die" through the withdrawal of life-sustaining treatment. However, the courts specifically distinguished any right involving active physician-assisted suicide. Before this Court is the request to obliterate this distinction.

Reviewing the people whom Jack Kevorkian assisted in committing suicide also demonstrates the potential for uncontrolled discrimination against people with disabilities, if this Court sanctions active physician-assisted suicide. Of the 40 people who died between June 4, 1990 and September 7, 1996 with the assistance of Kevorkian, at least 28 people had diseases that were not life-threatening and autopsies revealed they were not terminally ill.[11] For example, nine of them had multiple sclerosis. As the *New York Times* recently reported in connection with these people, multiple sclerosis is not a fatal disease. . . . [S]ervices are available to help every person with illness live a more productive and comfortable life and that whatever the state of a person's disability, life need not be worthless.[12]

Like those people who had multiple sclerosis, most of Kevorkian's other "patients" did not have terminal illnesses nor did they receive appropriate services to help make life meaningful. . . . These people represent the extent of discrimination that exists in our society; with appropriate treatment and services, many of them would be alive today. . . .

B. Denying People With Disabilities The State Benefit Of Suicide Prevention And Enforcement Of Abuse, Neglect And Homicide Laws Violates The ADA.

Lethal discrimination against people with severe disabilities and functional limitations is an integral and pervasive part of America's twentieth century history. The forms of this lethal discrimination include:

1. euthanasia, where nondisabled persons advocated for the involuntary euthanasia of 60,000 disabled persons in institutions and five times as many outside, since in these "hopeless" cases "we have no fear of error";[13]

2. eugenics "favoring the killing of defective children";[14]

3. involuntary sterilization of persons with developmental and physical disabilities;[15]

4. denial of life-saving medical assistance especially to children with severe physical disabilities; [16] and

5. withdrawal of medical treatment.[17]

. . . Congress clearly understood this history when, in 1990, it enacted the ADA, the basic civil rights statute for people with disabilities. After extensive hearings, Congress made extensive Findings: historically, society has tended to isolate and segregate individuals with disabilities, and despite some improvements, such forms of discrimination continue to be a serious and pervasive social problem; . . . individuals with disabilities continually encounter various forms of discrimination, including outright intentional exclusion . . . , segregation, and relegation to lesser . . . benefits. . . . To address and remedy this pervasive and relentless discrimination, Congress substantively required that "no qualified individual with a disability shall, by reason of such disability, be excluded from participation in or be denied the benefits of the services, programs, or activities of any public entity. . . ." 42 U.S.C. section 12132. . . . The states concluded that their fundamental interests in saving lives applied only to people without severe disabilities. . . .

Providing assisted suicide only for people with severe disabilities and conversely denying suicide prevention services only for people with severe disabilities violates the ADA in at least four respects:

1. The presence or absence of a severe disability determines whether state and local governments enforce laws requiring

health professionals to protect individuals who pose a danger to themselves. The disability, instead of the risk of suicide, determines the enforcement.

2. The presence or absence of a severe disability determines whether the state and medical practitioners respond to expressions of suicidal intent in people with disabilities with the application of lethal measures that are never applied to people without disabilities. The existence of a severe disability will be the reason for the denial of treatment that nondisabled persons routinely receive. Society's growing support of such discrimination is founded on inaccurate assumptions about the needs of persons with incurable health conditions, the role and authority of physicians, and the nature and significance of requests to die as they are understood and valued by physicians.[18]

3. The presence or absence of a severe disability determines whether state and local governments investigate or enforce potential medical malpractice, such as failure to provide pain medication, failure to establish an accurate diagnosis, prognosis and treatment plan, and failure to ensure informed consent. If one has a severe disability, each of these are treated differently than if one were nondisabled, resulting in a double standard that depends only on the existence of a severe disability.

4. The presence or absence of severe disability determines whether and the extent to which state and local governments investigate and enforce abuse and neglect and homicide statutes in cases reported as assisted suicides. Amici's experiences demonstrate that noninvestigation and nonenforcement are common practices when it comes to the death of people with disabilities.[19] The existence of a disability should never be the basis for these distinctions.

II. Adequate Safeguards Cannot Be Adopted To Protect People With Disabilities From Assisted Suicide Abuse And Therefore An Unequivocal Rule Must Be Established Prohibiting Assisted Suicide.

A. Any Purported Limitation Of The Right To Assisted Suicide To Terminally Ill Persons Will Not Protect People With Severe Disabilities.

Given the "history of purposeful unequal treatment" to which people with disabilities are subjected and the "continuing existence of unfair . . . discrimination and prejudice," 42 U.S.C. section 12101 (a)(7) & (9), adequate assisted-suicide safeguards cannot and will not prevent abuse against people with disabilities. History, contemporary attitudes and biases, the Netherlands, as well as prior judicial decisions, demonstrate that safeguards against abuse in assisted suicide cannot be developed. Amici discussed the current practices which demonstrate that assisted suicide has not and will not be limited to terminally ill persons. . . .[20]

At issue in the present case is nondisabled peoples' intense fear of becoming disabled. When a person with a disability states a desire to die, nondisabled people believe the request is natural and reasonable because they believe that living with a severe disability is a life of dependency, indignity and helplessness; in short, worse than death. The wish to die agrees with the nondisabled view that the primary problem for disabled people is the permanent disability and/or dependence on life aids. Medical professionals, jurists and the public consistently ignore underlying treatable depression, lack of health care or other supports, and exhaustion from confronting systemic discrimination. When medical professionals and the media use phrases like "imprisoned by her body," "helpless," "suffering needlessly," and "quality versus quantity of life," purportedly in a humanistic and compassionate way, they are really expressing very primitive human fears of severe disability and a very misguided condemnation, "I could never live like that." Society translates these primitive emotions into a supposedly rational social policy of assisted suicide. Whenever permanent disability is [defined] as the problem, death is the solution. . . . [T]he wish to die is transformed into a desire for freedom, not suicide. If it is suicide at all, it is 'rational' and, thereby, different from suicides resulting from [the same] emotional disturbance or illogical despair [that nondisabled persons face].[21]

The medical profession is not immune to these erroneous assumptions. Research shows that doctors frequently project the "quality of life of chronically ill persons to be poorer than patients themselves hold it to be, and give this conclusion great weight in inferring, incorrectly, that such persons would choose to forgo life-prolonging treatment."[22] . . . As long as physicians believe that a person with a severe disability has a "life unworthy of living,"[23] lethal errors and abuses will occur.

B. Any Purported Limitation Of A Right To Assisted Suicide Only In Cases Of "Voluntary" Requests Will Not Protect People With Disabilities From Abuse.

As long as people with disabilities are treated as unwelcome and costly burdens on society, assisted suicide is not voluntary but is a forced "choice." Amici are profoundly disturbed by the finding of a constitutional right for assisted suicide in a society which refuses to find a right to adequate and appropriate health care to stay alive. Until society is committed to providing life supports, including in-home personal assistance services, health care, and technological supports, then there is not voluntary choice. . . .

CONCLUSION

The circuit courts' conclusions that people with disabilities are not threatened by physician-assisted suicide is false, based on virtually every court decision to date, as well as on the actual practice in our society. The fact that proponents of assisted suicide continue to dismiss and marginalize the input of the disability rights community on this topic leads amici to believe that they may actually feel that their untimely deaths are ultimately acceptable in the interest of the "greater good," or even only in the interest of their individual need to maintain control in an uncertain and often cruel world.

People with disabilities request this Court protects their lives, to stand as perhaps the last barrier to the "right to die" juggernaut of the recent decade, to recognize that cloaked in the false rhetoric of "personal autonomy," physician assisted suicide threatens the remaining rights of a profoundly oppressed and marginalized people.

Respectfully submitted,

Stephen F. Gold
Diane Coleman

APPENDIX A

The following people were Kevorkin's "patients" through September 7, 1966:(45)

NAME, AGE, DATE DIED, STATUS AND CONDITION AT TIME OF DEATH

JANET AKINS, 54, 6/4/90. Not Terminal. Had Alzheimer's disease.

SHERRY MILLER, 43, 10/23/91. Not Terminal. Had multiple sclerosis with disorganization of motor control in legs and arms.

MARJORIE WANTZ, 58, 10/23/91.Not terminal. Had severe pelvic pain.

SUSAN WILLIAMS, 52, 5/15/92.Not terminal. Had multiple sclerosis and was blind.

LOIS HAWES, 52, 9/26/92. Terminal stages of lung cancer.

CATHERINE ANDREYEV, 46, 11/23/92. Terminal stages of breast cancer.

MARCELLA LAWRENCE, 67, 12/15/92. Not terminal. Had heart disease, emphysema and arthritis.

MARGUERITE TATE, 70, 12/15/92. Terminal stages of Lou Gehrig's disease.

JACK MILLER, 53, 1/20/93. Terminal stages of bone cancer. Also had emphysema.

STANLEY BALL, 82, 2/4/93. Not terminal. Had pancreatic cancer.

MARY BIERNAT, 73, 2/4/93. Had breast and chest cancer. Unclear whether terminal.

ELAINE GOLDBAUM, 47, 2/8/93. Not terminal. Had multiple sclerosis, was blind and used a wheelchair.

HUGH GALE, 70, 2/15/93. Unclear whether terminal. Had emphysema and congestive heart disease.

JONATHAN GRENZ, 44, 2/18/93. Terminal. Had throat cancer.

MARTHA RUWART, 41, 2/18/93. Terminal. Had duodenal and ovarian cancer.

RON MANSUR, 54, 5/16/93. Unclear whether terminal. Had lung and bone cancer.

THOMAS HYDE, 30, 8/4/93. Terminal. Had Lou Gehrig's disease.

DONALD O'KEEFE, 73, 9/9/93. Terminal. Had bone cancer.

MERIAN FREDERICK, 72, 10/22/93. Not terminal stage of Lou Gehrig's disease.

ALI KHALILI, 61, 11/22/93. Not terminal. Had progressive bone disease and multiple myeloma.

MARGARET GARRISH, 72, 11/26/94. Not terminal. Had double amputation from chronic degenerative joint disease.

JOHN EVANS, 77, 5/8/95. Not terminal. Had chronic lung disease.

NICHOLAS LOVING, 27, 5/12/95. Not terminal stage of Lou Gehrig's disease.

ERIKA GARCELLANO, 60, 6/26/95. Not terminal stage of Lou Gehrig's disease.

ESTHER COHAN, 46, 8/25/95. Not terminal. Had multiple sclerosis.

PATRICIA CASHMAN, 58, 11/8/95. Not terminal. Had breast cancer.

LINDA HENSLEE, 48, 1/29/96. Not terminal. Had multiple sclerosis.

AUSTIN BASTABLE, 53, 5/6/96. Not terminal. Had multiple sclerosis.

RUTH NEUMAN, 69, 6/10/96. Not terminal. Was overweight and had diabetes.

LONA JONES, 58, 6/18/96. Not terminal. Had a brain tumor.

BETTE LOU HAMILTON, 67, 6/20/96. Not terminal. Had a degenerative neurological disease.

SHIRLEY CLINE, 63, 7/4/96. Not terminal. Had colon cancer.

REBECCA BADGER, 39, 7/9/96. Not terminal. Had multiple sclerosis.

ELIZABETH MERCZ, 59, 8/6/96. Not terminal. Had Lou Gehrig's disease.

JUDITH CURREN, 42, 8/15/96. Not terminal. Had chronic fatigue syndrome and muscle disorder.

DORTHA SIEBENS, 76, 8/20/96. Not terminal. Had Lou Gehrig's disease.

PATRICIA SMITH, 40, 8/22/96. Not terminal. Had multiple sclerosis.

PAT DIGANGL, 66, 8/22/96. Not Terminal. Had debilitating muscle illness.

JACK LEATHERMAN, 73, 9/2/96. Terminal. Had pancreatic cancer.

ISABEL CORREA, 60, 9/7/96. Not terminal. Had severe pain from a spinal cord condition.

FOOTNOTES

1. All parties have consented in writing to filing of this brief. Copies of the written consents are on file with the Clerk of the Supreme Court.

2. U.S. Dep't. of Commerce, Statistical Abstract of the United States 1994 at 137 (114th ed. 1994) (Table

No. 202). Census data is not available for people with severe disabilities who are institutionalized.

3. See *infra* at 7–10.

4. Timothy Quill, et al, Sounding Board: Care of the Hopelessly Ill, New Eng. J. of Med. 1380, 1381, Nov. 5, 1992.

5. See Appendix A for a list of Kevorkian's "patients" by age, diagnosis and health status at the date of death.

6. Paul J. van der Maas, et al., Euthanasia and Other Medical Decisions Concerning the End of Life, 338 Lancet 669, 672 (1991).

7. See L. Hearn, It's More of a Struggle to Live than Die, Chi. Trib. Feb. 8, 1984, Sec. 51–53; Robert A. Bernstein, Accept the Disabled, N.Y. Times, Jan. 10, 1984, at A23; David.Gelman & Daniel Pedersen, The Most Painful Question, Newsweek, Jan. 16, 1984, at 72; Paul K. Longmore, Elizabeth Bouvia, Assisted Suicide and Social Prejudice, 3 Issues in Law & Med. 141, 153 (1987).

8. Much to the dismay of members of the disability community, including amici, death row prisoners receive more suicide prevention than Ms. Bouvia, Mr. Bergstedt and other persons with severe disabilities. See e.g., Autry v. McKaskle, 727 F.2d 358 (5th Cir. 1984).

9. Joseph Shapiro, Larry McAfee, Invisible Man: The Agonizing Fight to Prevent Legalized 'Suicide', U.S. News & World Rep., Feb.19, 1990, at 60.

10. See e.g., J.R. Bach & M.C. Tilton, Life Satisfaction and Well Being Measures in Ventilator Assisted Individuals with Traumatic Tetraplegia, 75 Arch. of Physical Med. & Rehab. 626 (1994).

11. Thomas Maier, Waiting at Death's Door, Newsday, Sept. 8, 1996, at A 4-5. See Appendix A.

12. Jane E. Brody, Putting Emphasis on Assisted Living with M.S., N.Y. Times, October 23, 1996 at C 11.

13. F. Kennedy, The Problem of Social Control of the Congenital Defective, 99 Am. J. Psych. 13–16 (1942). See also, The Right to Kill, Time, Nov. 18, 1935, at 53–54 (where a Nobel Prize winner at the Rockefeller Institute urged that "sentimental prejudice . . . not obstruct the quiet and painless disposition of incurable . . . and hopeless lunatics"); D. McKim, Heredity and Human Progress 189,193 (1900)(where a respected New York physician advocated the elimination of all severely handicapped children, including "idiots," most "imbeciles, and the greater number of epileptics, for society's protection, via a "gentle, painless death" by the inhalation of carbonic gas).

14. D.B. Shurtlett, Myelodysplasia: Management and Treatment, 10 Current Problems in Pediatrics 1, 8 (1980). See Nat Hentoff, Are Handicapped Infants

Worth Saving? Village Voice, Jan 8, 1991, at 18; Richard J. Neuhaus, The Return of Eugenics, Commentary, Apr. 1988, at 15–26.

15. Although the Court recognized the historical practice of "'putting away . . . the offspring of the inferior, or of the better when they chance to be deformed' [would]do . . . violence to both the letter and spirit of the Constitution," Meyer v. Nebraska, 262 U.S. 390, 401–02 (1923), three years later it upheld the constitutionality of sterilization imposed by a State because Carrie Buck was labelled "feeble-mindedness." Buck v. Bell, Superintendent of the Virginia Colony for Epileptics and Feeble Minded, 274 U.S. 200, 207 (1927). Buck ratified the view of the feebleminded as "a menace," holding: "It is better for all the world, if instead of waiting to execute degenerate offspring for crime, or to let them starve for their imbecility, society can prevent those who are manifestly unfit from continuing their kind." Id.

16. Studies reveal that many physicians, a majority in some specialities, oppose lifesaving surgery for babies with lifelong disabilities. A. Shaw, et al., Ethical Issues in Pediatric Surgery, 60 Pediatrics 588, 590 (1977); R.H. Gross, et al., Early Management and Decision-Making for the Treatment of Myelomeningocele, 72 Pediatrics 450, 456 (1983) . . . (documenting that surgeons at a teaching hospital were actually less likely to perform surgery on Down syndrome children with heart defects than survey studies would predict).

17. See e.g., Elizabeth Bouvia, Kenneth Bergstedt, David Rivlin and Larry McAfee, supra at 7–10.

18. The clinical aspects of such discrimination are explained in Appendix B, excerpts of Affidavit of Carol Gill, Ph.D. from the record in Lee v. Oregon, 869 F. Supp. 1491 (Ore.D., 1994)

19. There are already documented cases of discriminatory enforcement of homicide statutes. Myrna Lebov, a woman with nonterminal multiple sclerosis, was pressured and assisted to die by her husband, Mr. Delury who stated that he had repeatedly told his wife that she was a terrible burden on him, telling her that she was "a vampire sucking [his] life away." Herbert Hendin, Dying of Resentment, N.Y. Times, March 21, 1996 (Op-Ed Page). Mr. Delury plead guilty to a charge of attempted manslaughter and was sentenced to only 6 months in prison. . . . A mother recently killed her brain injured non-verbal teenage daughter. The judge said her actions were understandable, and other parents could be expected to react in the same way. She was sentenced to community service. B. Harris, Mom Freed in Mercy Killing, Spokesman-Review, Jan. 10, 1996 at A1, A7.

20. See infra at 7–10.

21. C.J. Gill, Suicide Intervention for People With Disabilities: A Lesson in Inequality, 8 Issues in Law & Med. 37, 39 (1992).

22. S. Miles, Physicians and Their Patients' Suicides, 271 J.A.M.A. 1786 (1994).

23. It was in Germany in the 1930s, preceding the well-known holocaust of Jewish people, that the Nazis instituted a program to eliminate approximately 200,000 persons with physical and mental disabilities because their lives were "unworthy of living." See e.g., H. Gallagher, By Trust Betrayed (1990); R. Proctor, Racial Hygiene—Medicine Under the Nazis (1988); R. Lifton, The Nazi Doctors—Medical Killing and the Psychology of Genocide (1986) (the medical profession was not coerced but were willing initiators); G. Aly, The Legalization of Mercy Killings in Medical and Nursing Institutions in Nazi Germany from 1938 Until 1941, Int. J. of Law And Psychiatry 145 (1984). The same attitude recently pervaded China's policies in the killing of children with disabilities. Human Rights Watch/Asia, Death by Default—A Policy of Fatal Neglect in China's State Orphanages (1996).

The Case of Helga Wanglie:
A New Kind of "Right to Die" Case

MARCIA ANGELL

HELGA WANGLIE, an 86-year-old Minneapolis woman, died of sepsis on July 4 after being in a persistent vegetative state for over a year. She was the focus of an extremely important controversy over the right to die that culminated in a court decision just three days before her death.[1] The controversy pitted her husband and children, who wanted her life maintained on a respirator, against doctors at the Hennepin County Medical Center, who wanted her removed from the respirator because they regarded the treatment as inappropriate. The judge decided in favor of Mr. Wanglie, and Helga Wanglie died still supported by the respirator.

The Wanglie case differed in a crucial way from earlier right-to-die cases, beginning with

Dr. Marcia Angell is the Executive Editor of the *New England Journal of Medicine*.

the case of Karen Quinlan 16 years ago [i.e., 1975]. In the earlier cases, the families wished to withhold life-sustaining treatment and the institutions had misgivings. Here it was the reverse; the family wanted to continue life-sustaining treatment, not to stop it, and the institution argued for the right to die. Mr. Wanglie believed that life should be maintained as long as possible, no matter what the circumstances, and he asserted that his wife shared this belief.

In one sense, the court's opinion in the Wanglie case would seem to be at odds with most of the earlier opinions in that it resulted in continued treatment of a patient in a persistent vegetative state. In another sense, however, the opinion was quite consistent, because it affirmed the right of the family to make decisions about life-sustaining treatment when the patient was no longer able to do so. By granting guardianship of

New England Journal of Medicine 325, 7 (August 15, 1991): 511–512. *Copyright 1991. Reprinted by permission of the Massachusetts Medical Society. All rights reserved.*

Mrs. Wanglie to her husband, the judge indicated that the most important consideration was who made the decision, not what the decision was. I believe that this was wise; any other decision by the court would have been inimical to patient autonomy and would have undermined the consensus on the right to die that has been carefully crafted since the Quinlan case.

What are the elements of that consensus and how should they be applied to the Wanglie case and others like it? There is general agreement that competent adults may refuse any recommended medical care. This right, based on principles of self-determination, has repeatedly been buttressed by the courts. When patients are no longer mentally competent, families are to act in accordance with what the patient would wish (a principle known as substituted judgment).[2-4] Disputes have arisen, however, when the patient had not, while competent, clearly expressed his or her preferences. This was the situation in the Wanglie case, as it was thought to be in the Cruzan case.[5]

To avoid these disputes, there is a growing movement to encourage all adults to prepare a document that would provide guidance, if necessary, for their families and doctors.[6] Such documents include living wills, durable powers of attorney, and other instruments that have been specially devised for the purpose. Congress recently mandated that as of December 1991, all health care facilities must provide an opportunity for patients to prepare such a document on admission.

We are still left with the problem of deciding for those who have nevertheless provided no guidance, including those who were unable to do so, such as children or profoundly retarded adults. In these cases as well, families usually make decisions on behalf of the patient, but since the patient's wishes are unknown, the consensus holds that the family's decision must be consistent with the patient's best interests.[2-4] A decision consistent with best interests is usually defined as a choice that reasonable adults might make if faced with the problem. This is a vague

but useful standard that, by definition, restricts the range of permissible decisions. It can, however, allow for more than one possible choice. For example, the decision to withdraw the respirator from Karen Quinlan was thought by the New Jersey Supreme Court to be consistent with her best interests, but her father was given the latitude to decide either way.[7]

The well-publicized legal disputes involving the right to die—such as the Quinlan case, the Brophy case in Massachusetts[8] and the Cruzan case in Missouri—have reached the courts either because the institution believed it improper to withhold life-sustaining treatment at the family's request or because the institution wanted legal immunity before doing so. Until the Wanglie case, there was only one well-publicized case of the reverse situation—that is, of a family wishing to persist in treatment over the objections of the institution. This was the poignant case of Baby L, described last year in the *Journal*.[9] The case involved a two-year-old child, profoundly retarded and completely immobile, who required repeated cardiopulmonary resuscitation for survival. Baby L's mother insisted that this be done as often as necessary, despite the fact that there was no hope of recovery. Representatives of the hospital challenged her decision in court on the grounds that the continued treatment caused great suffering to the child and thus violated its best interests. Before the court reached a decision, however, the mother transferred the child to a hospital that agreed to continue the treatment, and the case became legally moot.

Unlike the case of Baby L., the Wanglie case did not involve a course that would cause the patient great suffering. Because she was in a persistent vegetative state, Mrs. Wanglie was incapable of suffering. Therefore, a compelling case could not be made that her best interests were being violated by continued use of the respirator. Instead, representatives of the institution invoked Mrs. Wanglie's best interests to make a weaker case: that the use of the respirator failed to serve Mrs. Wanglie's best interests and should therefore not be continued. It was suggested that a victory for Mr. Wanglie would mean that patients or their families could demand whatever treatment they wished, regardless of its efficacy. Many commentators also emphasized the enormous expense of maintaining a patient on life support when those resources are needed to care for people who would clearly benefit. In the previous essay, Steven H. Miles, M.D., the ethics committee consultant at the Hennepin County Medical Center who was the petitioner in the Wanglie case, presents the arguments of the institution.[10] They are strong arguments that deserve to be examined, but I believe that they are on balance not persuasive.

It is generally agreed, as Miles points out, that patients or their surrogates do not have the right to demand any medical treatment they choose.[11,12] For example, a patient cannot insist that his doctor give him penicillin for a head cold. Patients' rights on this score are limited to refusing treatment or to choosing among effective ones. In the case of Helga Wanglie, the institution saw the respirator as "non-beneficial" because it would not restore her to consciousness. In the family's view, however, merely maintaining life was a worthy goal, and the respirator was not only effective toward that end, but essential.

Public opinion polls indicate that most people would not want their lives maintained in a persistent vegetative state. Many consider life in this state to be an indignity, and care givers often find caring for such patients demoralizing. It is important, however, to acknowledge that not everyone agrees with this view and it is a highly personal issue. For the decision to rest with the family is the most sensitive and workable approach, and it is the generally accepted one. Furthermore, a system in which life-sustaining treatment is discontinued over the objections of those who love the patient, on a case-by-case basis, would be callous. It can be argued on medical grounds that the definition of brain death should be legally extended to include a persistent vegetative state, but unless that is done universally we have no principled basis on which to override a family's decision in this kind of case. It

is dismaying, of course, that resources are spent sustaining the lives of patients who will never be sentient, but we as a society would be on the slipperiest of slopes if we permitted ourselves to withdraw life support from a patient simply because it would save money.

Since the Quinlan case it has gradually been accepted that the particular decision is less important than a clear understanding of who should make it, and the Wanglie case underscores this approach. When self-determination is impossible or an unambiguous proxy decision is unavailable, the consensus is that the family should make the decision. To be meaningful, this approach requires that we be willing to accept decisions with which we disagree. Only if a decision appears to violate the best interests of a patient who left no guidance or could provide none, as in the case of Baby L, should it be challenged by the institution. Thus, the sources of decisions about refusing medical treatment are, in order of precedence, the patient, the patient's prior directives or designated proxy, and the patient's family. Decisions from each of these sources should reflect the following standards, respectively: immediate self-determination, self-determination exercised earlier, and the best interests of the patient. Institutions lie outside this hierarchy of decision making and should intervene by going to court only if they believe a decision violates these standards. Although I am sympathetic with the view of the doctors at the Hennepin County Medical Center, I agree with the court that they were wrong to try to impose it on the Wanglie family.

NOTES

1. In re Helga Wanglie, Fourth Judicial District (Dist. Ct., Probate Ct. Div.) PX-91-283. Minnesota, Hennepin County.
2. Society for the Right to Die. The physician and the hopelessly ill patient: legal, medical and ethical guidelines. Now York: Society for the Right to Die, 1985.

3. Guidelines on the termination of life-sustaining treatment and the care of the dying: a report by the Hastings Center. Briarcliff Manor, N.Y.: Hastings Center, 1987.

4. President's Commission for the Study of Ethical Problems in Medicine and Biomedical and Behavioral Research. Deciding to forego life-sustaining treatment: a report on the ethical, medical, and legal issues in treatment decisions. Washington, D.C.: Government Printing Office, 1983.

5. *Cruzan v. Harmon,* 760 S.W.2d 408 (1988).

6. Annas, G.J. The health care proxy and the living will. *N Engl J Med* 1991;324:1210–3.

7. In re Quinlan, 70 NJ 10, 355 A.2d 647 (1976).

8. *Brophy v. New England Sinai Hospital, Inc.,* (Mass. Probate County Ct., Oct. 21, Nov. 29, 1985) 85E0009-G1.

9. Paris, J.J., Crone. R.K., Reardon F. Physicians' refusal of requested treatment: the case of Baby L. *N Engl J Med* 1990;322:1012–5.

10. Miles, S.H. Informed demand for "non-beneficial" medical treatment. *N Eng J Med* 1991;325:512–5.

11. Brett, A.S., McCullough, L.B. When patients request specific interventions: defining the limits of the physician's obligation. *N Engl J Med* 1986; 315:1347–51.

12. Blackhall, L.J. Must we always use CPR? *N Engl J Med* 1987;317:1281–5.

The Joint Centre for Bioethics Living Will Form

THE FOLLOWING IS the Joint Centre for Bioethics Living Will form. Be sure to discuss your wishes with your proxy. You can use the descriptions of the health situations and treatments, and the living will form, to help you with this discussion. This living will is a legal document. Although you can complete this form without a lawyer, it is a good idea to consult a lawyer with experience in this area.

The living will contains medical information to help you make decisions. If you have questions about the descriptions of health situations or treatments, or about your own medical conditions and what might happen to you in the future, you should discuss these with your doctor. Complete the living will using a black pen to make it easier to photocopy. When you have completed it, make copies to give to your proxy(ies), doctor, and lawyer. If you change

your mind about who you want to be your proxy, or about your wishes regarding treatment, change your living will and give copies of the new one to anyone who has a copy of the old one. Then, destroy all copies of your old living will.

THE PROXY DIRECTIVE

The proxy must follow the wishes of the person making the living will. In situations for which the person has not specified a wish, the proxy would make the decision based on the person's best interests, taking into consideration the person's value and beliefs.

If you name more than one person to act as your proxy, you should say how they will make decisions. There are three options:

Reprinted by permission of Peter Singer and the University of Toronto.

First, you can have your proxies make decisions individually, in the order that you list them in your living will. If the first named proxy is unavailable, or has died, then the next proxy listed in your living will would make the necessary decisions on your behalf, and so on.

Second, you can say in your living will that you want your proxies to make decisions as a group. If you want your proxies to make decisions as a group, you should indicate how you would like disagreements between your proxies to be resolved. This could be by majority vote or by giving your first-named proxy the final say.

Third, you can limit the authority of your proxies to make certain decisions. For example, you may have someone who you want to make decisions about your health care, and someone else to make other personal care decisions such as nutrition, clothing, hygiene or shelter.

The wishes contained in this living will are intended to help your proxy(ies) understand what you want. You can also say how much leeway your proxy should have in interpreting your wishes; i.e., do you want your instructions followed exactly or used only as a guideline?

I authorize the following person(s) to make health care and other personal care decisions on my behalf if I am no longer capable of making them for myself.

Proxy 1

Name:_____

Relationship:_____

Address:_____

Telephone:_____

If you want more than one person to be your proxy, add the additional name(s) below:

Proxy 2

Name:_____

Relationship:_____

Address:_____

Telephone:_____

Proxy 3

Name:_____

Relationship:_____

Address:_____

Telephone:_____

Do you want your proxies to make decisions individually (i.e., proxy 1 will make decisions if available; otherwise proxy 2 will make decisions etc.), or as a group?

☐ individually

☐ as a group

If you want your proxies to make decisions as a group, how do you want disagreements resolved?

☐ follow directions of proxy 1

☐ follow directions of the majority of my proxies

If you want particular proxies to make health care decisions, and others to make other personal care decisions, specify here:

How much leeway do you want to give your proxies in interpreting your wishes? Specify here:

THE INSTRUCTION DIRECTIVE

The first part of the instruction directive is the Treatment Table.

For each of the health situations (found in the first column of the table), imagine that you are in the situation described, and then you develop a further medical problem that requires some life-sustaining treatment (found in the top row of the table). If you do not receive this treatment,

	CPR	Ventilator	Dialysis	Life-saving surgery	Blood transfusion	Life-saving antibiotics	Tube feeding
Current health							
Mild stroke							
Moderate stroke							
Severe stroke							
Mild dementia							
Moderate dementia							
Severe dementia							
Permanent coma							
Terminal illness							

you would die. If you receive the treatment, the chance that you will live depends on the nature of the medical problem. Even if you recover fully from the medical problem, you would return to the health situation you were in before you developed the further medical problem.

As an example, imagine that, at some future time, you suffer from a severe stroke. Then, you develop pneumonia requiring life-saving antibiotics. Without the antibiotics, you would die. With the antibiotics, your chance of surviving depends on the nature and severity of the pneumonia. Of course, even if the antibiotics were successful in treating your pneumonia, you would still have severe stroke.

You should then decide whether or not you would want the particular treatment (antibiotics) if you were in this condition (severe stroke).

TO COMPLETE THE TABLE

Write your treatment decision ("YES", "NO", "UNDECIDED," or "TRIAL") in the box for every combination of health situation and treatment.

Take the example from the previous page and imagine again that you suffer from a severe stroke. If in that situation you would want life-saving antibiotics, if they were the only hope of saving your life, you would write "YES" in the box found where the column marked "Antibiotics" and the row marked "Severe Stroke" meet. If you would not want antibiotics in those circumstances, write "NO" in that box. If you are undecided, you would write "UNDECIDED."

One other option is possible. In some cases, it may be unclear initially whether a given treatment will be beneficial or not. In these cases, you may want to try the treatment for an appropriate period, usually a few days to a couple of weeks. During this time your doctors would monitor and assess the effectiveness of the treatment and determine how beneficial it was for you. If the treatment proved to be beneficial, it could be continued. If not, it could be stopped. If you wish such a treatment trial, then write "TRIAL" in the box. For CPR and surgery, a treatment trial is not appropriate because these treatments are given all at once in a short time.

Then, the rest of the boxes may be filled in, by imagining yourself in each health situation and that you require each of the life-sustaining treatments listed.

FURTHER INSTRUCTIONS ABOUT HEALTH CARE DECISIONS

The second part of the instruction directive allows you to express, in your own words, your wishes about health care decisions. It is not usually possible to foresee in advance all of the types of medical decisions which may have to be made for you.

Use this space to express any personal beliefs or values that you think make it easier for proxy decision makers or health care providers to understand and follow your wishes. Also, if there are any particular persons who should *not* take part in decision-making for you, this should also be recorded here.

INSTRUCTIONS ABOUT PERSONAL CARE DECISIONS

In this third part of the instruction directive, you may express, in your own words, your wishes about other personal care decisions, such as shelter, nutrition, hygiene, clothing and safety.

Statement by the Person Completing This Living Will

I have read and understood all sections of this living will.

All previous living wills made by me are to be revoked, and this directive is to be followed.

The person(s) whom I have named as a proxy(ies) is/are authorized to give directions and make decisions, on my behalf, concerning my personal care and to give or refuse consent on my behalf to treatment, in accordance with the instructions found in this living will.

Personal Information and Signature
(of person making this living will)

Name:_____

Address:_____

_____

Signature:_____

Date:_____

Sign in the presence of both witnesses.

Instructions for Witnesses

Although the requirements in different states/provinces vary, for greater certainty, use two witnesses. The witnesses must be present together and sign immediately after the living will is signed by the person completing it. Neither witness should be the proxy or the proxy's spouse.

Witness 1

Name:_____

Address:_____

_____

Signature:_____

Date:_____

Witness 2

Name:_____

Address:_____

_____

Signature:_____

Date:_____

AGREEMENT TO ACT AS PROXY

I agree to act as Proxy for _____
_____ in the event that he/she becomes incapable.

Proxy 1

Name:_____

Signature:_____

Date:_____

Proxy 2

Name:_____

Relationship:_____

Address:_____

Telephone:_____

Proxy 3

Name:_____

Relationship:_____

Address:_____

Telephone:_____

The Experiential Dimension

A Letter from a Patient's Daughter
[On Being a Patient]

ELISABETH HANSOT, PH.D.

MY MOTHER, GEORGIA HANSOT, died recently in the intensive care unit of a major hospital in the eastern United States. She was 87 years old. This is an account of the 5 days she spent in the hospital from the point of view of her daughter, a 57-year-old professional woman who was charged with her mother's power of attorney for health care. . . . This essay could as easily be entitled "There Are No Villains Here." Medical personnel, trained to save lives and not to let patients die, exerted themselves to that end. . . . Nonetheless, those 5 days were among the loneliest and most disorienting that I have ever experienced.

. . . I am astounded that I had so little inkling of how hard it would be to help my mother have the death she wanted. A widow of 6 years, my mother had retained the no-nonsense attitude of her Kansan farming origins. She lived in an affluent and stable community on the east coast, and she saw her physician of 25 years routinely

DR. ELISABETH HANSOT is a Senior Lecturer in the Department of Political Science at Stanford University.

for checkups. When we talked together about how she wanted to die, she was clear, consistent, and matter-of-fact. She hoped for a swift death and wanted no unnecessary prolongation of her life. Entrusted with a general power of attorney and a power of attorney for health care, I believed that I could make decisions on her behalf as she would want them made if she were to become incapacitated. As it turned out, I was woefully unprepared for what was in store for her and for me.

On a spring morning in April, my mother abruptly became ill and was promptly admitted to the local hospital. When I arrived in the late afternoon, she was resting comfortably. . . . Because she had been tired by the day's ordeal, I stayed only briefly. . . . At 2:00 the next morning, I was awakened by a call from the night nurse. My mother had suddenly taken a turn for the worse and was being transferred to intensive care. I arrived . . . just as the gurney was being wheeled into the unit. My mother's face was covered by an oxygen mask, but she was able to respond to my voice with an exclamation. It was

Annals of Internal Medicine *125 (1996): 149–151. Reprinted by permission of the American College of Physicians.*

the last time she would be able to do so. I tried to accompany her into the intensive care unit but could not. The physician in charge firmly instructed me to stay outside until my mother was "taken care of." An hour later, when I was allowed to see her, she was attached to a respirator and had a feeding tube inserted down her throat.

What had happened? My mother had left a carefully updated power of attorney for health care with her physician, her lawyer, and her offspring, reaffirming her determination not to have her life prolonged by artificial means. Exactly the opposite of what she had wished had occurred; the living will had become invisible just when it was needed most. My mother's physician, it turned out, had not notified the medical team of her advance directive, and the hospital, despite a 1990 federal law that mandates such inquiries, did not ask my mother whether she had such a document. And I, in turn, had neglected to check that the physicians and nurses knew about her desire not to have heroic measures used to prolong her life.

Over the ensuing 5 days, I came to understand how serious the results of these omissions were. I found that I was dealing with a bewildering array of medical specialists trained to prolong lives, not to let patients die. During the first day that my mother was in the intensive care unit, I asked her physician to make it clear to the attending medical personnel that she had given me durable power of attorney for health care. He readily complied. I was told that my mother had had a stroke and that she would not recover from her hemiparalysis. The physicians hoped to fit her with a tracheostomy tube and send her to a nursing home. From my many conversations with my mother about quality of life and medical care, I knew that she did not want such a life. Yet my mother's wishes, as they were understood by her family physician and her daughter, were now subject to the approval of strangers: the cadre of cardiologists, neurologists, and pulmonologists who attended her.

None of these specialists knew my mother, and they all had their convictions about how to do best by her. Most notably, they varied in the latitude with which they were willing to interpret her wishes. . . . The variance was widest between my mother's wishes and those of the attending pulmonologist. . . . He found it nearly impossible to accept that my mother would prefer death to living with hemiparalysis and a tracheotomy. Over the next several days, our conversations became terser and tenser. . . . I asked the family physician whether another pulmonologist could attend the case, only to be told that all of the pulmonologists accredited to the hospital shared similar beliefs.

My stress built . . . as my mother's distress was palpable. She successfully tore out her feeding tube only to have it reinserted and her restraints tightened. An attempt to remove my mother from the ventilator failed; her swollen larynx prevented her from breathing on her own. I had agreed to the removal on the condition that I be allowed to stay with her during the attempt. Afterward, the pulmonologist declared himself pleased that he had been able to reinsert her breathing tube . . . unaware of how agitated this process had left her. I asked that she be sedated, and an obliging nurse obtained permission for this. The hospital increasingly came to feel like alien territory, full of medical strangers intent on maintaining my mother's vital signs at all costs. During her ordeal, my mother became increasingly frantic. She continually leaned against her restraints, trying to get her hand close enough to her feeding tube to tear it out again. My sense of being trapped in a nightmare intensified. . . . One afternoon, she rapped her cuffed hand angrily against the bed bars to get my attention, then motioned toward the tubes that she clearly wished to have removed. The next day, when I was holding her hand, she squeezed mine so hard that I winced in pain, and after that a breakthrough came: We were able to devise a mode of talking to each other.

In response to a yes or no question, my mother nodded or shook her head. . . . I was able to ask my mother twice—with her nurse as a witness, and with 4 hours between each question—whether she wished to die. My very clearheaded and determined mother thus was able, finally, to assert herself. . . . The nurse informed the physicians of what she had seen. . . . The hours dragged by as the specialists were persuaded, one by one, to give their consent. Finally, a technician was allowed to pull the tube from my mother's throat. None of the physicians who had attended her was present.

In retrospect . . . there seems to be no simple explanation for what happened. Physicians are trained to save lives, and most of us would not have it otherwise. In their conversations with me, my mother's physicians related success stories. . . . These stories were intended to be helpful. . . . But in the end they turned into so many cautionary tales. Most of the stories seemed to define success as survival and ended with the patient's departure from the hospital. The quality of life after that departure was, at best, moot. . . . In the weeks that followed my mother's ordeal, I listened, with the rest of the United States, to accounts of the deaths of Richard Nixon and Jacqueline Onassis. Because both of them had living wills, the commentators explained, their lives would not be prolonged by mechanical means. Angry and frustrated at the way my mother had died, I wondered: Do you have to be notable to be heard in our society?

All told, I think that my mother was fortunate. In the long run, her wishes were followed; 5 days in the intensive care unit compares favorably with the experiences of many other elderly persons. But the experience was harrowing, for her and for me. What is routine for hospital staff is all too often the first experience of its kind for critically ill patients and their families. I had a very steep and painful learning curve. This essay is written in the hope that hospitals will devise procedures so that patients and their families can, with less pain and perplexity than I experienced, decide when and how death arrives.

Doing Everything
[On Being a Patient]

DAVID S. PISETSKY, M.D., PH.D.

I never knew what death was like until I watched my father die. He had Lou Gehrig's disease. I

DAVID S. PISETSKY, M.D., PH.D., is at the Durham Veterans Affairs Medical Center, Durham, NC.

learned about the meanness of this condition only as I saw what it did to him. Until he developed amyotrophic lateral sclerosis at 84 years of age, my father worked full time as a physician and was a robust man with a large belly and an

Annals of Internal Medicine 128 (1998): 869–870. *Reprinted by permission of the American College of Physicians.*

exuberant smile. After he got sick, he became immobile, despondent, and dependent on others. He had difficulty swallowing and, terrified of choking, restricted his diet to soft foods. He lost 100 pounds.

Toward the end of the summer, my mother phoned urgently to tell me that my father's condition had deteriorated. She said that he had suddenly lost the power of speech and refused food and water. . . . When I arrived at my family's home and saw my father, I was sure that he would die soon. He was in a hospital bed in the living room. He did not respond to my voice. His breathing was rapid and his gaze opaque. I went to the kitchen where my mother sat. . . . "He's very sick," I said. "What do you want to do?" "What can I do?" she said. . . . "We can go to the hospital." "He hates the ambulance. The sirens scare him. Suppose we don't go?" "He'll die today." "So soon?" she said. Her voice was strained. My father was 86 years old and had been miserably sick for 2 years. His death had lurked every day since a fateful electromyogram had led to his diagnosis; nevertheless, its imminence took her by surprise. "I'll take him myself in the car," I said. "Thank you," she said, crying. "I'm not ready for him to die."

I went to the living room to get my father. Anyone who says that caring for an old person is like caring for a baby is wrong. The flesh of babies is soft and buoyant. The flesh of old people is dense and dispirited. My father had no muscles. Coarse skin covered bones that were held together by tendons that seemed frayed and rigid. I was afraid that I would pull off a limb if I lifted him wrong. I put him over my shoulder the way I had been taught to remove hospitalized patients during a fire. I carried him part of the way to the car and stopped so that I could inspect his face. To my horror, he looked dead. . . .

I carried my father back to his bed and told my mother that he had said he wanted to be at home. "It's better this way. We can all be to-gether." During the next few hours, my sister, her husband, my niece, and my aunt all came to spend one last day with my father. "We're all here," my mother said into my father's ear and, for a instant, I thought his head moved in recognition. "Can he hear?" my aunt asked . . . "I think so," I said with authority. Once we were all assembled, we sat around my father's bed, linked by his presence. The room smelled of Vaseline and the perfume of baby wipes. Dust was thick in the air. I focused on the sound of my father's breath, straining to detect any clue that would signal his course, but his breathing was regular and like a whisper.

Throughout the morning, we all remained quiet by his bedside in anticipation of the end. I looked at my watch and realized that we had already spent 2 hours in the calm of the room. My mother, who had been awake the entire night, had not yet eaten, afraid that if she left my father's side he would die without her. I wanted her to take some food, so for a moment I became a physician again and assessed my father's condition. His skin was warm. His respiration rate was thirty breaths per minute, and through a stethoscope I could hear coarse sounds from his upper airways. I listened to his heart and was amazed by its strength. The sounds were forceful, pulsing against his chest defiantly. His heart mocked the name of his illness. His heart was the real Lou Gehrig. It was the iron horse, driven to a record of consecutive days on the field.

"His heart's good," I said to my mother. "You can take a break." "Life goes so fast," she said, distracted. While my mother went to the backyard to eat and sit in the sun, I took her place at my father's bedside. I stayed there for almost an hour, suspended in time. His breathing was steady, almost reassuring, but when I finally looked at his face, his skin seemed more lax and his lips were mottled.

I went to get my mother. "You should go back in," I said and took her by the arm to steady her for the walk back to the sickroom. We all came together in the living room and I announced, "It's time to say good-bye." One by one, my sister, my brother-in-law, my niece, my aunt, and I went to my father. We all cried. We all kissed him. We all said, "I love you." Because my wife and children had not made this trip, I added, "Ingrid and the kids say good-bye." For years, when I talked on the phone with my father, I would say, "Ingrid and the kids say hello," but this time the message had to change. My mother then spoke, and with words of power and stark eloquence, she recounted their life together. I heard of joy, love, injury, regret, and a wrenching wish to stay together. "We'll meet again," she said, and her tears came again, and then she was silent.

My medical judgment was wrong. My father would not die until later that night. When I look back on that day, I think that my father rallied briefly because these were probably among the richest moments he had ever spent. His family, whom he so cherished, infused him with their love, saying things that only the deathbed would allow. These were words he would have savored throughout his life, but only in his death did he have the chance. "This could go on all night," I said later that evening. . . . "What's the hurry?" my mother said, wistful and ironic.

I closed my eyes to the sound of the breathing as a calm descended on me and time passed without boundary. I must have fallen asleep because the next thing I can recall is my niece saying, "His breathing changed. What's wrong?" Instantly, I awoke. . . . It was 2:00 A.M. I looked at my father. He was agonal. Suddenly, the room became frantic with sound. I roused my mother, who had fallen asleep in a chair next to my father's bed, her hand on his. "You'd better wake up." "Is he dead?" "Not yet." "Did I miss it?" "You didn't. He's still alive. He waited for you." Gasp. Silence. Gasp. Silence. Silence, and then my mother's moan, shocked, wounded, and despairing. He was dead, and we all cried again and

said good-bye once more, this time to a body whose flesh had stiffened and whose mouth now gaped.

At 6:00 A.M., two men from the funeral home removed my father's body. . . . It was over.

Among the many feelings of that day that commingle in my mind—grief, sadness, guilt, longing, relief—there is also a surge of pride and even exhilaration. My family did not abandon my father at the time of his death. We did not cast him from his home and surrender him to the hospital and its fearsome machines. We kept him where he wanted to be, in a room where we had watched Ed Sullivan and Marshal Dillon, where we had celebrated graduations, marriages, and births. And just as death put my father under a spell that day, my family put death under its own spell.

Soon I will have to discuss end-of-life issues with the family of a patient who is old, near death, and defeated by illness. I will sit in a dreary alcove with pastel walls and plastic furniture. I will explain the meaning of cardiopulmonary resuscitation, intubation, cardioversion, and all of the options that are available when the heart stops, as if issues of such complexity can be distilled into a few sentences of approachable dimensions.

"What are the wishes of the family?" I will ask, as they look back and forth at each other to determine who will speak. And if anyone says, "Doctor, we want you to do everything," I know what I would like to say. I would like to say, "Family, only you can do everything. Only you can talk of your love and give kisses before the skin is cold. Only you can talk of the future and of dreams to be fulfilled. Only you can talk of the past when life was resplendent because time seemed infinite.

"Family, only you can oppose the flow of time and enjoy one last day together. Only you can give peace and sustenance for the next journey. Family, only you can do everything. I am only a physician. I can do nothing at all."

Case Study Exercises

1. A study of physician-assisted suicide in the Netherlands made a startling find: First, nearly half of all doctor-assisted deaths in the Netherlands in 1995 (2,844 out of 6,368) were not voluntary. This contradicted the Dutch government researchers' claim that 948 doctor-assisted deaths lacked the patient's *explicit* consent. Furthermore, the report, noted in the *New England Journal of Medicine,* indicated a related issue arose in 1995 regarding pain-control methods: 80 percent of the 1,896 opiate-induced deaths (caused by high doses of opiate drugs to treat pain) occurred without the patients' *explicit* consent. The authors of the study concluded that there has been a "striking increase in the number of cases terminated without request." Karen Orloff Kaplan, executive director of the New York-based Choice in Dying (which takes no position on physician-assisted suicide) declared this to be a "warning light" that "raises important questions that we as an ethical and humane society cannot afford to ignore." "The Dutch experience tells us that we have to go very carefully." (See Terence Monmaney, "Study Finds Disturbing Trend in Assisted Deaths," *Los Angeles Times,* 4 June 1997.)
   a. Given these numbers, do you think legalizing physician assisted death in the U.S. will lead down a slippery slope whereby patients' lives are terminated by doctors overlooking consent requirements?
   b. Set out the key concerns and then make your case.
2. In spring 1997, a twelve-member panel asserted that:

   Many Americans suffered preventable pain and stress at the end of life and that this leads to talk of assisted suicide. Dr. Cassel, chair of geriatrics and adult development at Mount Sinai Medical Center, said that too many are dying without the benefit of skillful and compassionate care. The panel said that American medicine focuses upon high-tech cures, surgery, and aggressive treatment and not what happens when death is inevitable. Furthermore, studies show that a majority of dying patients experience severe, undertreated pain. "No one should view suicide as their best option because they lack effective and compassionate care as they die," Dr. Cassel said. Panel member, Robert Burt, said that "There is a tension between the need to control illegal drugs and the need for palliative care to control pain." He recommends that controls could be much less rigid than currently is the case. (See Warren E. Leary, "Many in U.S. Denied Dignified Death," *New York Times,* 5 June 1997.)

   Assuming Robert Burt is right, what steps do you think we could take to make dying less agonizing?
3. In a survey of 2,700 physicians, it was found that doctors increasingly favor helping terminally ill patients end their lives but have misgivings about being able to do the job right. Sixty percent supported legalizing physician-assisted death, but 51% said they didn't know which drugs to prescribe to ensure a patient would die comfortably. (See Terence Monmaney, "2 Surveys Find Doctors Back Physician-Assisted Suicide," *Los Angeles Times,* 1 February 1996.) Should doctors receive such information as part of their medical training?
4. Share your reflections on the following questions about honesty and decision making:
   a. Should a patient with a terminal illness be told the truth?
   b. Should seriously ill patients make the decisions about their care, including those about the use of life-support systems?
5. A University of Southern California study of 800 elderly patients found that immigrants from South Korea and Mexico were far less willing to let individuals make decisions about medical care than were either black or white Americans. For such immigrants, the role of the family loomed larger and that of the individual patient was much smaller than in main-

stream American society. (See Seth Mydans, "Should Dying Patients Be Told? Ethnic Pitfall is Found," *New York Times,* 13 September 1995.) In the study, blacks and whites were about twice as likely as Korean-Americans and about one-and-a-half times as likely as Mexican-Americans to say yes to questions 4a and 4b, above. Discuss the degree to which cultural or religious background should be factors in resolving these issues.

6. To what extent should cultural diversity and religious beliefs play a role in the development of guidelines for handling patients with terminal illnesses?

7. Assuming we legalize physician-assisted death, are there any compelling reasons to require that the requesting patient be *competent?* Given that the family of an incompetent patient may raise legitimate concerns, what sorts of guidelines might be developed to deal with this issue?

8. Discuss the ethical issues raised by neonatal euthanasia. What do you think is the most compassionate way for us to deal with parents facing a decision regarding a seriously ill infant with a dim prognosis for a meaningful life or one free of suffering?

9. Should physicians, in the absence of advance directives, be required to "err on the side of life"? Set out three reasons in support of your position. Can you conceive of any situation that would cause you to reassess your point of view?

10. If a patient cannot speak for him or herself and has left no advance directives, but the hospital knows the patient's religious affiliation, should doctors be allowed to turn to a representative of that religion (e.g., priest, rabbi, or minister) for guidance in decision making about the ending of the patient's life?

11. A British study reported in July 1996 said that 43% of patients diagnosed as being in a persistent vegetative state were later found to be alert and aware and could make sense of the spoken word. It was further reported that:

    The American Neurological Assn. claims a person in a vegetative state betrays no awareness of self or surroundings and does not respond to questions or physical stimuli, in contrast to a coma victim who rarely opens the eyes and doesn't appear to have a sleep-wake cycle. The study suggested that a significant number of the estimated 14,000 to 35,000 Americans said to be in a vegetative state may not be so profoundly incapacitated after all. Dr. Helena Chui, neurologist, asserted that, "Since consideration is often given in the United States to withholding treatment from persons in a persistent vegetative state, the possibility of misdiagnosis of this condition would be disconcerting." Ronald Cranford, a leading authority on the persistent vegetative state, suggested that the British findings may indicate these patients could be enduring pain (contrary to the current neurological assumption) and, therefore, some people are going to want more doctor-aided suicide. (See Terence Monmaney, "Many So-Called Vegetative Patients Aware, Study Finds," *Los Angeles Times,* 6 July 1996.)

    a. Do you agree with Cranford that the possibility that these patients have a vital consciousness trapped in an unresponsive body may add fuel to the movement for physician-assisted death?

    b. Share your ideas as to what ought to be done in such cases.

12. In a letter to the *New England Journal of Medicine* in May 1997, a story was told about a Dutch gynecologist who gave a lethal injection to a 3-day old girl with severe birth defects. The doctor was cleared of murder charges because the baby's parents had consented and he had followed the country's guidelines for assisted euthanasia. (See Gina Kolata, "Ethicists Struggle Against 'the Tyranny of the Anecdote'," *New York Times,* 24 June 1997.) When people talk about euthanasia, they tend to think of the elderly or the terminally ill who are suffering terrible agony. The infant with birth defects is not usually the image of the patient

who gets doctor-assisted death. Ought parents be allowed to decide to have active euthanasia for a child who is not terminally ill and not suffering pain?

13. What sort of ethical guidelines should there be to deal with any moral objections that doctors or nurses have to assisting in either active or passive euthanasia? Should they be able to refuse to participate in either directly or indirectly ending a life?

14. Since Oregon has legalized physician-assisted death, there was some worry that it would cause a flood of patients seeking help from doctors to kill themselves. However, in the first year under the assisted suicide law, only 15 deaths were reported and state officials found no evidence of abuse. (See Sam How Verhover, "Oregon Reporting 15 Deaths in Year Under Suicide Law," *New York Times,* 18 February 1999.) Oregon permits only assisted *suicide,* however — not lethal injections. Do you think Oregon should have permitted doctors to use lethal injections to assist a patient who wants to die? Set out the issues and concerns and share your thoughts on this issue.

15. After years of helping individuals die and surviving numerous legal hurdles and four trials, Jack Kevorkian was convicted of murder. He gave a lethal injection (which he videotaped) to Thomas Youk, suffering from Lou Gehrig's disease. The tape was broadcast on the TV show *60 Minutes* in November 1998. Since Kevorkian injected Youk himself, rather than assist the man in committing suicide, it was much easier for the prosecution to make its case. Some ethicists, however, see no moral distinction between active killing (as with a lethal injection) and letting die (as a DNR order). The question is: Is there a moral distinction between active killing (e.g., a lethal injection) and providing another person the means to kill him or herself (e.g., sleeping pills, carbon monoxide poisoning)?

16. Your neighbor comes over with the following dilemma: His cousin Ralph was hit by a train while trying to cut across the tracks coming home from work. Ralph is now on a respirator with multiple internal injuries. His prognosis is very grim. Ralph left no advance directives, but he was thought not to favor allowing people to linger when a medical situation seemed futile. The family wonders whether or not to remove the respirator and asks for some guidance.
    a. What is the strongest case that could be made for passive euthanasia?
    b. What is the strongest case that could be made for physician-assisted death?
    c. What are the key differences between your answers to (a) and (b)?
    d. What is the strongest argument for leaving Ralph on the respirator and not turning to either passive euthanasia or physician-assisted death?

17. Do you think there is a moral distinction between neonatal euthanasia and adult euthanasia? Share your reflections. To what degree is the competence of the adult a factor in assessing the moral permissibility of euthanasia for an adult patient?

18. It appears that the Dutch are likely to legalize euthanasia by the fall of 2000. According to *The New York Times,* "The new law, which almost everyone here expects will be passed in the fall, could allow help to die for people ranging from Alzheimer's disease sufferers to perhaps even terminally ill children as young as 12." (See Suzanne Daley, "The Dutch Seek to Legalize Long-Tolerated Euthanasia," *New York Times,* 20 June 2000.) Do you think North Americans should follow suit?

19. A great deal more discussion in bioethics is focused on the pros and cons of physician-assisted death than on hospice and the alleviation of pain and suffering. Set out the strongest case for turning to a hospice rather than to euthanasia. You might want to take into consideration the remarks of Peter Fish about the use of hospice care for his terminally ill mother:

Serious illness is a journey to a foreign country. You don't speak the language, the inhabitants are strangers, you cannot know how you will behave until you arrive. St. Thomas

Aquinas condemned suicide because it violates God's authority over life. I believed that. And one of my favorite writers, Flannery O'Connor—herself the victim of a slow death at a young age—wrote, "Sickness before death is a very appropriate thing and I think those who don't have it miss one of God's mercies." I believed that, too. Now I believe that there is suffering that is ennobling but also suffering that strips the humanity from a person, that is so unendurable you would be wise not to predict your reaction to it until you confront it.

But inner strength, too, is unpredictable. Often during the past few years of heated debate over assisted suicide, I have listened to people plead that they could not possibly endure the final illness of someone they love—or endure their own final illness. And I find myself thinking, Don't sell yourself short. Don't be so sure. It will be bad. But perhaps not as bad as your worst fears. I have reached an age where people I know—parents of friends, aging relatives—are receiving terminal diagnoses with some regularity. I find that once I hear the grim news, the second or third sentence out of my mouth is "You'll want to find a hospice program." For after I stopped by the side of the road and thought I couldn't go on, we went on. That could not have happened without hospice. (See Peter Fish, "A Harder Better Death," *Health,* Nov.–Dec 1997, vol. 11, no. 8.)

InfoTrac College Edition

1. David Lester, "Psychological Issues in Euthanasia, Suicide and Assisted Suicide"
2. Thomas W. Clark, "Thou Shalt Not Play God"
3. Peter J. Bernardi, "Is Death a Right? What Begins as a Right Can Soon Become an Obligation"
4. Yueh-Yang Chen, "Cross-Cultural Research on Euthanasia and Abortion"
5. Carol A. Wesley, "Social Work and End-of-Life Decisions: Self-Determination and the Common Good"
6. Ronald E. Cranford, "Withdrawing Artificial Feeding from Children with Brain Damage: Is not the Same as Assisted Suicide or Euthanasia"
7. Wesley J. Smith, "Eating His Words"
8. Nancy J. Osgood, "Assisted Suicide and Older People—A Deadly Combination: Ethical Problems in Permitting Assisted Suicide"
9. Hugh Gregory Gallagher, "'Slapping Up Spastics': The Persistence of Social Attitudes Toward People with Disabilities"
10. Courtney S. Campbell, "Give Me Liberty and Give Me Death: Assisted Suicide in Oregon"
11. John Deigh, "Physician-Assisted Suicide and Voluntary Euthanasia: Some Relevant Differences"
12. Adam Wolfson, "Killing Off the Dying?"
13. Peter Fish, "A Harder Better Death"
14. Frederique Zwart, "A Very Special Dying"
15. Nathan I. Cherny, "The Problem of Inadequately Relieved Suffering"
16. Carl Elliott, "Philosopher Assisted Suicide and Euthanasia"

Web Connections

For links to Death and Dying Web sites, articles, cases, and more exercises go to our Euthanasia page at www.philosophy.com/teays.purdy/euthanasia

Chapter 6

Abortion and Reproductive Freedom

REPRODUCTIVE ISSUES are among the most heated and controversial in bioethics. We need only look at the range of opinions on minors seeking abortion and the political maneuvering on legislation regarding late-term abortions to realize just how many people hold strong sentiments in this area. The ethical issues surrounding contraception, abortion, and maternal-fetal conflicts are wide-ranging and have touched the lives of a vast number of women and men.

There is a broad range of concerns here, such as the moral status of the fetus, disagreements about who should control access to reproductive services, and the proper resolution of conflicts of interest (real or apparent) between the pregnant woman and fetus. The readings in this chapter address some of the most pressing underlying questions:

- Is there a right to control reproduction?

- Who can exercise this right?

- What moral issues are raised by controlling reproduction?

- What rights, if any, do fetuses have?

- How can we resolve conflicts between maternal and fetal rights?

Abortion is the focus of powerful disagreement in the United States and many other countries. The 1973 Supreme Court *Roe v. Wade* ruling that laws prohibiting abortion in the first trimester of pregnancy are unconstitutional intensified the struggle about access to abortion. Among its current manifestations are the political fights over availability of the abortifacient drug RU–486, and violence against abortion clinics and physicians who do abortions. Moreover, the decision by the Supreme Court not to ban late-term ("partial-birth") abortions ensures that the abortion debate is far from dead.

However, many of the questions raised by abortion are also relevant to the practice of contraception. Among them are whether women's right to self-determination includes a right to control their bodies, and if not, who does (men, the church, the state?). Also relevant are the rights of humans, possible persons, potential persons, and future persons.

It has been argued that anything possessing the human genetic code, such as a newly fertilized egg, is human, and that being human is the ground for various rights, including the right to life. Some reject this position in favor of the view that it is not the human genetic code that is morally relevant, but rather certain characteristics — like self-consciousness — possessed by competent, adult humans. Thus nonhuman organisms, such as chimpanzees, may well possess rights usually attributed only to genetic humans. Also, an individual may have a human genetic code without necessarily possessing full human rights.

Many philosophers use the word "person" as a synonym for organisms that have a right to life, even though they may have very different views about what makes someone a person. Possible persons are individuals who do not now exist, but who might exist at some time in the future. Potential persons are individuals who exist but who are not yet persons. Future persons may or may not now exist, but will exist someday. Possible persons are not yet conceived; potential persons are conceived but do not yet have the status of persons. Various views about the status and rights of fetuses are embodied in judgments about human beings, potential persons, and may be embodied in judgments about future persons (e.g., minors, prisoners, the comatose, the mentally retarded).

We believe that the issue of contraception is interesting in its own right and examining it is useful for analyzing concerns about abortion. It may be useful to attempt to resolve those issues before dealing with questions about the moral status of the fetus, which weighs so heavily on the abortion decision. Furthermore, there is a gray area between contraception and abortion that cries out for clarification. For example, we might ask whether the IUD, which prevents the fertilized egg from implanting itself in the uterus, is a contraceptive or an abortifacient, and whether the use of RU–486, or the "morning after pill," creates the same sort of moral problems as abortion.

CONTRACEPTION

So much controversy is generated by abortion and more recent, related topics like "wrongful birth" and "fetal abuse" that contraception is rarely considered a significant bioethical issue. Nevertheless, contraception creates moral problems for those, like Catholics, whose religion prohibits or otherwise regulates it. In the early 1980s, for example, there were powerful political pressures to limit federal funding of family planning agencies, both nationally and internationally, to "natural birth control."

With rising infertility, it is easy to imagine a scenario in which this issue could rise to the political forefront again, and contraception be made illegal. For instance, picture some variation on Canadian author Margaret Atwood's futuristic novel *The Hand-maid's Tale* (after a violent takeover of the U.S. Congress a fascist society is set up in which young, fertile women are forced to be reproductive slaves—"handmaids"—for the ruling class). Moreover, we must not forget that the most effective means of birth control (the Pill, sterilization) are still medically controlled and that teenagers may have limited access to birth control measures.

Contraceptive devices could be—and were—banned in many parts of the United States until quite recently. It was just thirty-five years ago, in *Griswold v. Connecticut* (1965), that the Supreme Court ruled that it was unconstitutional to outlaw the use of contraceptives by married couples. The Connecticut law had prohibited the use of contraceptives, providing them for others, and even counseling about contraception. And it was not until 1972 that the Court (in *Eisenstadt v. Baird*) prevented states from criminalizing the distribution of contraceptives to unmarried persons.

Restricted access to contraception is rooted in both religious values and eugenic concerns. Although these are dubious grounds for legal prohibitions, especially in a pluralistic society like the United States, laws are at least as much about power as about justice. Furthermore, judges tend to be reluctant to deviate too far from the dominant religious values of the country, despite the constitutional wall between church and state.

We might ask who should take responsibility for contraception when pregnancy is not desired. The most effective and convenient methods now mostly require action on the part of the female. Boys and men who do not wish to become fathers may take the lead in using birth control, but many assume, without any real discussion, that the woman is "taking care of it." Girls and women, constricted by social norms that disapprove of females preparing for sex, may not protect themselves. The outcome—unintended pregnancy—is in the interest of neither party.

Education is clearly the first step in avoiding undesired outcomes. People of both sexes need to see that when they engage in sexual behavior they must do it responsibly, recognizing what they want out of it, taking steps to avoid what they don't want, and taking responsibility for the mishaps when they occur. In particular, we must eradicate the double-bind that says a "good" woman does not prepare for sexual encounters even though she is responsible for unwanted outcomes.

These social changes are doubly important now that contraception must also protect against life-threatening sexually transmitted diseases (STDs) like AIDS and syphilis. Developing a broader array of safe, effective contraceptives that can be used by both sexes would also help sexually active persons stay healthy and avoid unwanted pregnancies. Women's groups, however, are not uniformly positioned on the issue of birth control.

Unfortunately the birth control movement has a checkered history, with the politics of race and class leaving its effect. Some leaders have focused primarily on the needs and desires of white, middle-class women, ignoring those of other groups like the poor, ethnic minorities, or the disabled. Worse still, some have been downright racist; consequently blacks and Latinas have justifiably been skeptical of a movement that could so easily turn birth control options into attempts to limit their numbers. For instance, we ought not forget the obstetrics experiments conducted on black slave women and the birth control experiments conducted on Latinas, where one group was given a placebo, resulting in no birth control and, thus, many unwanted births.

The recent introduction of long-acting contraceptives like Norplant and Depoprovera that cannot be controlled by the user without medical cooperation seems to lend additional substance to such worries. Norplant is surgically inserted under the skin and remains there, preventing pregnancy for five years or until it is surgically removed. Like all devices that influence women's hormonal function, it raises questions about "side-effects," as well as safety. Depoprovera, another long-term contraceptive, has already been required in places like Thailand as a term of employment. The specter of authoritarian population control and race genocide is a real concern.

Another major concern is the ease with which such drugs can be used on women without clear-cut and informed consent. Indeed, some judges have offered Norplant to women convicted of certain crimes, like child abuse, as an alternative to jail. This we saw in the Darlene Johnson case, in which a Fresno, California, judge instructed Johnson to choose between Norplant and jail after she was convicted of child abuse and neglect. There is considerable debate, even among those sensitive to women's welfare, as to whether this option is harmful or beneficial and whether women like Johnson are thereby deprived of their civil liberties and the right to self-determination.

In evaluating this matter it is important to consider whether limits on reproductive rights have a disproportionate impact on minority women. For example, critics of the Johnson case were not surprised by the fact that Johnson is black. Complicating the situation here is the truly debilitating social reality many such women (and girls) face. Having children at an early age may be one of the few sources of gratification to which they have access and one of the ways they exercise their reproductive freedom. Clearly, the idea of using reproductive controls as punishment needs to be carefully examined.

ABORTION

Whether an induced abortion (as opposed to a miscarriage, where the pregnant woman has no control) is morally permissible or not is one of the most pressing and contested moral questions of our day. Key moral questions pertaining to it and addressed in the readings are:

- Do embryos and fetuses have rights?

- Are fetuses persons?

- Is it wrong to kill fetuses?

- What other features of the situation are morally relevant?

Historical attitudes toward abortion are much more lenient than we might expect, given the present contentiousness of the issue. In ancient Greece and Rome, for example, abortion was widely performed and easily obtainable. In part because of this, Hippocrates (in the Hippocratic Oath) sought more stringent ethical guidelines to discourage the practice. English common law generally permitted abortion before "quickening," when the pregnant woman could feel the fetus move. Even where the law judged such abortions as misdemeanors, its main concerns were the man's perceived rights over his offspring, or maternal health.

Many people will be surprised to learn that abortion was widely accepted in the United States as well. Indeed, the history of abortion legislation should be eye-opening: Abortion was not regulated until the early to mid-nineteenth century, and there is reason to believe that alleged harm to the fetus was not at the center of the debate. Although this history does not determine whether abortion is immoral or not (moral argumentation is required), setting the question in historical context will help us understand it.

Understanding the contemporary debate also requires of us some familiarity with the 1973 landmark Supreme Court case, *Roe v. Wade. Roe v. Wade* set the stage for over-turning most state laws restricting access to abortion. Opponents of abortion, appalled by the decision, have since fought to reverse its consequences. The courts and Congress continue to be a central battleground. Republican presidents Reagan and Bush attempted to make sure that new judicial appointees, including Supreme Court appointees, opposed abortion. Since 1980, access to abortion services has been limited by a variety of cases, such as *Webster v. Reproductive Health Services* and *Casey v. Planned Parenthood,* which have modified but not reversed *Roe v. Wade.*

Access to abortion services has also been limited by legislation, such as the Hyde Amendment that now prevents federal tax dollars from funding abortions. Although the principle that citizens should not have to pay for federal activities of which they disapprove has some appeal, it does not enjoy widespread support.

Women's access to abortion services is also limited by the inequitable distribution of medical personnel between urban and rural areas. This problem is exacerbated by the failure of medical training programs to ensure that all physicians in the relevant specialties are trained to do abortions. Finally, access to abortion services has been limited by terrorist acts against clinics that provide abortions, including the murder of physicians who do abortions. A recent example of this was the Paul Hill case. The Supreme Court has not eliminated the possibility of potential volatile confrontations in front of abortion clinics. For instance the 1997 decision that gave protection to "in your face" anti-abortion protests as constitutionally protected free speech means that we will continue to see at least verbal conflicts in front of the clinics.

Rust v. Sullivan held that family planning programs receiving federal monies were banned from mentioning that abortion is available, recommending that a woman consider abortion, or helping her find abortion services. This so-called "gag rule" was dropped when President Clinton was elected in 1992.

Some people consider abortion morally unacceptable. One justification of this position is that fetuses should not be killed because of their moral status as persons. Thus the moral status of the fetus is taken to be the central and overriding issue posed by the practice of abortion. This position is primarily based in theology, as is the Catholic prohibition of abortions (other than those intended to relieve ectopic pregnancies or ovarian cancers). Yet the Catholic Church has not always prohibited abortion.

St. Thomas Aquinas, a leading Catholic moral philosopher, believed, like St. Augustine, that abortion was acceptable until ensoulment (when the soul was said to enter the body). Ensoulment was thought to occur at 40 days for males and 80 days for females. Even now, a few abortions are considered acceptable, under the doctrine of double effect. The issue turns on whether the intention is evil, or whether evil (such as the death of the fetus) must intend to bring about good. Thus, an abortion intended to kill the fetus is wrong, since intentional killing is morally prohibited. However, if the death of the fetus is not intended, a medical procedure necessary to save a woman's life, as with an ectopic pregnancy, is morally tolerated.

Common reasons for believing that a fetus should not be killed are that it is alive, that it is a distinct individual, that it looks human, that it is human, or that it is a person. Some believe that it is wrong to kill fetuses because they potentially have a right to life. Many find the "personhood" objection to such positions appealing. This view holds that all and only persons have a right to life. Fetuses aren't persons because they lack one or more crucial characteristics and, consequently, have no right to life. This view is set out by Mary Anne Warren, who argues that persons must have at least some of these characteristics: namely, consciousness or the ability to feel pain, self-aware-ness, self-motivated activity, reasoning, and the ability to communicate. She argues that fetuses have none of these. However, this position implies that abortion is accept-able any time before birth, and also that infants have no right to life for some time after birth. Since many who believe abortion to be morally permissible judge infanticide to be unacceptable, it is helpful to consider whether there are morally relevant differences between the two.

The status of the fetus continues to be hotly debated, both in the public arena and in an increasingly subtle and sophisticated philosophical literature. Some despair of finding common ground here, so they focus on other aspects of the question. Others believe that the status of the fetus fails, in any case, to determine whether abortion is morally wrong.

Given the emotional context of the abortion debate, and competing arguments on all sides, it is hard to picture a social consensus on abortion in the United States any time soon. However, there are defensible moral arguments that abortion is permissible and the procedure is constitutionally protected. In light of this, we need to consider whether some people are unjustifiably prevented from access to it. For example, are the poor deprived of their right to abortion by lack of Medicaid funding? Do minors have a right to abortion that is violated by laws mandating parental notification or consent? Are women in general deprived of the right to control their bodies by male violence? Anyone concerned about social justice must examine these important questions.

MATERNAL-FETAL CONFLICTS

The issue of control arises in the context of pregnancy in other ways. On the one hand, the decision whether to continue a pregnancy weighs upon women who do not enjoy the economic and social security to have children. On the other hand, pregnant women increasingly face threats to their bodily autonomy in the name of fetal welfare. Distressed fetuses sometimes are at risk of serious harm from vaginal delivery. Women who refuse cesarean sections risk that the physician will seek a court order to operate anyway.

An infamous example of this kind of case was Angela Carder, a twenty-four week pregnant woman with leukemia. She was ordered by the court to undergo a cesarean (against her own wishes and those of her husband and her parents). Both Carder and the fetus died shortly after the surgery. Although the hospital subsequently developed guidelines that would prevent such cases, forced caesarians still take place elsewhere. The question is whether they are justifiable. It has been argued that a woman abdicates her right to self-determination by continuing her pregnancy, whereas others believe that it is an inalienable right. Bonnie Steinbock, writing on compulsory medical treatment of pregnant women, considers whether or not cases like *McFall vs. Shimp*—in which it was determined that there is no obligation of family members to donate organs to relatives—ought to be applied to pregnant women in relation to the needs of their fetuses.

As fetal medicine develops new and potentially beneficial treatments that promise to prevent harm and save lives, the pressures on women to consent to prebirth treatments will grow. More worrisome still, women's lifestyle choices, such as smoking, drinking alcohol, or using illicit drugs, can seriously harm fetuses. At issue here is whether fetal welfare is more important than women's autonomy. Many people believe that fetal welfare should have priority, and there have already been convictions of drug-abusing pregnant women as a result of the novel argument that the umbilical cord is a drug-delivery system.

Reaching a consensus about these situations will be difficult, as they embody widely differing views of women's nature and value. Those who see women primarily as nurturers will tend to favor the fetus in the event of a conflict. Feminists who argue that women should be equal partners in human endeavors oppose discounting of women's welfare and argue that her rights should normally prevail over any presumed fetal rights.

Furthermore, some conflicts between woman and fetus are only apparent, since the two have many interests in common. Many of these common interests could be more humanely and efficiently met by a variety of social supports, like accessible prenatal care, feeding programs, or drug treatment programs. These would be preferable to coercion or punishment for allegedly irresponsible behavior on the part of pregnant women. These claims are plausible. They also raise basic questions about the rationality of some of our fundamental social arrangements. However, in cases in which the interests of the pregnant woman and the fetus may conflict, we must make a decision about how to assess the competing interests and determine whose rights prevail.

The readings in this chapter are divided into two sections: the first focuses on contraception and abortion, and the second focuses on maternal-fetal conflicts. The first section contains the following articles:

1. Angela Davis writes on racism, birth control, and reproductive rights; arguing that the history of the birth control movement reveals both classism and racism. She discusses failures on the part of abortion-rights activists to seriously appraise the attitudes (and fears) of African Americans.

2. Bonnie Steinbock looks at coercion and long-term contraceptives such as Norplant and the potential for abuse.

3. Bob Herbert reports on antiabortion terrorists who target abortion doctors, discussing the personal impact of death threats.

4. Rebecca S. Dresser examines the lessening access to abortion in the United States and the decrease in the number of doctors willing to perform abortion, as well as the conflict between doctors' First Amendment rights to refuse to do abortions and women's reproductive health choices and needs.

5. In his opposition to abortion, save in self-defense, John T. Noonan, Jr. sets out an argument based on the notion of what it means to be a human being. Noonan uses a genetics-based rights approach to make his case.

6. Mary Anne Warren, taking the opposite side from Noonan, offers a different perspective on abortion rights by seeing birth, not conception, as the morally defining moment in assigning rights.

7. Laura Purdy uses the analogies of forced labor and war to examine societal attitudes (and opposition) to abortion, arguing that the logical inconsistencies are sufficient to require us to reconsider our assessment of abortion rights.

8. Allison Beth Hubbard discusses minors' abortion rights and the erosion of those rights. She draws from court decisions to make her case.

In the second section, we look at maternal-fetal conflicts.

1. Robert Blank discusses court decisions and social policies regarding maternal-fetal conflicts, offering suggestions for a dialogue on the issue.

2. Nancy K. Rhoden discusses court-ordered caesarians, arguing that competent women should have the right to refuse such caesarians, even at the risk of tragic consequences to the fetus.

3. Bonnie Steinbock examines the moral issues surrounding compulsory treatment of pregnant women and the question of applying such cases as *McFall v. Shimp* to pregnant women and their fetuses.

4. Margaret E. Goldberg examines the needs of substance-abusing women and offers suggestions regarding treatment and services.

Contraception and Abortion

Racism, Birth Control, and Reproductive Rights[1]

ANGELA DAVIS

BIRTH CONTROL—individual choice, safe contraceptive methods, as well as abortions when necessary—is a fundamental prerequisite for the emancipation of women. Since the right of birth control is obviously advantageous to women of all classes and races, it would appear that even vastly dissimilar women's groups would have attempted to unite around this issue. In reality, however, the birth control movement has seldom succeeded in uniting women of different social backgrounds, and rarely have the movement's leaders popularized the genuine concerns of working-class women. Moreover, arguments advanced by birth control advocates have sometimes been based on blatantly racist premises. The progressive potential of birth control remains indisputable. But in actuality, the historical record of this movement leaves much to be desired in the realm of challenges to racism and class exploitation.

ANGELA DAVIS, the author of numerous works, who has taught philosophy at UCLA and UC Santa Cruz, is an activist and speaker on prisoners' rights.

The most important victory of the contemporary birth control movement was won during the early 1970s when abortions were at last declared legal. Having emerged during the infancy of the new women's liberation movement, the struggle to legalize abortions incorporated all the enthusiasm and the militancy of the young movement. By January 1973, the abortion rights campaign had reached a triumphant culmination. In *Roe v. Wade* (410 U.S.) and *Doe v. Bolton* (410 U.S.), the U.S. Supreme Court ruled that a woman's right to personal privacy implied her right to decide whether or not to have an abortion.

The ranks of the abortion rights campaign did not include substantial numbers of women of color. Given the racial composition of the larger women's liberation movement, this was not at all surprising. When questions were raised about the absence of racially oppressed women in both the larger movement and in the abortion rights campaign, two explanations were commonly proposed in the discussions and literature of the period: women of color were overburdened by their people's fight against racism, and/or they had not yet become conscious of the centrality of sexism. But the real meaning of the almost lily-white complexion of the abortion rights campaign was not to be found in ostensibly myopic or underdeveloped consciousness among women of color. The truth lay buried in the ideological underpinnings of the birth control movement itself.

The failure of the abortion rights campaign to conduct a historical self-evaluation led to a dangerously superficial appraisal of Black people's suspicious attitudes toward birth control in general. Granted, when some Black people unhesitatingly equated birth control with genocide, it did appear to be an exaggerated — even paranoiac — reaction. Yet white abortion rights activists missed a profound message, for underlying these cries of genocide were important clues about the history of the birth control movement. This movement, for example, had been known to advocate involuntary sterilization — a racist form of mass "birth control." If ever women would enjoy the right to plan their pregnancies, legal and easily accessible birth control measures and abortions would have to be complemented by an end to sterilization abuse.

As for the abortion rights campaign itself, how could women of color fail to grasp its urgency? They were far more familiar than their white sisters with the murderously clumsy scalpels of inept abortionists seeking profit in illegality. In New York, for instance, during the several years preceding the decriminalization of abortions in that state, some 80 percent of the deaths caused by illegal abortions involved Black and Puerto Rican women.[2] Immediately afterward, women of color received close to half of all the legal abortions. If the abortion rights campaign of the early 1970s needed to be reminded that women of color wanted desperately to escape the back-room quack abortionists, they should also have realized that these same women were not about to express pro-abortion sentiments. They were in favor of *abortion rights,*

which did not mean that they were proponents of abortion. When Black and Latina women resort to abortions in such large numbers, the stories they tell are not so much about the desire to be free of their pregnancy, but rather about the miserable social conditions which dissuade them from bringing new lives into the world.

Black women have been aborting themselves since the earliest days of slavery. Many slave women refused to bring children into a world of interminable forced labor, where chains and floggings and sexual abuse for women were the everyday conditions of life. A doctor practicing in Georgia around the middle of the last century noticed that abortions and miscarriages were far more common among his slave patients than among the white women he treated. . . .

During the early abortion rights campaign, it was too frequently assumed that legal abortions provided a viable alternative to the myriad problems posed by poverty. As if having fewer children could create more jobs, higher wages, better schools, etc. This assumption reflected the tendency to blur the distinction between *abortion rights* and the general advocacy of *abortions.* The campaign often failed to provide a voice for women who wanted the *right* to legal abortions while deploring the social conditions that prohibited them from bearing more children.

The renewed offensive against abortion rights that erupted during the latter half of the 1970s has made it absolutely necessary to focus more sharply on the needs of poor and racially oppressed women. By 1977, the passage of the Hyde Amendment in Congress had mandated the withdrawal of federal funding for abortions, causing many state legislatures to follow suit. Black, Puerto Rican, Chicana, and Native American Indian women, together with their impoverished white sisters, were thus effectively divested of the right to legal abortions. Since surgical sterilizations, funded by the Department of Health, Education and Welfare [now the Department of Health and Human Services], remained free on demand, more and more poor women have been forced to opt for permanent infertility. What is urgently required is a broad campaign to defend the reproductive rights of all women—and especially those women whose economic circumstances often compel them to relinquish the right to reproduction itself. . . .

Toward the end of the 19th century the white birth rate in the United States suffered a significant decline. Since no contraceptive innovations had been publicly introduced, the drop in the birth rate implied that women were substantially curtailing their sexual activity. By 1890, the typical native-born white woman was bearing no more than four children.[3] Since U.S. society was becoming increasingly urban, this new birth pattern should not have been a surprise. While farm life demanded large families, they became dysfunctional within the context of city life. Yet this phenomenon was publicly interpreted in a racist and anti-working-class fashion by the ideologues of rising monopoly capitalism. Since native-born white women were bearing fewer children, the specter of "race suicide" was raised in official circles.

In 1905, President Theodore Roosevelt concluded his Lincoln Day Dinner speech with the proclamation that "race purity must be maintained."[4] By 1906, he blatantly equated the falling birth rate among native-born whites with the impending threat of "race suicide." In his State of the Union message that year, Roosevelt admonished the well-born white women who engaged in "willful sterility—the one sin for which the penalty is national death, race suicide."[5] These comments were made during a period of accelerating racist ideology and of great waves of race riots and lynchings on the domestic scene. . . .

The acceptance of the race-suicide thesis, to a greater or lesser extent, by women such as Julia Ward Howe and Ida Husted Harper reflected the suffrage movement's capitulation to the racist posture of Southern women. If the suffragists acquiesced to arguments invoking the extension of the ballot to women as the saving grace of white supremacy, then birth control advocates either acquiesced to or supported the new arguments invoking birth control as a means of preventing the proliferation of the "lower classes" and as an antidote to race suicide. Race suicide could be prevented by the introduction of birth control among Black people, immigrants, and the poor in general. In this way, the prosperous whites of solid Yankee stock could maintain their superior numbers within the population. Thus class bias and racism crept into the birth control movement when it was still in its infancy. More and more, it was assumed within birth control circles that poor women, Black and immigrant alike, had a "moral obligation to restrict the size of their families."[6] What was demanded as a "right" for the privileged came to be interpreted as a "duty" for the poor. . . .

NOTES

1. This article is excerpted from Angela Y. Davis, *Women, Race, & Class,* Chapter 12, (New York: Random House, 1981). Reprinted by permission.

2. Edwin M. Gold *et al.,* "Therapeutic Abortions in New York City: A Twenty-Year Review," *American Journal of Public Health,* Vol. LV (July, 1965), pp. 964–972. Quoted in Lucinda Cisler, "Unfinished Business: Birth Control and Women's Liberation," in Robin Morgan, ed., *Sisterhood Is Powerful: An Anthology of Writings From the Women's Liberation Movement* (New York: Vintage Books, 1970), p. 261. Also quoted in Robert Staples, *The Black Woman in America* Chicago: Nelson Hall, 1974), p. 146.

3. Mary P. Ryan, *Womanhood in America from Colonial Times to the Present* (New York: Franklin Watts, Inc., 1975), p. 162.

4. Melvin Steinfeld, *Our Racist Presidents* (San Ramon, California: Consensus Publishers, 1972), p. 212.

5. Bonnie Mass, Population Target: *The Political Economy of Population Control in Latin America* (Toronto, Canada: Women's Education Press, 1977), p. 20.

6. Linda Gordon, *Woman's Body, Woman's Right: A Social History of Birth Control in America* (New York: Penguin Books, 1976), p. 15–18.

Coercion and Long-Term Contraceptives

BONNIE STEINBOCK

PRECISELY THOSE FEATURES of long-acting contraceptives that make them nearly ideal — their effectiveness and the fact that they work without having to think about them — also open the potential for their coercive use. As an article in *The New York Times* noted in regard to Norplant®:

> The same qualities that make Norplant a boon to women may be a two-edged sword: some public health groups and women's advocates worry that the contraceptive could easily become an instrument of social control, forced on poor women and others whose fertility is seen as more of a threat to society than a blessing.[1]

Yet, it is often far from clear whether a given policy or program is coercive because the concept is complex, controversial, and often difficult to apply. For example, should we understand coercion narrowly, as involving only physical threats or force? Or can the offering of benefits and incentives to get people to do things they otherwise would not do be coercive? Intuitions differ as to whether a proposal *expands* or *constricts* a person's options, and so enhances or limits its freedom. Moreover, the essentially normative nature of claims of coercion entails that judgments about whether a policy is coercive embody substantive moral arguments, about which

BONNIE STEINBOCK is Professor and Chair in the Department of Philosophy at the State University of New York, Albany, with joint appointments in Public Policy and Public Health.

reasonable people can disagree. Thus the concept calls for further exploration.

OFFERS, THREATS, AND INCENTIVES

Coercion plays an important role in morality and the law because it typically acts as a *disclaimer of responsibility* in that it deprives people of free choice and thus makes what they do, to some extent, nonvoluntary.

In the paradigmatic coercion situation, A says to B, brandishing a pistol, "Your money or your life." In what sense is B not acting according to his own free will? When B gives A his money, he does so deliberately and intentionally. He does what he most wants to do, given the situation. The coercion in this example is not the absence of volition, but rather *constrained volition*. Although intentional and deliberate, B's action is not done freely or autonomously.

The mere existence of external pressure or influence does not establish coercion. The influence or pressure exerted must be of a kind and amount that diminishes free choice. The central question, then, for understanding the concept of coercion is, *How much, and what kind of, influence or pressure deprives actions and decisions of their autonomous character?*

While the highwayman example is a clear case of coercion, we need a general theory of coercion to help us decide more controversial cases. Alan Wertheimer proposes two independent tests for

The Hastings Center Report 25, 1(1995) (Supplement): S19–S22. *Reprinted by permission of Bonnie Steinbock and The Hastings Center. Copyright 1995, The Hastings Center.*

coercion or duress, each of which is necessary and which are together jointly sufficient:[2]

1. The choice prong. A's proposal is coercive only if B has *no reasonable alternative but to succumb* to A's proposal.

2. The proposal prong. A's proposal is coercive only if it is *wrongful*. In general, if A has a right to do what he proposes, then his proposal is not wrongful (although it may be morally objectionable on other grounds).

Both offers and threats are proposals that provide an external influence or impetus to action. Yet threats coerce, whereas offers generally do not. How can threats be distinguished from offers? The intuitive answer is that threats limit freedom, whereas offers enhance it; that one acts involuntarily in response to a threat, whereas one voluntarily accepts an offer, that the recipient of a threat is not free to decline, whereas the recipient of an offer is. Wertheimer characterizes the distinction between threats and offers this way: A threatens B by proposing to make B worse off relative to some baseline. A makes an offer when, if B does not accept A's proposal, B will be no worse off than in the relevant baseline position.

However, sometimes it seems that A's proposal can make B better off than he would have been, relative to his baseline situation, and still be coercive. Consider this example from Robert Nozick:

The Slave Case. A beats B, his slave, each morning, for reasons having nothing to do with B's behavior. A proposes not to beat B the next morning, if B will do X, which is distasteful to him.

Assume that B would rather do X than get beaten. If we think of B's baseline as being set by what *normally happens* (call this the "statistical test"), A is making an offer (noncoercive). B expects to be beaten each morning, and relative to that expectation, A is proposing to make B better off. However, we can also think of the baseline as being set by what is *morally required* (call this the "moral test"). Under the moral test, A is making a threat (coercive). For A is morally required not to beat B, indeed, not to own slaves at all, and relative to that baseline, A is proposing to make B worse off. In addition to the statistical and moral tests, Wertheimer says there is also a "phenomenological test": how it seems to B. A's proposal may *feel like* a threat to B. Consider the following example:

> Each week, A calls B and asks her for a date. They have grown fond of each other, but they have not had sexual intercourse. After three months, A tells B that unless she has sexual intercourse with him, he will stop dating her.

Wertheimer comments that under the statistical and phenomenological tests, B may or may not regard A's proposal as a threat. "That would depend upon the history of their relationship and B's expectations."[3] Applying the moral test is complicated, but Wertheimer thinks that it is clear that B has no right that A continue to date her, and on B's preferred terms. Relative to that moral baseline, A's proposal is an offer.

It is by no means clear that Wertheimer has applied the moral test correctly. One might equally argue that A is not entitled to expect sexual intercourse from B, and is wrong to insist on sex as a condition of the relationship continuing. Relative to that moral baseline, A's proposal is a threat. The correct application of the moral test would depend on factual details not given, such as the age of the parties, their views on the morality of extramarital sexual intercourse, and so forth.

Wertheimer maintains that it is because there are these different tests, all of which can be used to characterize A's proposal as an offer or a threat, that intuitions about coerciveness of proposals often conflict. What looks like an offer may really be a threat. It depends on what test is used — and, I would add, how the test is applied — to set the baseline. Moreover, Wertheimer doesn't think there's any way to decide which is *the* correct test to determine the baseline. This often makes it difficult to say, with any certitude, that a proposal is coercive (and so objectionable).

Some philosophers argue that offers, as well as threats, can be "coercive." Consider the following intriguing example:

> *The Lecherous Millionaire.* B's child will die without expensive surgery, which her insurance doesn't cover, and for which the state will not pay. A, a millionaire, offers to pay for the surgery if B will agree to become his mistress.

Joel Feinberg argues that the Lecherous Millionaire's proposal is a "coercive offer" because it manipulates B's options in such a way that B has no choice but to comply, or else suffer an unacceptable alternative. Wertheimer responds that A also "manipulates" B's options when he offers him a job at three times his present salary. This may well be "an offer he cannot refuse," yet surely such an offer is not coercive. Moreover, what if it was the child's mother who proposed to the millionaire, knowing of his lecherous propensities, that she become his mistress if he will pay for the surgery? Surely that wouldn't be a coercive offer, Wertheimer says, so why is it coercive when A makes the offer to B? A's proposal may be "unseemly," according to Wertheimer, but it is not coercive, because it expands rather than reduces B's options.

Can an offer which expands one's options nevertheless be coercive? Consider the proposal made in the fairy tale, *Rumpelstiltskin*. According to the story, the miller's daughter will be put to death if she doesn't spin a roomful of straw into gold. Twice Rumpelstiltskin saves her by spinning the straw into gold in return for trinkets she gives him. The third time, however, the miller's daughter has nothing left to give him. Rumpelstiltskin then offers to spin the straw into gold in return for her firstborn child. The girl reluctantly accepts.

Has the miller's daughter been coerced? Feinberg would say yes. The decision to give up her child is not one she makes freely or willingly or voluntarily. She makes it because otherwise she will be killed. Admittedly, the miller's daughter prefers relinquishing her child to being put to death,[4] but the fact that she prefers one alternative to the other doesn't prevent the offer from being coercive. The robbery victim also prefers giving up his money to being killed. What makes both of these cases of coercion is that the choosers reasonably see themselves as having no choice.

Is there a way to reconcile the persuasive intuition that there can be "coercive offers" with Wertheimer's analysis of coercion? One possibility is to reconsider the moral baseline. If we think of the baseline as being set by what is morally required, as opposed to simply what normally happens, whether Rumpelstiltskin is making an offer or a threat will depend on whether Rumpelstiltskin has an obligation to spin the straw into gold for the miller's daughter. It might seem that he has no such obligation. Individuals are not generally obligated to do work for others, especially without compensation. However, morality requires that we help others when they will die otherwise, and when giving the help is not terribly onerous. We might not want such moral obligations to be made into law, but it is certainly plausible that there are such obligations. On this basis, it could be argued that Rumpelstiltskin ought to help the miller's daughter, even though she has nothing left to give him, because she needs his help so desperately, and helping her isn't terribly burdensome to him. Relative to that moral baseline, he is proposing to make her worse off. His proposal is therefore a threat, and by definition coercive.

However, this move will not help us with the Lecherous Millionaire. His offer can be seen as a threat only if we maintain that the millionaire has a moral obligation to pay for the child's expensive surgery. It does not seem plausible to maintain that a person—even a very wealthy person—is morally required to lay out large sums of money to meet the medical expenses of strangers. What's objectionable about the millionaire's behavior is not that he fails to help someone he could have helped; rather, it is that he exploits the woman's desperate situation in a particularly nasty way. That his offer is exploitive is unquestionable. The question is whether such exploitation should be regarded as coercive (because under the circumstances, the child's mother has "no choice") or whether it should be regarded as noncoercive (because the millionaire does not create, but merely takes advantage of, the woman's plight). In my opinion, this is an example of a difference that does not make a moral difference, since—as the examples show—an exploitive (but not coercive) offer can be as morally reprehensible as a coercive one.

Incentives, like threats, are ways of trying to get people to do things. Unlike threats, incentives are typically welcome offers that seem morally unobjectionable. Yet sometimes inducements and incentives are alleged to be coercive. For example, A offers B, who is desperately poor, a large sum of money for his kidney. Why is this thought to be coercive? It isn't just that B is being offered a lot of money; generous offers are not coercive. Perhaps the objection is that B's impoverished situation may make him unable fully to weigh the costs and benefits of the proposal. He may be inclined to weigh too heavily the short-term benefits of having the money, versus the long-term risks of not having an extra kidney. Offering a poor person money for a body part exploits or takes advantage of his poverty, but it is not clear that it forces or coerces him.

Incentives to do things that people ordinarily would not consider doing appear to be in the same category as exploitive offers. Whether they are coercive is unclear. However, even if they are not coercive, they may be morally impermissible. Only a detailed substantive analysis can determine this. We have to ask other questions, such as, Can persons in such conditions make intelligent judgments about their interests? Does society have an obligation to provide them with better alternatives? If society has not provided them with better alternatives, should such persons be allowed to improve their situations anyway?

FINANCIAL INCENTIVES FOR USING BIRTH CONTROL

After Norplant was approved in December 1990, states moved rapidly to add it to their Medicaid programs. In 1991, a new kind of assistance program appeared: offering a cash bonus to women on public assistance if they use birth control (usually Norplant). In Kansas, for example, a bill was introduced that would have provided any woman on public assistance with a one-time grant of $500 for getting Norplant implanted, as well as $50 a year for each year she kept it in. Representative David Duke introduced a bill in 1991 that would have given Louisiana women on public assistance $100 a year if they used Norplant. (The final version of the bill simply provided that Norplant would be given free of charge to women on public assistance.) And in Mississippi, a bill introduced in 1992 would have required women with four or more biological children to have Norplant implanted in order to be eligible to receive state assistance.

Are Norplant bonus programs in general coercive? Or are they a logical extension of other kinds of incentive programs, such as those that offer incentives for welfare recipients to stay in school?[5]

Most commentators have no objection to educational incentives. It is pointed out that financial gain motivates the poor like everyone else, and that there is nothing wrong with such incentives. If it is acceptable to offer tax breaks to the rich to get them to act in socially responsible ways (for example, donating their art to museums rather than selling it), it is equally acceptable to offer cash incentives to young mothers to get them to stay in school.

By contrast, many regard incentives to persuade women on public assistance not to get pregnant as coercive. They argue that women are not free to reject the extra money and that it is intrinsically wrongful to ask them to curb their fertility. Let us look more closely at the arguments against this kind of incentive.

It might be argued that Norplant bonus programs do not make anyone worse off, since while those who choose to participate are given extra benefits, the benefits of those who opt not to take the offer are not reduced. They remain in the same economic position they had prior to the offer.

David Coale argues that offering such a bonus *does* make those who do not take it worse off, however, and thus burdens the constitutional right not to take Norplant. He writes:

> Poor women who do not take Norplant must forego $1000 in consumption possibilities. Women who do not take Norplant then suffer the harm of a reduction in economic status compared to women who do take the drug. That reduction affects their self-esteem, which then changes almost every aspect of their lives.[6]

Unless women agree to waive their constitutional right to reproduce, they are threatened with economic loss, compared to what others receive. Put this way, Norplant bonuses look coercive. But is this a plausible interpretation? It seems to prove too much. The government attempts to influence behavior of various kinds through tax breaks and incentives: to get people to donate to charity, to save money, to join retirement plans. Such plans make some people comparatively better off than those who opt not to participate, but it is not plausible that the nonparticipants are thereby harmed or made worse off by the program.[7]

What are the state's interests in offering Norplant bonuses? Obviously, saving the state money by reducing the number of children on welfare is a prime motivation.[8] The attempt to help people out of poverty is certainly a legitimate, perhaps even a compelling, state interest. It can be argued that linking Norplant to welfare

benefits goes beyond legitimate attempts toward helping the poor improve their lives. Providing people with information about birth control, making contraceptives accessible and affordable (or even free), paying for abortion as well as childbirth—all of these activities are acceptable because they enhance individual choice. Offering fairly large sums of money to use Norplant is a different matter.

Does this mean that financial incentives for procreative decisions are always improper? Not necessarily. Consider the "Dollar-a-Day" program sponsored by Planned Parenthood in Denver, whose goal is to reduce the repeat pregnancy rate for teens, mostly black and Hispanic, who have become pregnant before the age of sixteen. The program requires girls to come to one meeting a week, where they receive their $7, paid out for symbolic reasons in one dollar bills. Girls who become pregnant must drop out of the group.

After five years, the program was judged a success. Only 17 percent of the girls in the program became pregnant; this compares very favorably to a 50 percent risk of repeat pregnancy within two years for girls who have become pregnant before age sixteen. In addition, the program is claimed to have saved Colorado in excess of a quarter of a million dollars in welfare and Medicaid payments.

Is the "Dollar-a-Day" program coercive? It seems clear that Wertheimer's choice prong is not satisfied. The girls are not threatened or forced or pressured into avoiding pregnancy. Rather, a small financial incentive is offered—enough to get the girls into the program, but not so much that they have no reasonable alternative but to join. If they decide not to join, they are not thereby made worse off.

Nor can the program be considered exploitive, because, whatever financial benefits it has for the state, its primary benefit is to the girls themselves, who are likely to remain in poverty if they have a child, or especially two children, before the age of twenty. Getting teenage girls to delay pregnancy is not like getting them to give up kidneys or become contract birthgivers—something they might choose under the pressure of poverty and regret later on.

The second proposal prong is satisfied if offering financial incentives to get people to avoid pregnancy is wrongful, that is, something the state has no right to do. It is doubtful that small financial incentives infringe on self-determination, or compromise the individual's voluntary choice. Moreover, to oppose monetary incentives on the ground that they illegitimately influence teens to avoid pregnancy is to ignore the psychological and peer pressures to *get* pregnant placed on the girls targeted by the program.

While the use of financial incentives raises the potential for coercion or improper influence, the facts suggest that the Dollar-a-Day program is more reasonably seen as liberty enhancing than as liberty limiting. Characterizing the program as "coercive" is inaccurate and misleading.

BEYOND COERCION

Long-acting contraceptives like Norplant, which are easy to monitor and do not require user compliance, clearly have a potential for coercive use. That potential for coercion is greater where there are financial incentives, as in the "Dollar-a-Day" program, because there is the risk that financial pressures will force individuals to make reproductive choices contrary to their own values and preferences. However, it seems extremely unlikely that small amounts of money could constitute such pressure. In addition, the psychosocial pressures *toward* teenage pregnancy are very strong among some groups, despite the fact that teenage childbearing has a very negative impact on the lives of the young women and their children. Small financial incentives, combined with

other sorts of encouragement, can counteract these harmful influences.

It is more difficult to determine whether incentives paid to women on public assistance who get Norplant are coercive. Those who think they are not coercive point to the fact that the women who opt not to have Norplant are no worse off for refusing than they would be if there were no incentive program. The program thus expands, rather than contracts, their options. Those who think they are coercive maintain that poor women have no choice but to accept Norplant, or else suffer an unacceptable alternative, that is, go without desperately needed money.

It should be remembered, however, that coercion is not always unjustified or improper. Some socially desirable ends can only be achieved through mutually agreed-upon coercive policies, such as taxation and immunization. Too often coercion is used as a generalized term of abuse. Incentives for birth control, for example, might be criticized as violating autonomy, equal protection, or informed consent, even if offering such incentives is not coercive. And focusing entirely on whether programs like those to encourage contraception are coercive may mask other important objections to such programs, such as their targeting of vulnerable groups, creating and reinforcing inequality.

REFERENCES

1. Tamar Lewin, "5-Year Contraceptive Implant Seems Headed for Wide Use," *The New York Times,* 29 November 1991.
2. Alan Wertheimer, *Coercion* (Princeton: Princeton University Press, 1987).
3. Wertheimer, *Coercion,* p. 21.
4. More precisely, she prefers promising to relinquish her firstborn child to being put to death. That promise will not have to be fulfilled until some time in the future, and anything could happen. She might not have a child, Rumpelstiltskin might die, or he might forget her promise. Admittedly, it is possible

that the king might not carry out his threat to put her to death if the straw isn't spun into gold, but the king's threat is much more immediate and, for that reason, more certain.

5. See, for example, Jason DeParle, "Ohio Welfare: Bonuses Keep Teenage Mothers in School," *New York Times,* 12 April 1993.

6. David S. Coale, "Norplant Bonuses and the Unconstitutional Conditions Doctrine," *Texas Law Review* 71 (1992): 189–215, at 208.

7. Kathleen Sullivan, "Unconstitutional Conditions," *Harvard Law Review* 102 (1989): 1413–1506, at 1415.

8. Coale, "Norplant Bonuses," pp. 196–97.

In the War Zone

BOB HERBERT

THERE ARE TIMES when Dr. Warren Hern feels more like a combat veteran than a physician. Here is what he says about a normal workday: "I walk out of my office and the first thing I do is look at the parking garage that the hospital built two doors away and see if there is a sniper on the roof. I basically expect to be shot any day."

Two of his close friends have been shot. "My dear friend, Garson Romalis in Vancouver—he was the first of the Canadian doctors to be shot. They almost shot off his leg. He nearly died on his kitchen floor."

That was in the fall of 1994. Dr. George Tiller was another friend. He was shot in both arms in Wichita, Kan., in 1993.

Other doctors have fallen. Dr. David Gunn was shot to death in Pensacola, Fla., in 1993, and

BOB HERBERT is a journalist who regularly publishes op-ed pieces in *The New York Times.*

Dr. John Britton was shot to death, also in Pensacola, in 1994. Dr. Barnett Slepian was shot to death in the Buffalo suburb of Amherst a little over two weeks ago.

There are big headlines whenever a doctor who performs abortions is killed, but the relentless terror and gruesome violence that continue to plague abortion providers and the people who assist them take place below the level of consciousness of most Americans.

Few people know about Robert Sanderson, the Birmingham, Ala., police officer moonlighting as a security guard whose body literally was blown to pieces in the bombing of a clinic last January. Or about the widely circulated "Army of God" manual that gives detailed information on the construction and use of bombs and other murderous devices, and recommends that if you don't kill doctors who perform abortions you should at least render their hands useless.

"It's a war zone," said Dr. Hern, who runs the Boulder Abortion Clinic in Boulder, Colo. "It's very frightening and it ruins your life."

The terror frightens everyone. Dr. Hern said: "We had this absolutely fantastic candidate for a front-desk job in my office. She was ready to accept, but because of the assassination of Dr. Slepian she decided not to work here. She talked to her friends and family and decided she could not live with that kind of fear. I didn't blame her. That has happened on numerous occasions. We've had people leave here because of the violence."

What that means, said Dr. Hern, is that the violence and the terror are working.

"How do we provide these services to women," he asked, "if those who would help us are terrified?"

The anti-abortion terrorists get much aid and comfort—sometimes openly, sometimes covertly—from various right-wing political elements, including members of the Christian right, the militia movement and the white supremacy movement. The moral fervor of the right, so loudly proclaimed, is selective indeed.

The feeling of many on the right is that if violence and terror result in the curtailment of abortion, so be it.

Dr. Hern is the author of "Abortion Services," the principal textbook on abortion for doctors in the U.S. and a number of other countries. He is also an associate clinical professor of obstetrics and gynecology at the University of Colorado.

He lost count of the death threats against him many years ago. They started as soon as he began doing abortions back in the early 1970's. "I slept with a rifle beside my bed," he said, "because I lived up in the mountains and was afraid I would be attacked."

He wears a bulletproof vest at some of his public appearances. In 1988 someone fired five shots into his office. "I had to install bulletproof windows," he said. He'd already hired private, armed security guards. The harassment, the demonstrations and the terror continued. The office at times was surrounded by 50 to 100 peace officers of one kind or another.

"It was," said Dr. Hern, "a nightmare." . . .

Freedom of Conscience, Professional Responsibility, and Access to Abortion

REBECCA S. DRESSER

ACCESS TO ABORTION is becoming increasingly restricted for many women in the United States. Besides the longstanding financial barriers facing low-income women in most states, a newer source of scarcity has emerged. The relatively small number of physicians willing to perform the procedure is compromising the ability of women in certain parts of the country to obtain an abortion.

Do physicians have a duty to respond to this situation? Do they have a professional responsibility to ensure that abortions are reasonably available to the women who want to terminate their pregnancies? Or, is abortion so morally and socially controversial as to remove any professional obligation to provide reasonable access?

Both law and medical ethics have traditionally protected physicians' freedom to refuse to perform any procedure, including abortion, that conflicts with their religious or other moral beliefs. The right of "conscientious objection" to performing abortion is enshrined in many statutes;[1] moreover, the First Amendment's religious freedom provision arguably would prevent health officials from requiring individual physicians who are ethically opposed to abortion to participate in the procedure.[2] Freedom of conscience is one of the most respected values in our

REBECCA S. DRESSER is a Professor of Law and Medicine at Indiana University-Bloomington.

culture, and most people would find repugnant any proposal to coerce or pressure physicians into performing abortions.

Yet, the current scarcity of abortion providers also has serious ethical implications. When a substantial number of qualified members of the medical profession refrain from performing a procedure that many women deem a critical reproductive health need, we may question whether the profession is fulfilling its responsibilities in this area. Moreover, the current situation is troubling in light of the burdens it imposes on the relatively small group of physicians who are now willing to provide women with abortions. These concerns make it incumbent on both the profession and the broader society to consider whether the present policies should be altered in any way.

THE EXISTING SHORTAGE

With its decision in *Planned Parenthood v. Casey*,[3] the United States Supreme Court reaffirmed its basic commitment to preserving a woman's right to choose abortion. States are prohibited from enacting laws that place an "undue burden" on women seeking to terminate their pregnancies before viability. Although the undue burden standard permits some state interference, such as the imposition of waiting periods in certain cir-

From Journal of Law, Medicine & Ethics *22 (1994): 280–85. Copyright 1994. Reprinted by permission of Rebecca Dresser and the American Society of Law, Medicine, & Ethics. All rights reserved.*

cumstances, states may not impose significant barriers to women's access.

But, to obtain an abortion, women need more than constitutional protection from state interference. Women need a physician or other competent health care professional who is willing to perform the procedure. And some women face considerable difficulty in reaching such an individual. The need for lengthy travel may pose material financial and other personal obstacles in states, such as Pennsylvania, where waiting periods are required between the time a woman is informed about the abortion procedure and the time she may undergo it.[4] Without reasonable access, the right to terminate a pregnancy becomes an empty right.

Here are some of the statistics. A 1993 survey of U.S. counties found that 84 percent had no abortion provider. At that time, 30 percent of women of reproductive age in the United States lived in those counties.[5] The same study found that just over half of American metropolitan counties (defined as counties including or adjacent to cities of at least 50,000 people) lacked an abortion provider. According to this study, certain states in the west and south have very few providers; North Dakota and South Dakota, for example, each have only one facility in which abortions are available. An earlier study suggested that the distance from an abortion provider is inversely related to abortion rates.[6]

Although many physicians in principle support women's access to abortion, relatively few offer this service. In a 1985 survey conducted by the American College of Obstetricians and Gynecologists (ACOG), 84 percent of a representative sample of members agreed that "elective abortions should be performed under some circumstances," but only 34 percent of those physicians reported that they themselves performed such procedures.[7] A 1983 survey of private general/family physicians, general surgeons, and obstetrician-gynecologists found that just 12 percent of those surveyed performed abortions.

Thirty-five percent of respondents not performing abortions cited moral or religious reasons as the basis for omitting this service. Others attributed the exclusion to the cost and inconvenience of obtaining proper training and to a lack of access to equipment or facilities, which sometimes was due to hospital policies forbidding abortions on the premises.[8]

Indications are that the current physician scarcity is likely to intensify, unless efforts are made to alter it. According to a 1985 survey of American residency programs listed by the Council on Resident Education in Obstetrics and Gynecology, abortion techniques often are regarded as outside the realm of training given routinely to obstetrics-gynecology residents. Just 23 percent of the responding programs included abortion training as a standard part of the education provided to residents. (These programs did permit individuals objecting on moral or religious grounds to be excused from this portion of their training.) Fifty percent of residency programs offered abortion training as an option, and 28 percent excluded it completely. The latter represented a fourfold increase over a survey performed ten years previously.[9] More recent surveys indicate that training opportunities have declined even further since 1985. According to one study, by 1992, the percentage of programs routinely offering training in first-trimester abortions had fallen to 12 percent, with only 7 percent of programs including instruction on second-trimester abortion techniques as part of routine training.[10] In a 1992 survey of 184 of the 271 American obstetrics-gynecology residency programs, 47 percent of graduating chief residents reported that they had never performed a first-trimester abortion.[11]

The current access problem could be reduced if RU–486 becomes available in this country as an alternative to surgical abortion. Some physicians in the United States who do not perform surgical abortions have stated that they would be willing to prescribe RU–486 to their pregnant patients.[12] But, RU–486 is only effective during the earliest weeks of pregnancy, is not medically indicated for many women, and, in some cases, does not result in pregnancy termination.[13] Moreover, experience in other countries suggests that when the medical and surgical abortion procedures are both available, many women prefer the surgical procedure, because it is shorter, often less painful, and requires fewer follow-up visits.[14] Thus, although the existing problem of abortion provider scarcity could be lessened by the availability of RU–486, it is unlikely that the problem will disappear.

IMPLICATIONS OF BARRIERS TO ACCESS

I will not present here the arguments on the morality of abortion. The subject has produced some of the most heated and fundamental moral disagreement that exists among people in this country. Yet, even those opposed to abortion generally believe it is a medical procedure that should be available in certain situations: if pregnancy presents a serious risk to the life or health of the woman or, possibly, if the case involves rape, incest, or serious fetal abnormality.[15]

Many others take a more liberal view, and include so-called "elective" abortions within the scope of medical services that should be available to women. These individuals support availability of abortion for a broader array of reasons, such as maintaining employment demands and meeting responsibilities to existing family members. Many in this group believe that barriers to abortion have a discriminatory impact on women, reducing women's opportunity for full participation in the larger society.[16] The high number of abortions each year in this country indicates that many women define abortion as a necessary surgical procedure at some point in their lives.[17]

Both the conservative and the more liberal views support the argument that the abortion provider shortage impairs at least some women's access to appropriate medical care. Women seeking care may be substantially burdened by the costs, the travel, and the time away from their jobs and families that can accompany performance of the service. Some commentators also have expressed concern that women who cannot assume these burdens will increasingly seek abortions from unqualified persons, thus exposing themselves to serious health risks.[18] In sum, the scarcity of physicians willing to perform abortions has significant implications for the health and well-being of American women.

The current scarcity also imposes burdens on the relatively small group of physicians who now offer the procedure. Stories of physicians spending long hours working in and journeying between widely dispersed abortion clinics are becoming increasingly commonplace.[19] Doctors personally committed to maintaining women's access to abortion may find themselves spending more time at this task than they would prefer, due to the void that would result from any cutback on their part.

PROFESSIONAL DUTIES AND ACCESS

The current scarcity of abortion providers is a troubling situation for persons supporting a woman's freedom to choose against continuing a pregnancy, as well as for those concerned with the heavy burdens borne by physicians now providing abortion services. Does the medical profession have a special duty to respond to this situation? An analysis of the professionalism concept suggests that it does.

Physicians and other professionals traditionally have enjoyed relatively high financial rewards, social standing, and substantial freedom from external regulation, as compared to individuals in other types of occupations. The professions are assumed capable of self-regulation, able to exercise internal monitoring of their members' activities to ensure that the public is adequately served. In return for the rewards of professional status, professions and their members are expected to exhibit a strong commitment to the needs and welfare of the people they serve.[20]

This "social bargain" model of the professions suggests that, although every individual member of the medical profession might not have a duty to perform every procedure within his or her competence, society expects the broader profession to adopt reasonable measures to promote patient access to medically acceptable procedures.[21] Traditional rules governing the individual physician's freedom to withdraw from a patient's care rest on the assumption that the patient will be able to secure care from another qualified professional.[22] The broader profession would seem to have some responsibility to undertake efforts to ensure that such alternative care is reasonably available.

Several medical organizations have publicly articulated their disagreement with state-imposed impediments to obtaining an abortion. The American Medical Association (AMA), the ACOG, and the American Medical Women's Association have issued resolutions and policies opposing legal requirements that impair patients' access to abortion, such as parental consent requirements or restrictions on public funding of abortion.[23] These statements, as well as other organizational actions portraying abortion as properly a medical matter, would seem to commit the profession to some role in preserving women's access to the procedure. For example, the AMA policy asserts that "abortion is a medical procedure that should be performed only by a duly licensed physician."[24] Professional claims that physicians are the sole individuals qualified to perform

abortion support the existence of an accompanying responsibility to address the current scarcity.

But, to date, the profession has been reluctant to engage in organizational efforts to reduce the access problem. Instead, in strongly affirming their members' freedom of conscience on this matter, medical organizations have appeared to disavow the responsibility to safeguard access. For example, the AMA policy states that "the issue of support of or opposition to abortion is a matter for members of the AMA to decide individually, based on personal values or beliefs. The AMA will take no action that may be construed as an attempt to alter or influence the personal views of individual members regarding abortion procedures."[25] This pledge seems unnecessarily overbroad, and could be interpreted to rule out any educational or other organizational commitment to address the current access problem.

It would be possible for professional organizations to respond constructively to the current abortion provider shortage without infringing on their members' personal values or beliefs. In the present climate, physicians' decisions not to perform abortions may reflect not only their positions on the moral status of the human fetus, but also their concerns about personal safety, the safety of their families, economic well-being, professional prestige, and an understandable desire to avoid the controversy and public exposure that frequently accompany the life of today's abortion provider. As one medical student put it, "[m]any people would like to provide [abortion] as a service. . . . But there's so much controversy now, there's a feeling that 'it should be done, but let someone else do it.'"[26] The diverse considerations that may be influencing many physicians-in-training, as well as obstetrician-gynecologists and primary care physicians who now omit abortion from the services they offer their women patients, suggest directions for professional as well as societal action to address the abortion provider shortage.

BALANCING WOMEN'S AUTONOMY AND PROFESSIONAL CONSCIENCE

Problematic Approaches

The decreasing availability of abortions presents the medical profession with a significant challenge. Care must be taken to avoid any element of coercion or pressure on residents and practicing physicians to perform a procedure that they believe is morally wrong. Besides infringing on the individual's freedom of conscience, such a practice would pose risks to patients. Physicians reluctant to perform the procedure could communicate this to their patients, both expressly and indirectly, which would have a negative effect on their interaction and perhaps even on the quality of care that patients received.[27]

For these reasons, I disagree with the idea of turning residency faculty into "draft boards" who scrutinize the authenticity of residents' claimed moral or religious opposition to participating in abortion. Chervenak and McCullough recommend that residency policies "require residents to document the basis of their objections to performing abortions in a rigorous way, analogous to the requirement imposed on citizens who seek conscientious objector status regarding military service."[28] Admittedly, a failure to cross-examine residents about the sources of their desires to avoid training in abortion techniques will enable some residents to be excused for less worthy reasons. Yet, the negative effects of the draft board approach on patient care, as well as on the morale of those participating in the residency program, would, in my view, outweigh its benefits.

Another possible way to increase the number of residents receiving training in abortion techniques would be to set an explicit entry requirement for those areas of medicine typically involving reproductive and primary health care for women. Individuals considering these fields would be informed that abortion is among the standard package of services that physicians in these areas are expected to offer. Medical school graduates opposed to abortion would be free to choose other practice areas, but, if they chose obstetrics-gynecology or family practice, for example, they would not be permitted to opt out of learning and subsequently offering the procedure.

Although this approach would incorporate explicit consent as the basis for restricting physicians' subsequent freedom, it remains ethically questionable. Some residents who agreed to the condition could, after further experience and thought, come to oppose their involvement in abortion. The opportunity to withdraw consent is an important element of informed decision making that ought to be preserved in this context. Yet, if individuals were permitted to change their minds about performing abortions, the effectiveness of this approach would be undermined. On the other hand, requiring these individuals to change their areas of training and practice to avoid further involvement in performing abortion would impose on them substantial personal burdens and deprive society of their services during the period of retraining. In light of such moral and practical problems with the consent model, it would be better to address the access barriers through alternative methods.

Fortunately, the medical profession has available a number of less drastic measures that could succeed in reducing the existing barriers to abortion access. Adopting these measures would enable the profession to meet its responsibility to address women's needs for full reproductive health services without forcing individual members to compromise their moral and religious beliefs.

Potential Training Program Modifications

Residency training perhaps offers the greatest opportunity for change. The 1985 study of obstetrics-gynecology residency programs found that residents were much more likely to accept training in abortion techniques when it was routinely included as part of residency education. When training was optional, participation rates declined.[29] Since residents in both groups could decline training on religious and moral grounds, it appears that making training optional discourages an additional group of residents from participating. Taking advantage of optional training may require residents to assume duties beyond those normally assigned, which can be a powerful disincentive to many residents struggling to cope with their ordinary tasks.[30] Altering the standard curriculum of obstetrics-gynecology and primary care residencies to include training in abortion techniques would have a salutary effect on the number of physicians qualified to offer their patients this service. Programs also could arrange for substitute duties to be assigned to residents who forgo such training.[31] Accreditation and certification bodies could consider adopting standards to encourage this approach.

Residency programs may encounter several practical obstacles to integrating abortion techniques into the customary residency education, however. Few abortions are now performed in the hospitals where most of the residency training occurs. Instead, most abortions are performed in freestanding clinics, which are able to offer the service at a lower cost to patients.[32] To increase training opportunities, many residency programs will need to establish rotations at local abortion clinics, or, alternatively, to arrange for hospital clinics to offer abortion services on an outpatient basis.[33] If more hospital-based clinics provided the proper equipment for abortion services, more established physicians might be willing to perform the procedure as well.[34] The latter approach also offers a means of reducing the isolation and harassment experienced by many physicians now performing abortions in freestanding facilities, though the problem of higher costs could reduce its feasibility.

Certain hospitals could resist proposals to include abortion among the procedures that physicians perform on the premises. Facilities affiliated with particular religious denominations, as well as some nonsectarian institutions, may have policies prohibiting elective abortions. Although it is legally permissible for health care institutions to promulgate and enforce policies adopting distinctive moral positions on the care patients may receive, the scope of this institutional prerogative has not been clearly established and probably varies from state to state.[35] Residency program faculty seeking to establish training programs should examine and perhaps question their hospital's stance on the matter; if the institution's policy is firm, then faculty should seek training opportunities for their residents at other sites.

Last, members of the larger community could be enlisted to join medical professionals in conveying to physicians-in-training the importance of preserving women's access to safe abortion procedures. Although many older physicians remember when women died or suffered serious injury due to complications from illegal abortions, such occurrences fortunately have become quite rare. Today's young physicians are much more likely to be familiar with the personal risks and burdens accompanying the decision to offer abortion services. Older physicians and nonprofessional groups committed to preserving women's access could work together to educate medical students and residents on the health and other benefits flowing from the availability of safe abortion.[36] Hearing a more positive message on the value of providing abortion services could affect the decision making of young physicians training to become primary health care providers to women.

Changing the Social Context of Providing Abortion

Producing more physicians trained in abortion techniques will not necessarily lead to greater access for women. The existing provider shortage will persist unless those who obtain training are also willing to offer the service when they enter practice. Physicians working in small towns and rural areas, where the availability of abortion is most restricted, are more likely to encounter political and religious opposition to the procedure than physicians in many metropolitan areas.[37] Even in urban areas, physicians performing abortions in freestanding facilities may be exposed to organized protests, vandalism, hate mail, death threats, property damage, and physical violence.[38] Antiabortion groups have identified physicians as the "weak link" in the availability of abortions; doctors have reportedly been targeted for "expos[ure]" and "humiliat[ion]."[39] Moreover, physicians' compensation for abortion is relatively low, and abortion clinic work can be regimented and repetitive. Abortion providers typically do not enjoy the high esteem of their professional colleagues, due to the procedure's controversial nature and lack of technical challenge.[40]

Both the medical profession and the broader community have several options available for responding more effectively to the ordeals of today's abortion providers. Professional organizations could take symbolic and practical measures to extend support to their members committed, indeed, courageous enough, to undergo personal hardship to safeguard the availability of safe abortion. Physicians who support preservation of women's access, but do not themselves offer abortion services, could publicly acknowledge the important benefit their colleagues provide. Members of the medical profession also could thoughtfully evaluate regulatory proposals to expand the pool of health professionals permitted to provide abortion services. In the few states that now permit specially trained, physician-supervised nurse-practitioners, nurse-midwives, and physician's assistants to perform first-trimester abortions, the nonphysicians have safety records comparable to those of physicians.[41]

Medical organizations also could solicit public and private assistance in the effort to protect women's access. In many areas, local community law enforcement and government officials could do more to protect abortion clinics and their staffs. Efforts could be initiated to modify the low fees physicians now receive for abortion, with the goal of making compensation equal to what is assigned to other comparable procedures. Finally, it is time for the many individuals and community groups who support women's continued access to voice publicly their appreciation of the medical profession's contribution. To date, the medical community has received the most powerful signals from groups and individuals opposed to women's freedom to choose abortion. Pro-choice advocates must deliver a more positive message of gratitude and encouragement to the physicians playing such a crucial role in protecting women's access.

Some signs from the profession and the community suggest that they are ready to confront the access problem. ACOG and the National Abortion Federation recently sponsored a symposium to address the existing disincentives to providing abortion services.[42] When a Massachusetts hospital joined with Planned Parenthood to offer training in abortion techniques, fifteen of seventeen obstetrics-gynecology residents volunteered to participate.[43] Congress recently enacted the Freedom of Access to Clinic Entrances Act, which makes harassment and violence toward reproductive health care providers a federal offense.[44] In some states, courts and legislatures have taken legal action to protect abortion patients, providers, and the facilities in which abortions are performed.[45] During the summer of 1993, when abortion opponents embarked on an organized effort to disrupt abortion services in many cities, local community officials and pro-choice supporters were largely successful in preserving clinic access during that period.[46]

I do not mean to suggest that the abortion access problem will be solved easily. The medical profession will have to make a substantial commitment to reducing the provider shortage, and society will have to do its share as well. Preserving access to safe abortion poses a considerable challenge to a profession and a populace as diverse as that of the United States. Abortion is undeniably one of the most hotly contested issues of our time, and most physicians as well as nonphysicians might prefer to avoid personal involvement in the controversy. Yet, it would be unfortunate if the harassment and violence exhibited by a small group of abortion opponents kept physicians who support women's access from providing their patients with full reproductive services. With heightened attention and cooperation among professional and community groups, it should be possible to ameliorate the abortion access problem without intruding on the religious and moral convictions of individual physicians.

REFERENCES

1. Judith F. Daar, "A Clash at the Bedside: Patient Autonomy v. a Physician's Professional Conscience," *Hastings Law Journal*, 44 (1993): 1241–89.
2. Irene P. Loftus, "I Have a Conscience, Too: The Plight of Medical Personnel Confronting the Right to Die," *Notre Dame Law Review*, 65 (1990): 699–730.
3. 112 S. Ct. 2791 (1992).
4. *Planned Parenthood v. Casey*, 114 S. Ct. 909 (1994) (refusing to issue a stay on enforcing waiting period in Pennsylvania law).
5. Stanley K. Henshaw and Jennifer Van Vort, "Abortion Services in the United States, 1991 and 1992," *Family Planning Perspectives*, 26, no. 3 (1994): 112.
6. James D. Shelton, Edward A. Brann, and Kenneth F. Schulz, "Abortion Utilization: Does Travel Distance Matter?," *Family Planning Perspectives*, 8, no. 6 (1976): 260–62. See also Archon Fung, "Making Rights Real: *Roe*'s Impact on Abortion Access," *Politics & Society*, 21, no. 4 (1993): 465–504.
7. "ACOG Poll: Ob-Gyns' Support for Abortion Unchanged Since 1971," *Family Planning Perspectives*, 17, no. 6 (1985): 275.
8. Margaret T. Orr and Jacqueline D. Forrest, "The Availability of Reproductive Health Services from U.S. Private Physicians," *Family Planning Perspectives*, 17, no. 2 (1985): 63–69.
9. Philip D. Darney, Uta Landy, Sara MacPherson, et al., "Abortion Training in U.S. Obstetrics and Gynecology Residency Programs," *Family Planning Perspectives*, 19, no. 4 (1987): 158–62.
10. Helene Cooper, "Medical Schools, Students

Shun Abortion Study," *The Wall Street Journal*, Mar. 12, 1993, sec. B1.
11. Carolyn Westoff, Frances Marks, and Allan Rosenfeld, "Residency Training in Contraception, Sterilization, and Abortion," *Obstetrics & Gynecology*, 81, no. 2 (1993): 311–14.
12. Katherine Q. Seelye, "Enter RU–486, Exit Hype," *The New York Times*, May 22, 1994, sec. 4, 16.
13. *Id.* See also Louise Silvestre, Catherine Dubois, Maguy Renault, et al., "Voluntary Interruption of Pregnancy With Mifepristone (RU–486) and a Prostaglandin Analogue," *New England Journal of Medicine*, 322, no. 10 (1990): 645–48.
14. Nina Darnton, "Surprising Journey for Abortion Drug," *The New York Times*, Mar. 23, 1994, sec. B6.
15. Robert J. Blendon, John M. Benson, and Karen Donelan, "The Public and the Controversy over Abortion," *JAMA*, 270 (1993): 2871–75.
16. *Planned Parenthood v. Casey*, 112 S. Ct. at 2807; and Ruth B. Ginsberg, "Some Thoughts on Autonomy and Equality in Relation to *Roe v. Wade*," *North Carolina Law Review*, 63 (1985): 375–86.
17. Henshaw and Van Vort, *supra* note 5, at 101.
18. Janet Benshoof, "*Planned Parenthood v. Casey*: The Impact of the New Undue Burden Standard on Reproductive Health Care," *JAMA*, 269 (1993): 2249–57.
19. Sara Rimer, "Forceps and Fear on Abortion Circuit," *The New York Times*, Sept. 3, 1993, sec. A1.
20. David M. Mirvis, "Physicians' Autonomy— The Relation Between Public and Professional Expectations," *New England Journal of Medicine*, 328, no. 18 (1993): 1346–49.
21. Norman Daniels, "Duty to Treat or Right to Refuse?," *Hastings Center Report*, 21, no. 2 (1991): 36–46.
22. Darr, *supra* note 1. See also Jeffrey Blustein, "Doing What the Patient Orders: Maintaining Integrity in the Doctor-Patient Relationship," *Bioethics*, 7, no. 4 (1993): 289–314.
23. Council on Ethical and Judicial Affairs, American Medical Association, "Mandatory Parental Consent to Abortion," *JAMA*, 269 (1993): 82–86; American Medical Association, "Public Funding of Abortion Services," *Policy Compendium* (1992): sec. 5.998; American College of Obstetricians and Gynecologists, "Confidentiality in Adolescent Health Care," *ACOG Statement of Policy* (1988); American College of Obstetricians and Gynecologists, "ACOG Policy on Abortion," *ACOG Statement of Policy* (1993); and American Medical Women's Association, "Abortion," *AMWA Resolutions Booklet*, (1960–1992): secs. 1989.3, 1991.1, 1991.3.
24. Janet E. Gans, Robert C. Rinaldi, and Jerod Loeb, "Abortion Mortality Trends," *JAMA*, 269, no. 17 (1993): 2211–12.

25. *Id.*

26. Maureen Dezell, "Stalked by Fear," *Boston Phoenix,* Apr. 23, 1993, sec. 1, 22.

27. Edmund G. Howe, "On Expanding the Parameters of Assisted Suicide, Directive Counseling, and Overriding Patients' Cultural Beliefs," *Journal of Clinical Ethics,* 4, no. 2 (1993): 107–11.

28. Frank A. Chervenak and Laurence B. McCullough, "Does Obstetric Ethics Have Any Role in the Obstetrician's Response to the Abortion Controversy?," *American Journal of Obstetrics and Gynecology,* 163, no. 5 (1990): 1425–29.

29. Darney, Landy, MacPherson, et al., *supra* note 9.

30. David A. Grimes, "Clinicians Who Provide Abortions: The Thinning Ranks," *Obstetrics & Gynecology,* 80, no. 4 (1992): 719–23.

31. Chervenak and McCullough, *supra* note 28.

32. Henshaw and Van Vort, *supra* note 5.

33. Darney, Landy, MacPherson, et al., *supra* note 9.

34. Orr and Forrest, *supra* note 8.

35. Steven H. Miles, Peter A. Singer, and Mark Siegler, "Conflicts Between Patients' Wishes to Forgo Treatment and the Policies of Health Care Facilities," *New England Journal of Medicine,* 321, no. 1 (1989): 48–50.

36. Grimes, *supra* note 30.

37. Darney, Landy, MacPherson, et al., *supra* note 9.

38. Benshoof, *supra* note 18; Ronald Smothers, "Abortion Doctor and Bodyguard Slain in Florida," *The New York Times,* July 30, 1994, sec. A1; and Tamar Lewin, "Clinic Firebombed in Pennsylvania," *The New York Times,* Sept. 30, 1993, sec. A16.

39. Larry Rohter, "Doctor is Slain During Protest over Abortions," *The New York Times,* Mar. 11, 1993, sec. A1.

40. Grimes, *supra* note 30.

41. *Id.;* and Mary A. Freedman, David A. Jillson, Roberta R. Coffin, et al., "Comparison of Complication Rates in First Trimester Abortions Performed by Physician Assistants and Physicians," *American Journal of Public Health,* 76, no. 5 (1986): 550–54.

42. Grimes, *supra* note 30.

43. "The Unfinished Abortion Battle (editorial)," *The New York Times,* May 12, 1993, sec. A18.

44. Pub. L. No. 103–259, 108 Stat. 694 (1994).

45. Center for Reproductive Law & Policy, "A Woman's Right to Choose After *Planned Parenthood v. Casey,*" July 20, 1994.

46. Michael D. Hinds, "Anti-Abortion Drive Surprisingly Quiet," *The New York Times,* July 15, 1993, sec. A16.

An Almost Absolute Value in History

JOHN T. NOONAN, JR.

THE MOST FUNDAMENTAL QUESTION involved in the long history of thought on abortion is: How do you determine the humanity of a

JOHN T. NOONAN is a Judge on the 9th Circuit Court of Appeals and is an author.

being? To phrase the question that way is to put in comprehensive humanistic terms what the theologians either dealt with as an explicitly theological question under the heading of "ensoulment" or dealt with implicitly in their treatment of abortion. The Christian position as it originated did not depend on a narrow theological or philosophical concept. It had no relation to theories of infant baptism. It appealed to no special theory of instantaneous ensoulment. It took the world's view on ensoulment as that view changed from Aristotle to Zacchia. There was, indeed, theological influence affecting the theory of ensoulment finally adopted, and, of course, ensoulment itself was a theological concept, so that the position was always explained in theological terms. But the theological notion of ensoulment could easily be translated into humanistic language by substituting "human" for "rational soul"; the problem of knowing when a man is a man is common to theology and humanism.

If one steps outside the specific categories used by the theologians, the answer they gave can be analyzed as a refusal to discriminate among human beings on the basis of their varying potentialities. Once conceived, the being was recognized as man because he had man's potential. The criterion for humanity, thus, was simple and all-embracing: if you are conceived by human parents, you are human.

The strength of this position may be tested by a review of some of the other distinctions offered in the contemporary controversy over legalizing abortion. Perhaps the most popular distinction is in terms of viability. Before an age of so many months, the fetus is not viable, that is, it cannot be removed from the mother's womb and live apart from her. To that extent, the life of the fetus is absolutely dependent on the life of the mother. This dependence is made the basis of denying recognition to its humanity.

There are difficulties with this distinction. One is that the perfection of artificial incubation may make the fetus viable at any time: it may be removed and artificially sustained. Experiments with animals already show that such a procedure is possible. This hypothetical extreme case relates to an actual difficulty: there is considerable elasticity to the idea of viability. Mere length of life is not an exact measure. The viability of the fetus depends on the extent of its anatomical and functional development. The weight and length of the fetus are better guides to the state of its development than age, but weight and length vary. Moreover, different racial groups have different ages at which their fetuses are viable. Some evidence, for example, suggests that Negro fetuses mature more quickly than white fetuses. If viability is the norm, the standard would vary with race and with many individual circumstances.

The most important objection to this approach is that dependence is not ended by viability. The fetus is still absolutely dependent on someone's care in order to continue existence; indeed a child of one or three or even five years of age is absolutely dependent on another's care for existence; uncared for, the older fetus or the younger child will die as surely as the early fetus detached from the mother. The unsubstantial lessening in dependence at viability does not seem to signify any special acquisition of humanity.

A second distinction has been attempted in terms of experience. A being who has had experience, has lived and suffered, who possesses memories, is more human than one who has not. Humanity depends on formation by experience. The fetus is thus "unformed" in the most basic human sense.

This distinction is not serviceable for the embryo which is already experiencing and reacting. The embryo is responsive to touch after eight weeks and at least at that point is experiencing. At an earlier stage the zygote is certainly alive and responding to its environment. The distinction may also be challenged by the rare case where aphasia has erased adult memory: has it erased humanity? More fundamentally, this distinction leaves even the older fetus or the younger child to be treated as an unformed inhuman thing. Finally, it is not clear why experience as such confers humanity. It could be argued that certain central experiences such as loving or learning are necessary to make a man human. But then human beings who have failed to love or to learn might be excluded from the class called man.

A third distinction is made by appeal to the sentiments of adults. If a fetus dies, the grief of the parents is not the grief they would have for a living child. The fetus is an unnamed "it" till birth, and is not perceived as personality until at least the fourth month of existence when movements in the womb manifest a vigorous presence demanding joyful recognition by the parents.

Yet feeling is notoriously an unsure guide to the humanity of others. Many groups of humans have had difficulty in feeling that persons of another tongue, color, religion, sex, are as human as they. Apart from reactions to alien groups, we mourn the loss of a ten-year-old boy more than the loss of his one-day-old brother or his 90-year-old grandfather. The difference felt and the grief expressed vary with the potentialities extinguished, or the experience wiped out; they do not seem to point to any substantial difference in the humanity of baby, boy, or grandfather.

Distinctions are also made in terms of sensation by the parents. The embryo is felt within the womb only after about the fourth month. The embryo is seen only at birth. What can be neither seen nor felt is different from what is tangible. If the fetus cannot be seen or touched at all, it cannot be perceived as man.

Yet experience shows that sight is even more untrustworthy than feeling in determining humanity. By sight, color became an appropriate index for saying who was a man, and the evil of racial discrimination was given foundation. Nor can touch provide the test: a being confined by sickness, "out of touch" with others, does not thereby seem to lose his humanity. To the extent that touch still has appeal as a criterion, it appears to be a survival of the old English idea of "quickening"—a possible mistranslation of the Latin *animatus* used in the canon law. To that extent touch as a criterion seems to be dependent on the Aristotelian notion of ensoulment, and to fail when this notion is discarded.

Finally, a distinction is sought in social visibility. The fetus is not socially perceived as human. It cannot communicate with others. Thus, both subjectively and objectively, it is not a member of society. As moral rules are rules for the behavior of members of society to each other, they cannot be made for behavior toward what is not yet a member. Excluded from the society of men, the fetus is excluded from the humanity of men.

By force of the argument from the consequences, this distinction is to be rejected. It is more subtle than that founded on an appeal to physical sensation, but it is equally dangerous in its implications. If humanity depends on social recognition, individuals or whole groups may be dehumanized by being denied any status in their society. Such a fate is fictionally portrayed in *1984* and has actually been the lot of many men in many societies. In the Roman empire, for example, condemnation to slavery meant the practical denial of most human rights; in the Chinese Communist world, landlords have been classified as enemies of the people and so treated as nonpersons by the state. Humanity does not depend on social recognition, though often the failure of society to recognize the prisoner, the alien, the heterodox as human has led to the destruction of human beings. Anyone conceived by a man and a woman is human. Recognition of this condition by society follows a real event in the objective order, however imperfect and halting the recognition. Any attempt to limit humanity to exclude some group runs the risk of furnishing authority and precedent for excluding other groups in the name of the consciousness or perception of the controlling group in the society.

A philosopher may reject the appeal to the humanity of the fetus because he views "humanity" as a secular view of the soul and because he doubts the existence of anything real and objective which can be identified as humanity. One answer to such a philosopher is to ask how he reasons about moral questions without supposing that there is a sense in which he and the others of whom he speaks are human. Whatever group is taken as the society which determines who may be killed is thereby taken as human. A second answer is to ask if he does not believe that there is a right and wrong way of deciding moral questions. If there is such a difference, experience may be appealed to: to decide who is human on the basis of the sentiment of a given society has led to consequences which rational men would characterize as monstrous.

The rejection of the attempted distinctions based on viability and visibility, experience and feeling, may be buttressed by the following considerations: Moral judgments often rest on distinctions, but if the distinctions are not to appear arbitrary fiat, they should relate to some real difference in probabilities. There is a kind of continuity in all life, but the earlier stages of the elements of human life possess tiny probabilities of development. Consider for example, the spermatozoa in any normal ejaculate: There are about 200,000,000 in any single ejaculate, of which one has a chance of developing into a zygote. Consider the oocytes which may become ova: there are 100,000 to 1,000,000 oocytes in a female infant, of which a maximum of 390 are ovulated. But once spermatozoon and ovum meet and the conceptus is formed, such studies as have been made show that roughly in only 20 percent of the cases will spontaneous abortion occur. In other words, the chances are about 4 out of 5 that this new being will develop. At this stage in the life of the being there is a sharp shift in probabilities, an immense jump in potentialities. To make a distinction between the rights of spermatozoa and the rights of the fertilized ovum is to respond to an enormous shift in possibilities. For about twenty days after conception the egg may split to form twins or combine with another egg to form a chimera, but the probability of either event happening is very small.

It may be asked, What does a change in biological probabilities have to do with establishing humanity? The argument from probabilities is not aimed at establishing humanity but at establishing an objective discontinuity which may be taken into account in moral discourse. As life itself is a matter of probabilities, as most moral reasoning is an estimate of probabilities, so it seems in accord with the structure of reality and the nature of moral thought to found a moral judgment on the change in probabilities at conception. The appeal to probabilities is the most

commonsensical of arguments, to a greater or smaller degree all of us base our actions on probabilities, and in morals, as in law, prudence and negligence are often measured by the account one has taken of the probabilities. If the chance is 200,000,000 to 1 that the movement in the bushes into which you shoot is a man's, I doubt if many persons would hold you careless in shooting; but if the chances are 4 out of 5 that the movement is a human being's, few would acquit you of blame. Would the argument be different if only one out of ten children conceived came to term? Of course this argument would be different. This argument is an appeal to probabilities that actually exist, not to any and all states of affairs which may be imagined.

The probabilities as they do exist do not show the humanity of the embryo in the sense of a demonstration in logic any more than the probabilities of the movement in the bush being a man demonstrate beyond all doubt that the being is a man. The appeal is a "buttressing" consideration, showing the plausibility of the standard adopted. The argument focuses on the decisional factor in any moral judgment and assumes that part of the business of a moralist is drawing lines. One evidence of the nonarbitrary character of the line drawn is the difference of probabilities on either side of it. If a spermatozoon is destroyed, one destroys a being which had a chance of far less than 1 in 200 million of developing into a reasoning being, possessed of the genetic code, a heart and other organs, and capable of pain. If a fetus is destroyed, one destroys a being already possessed of the genetic code, organs, and sensitivity to pain, and one which had an 80 percent chance of developing further into a baby outside the womb who, in time, would reason.

The positive argument for conception as the decisive moment of humanization is that at conception the new being receives the genetic code. It is this genetic information which determines his characteristics, which is the biological carrier of the possibility of human wisdom, which makes him a self-evolving being. A being with a human genetic code is man.

This review of current controversy over the humanity of the fetus emphasizes what a fundamental question the theologians resolved in asserting the inviolability of the fetus. To regard the fetus as possessed of equal rights with other humans was not, however, to decide every case where abortion might be employed. It did decide the case where the argument was that the fetus should be aborted for its own good. To say a being was human was to say it had a destiny to decide for itself which could not be taken from it by another man's decision. But human beings with equal rights often come in conflict with each other, and some decision must be made as to whose claims are to prevail. Cases of conflict involving the fetus are different only in two respects: the total inability of the fetus to speak for itself and the fact that the right of the fetus regularly at stake is the right to life itself.

The approach taken by the theologians to these conflicts was articulated in terms of "direct" and "indirect." Again, to look at what they were doing from outside their categories, they may be said to have been drawing lines or "balancing values." "Direct" and "indirect" are spatial metaphors; "line-drawing" is another. "To weigh" or "to balance" values is a metaphor of a more complicated mathematical sort hinting at the process which goes on in moral judgments. All the metaphors suggest that, in the moral judgments made, comparisons were necessary, that no value completely controlled. The principle of double effect was no doctrine fallen from heaven, but a method of analysis appropriate where two relative values were being compared. In Catholic moral theology, as it developed, life even of the innocent was not taken as an absolute. Judgments on acts affecting life issued from a process of weighing. In the weighing, the fetus was always given a value greater than zero, always a value separate and independent from its parents. This valuation was crucial and fundamental in all Christian thought on the subject and marked it off from any approach which considered that only the parents' interests needed to be considered.

Even with the fetus weighed as human, one interest could be weighed as equal or superior: that of the mother in her own life. The casuists between 1450 and 1895 were willing to weigh this interest as superior. Since 1895, that interest was given decisive weight only in the two special cases on the cancerous uterus and the ectopic pregnancy. In both of these cases the fetus itself had little chance of survival even if the abortion were not performed. As the balance was once struck in favor of the mother whenever her life was endangered, it could be so struck again. The balance reached between 1895 and 1930 attempted prudentially and pastorally to forestall a multitude of exceptions for interests less than life.

The perception of the humanity of the fetus and the weighing of fetal rights against other human rights constituted the work of the moral analysts. But what spirit animated their abstract judgments? For the Christian community it was the injunction of Scripture to love your neighbor as yourself. The fetus as human was a neighbor; his life had parity with one's own. The commandment gave life to what otherwise would have been only rational calculation.

The commandment could be put in humanistic as well as theological terms: Do not injure your fellow man without reason. In these terms, once the humanity of the fetus is perceived, abortion is never right except in self-defense. When life must be taken to save life, reason alone cannot say that a mother must prefer a child's life to her own. With this exception, now of great rarity, abortion violates the rational humanist tenet of the equality of human lives.

For Christians the commandment to love had received a special imprint in that the exemplar proposed of love was the love of the Lord for his disciples. In the light given by this example, self-sacrifice carried to the point of death seemed in the extreme situations not without meaning. In the less extreme cases, preference for one's own interest to the life of another seemed to express cruelty or selfishness irreconcilable with the demands of love.

The Moral Significance of Birth

MARY ANNE WARREN

. . . I HAVE DEFENDED what most regard as needing no defense, i.e., the ascription of an equal right to life to human infants. Under reasonably favorable conditions that policy can protect the rights and interests of all concerned, including infants, biological parents, and potential adoptive parents.

But if protecting infants is such a good idea, then why is it not a good idea to extend the same strong protections to sentient fetuses? The question is not whether sentient fetuses ought to be protected: of course they should. Most women readily accept the responsibility for doing whatever they can to ensure that their (voluntarily continued) pregnancies are successful, and that no avoidable harm comes to the fetus. Negligent or malevolent actions by third parties which result in death or injury to pregnant women or their potential children should be subject to moral censure and legal prosecution. A just and caring society would do much more than ours does to protect the health of all its members, including pregnant women. The question is whether the law should accord to late-term fetuses *exactly the same* protections as are accorded to infants and older human beings.

The case for doing so might seem quite strong. We normally regard not only infants, but all other postnatal human beings as entitled to strong legal protections *so long as they are either sentient or capable of an eventual return to sentience*. We do not also require that they demonstrate a capacity for thought, self-awareness, or social re-

MARY ANNE WARREN is a Professor of Philosophy at San Francisco State University.

lationships before we conclude that they have an equal right to life. Such restrictive criteria would leave too much room for invidious discrimination. The eternal propensity of powerful groups to rationalize sexual, racial, and class oppression by claiming that members of the oppressed group are mentally or otherwise "inferior" leaves little hope that such restrictive criteria could be applied without bias. Thus, for human beings past the prenatal stage, the capacity for sentience — or for a return to sentience — may be the only pragmatically defensible criterion for the ascription of full and equal basic rights. If so, then both theoretical simplicity and moral consistency may seem to require that we extend the same protections to sentient human beings that have not yet been born as to those that have.

But there is one crucial consideration which this argument leaves out. It is impossible to treat fetuses *in utero* as if they were persons without treating women as if they were something less than persons. The extension of equal rights to sentient fetuses would inevitably license severe violations of women's basic rights to personal autonomy and physical security. In the first place, it would rule out most second-trimester abortions performed to protect the woman's life or health. Such abortions might sometimes be construed as a form of self-defense. But the right to self-defense is not usually taken to mean that one may kill innocent persons just because their continued existence poses some threat to one's own life or health. If abortion must be justified as self-defense, then it will rarely be performed until the woman is already in extreme danger, and perhaps not

Hypatia *4.3: 46–65. Permission granted by Indiana University Press and Mary Anne Warren.*

even then. Such a policy would cost some women their lives, while others would be subjected to needless suffering and permanent physical harm.

Other alarming consequences of the drive to extend more equal rights to fetuses are already apparent in the United States. In the past decade it has become increasingly common for hospitals or physicians to obtain court orders requiring women in labor to undergo cesarean sections, against their will, for what is thought to be the good of the fetus. Such an extreme infringement of the woman's right to security against physical assault would be almost unthinkable once the infant has been born. No parent or relative can legally be forced to undergo any surgical procedure, even possibly to save the life of a child, once it is born. But pregnant women can sometimes be forced to undergo major surgery, for the supposed benefit of the fetus. As George Annas (1982, 16) points out, forced cesareans threaten to reduce women to the status of inanimate objects—containers which may be opened at the will of others in order to get at their contents.

Perhaps the most troubling illustration of this trend is the case of Angela Carder, who died at George Washington University Medical Center in June 1987, two days after a court-ordered cesarean section. Ms. Carder had suffered a recurrence of an earlier cancer, and was not expected to live much longer. Her physicians agreed that the fetus was too undeveloped to be viable, and that Carder herself was probably too weak to survive the surgery. Although she, her family, and the physicians were all opposed to a cesarean delivery, the hospital administration—evidently believing it had a legal obligation to try to save the fetus—sought and obtained a court order to have it done. As predicted, both Carder and her infant died soon after the operation.[1] This woman's rights to autonomy, physical integrity, and life itself were forfeit—not just because of her illness, but because of her pregnancy.

Such precedents are doubly alarming in the light of the development of new techniques of fetal therapy. As fetuses come to be regarded as

patients, with rights that may be in direct conflict with those of their mothers, and as the *in utero* treatment of fetuses becomes more feasible, more and more pregnant women may be subjected against their will to dangerous and invasive medical interventions. If so, then we may be sure that there will be other Angela Carders.

Another danger in extending equal legal protections to sentient fetuses is that women will increasingly be blamed, and sometimes legally prosecuted, when they miscarry or give birth to premature, sick, or abnormal infants. It is reasonable to hold the caretakers of infants legally responsible if their charges are harmed because of their avoidable negligence. But when a woman miscarries or gives birth to an abnormal infant, the cause of the harm might be traced to any of an enormous number of actions or circumstances which would not normally constitute any legal offense. She might have gotten too much exercise or too little, eaten the wrong foods or the wrong quantity of the right ones, or taken or failed to take certain drugs. She might have smoked, consumed alcohol, or gotten too little sleep. She might have "permitted" her health to be damaged by hard work, by unsafe employment conditions, by the lack of affordable medical care, by living near a source of industrial pollution, by a physically or mentally abusive partner, or in any number of other ways.

Are such supposed failures on the part of pregnant women potentially to be construed as child abuse or negligent homicide? If sentient fetuses are entitled to the same legal protections as infants, then it would seem so. The danger is not a merely theoretical one. Two years ago in San Diego, a woman whose son was born with brain damage and died several weeks later was charged with felony child neglect. It was said that she had been advised by her physician to avoid sex and illicit drugs, and to go to the hospital immediately if she noticed any bleeding. Instead, she had allegedly had sex with her husband, taken some inappropriate drug, and delayed getting to the hospital for what might have been several hours after the onset of bleeding.

In this case, the charges were eventually dismissed on the grounds that the child protection law invoked had not been intended to apply to cases of this kind. But the multiplication of such cases is inevitable if the strong legal protections accorded to infants are extended to sentient fetuses. A bill recently introduced in the Australian state of New South Wales would make women liable to criminal prosecution if they are found to have smoked during pregnancy, eaten unhealthful foods, or taken any other action which can be shown to have adversely affected the development of the fetus (*The Australian*, July 5, 1988, 5). Such an approach to the protection of fetuses authorizes the legal regulation of virtually every aspect of women's public and private lives, and thus is incompatible with even the most minimal right to autonomy. Moreover, such laws are apt to prove counterproductive, since the fear of prosecution may deter poor or otherwise vulnerable women from seeking needed medical care during pregnancy. I am not suggesting that women whose apparent negligence causes prenatal harm to their infants should always be immune from criticism. However, if we want to improve the health of infants we would do better to provide the services women need to protect their health, rather than seeking to use the law to punish those whose prenatal care has been less than ideal.

There is yet another problem, which may prove temporary but which remains significant at this time. The extension of legal personhood to sentient fetuses would rule out most abortions performed because of severe fetal abnormalities, such as Down syndrome or spina bifida. Abortions performed following amniocentesis are usually done in the latter part of the second trimester, since it is usually not possible to obtain test results earlier. Methods of detecting fetal abnormalities at earlier stages, such as chorion biopsy, may eventually make late abortion for reasons of fetal abnormality unnecessary; but these methods are not yet widely available.

The elimination of most such abortions might be a consequence that could be accepted, were the society willing to provide adequate support for the handicapped children and adults who would come into being as a result of this policy. However, our society is not prepared to do this. In the absence of adequate communally-funded care for the handicapped, the prohibition of such abortions is exploitative of women. Of course, the male relatives of severely handicapped persons may also bear heavy burdens. Yet the heaviest portion of the daily responsibility generally falls upon mothers and other female relatives. If fetuses are not yet persons (and women are), then a respect for the equality of persons should lead to support for the availability of abortion in cases of severe fetal abnormality.[2]

Such arguments will not persuade those who deeply believe that fetuses are already persons, with equal moral rights. How, they will ask, is denying legal equality to sentient fetuses different from denying it to any other powerless group of human beings? If some human beings are more equal than others, then how can any of us feel safe? The answer is twofold.

First, pregnancy is a relationship different from any other, including that between parents and already-born children. It is not just one of innumerable situations in which the rights of one individual may come into conflict with those of another; it is probably the *only* case in which the legal personhood of one human being is necessarily incompatible with that of another. Only in pregnancy is the organic functioning of one human individual biologically inseparable from that of another. This organic unity makes it impossible for others to provide the fetus with medical care or any other presumed benefit, except by doing something to or for the woman. To try to "protect" the fetus other than through her cooperation and consent is effectively to nullify her right to autonomy, and potentially to expose her to violent physical assaults such as would not be legally condoned in any other type of case. The uniqueness of pregnancy helps to explain why the toleration of abortion does not lead to the disenfranchisement of other groups of human beings, as opponents of abortion often claim. For biological as well as psychological reasons, "It is all but impossible to extrapolate from attitudes towards fetal life attitudes toward [other] existing human life" (D. Callahan 1970, 474).

But, granting the uniqueness of pregnancy, why is it *women's* rights that should be privileged? If women and fetuses cannot both be legal persons then why not favor fetuses, e.g., on the grounds that they are more helpless, or more innocent, or have a longer life expectancy? It is difficult to justify this apparent bias towards women without appealing to the empirical fact that women are already persons in the usual, nonlegal sense—already thinking, self-aware, fully social beings—and fetuses are not. Regardless of whether we stress the intrinsic properties of persons, or the social and relational dimensions of personhood, this distinction remains. Even sentient fetuses do not yet have either the cognitive capacities or the richly interactive social involvements typical of persons.

This "not yet" is morally decisive. It is wrong to treat persons as if they do not have equal basic rights. Other things being equal, it is worse to deprive persons of their most basic moral and legal rights than to refrain from extending such rights to beings that are not persons. This is one important element of truth in the self-awareness criterion. If fetuses were already thinking, self-aware, socially responsive members of communities, then nothing could justify refusing them the equal protection of the law. In that case, we would sometimes be forced to balance the rights of the fetus against those of the woman, and sometimes the scales might be almost equally weighted. However, if women are persons and fetuses are not, then the balance must swing towards women's rights.

CONCLUSION

Birth is morally significant because it marks the end of one relationship and the beginning of others. It marks the end of pregnancy, a relationship so intimate that it is impossible to extend the equal protection of the law to fetuses without severely infringing women's most basic rights. Birth also marks the beginning of the infant's existence as a socially responsive member of a human community. Although the infant is not instantly transformed into a person at the moment of birth, it does become a biologically separate human being. As such, it can be known and cared for as a particular individual. It can also be vigorously protected without negating the basic rights of women. There are circumstances in which infanticide may be the best of a bad set of options. But our own society has both the ability and the desire to protect infants, and there is no reason why we should not do so.

We should not, however, seek to extend the same degree of protection to fetuses. Both late-term fetuses and newborn infants are probably capable of sentience. Both are precious to those who want children; and both need to be protected from a variety of possible harms. All of these factors contribute to the moral standing of the late-term fetus, which is substantial. However, to extend equal legal rights to fetuses is necessarily to deprive pregnant women of the rights to personal autonomy, physical integrity, and sometimes life itself. *There is room for only one person with full and equal rights inside a single human skin.* That is why it is birth, rather than sentience, viability, or some other prenatal milestone that must mark the beginning of legal personhood.

NOTES

1. See *Civil Liberties,* 363 (Winter 1988), 12, and Lawrence Lader, "Regulating Birth: Is the State Going Too Far?" *Conscience* IX: 5 (September/October, 1988), 5–6.

2. It is sometimes argued that using abortion to prevent the birth of severely handicapped infants will inevitably lead to a loss of concern for handicapped persons. I doubt that this is true. There is no need to confuse the question of whether it is good that persons be born handicapped with the very different question of whether handicapped persons are entitled to respect, support, and care.

REFERENCES

Annas, George. 1982. Forced cesareans: The most unkindest cut of all. *Hastings Center Report* 12(3): 16–17;45.

The Australian, Tuesday, July 5, 1988, 5.

Callahan, Daniel. 1970. *Abortion: Law, choice and morality.* New York: Macmillan.

Abortion, Forced Labor, and War

LAURA PURDY

OPPONENTS OF ABORTION often assert that most abortions are carried out just for women's "convenience." Suppose that, for the sake of argument, one were to concede this claim. Would it follow, as opponents of abortion assume, that these abortions are immoral and ought to be prohibited? No. Attention to consistent social policy requires us first to determine whether similar deaths are condoned in other contexts. If so, then abortion cannot justifiably be prohibited unless some morally relevant difference is found between these cases.[1]

A careful look at social policy reveals a surprisingly high tolerance for practices that routinely cause deaths. Some, like building bridges to speed traffic, are appropriately described as a matter of convenience. Others, like growing tobacco for profit, are only charitably so de-

scribed. . . . In such mortal tradeoffs, education alone could prevent deaths; in others, changing the situation would require that resources be allocated differently. We, as a society, often prefer to keep costs low even if that results in more deaths. Yet in the case of abortion, it is argued that preventing fetal deaths is worth any price. . . . The morally troubling point here is that these deaths are excused by pointing to a justifying context. Yet when the same kind of justifying context is proposed for abortion, it is rejected because life is so sacred that no competing values outweigh it. This state of affairs constitutes a costly double standard for women who bear most of the resulting burdens.

Now many abortions would be unnecessary if society were organized somewhat differently. Some of these alternative arrangements would be expensive, although all would provide worthwhile benefits on top of their power to reduce the need for abortions. But opponents of abortion can prohibit abortion and shift its burdens to women by rejecting the alternatives as "too

LAURA PURDY, recently a visiting Bioethicist and Professor of Philosophy at the University of Toronto Joint Centre for Bioethics, University Health Network, Department of Philosophy, is a Professor of Philosophy at Wells College, NY.

expensive." . . . If they, instead of women, bore the burden, one wonders whether they would judge the benefit to be worth the cost. For the real social perception of the value of life emerges every time a safety standard or a vaccination program is rejected as "too expensive."

Until this double standard is eradicated, it would be inconsistent to call for an end to abortions for convenience. But suppose society set itself the goal of preventing other convenience based deaths? It seems reasonable to suppose that this turn of events would include a new willingness to undertake changes that would substantially lessen women's need for abortions.[2] So there would be relatively few cases where women would want abortions for the kinds of reasons that are now labeled matters of convenience. . . . I will argue here that the values preserved by full access to abortion are not of the relatively trivial sort implied by the word "convenience" that has been attached to them by opponents of abortion. They are, in fact, much more significant.

TYPES OF ABORTION

Many people are prepared to concede that some abortions are justifiable. Among them are those that avert or remedy threats to a woman's life or health, or that result from rape or incest. More liberal moderates may also countenance abortion for fetal deformity, poverty, or heavy family responsibilities. It is generally understood that these are not mere matters of convenience. Just what principles permit these cases to slip by the gatekeepers?

What they seem to have in common is that a woman's access to abortion has important benefits for others. Rape looks quite different. Reasonable people agree that rape is a particularly horrible form of assault, although many still believe that women themselves are at fault when they are raped. Why then is the exception for rape so widely accepted? One plausible line of reasoning is that rape followed by pregnancy embarrasses the man who is supposed to be in charge of a particular woman. Incest may also involve rape; in addition, it may produce children with serious problems; the same is true of fetuses thought to have biological defects. They, like the children of women in extreme poverty, may well become costly social burdens.

Focusing on the benefits, not for women, but for those around them, is characteristic of "moderate" treatments of abortion. As Rosalind Petchesky points out, even feminist positions tend to be influenced by "the association of fetus with 'baby' and the aborting woman with 'bad mother,' . . . and the assumption that sex for pleasure is 'wrong' (for women) and the women who indulge in it have to pay a price. . . ."[3] These ways of looking at women and sex "obscure the ways in which abortion is a basic need of women, which is different from either a 'necessity' (unchosen) or a 'choice' (unnecessary)."[4]

Even a feminist utopia would not eradicate the women's desire for abortions. As I have argued elsewhere,[5] it is a mistake to think that only patriarchy and capitalism stand in the way of women rearing every child they conceive. Although women clearly need much more help than they are getting, and they do often abort or give up their babies because they cannot cope with existing social conditions, the way these claims creates a standard that could make it quite difficult for a pregnant woman to refuse motherhood.

However, not even an unimaginably supportive society will take all the burden of motherhood from women. . . . There will always be women whose other projects are incompatible with the demands of motherhood, and it is surely best for both woman and child if such a reluctantly pregnant woman either aborts or lets others do the rearing. Even if the perfect contraceptive may considerably reduce this problem, it will not, given human nature, make it go away altogether. In any case, do we really want a society where women cannot change their minds about a given pregnancy?

As Kristen Luker notes, "this round of the abortion debate is so passionate and hard-fought *because it is a referendum on the place and meaning of motherhood.*"[6] But is the issue motherhood? Or womanhood? Nancy (Ann) Davis writes: "both sets of women seemed to accept the conventional wisdom that it is the special capacity to nurture that sets females apart . . . once one considers the possibility that the 'essential female characteristic' (that is, nurturance) is not strongly tied to biological reproduction . . . the question "Why should nurturance — or indeed, any particular characteristic or set of allegedly female, cultural characteristics — be seen as the basis of female gender-identity?" seems inescapable.[7] . . .

As feminists have been pointing out for some time, much of women's oppression can be traced to their nurturing role.[8] If this kind of essentialism were true, then justice would require that society reward female nurturing as much as more traditionally masculine activities. But that approach ignores the vast psychological differences among women, and assumes human women have more in common with females of other species than with human men.[9] That these assumptions are widespread helps explain why the notion of equal rights for women still seems so alien to most people. Yet it is only in this context of equality that the full consequences of unwanted childbearing can be evaluated. For only such a perspective makes it possible to compare the sacrifices required by it with men's expectations of freedom. In this light, unwanted childbearing looks a lot less like a labor of love than the kind of threat that impels men to war.

Because public life is still so male centered, there is little social recognition of what it means to become a mother. Laurence Tribe puts it beautifully: "Pregnancy does not merely 'inconvenience' the woman for a time; it gradually turns her into a mother and makes her one for all time."[10] Indeed, "Having a child is a permanent commitment. Yet the decision is often a blind one, and the outcome is unpredictable . . . there is no way of knowing whether a child will be a source of love, comfort, and inexpressible joy or worry, pain, and torment. . . ."[11] For poor women, of course, having children has still more fundamental consequences, as Surgeon General Jocelyn Elders notes.[12] The financial cost of children is suggestive of the demands of childrearing. According to the U.S. Dept. of Agriculture, raising a "no-frills" kid to the age of eighteen costs some \$100,000; college adds another \$100,000.[13] Middle class children cost more still, and neither of these figures includes opportunity costs for women who choose to be housewives.[14] Other costs are substantial.[15]

Some human rights legislation addresses the question of how such social burdens should be allocated. Consider the ILO Forced Labor Convention of 1930.[16] It prohibits forced labor except in a series of narrowly restricted cases.[17] In particular, forced labor is not to be used as a means of political repression, economic development, or "as a means of racial, social, national or religious discrimination."[18] Forced labor cannot be used to benefit private parties. Furthermore, . . . the work or service must be "of present or imminent necessity," it must not "lay too heavy a burden upon the present population," and it must have "been impossible to obtain voluntary labor for carrying out the work or rendering the service by the offer of rates of wages and conditions of labor not less favorable than those prevailing in the area concerned for similar work or service."[19]

It is instructive that "the maximum period for which any person may be taken for forced or compulsory labor of all kinds in any one period of twelve months shall not exceed sixty days," that "the normal working hours of any person from whom forced or compulsory labor is exacted shall be the same as those prevailing in the case of voluntary labor, and the hours worked in excess of the normal working hours shall be remunerated at the rates prevailing in the case of overtime for voluntary labor," and that "a weekly day of rest shall be granted to all persons from whom forced or compulsory labor of any kind is exacted."[20] Furthermore, wages are to be paid "to each worker individually and not to his tribal chief or to any other authority."[21]

Those responsible for this document would, no doubt, be shocked at the suggestion that it might have some relevance for women's child-related labor. Forced labor seems to be a well-defined notion, and the authors are quick to exclude women from its demands altogether. [Although] . . . from an egalitarian perspective, much of what women experience might fall squarely under its purview.[22] Perhaps they would, if pressed, include women's child-related work with "the work or service which forms part of the normal civil obligations of the citizens of a fully self-governing country," or "minor communal services of a kind which, being performed by the members of the community in the direct interest of the community. . . ."[23]

The authors of the ILO Convention on Forced Labor would no doubt be inclined to compare women's child-related labor to military service expected of men, or perhaps even men's productive labor. But these comparisons are not successful. It is true that most societies have expected men to be available for military service. Such service has often severely limited men's liberty and sadly, has cost many their lives.[24] However, periods of service are usually limited, well short of the twenty years or so it takes to raise a child. . . . Furthermore, men often enjoy special privileges like free medical care or veteran's points in civil service exams, in return for their military service.[25]

Today studies show that women generally work more hours than men, since they do both productive and reproductive labor. . . . Furthermore, men, except again for those on the bottom, have many more options about what work they will undertake, and are far more often rewarded for their work with privilege, money, and power.[26] Attempts to fend off uncomfortable comparisons of women's child-related work to forced labor would face additional serious difficulties. . . . It is surely doubtful that women as a group or their representatives agree to compulsory pregnancy and its attendant childrearing duties.[27] Nor would they agree that this unequal division of labor would be in the interest of the community as a whole. . . . So while reproductive service may very well be viewed as part of "the normal civic obligations of the citizens of a fully self-governing country," the burning question is whether that assumption is morally tenable, especially where overpopulation is more of a problem than underpopulation.

It is instructive to compare the conditions under which forced labor is considered acceptable by the 1930 Convention with those under which most women rear children. First, forced labor is prohibited where it is used as a means of discrimination. It is true that sexual discrimination is not included in the list of unacceptable discriminations, but that just demonstrates how widely accepted is women's second class status. If sexual discrimination were included, compulsory childbearing and rearing would have to be illegal, given their consequences.[28] Second, forced labor is not supposed to benefit private parties, yet forcing women to bear and rear children against their will often benefits men who want children without taking full responsibility for them.[29] Otherwise women could choose to conceive only by men who can be trusted to share the burdens of reproduction as fully as possible.[30]

Third, compulsory pregnancy and childrearing does not meet the requirement that forced labor be of important and direct interest to the community. Although it is true that once children are born their care is of . . . direct interest to the community, the same is not true of compulsory pregnancy itself unless a community is threatened with extinction. . . . Furthermore, there is little discussion about whether forced childbearing and rearing imposes "too heavy" a burden on women, but consider the outcry if state-imposed mandates placed the same constraints on men in the name of community service.

Last, but not least, mothering, especially mothering in poverty, violates the time limitations placed on acceptable forced labor. Remember that forced labor can be required no more than sixty days a year, but women rearing children they did not want must often labor on their behalf 365 days a year. Forced labor is to be limited to normal working hours, with overtime for extra hours. But most women work, directly or indirectly, on behalf of their children for more than forty hours a week; nor do they receive pay of any kind for their direct labor, no matter how long their hours.[31] Remember, too, that there is to be a weekly day of rest; but there is no day of rest for most women raising children.

This kind of comparison suggests that despite many social changes, the situation for many women today isn't so different from the one that prompted John Stuart Mill to comment: "The general opinion of men is supposed to be, that the natural vocation of a woman is that of a wife and mother. . . . I should like to hear somebody openly enunciating the doctrine . . . 'It is necessary to society that women should marry and produce children. They will not do so unless they are compelled. Therefore it is necessary to compel them.' The merits of the case would then be clearly defined." He compares this case with the argument for slavery, which ran thus: "It is necessary that cotton and sugar should be grown. White men cannot produce them. Negroes will not, for any wages which we choose to give. *Ergo* they must be compelled."[32]

The core of what Mill has to say here is still relevant. Of course despotic husbands may now be divorced, but the existence of children often leads women to stay with abusive men. Single parenthood places enormous burdens on most women, and is likely to be comfortable only for the wealthiest women. But few women are wealthy. The application of Mill's moral here is that if having children were properly respected and remunerated, then many women would undoubtedly choose to have them even if they were free not to do so. Forcing pregnant women to choose between life-threatening illegal abortions or childbearing suggests that people are well aware that if women had other choices they would be much less likely to choose motherhood under the current circumstances.

Revolutionary theory, just war theory, and even international law recognize certain threats to life as a defense of violence. One common defense of abortion draws upon this appeal to self-defense by arguing that women have a right to kill fetuses which threaten their lives. But it is erroneously assumed that the defense of violence is limited to threats to life, whereas a variety of different threats are widely recognized as such a defense.

Self-determination plays a central role in international law. In 1984, the Human Rights Committee adopted a special comment on article 1 of the International Covenant on Civil and Political Rights, declaring that "the right of self-determination is often of particular importance because its realization is an essential condition for the effective guarantee and observance of individual human rights and for the promotion and strengthening of those rights."[33] Furthermore, the same document emphasizes that . . . "the self-determination of citizens, individually, on the basis of the recognition of their political rights, is a prerequisite of the effective realization of self-determination as the people's collective right."[34] The document recognizes this right only for peoples who are under "colonial and alien" domination, not ones already organized in the form of a free state, since it does not wish to promote the disruption of countries. It comments, however, that such a government must represent "the whole people belonging to the territory without distinction as to race, creed or colour," a standard which is, of course, conspicuous for the absence of sex.

In 1979, the United Nations issued a further study of self-determination, entitled *The Right to Self-Determination: Implementation of United Nations Resolutions.*[35] This document elaborates the notions of political, economic, social, and cultural factors inherent in the concept of self-determination. It holds that peoples have a right to determine their economic system, and that

they enjoy permanent sovereignty over their natural resources. It also holds that "the social aspects of the right of peoples to self-determination are related, in particular, to the promotion
of social justice, to which every people is entitled
and which, in its broadest sense, implies the
right to the effective enjoyment by all the individual members of a particular people of their
economic and social rights without any discrimination whatsoever. Cultural self-determination,
in its turn, implies a right to determine and establish the cultural regime or system under
which it is to live.[36] . . .

If self-determination is so highly valued, what
role does it play in contemporary thinking about
war? Michael Walzer writes that the defense of
rights is the only reason for fighting, and that
"the wrong the aggressor commits is to force
men and women to risk their lives for the sake of
their rights."[37] The central rights he emphasizes
are territorial integrity and political sovereignty.[38] Using what he calls the "legalist paradigm" that sees the realm of states as a society of
individuals writ large, these threats can reasonably be translated as bodily control and some degree of control over one's resources.[39]

Those who find my comparison of women's
and men's rights to self-determination perverse
will no doubt be distressed by my attempt to
conflate individual rights and those of nations.
They will attempt to distinguish them by laying
out morally relevant distinctions between the situation of women and that of wronged nations.
The central political problem for women, as I see
it, is that for various reasons, women are likely to
remain spread among national groups rather
than gathering together in such a way that their
special interests could be protected. But the
moral — as opposed to the political — significance
of this state of affairs is questionable. What matters morally, and what ought to matter politically, is that the rights at issue for them are those
for which men are often ready to die.

Compulsory pregnancy would violate
women's self-determination even if they had no

qualms about adopting out their infants. But
women are rarely willing to do that. . . . Although it seems clear that we need to rethink the
importance of biological relationships, children
would be even worse off than they are now if
more individuals rejected responsibility for the
welfare of their children.

The upshot is that few women seriously entertain the notion of giving up a child. Unwanted pregnancy therefore drafts women into
motherhood. But even if such motherhood does
not threaten a woman's life or health, her choices
become much more limited, as most of her resources must now be committed to those children. This state of affairs usually excludes full
participation in the social, cultural, and political
life of society, and, under current arrangements,
often leads to impoverishment and lack of respect for her as a person. In short, motherhood,
especially responsible motherhood, forecloses
many worthwhile options.

The options in question are ones men take for
granted. Although class and race make a big difference in the goods a person enjoys, men generally have — and expect to have — a great deal
more freedom to determine the conditions
under which they will live than similarly situated
women. Men are willing to go to great lengths
to protect these same values. Only a world view
that sees women as less than Kantian persons
could acquiesce in the same judgment on their
behalf. . . .

NOTES

1. I have argued this issue more at length elsewhere. See "Abortion and the Argument from
Convenience."
2. As I argue in "Abortion and the Argument from
Convenience," measures that could reduce the need
for these abortions include universal access to contraception, and the kind of gender equality that empow-
ers to say "no" to sex they don't want and to make sure
that contraception is used in sexual encounters they do
want. These are changes incompatible with the value
systems of many anti-abortion activists, naturally.
Likewise, reducing pregnancies due to contraceptive

failure requires making the development of safe, convenient, and effective contraceptives a priority. And, to reduce the number of abortions necessary for women's health, it would be necessary to take expensive measures to improve women's health in the first place. Addressing the need for abortion for fetal defect would require society to provide universal pre-conception counseling, and care for impaired children and adults. Finally, providing the financial and social support women need to raise more children well would require enormous social changes.

3. Rosalind Pollack Petchesky, *Abortion and Woman's Choice: The State, Sexuality, and Reproductive Freedom* (Boston: Northeastern University Press, 1985), p. 386.

4. Rosalind Pollack Petchesky, *Abortion and Woman's Choice: The State, Sexuality, and Reproductive Freedom* (Boston: Northeastern University Press, 1985), p. 384–5.

5. "Another Look at Contract Pregnancy," *Issues in Reproductive Technology I: An Anthology,* ed., Helen B. Holmes (New York: Garland Press, 1992), pp. 308–9.

6. Kristen Luker, *Abortion and the Politics of Motherhood* (Berkeley: University of California Press, 1984), p. 192.

7. Nancy (Ann) Davis, "The Abortion Debate: The Search for Common Ground, Part I," *Ethics* 103 (April 1993): 516–39; p. 534.

8. See John Stuart Mill, *The Subjection of Women,* . . . Nurturing is by no means the only source of oppression, as psychological studies have been showing for some time. (Studies that show that "healthy" females have what would be considered "unhealthy" human (e.g., male) traits.

9. Not that it is always the females of other species that do most of the nurturing, as feminist biologists have been noticing lately. But, of course, in many species it is the female who bears most of this burden.

10. Laurence H. Tribe, *Abortion: The Clash of Absolutes* (New York: Norton, 1990), p. 104.

11. Susan S. Lang, *Women Without Children: The Reasons, the Rewards, the Regrets* (New York: Pharos Books, 1991), pp. 3–4. She goes on to point out that studies show that "parenthood . . . tends to wreak havoc on a marriage. . . . Study after study confirms that the negative impact of children on marital happiness is pervasive, regardlessof race, religion, education, and wives' employment" (p. 81).

12. ". . . if you're poor and ignorant, with a child, you're a slave. Meaning that you're never going to get out of it. These women are in bondage to a kind of slavery that the 13th Amendment just didn't deal with. . . . You can't control your life." Quoted in "Joce-lyn Elders Toughs It Out," *New York Times Magazine,* January 30, 1994, p. 18.

13. Lang, p. 206.

14. Lang, p. 207.

15. See *In Their Best Interest?*

16. Edward Lawson, *Encyclopedia of Human Rights* (New York: Taylor and Francis, 1991), pp. 802ff.

17. Excluded from the prohibition are 1) work exacted in the course of compulsory military service laws for work of a purely military nature, 2) work that "forms part of the normal civic obligations of the citizens of a fully self-governing country," 3) public work resulting from criminal conviction, 4) work required by a major emergency, and 5) "minor communal services of a kind which, being performed by the members of the community in the direct interest of the said community, can therefore be considered as normal civic obligations incumbent upon the members of the community, provided that the members of the community or their direct representatives shall have the right to be consulted in regard to the need for such services" (Lawson, p. 802).

18. Lawson, *Encyclopedia of Human Rights,* p. 1351.

19. Lawson, *Encyclopedia of Human Rights,* p. 803.

20. Lawson, *Encyclopedia of Human Rights,* p. 803.

21. Interestingly, although "ordinary rations [may be] given as a part of wages, . . . deductions from wages shall not be made either for the payment of taxes or for special food, clothing or accommodation supplied to a worker for the purpose of maintaining him in fit condition to carry on his work . . . or for the supply of tools" (Lawson, p. 804).

22. That authors of human rights documents (most of whom are, after all, men) write from traditional rather than egalitarian perspectives is evident after even a cursory examination of the *Encyclopedia of Human Rights.* Of particular relevance here are the 1957 additions to the ILO Convention on Forced Labor, the ILO Abolition of Forced Labor Convention. The latter asserts that forced labor is prohibited "as a means of racial, social, national or religious discrimination" (1334). Notice the glaring absence of sexual discrimination. Another important example is the comment of the Human Rights committee on article 1 of the International Covenant on Civil and Political Right, which proposes that governments must represent "the whole people belonging to the territory without distinction as to race, creed or colour" 1334). Once again, the potential for lack of representation on the basis of sex either never enters the picture or is dismissed altogether. Presumably the justification for such dismissal is that women's interests are represented by those of the men to whom they are attached.

For trenchant critiques of this notion, see recent feminist scholarship, most notably Susan Okin.

23. Lawson, *Encyclopedia of Human Rights,* p. 802.

24. As has childbearing for women.

25. None of this is to deny that men have often been unjustly robbed by military service or war itself, of their self-determination. But that fact does not imply that women also deserve such ill-treatment. The right response is to attempt to eradicate militarism.

26. Once again, the fact that many men are deprived of significant choices about their work and enjoy few rewards does not justify the same conditions for women. The right response is greater egalitarianism with respect to these matters.

27. By "compulsory pregnancy" I refer to the situation where a pregnant woman is refused an abortion she desires.

28. One might want to distinguish here between intentionally discriminatory actions and those which merely have discriminatory consequences. But if discrimination is the evil, once the causal relationship is known, consequences are what count.

29. This is a particularly interesting issue, as the question of who is benefitted by child-related labor is as yet unresolved. Common arguments against the provision of benefits for individuals who are rearing children are predicated on the assumption that children are a private luxury. It would follow from this position that child-rearing labor does indeed benefit private parties. However, it does seem clear that society as a whole does benefit from having some number of children, assuming it wants a future. But whether it now benefits from the existence of unwanted children is questionable.

30. This raises the question of why women have sexual intercourse with men who are not likely to be reliable partners. Sometimes they have little choice in the matter. The rest of the time such behavior is no doubt voluntary, even if often uninformed. In any case, it is hard to see why women must be held responsible for the full consequences of unwise sexual attraction when men so often go scot free.

31. Some years ago economists began to compile statistics on market rates for the kinds of work undertaken by typical housewives.

32. Mill, "The Subjection of Women," p. 155.

33. Lawson, *Encyclopedia of Human Rights,* p. 1332. The document is UN Doc. A/39/40, Annex VI, para. 1–8.

34. Lawson, *Encyclopedia of Human Rights,* p. 1334.

35. This report was prepared by Mr. Hector Gros Espiell, special rapporteur of the U.N. SubCommission on Prevention of Discrimination and Protection of Minorities. U.N. Publication, Sales No. r/79.XIV.5.

36. Lawson, *Encyclopedia of Human Rights,* p. 1335.

37. Michael Walzer, *Just and Unjust Wars* (New York: Basic Books, 1977), p. 51. Of course, rights violations do not, by themselves, justify war. First, war must be fought according to certain rules, for example those that protect civilians. Secondly, to be just, the decision to go to war must be made by the right authority, with the right intention, and only as a last resort. The war must also be likely to result in peace, and the total evil of the acts done under its name must be proportionate to the good achieved. See Duane L. Cady, *From Warism to Pacifism: A Moral Continuum* (Philadelphia: Temple University Press, 1989), p. 24. These criteria could quite well be applied to decisions about abortion. Notice that abortions are, overall, much less destructive than the average war.

38. Walzer, *Just and Unjust Wars,* p. 52.

39. Walzer, *Just and Unjust Wars,* chap. 4. It is true that he sees these threats as more serious on the international level than he does at the individual level, because there they cannot be countered without risking loss of life. But if the rights in question are considered sufficiently important to kill for at the international level, it is hard to see why they shouldn't be defended with equal vigor at the personal level. After all, Walzer believes that the rights involved in territorial integrity and political sovereignty are based on the rights of individuals, "and from them they take their force" (p. 53). He goes on to assert that "when states are attacked; it is their members who are challenged, not only in their lives, but also in the sum of things they value most, including the political association they have made. If they were not morally entitled to choose their form of government and shape the policies that shape their lives, external coercion would not be a crime; nor could it so easily be said that they had been forced to resist in self-defence. Individual rights (to life and liberty) underlie the most important judgments that we make about war. . . . States rights are simply their collective form" (pp. 53–54).

The Erosion of Minors' Abortion Rights

ALLISON BETH HUBBARD

INTRODUCTION

In the summer of 1988, Becky Bell, a seventeen year old from Massachusetts, died from complications from an illegal abortion.[1] When she first realized she was pregnant, she turned to her boyfriend for help. He "threw her out of his car,"[2] forcing her to face the prospect of her pregnancy alone. She went to Planned Parenthood where she discovered that Massachusetts is one of fourteen states that require notification or consent of the minor's parents before her pregnancy can be terminated.[3] Although Becky had a close relationship with her parents, she was afraid of disappointing them by revealing that she was pregnant.[4] Becky was also convinced that a judge would refuse to grant her an exemption, and her parents would ultimately be notified.[5] Consequently, Becky obtained an illegal abortion. She died shortly thereafter.[6]

Becky's story illustrates the tragic consequences that can result from parental notification statutes. These laws are so oppressive that they induce minors to take incredible risks to avoid their parents' disappointment, anger, or abuse. Parental notification statutes should not be constitutionally permissible because they impose a severe burden on the minor's right to abortion, and can lead to disastrous results.

ALLISON BETH HUBBARD, now Alison Hubbard Ashton, is an Associate Professor at the University of Texas, Austin, with an expertise in behavioral decision theory and information, describing and costing surgical procedures.

The Supreme Court established nineteen years ago that women have the right to abortion.[7] In *Roe v. Wade,* the Court held that the right to privacy encompasses a woman's decision whether to terminate her pregnancy.[8] The Court further held that a state cannot prohibit abortion during the first two trimesters of a woman's pregnancy.[9] In *Planned Parenthood of Central Missouri v. Danforth,*[10] the Court extended the fundamental right of abortion to minors. The Court denied a state the right to confer on parents an absolute veto power over the minor's decision to terminate her pregnancy. Later in *Bellotti v. Baird,* Justice Powell stated in dicta that although a state may require parental consent prior to a minor's abortion, the state must also provide a judicial-bypass procedure whereby a minor has an opportunity to prove she is mature enough to decide to obtain an abortion, or in the alternative, that the abortion is in her best interest.[11]

The Court has thus established that minors have a right to abortion. In *Hodgson v. Minnesota*[12] and *Ohio v. Akron Center for Reproductive Health,*[13] however, the Court upheld statutes which impose severe burdens on a minor's right to procure an abortion. The Minnesota statute in *Hodgson* requires that both parents receive notification forty-eight hours before a female under the age of eighteen may obtain an abortion.[14] The statute also provides an escape clause in the event a court holds the two-parent notification requirement unconstitutional. This escape clause consists of a judicial-bypass procedure.[15] This procedure allows the minor to receive a court's permission to circumvent the required notification of her parents.

Originally published in UCLA Women's Law Journal *1, 1(1991): 227–44. Copyright 1991, The Regents of the University of California. All Rights Reserved.*

The Court was extremely fractured in upholding the Minnesota statute. Four Justices would have upheld the statute even without the judicial-bypass procedure.[16] Another four indicated that they would have invalidated the two-parent notification requirement even when it included a judicial-bypass provision.[17] Justice O'Connor, who cast the deciding vote, held that the two-parent notification requirement is only constitutional when it is supplemented with the judicial-bypass provision. The Minnesota statute was, therefore, upheld because the bypass procedure provides the minor an alternative to parental notification, and, in Justice O'Connor's view, is not unduly burdensome on the minor's right to abortion.[18]

This rationale undervalues the extreme burden on the minor's privacy rights when she is forced to divulge sensitive and personal information about herself during an intimidating court procedure. Justice O'Connor's holding also recognizes parental notification requirements as valid state legislation, which conflicts with well-established constitutional doctrine that a state cannot interfere with a female's decision to terminate her pregnancy before the third trimester.[19] The Court further curtailed a minor's access to abortion in *Ohio v. Akron Center for Reproductive Health*.[20] Under the Ohio law, it is a crime for a physician to perform an abortion on an unmarried woman under eighteen years of age without notifying one of her parents.[21] While the minor also has the option of obtaining judicial authorization in lieu of parental notification,[22] this option is severely limited by the various procedural traps in the Ohio bypass procedure.

From the moment the minor files the complaint, she is subjected to complicated procedures, a lack of anonymity, and a heightened burden of proof standard. Additionally, the process could take days or weeks, yet the state provides no practical recourse for the minor if the court fails to make a ruling. The length of the process will prohibit some minors from obtaining an abortion until later in their pregnancies, thereby increasing the costs and health risks of the surgical procedure.[23]

This Recent Development will illustrate how the Court, in both *Hodgson* and *Akron Center*, overlooked the practical effects of the statutes involved. Specifically, the Court failed to appreciate the position of minors in modern families and the extent to which notification statutes and judicial-bypass procedures burden their right to privacy. The Court upheld these parental notification statutes even though the states failed to prove any resulting benefits to minors, parents, or families. Under a traditional fundamental rights analysis, a state cannot impose burdens on minors' abortion rights without effectively furthering a compelling state interest. The Court, however, applied only a rational basis review in examining these statutes. The Court was unwilling to speculate on the underlying intentions of the parental notification statutes, even though the purported intentions of the statutes were not being furthered by the statutes. Under this lower standard of scrutiny, these statutes should be held unconstitutional because Minnesota and Ohio failed to prove that their laws are even rationally related to their purported interests. The Court's application of a lower standard of review when examining these abortion statutes raises serious questions about the future of abortion rights of all women.

I. THE BURDENS OF A PARENTAL NOTIFICATION REQUIREMENT

Although *Hodgson* appeared at first glance to be a victory for abortion rights because the Court declared the two-parent notification statute unconstitutional without a judicial-bypass procedure, the Court's reasoning reveals an undervaluation of minors' abortion rights.

This reasoning led to the Court's subsequent upholding of the one-parent notification statute in *Akron Center.* Several members of the Court believe that a woman's decision to control her own reproduction is a "liberty interest" not a "fundamental right" protected by the fourteenth amendment.[24] This change in terminology is significant because a state can subject a liberty interest to regulation that would be impermissible under a traditional fundamental rights analysis.[25]

Under a traditional fundamental rights analysis, state laws which regulate abortion must be necessary to further a compelling state interest.[26] Nevertheless, a majority of the Court is now willing to allow states to regulate abortion, if the state's means are reasonably related to a legitimate state interest.[27] Thus, statutes that abridge abortion rights will only be given a rational basis examination.[28] In *Hodgson,* the state purported to have three interests in implementing a parental notification statute: (1) an interest in the pregnant minor's welfare; (2) an interest in preserving parents' right to raise their children; and (3) an interest in protecting the family unit.[29] . . .

A. The Welfare of the Pregnant Minor

Justices Kennedy, Rehnquist, White, and Scalia held that the state has a legitimate interest in ensuring that minors have the assistance of their parents when deciding whether to obtain an abortion.[30] Justice Stevens also maintained that the state has a legitimate interest in the protection of minors whose "immaturity, inexperience, and lack of judgment may sometimes impair their ability to exercise their rights wisely."[31] The failure in Justice Stevens's analysis is that it is precisely this immaturity that supports enabling minors to obtain an abortion without parental notification. The younger and more immature the minor, the less equipped she will be to cope with an unintended child.

Older minors, on the other hand, are better able to determine, without state interference, whether the abortion is in their best interest.

Forced notification will also deter minors who fear revealing their pregnancy to their parents from obtaining an abortion as soon as they are aware of the pregnancy. The resulting delay is potentially dangerous to the minor's health,[32] and in extreme cases the minor may choose to obtain an illegal abortion[33] to avoid parental notification.[34]

Moreover, many parental notification statutes require that a minor wait a certain period of time after both parents have been notified before terminating her pregnancy, which will cause even greater delay. Minnesota's statute requires that the minor wait forty-eight hours, while the Ohio statute imposes a twenty-four hour waiting period on the minor.[35] According to the Court, this requirement serves the state's interest in ensuring informed decision making while imposing only a minimal burden on the minor's right.[36] This reasoning, however, overlooks the increased health risks caused by the delay.[37] Such an increase in the health risks of the abortion procedure imposes a severe—not a minimal—burden on the minor's rights. . . .

Besides the health risks, waiting periods combined with parental notice requirements like those found in both *Hodgson* and *Akron Center* will severely limit certain minors' access to abortion. The waiting period enables parents who have religious or personal beliefs opposing abortion the opportunity to interfere with the minor's personal decision. To hold that mere notification does not burden the minor's choice is misguided and disregards the extent to which parents exert control over their children's lives. . . . Parents usually exert a great amount of economic control over their children, and many could even physically prevent their daughters from asserting their abortion rights.

Thus, parental notification requirements deprive minors of their established constitutional right to abortion.[38] . . . Furthermore, under Justice O'Connor's "unduly burdensome" analysis, parental notification requirements are unconstitutional because they unduly infringe upon minors' abortion rights; and these requirements are not necessary to advance the states' interest in pregnant minors' welfare.

B. The Interest in Protecting Parental Authority

According to Justice Stevens, the state's purported interest in protecting parental rights directly conflicts with the right of one parent to assert his or her authority without the interference of the other parent.[39] Justice Stevens viewed this intrusion on the parents' rights as unjustified, particularly in the case of the divorced family.[40] . . . He believed that forcing notification of both parents unreasonably burdens parental rights. . . . It is clear from other Supreme Court opinions that Justice Stevens believes that one-parent notification is constitutionally acceptable.[41] Therefore, Justice Stevens's concern for parental rights—not his concern for minors' abortion rights—persuaded him to hold the two-parent requirement unconstitutional.

. . . To ignore the minor's rights is to ignore the severe financial, emotional, and physical strains that can occur when a minor is forced to bear a child. It is precisely this disregard for the abortion rights of minors that led the Court to uphold the one-parent notification statute in *Akron Center.* Even more disturbing is the Court's implication that it may be willing to allow a one-parent notification requirement even in the absence of a judicial-bypass procedure.[42] Justice Stevens's reasoning in *Hodgson,* therefore, could result in a law which gives the minor no alternative to parental notification.

C. An Interest in Protecting the Family Unit

Parental notification statutes also fail to further any state interest in protecting the family unit.[43] Forced notification is potentially devastating in dysfunctional families[44] and could spark violence and abuse.[45] Although Justice Stevens views this as a problem with two-parent notification requirements, he fails to recognize the same difficulties with a one-parent notification requirement.[46] It is doubtful that familial communications will improve in dysfunctional families as a result of parental notification of even one parent. In functional families where minors would probably consult with their parents regardless of any notification requirement, the parental notification statutes will have no effect.

Furthermore, Becky Bell's death illustrates that even in functional families forcing notification could be devastating.[47] Any interest in protecting the family unit by fostering familial communications is not effectively furthered by parental notification requirements. Moreover, by interfering with the family the states are actually threatening the family unit.[48] Therefore, the statutes are not rationally related to the state's purported goal of protecting the family unit.

II. THE INADEQUACIES AND BURDENS OF A JUDICIAL-BYPASS PROCEDURE

Justice O'Connor, who cast the deciding vote in *Hodgson,* was the only justice to hold that the two-parent notification requirement is constitutional when coupled with the judicial-bypass procedure.[49] She reasoned that, although the statute lacks a sufficient justification for the state's interference with family decision making, a judicial-bypass provision rescues the statute because requiring the minor to appear before a court does not unduly burden the minor's right.[50] In Justice O'Connor's view, if the statute is not unduly burdensome, then it need only be rationally related to a legitimate state purpose.[51]

In *Hodgson,* none of the judges who testified at the District Court level identified any positive effects of the bypass procedure.[52] These judges testified that the bypass procedure produced "fear, tension, anxiety, and shame among minors, causing some who were mature, and some whose best interests would have been served by an abortion" to notify their parents or to continue the pregnancy.[53] The bypass procedure sometimes caused delays of over one week, which increased the medical risks "to a statistically significant degree."[54]

Other considerations support these judges' testimony that a judicial-bypass procedure is oppressive. A court proceeding could be so frightening and confusing for the minor, that she may choose to forgo asserting her right simply to avoid the uncomfortable and potentially humiliating situation.[55] In a judicial-bypass procedure the minor must admit to a total stranger that she is sexually active, that perhaps she did not take any precautions to avoid pregnancy, and that she is pregnant. This type of experience could be extremely traumatic. Moreover, in large cities, the ability of minors, especially economically disadvantaged minors, to get transportation to the courthouse could be extremely limited. Thus, a teenager, who is incapable of raising a child emotionally and financially, may be forced to bear a child, precisely because of a lack of resources, confusion, or her fear of the judicial process. It is difficult to imagine why the Court would not view the above procedures as unduly burdensome on minors' abortion rights.

[EDITORS' NOTE: The author's discussion of *City of Akron v. Akron Center for Reproductive Health* is not included here. For the full text, please refer to the longer version in the *UCLA Women's Law Journal*.]

NOTES

1. *Wash. Post,* Aug. 8, 1990, at A3, col. 1.

2. English, Mindless Law, Needless Death, *Boston Globe,* Aug. 22, 1990, at 29, col. 1.

3. *Wash. Post,* Aug. 8, 1990, at A3, col. 1. These states are Alabama, Arkansas, Indiana, Louisiana,

Massachusetts, Minnesota, Missouri, North Dakota, Ohio, Rhode Island, South Carolina, Utah, West Virginia, and Wyoming. Id.

4. Id.

5. The Minnesota law provided for a judicial-bypass procedure so that minors could go to court and ask a judge's permission to obtain an abortion without their parents' knowledge.Id. . . .

6. Id.

7. *Roe v. Wade,* 410 U.S. 113 (1973).

8. Id. at 153.

9. Id. at 164. In *Webster v. Reproductive Health Servs.,* 109 S. Ct. 3040 (1989), the court replaced the trimester framework with a viability standard. Therefore, after *Webster* the state cannot regulate abortion in a way that unduly burdens the right of the female before viability of the fetus.

10. 428 U.S. 52 (1976).

11. 443 U.S. 622 (1979). The validity of Powell's dicta is questionable. A judicial-bypass procedure does very little to ease the burdens of a parental-notification or consent requirement. For a discussion on the problems of judicial-bypass procedures see infra section II.

12. 110 S. Ct. 2926 (1990).

13. 110 S. Ct. 2972 (1990).

14. *Hodgson,* 110 S. Ct. at 2931. This notice is mandatory unless (1) the attending physician certifies that an immediate abortion is necessary to prevent the woman's death, and there is insufficient time to provide the required notice; (2) both of her parents have consented in writing; or (3) the woman declares that she is a victim of parental abuse or neglect, in which case notice of her declaration must be given to the proper authorities. Id. at 2932.

15. Id. Therefore, if the notice provision of the statute were declared unconstitutional by the courts, the judicial-bypass procedure would take effect to preserve the statute's constitutionality. . . .

16. Justices Kennedy, Scalia, White, and Rehnquist would have upheld the law out of paternalistic notions that a "girl of tender years" needs guidance from her parents. See Id. at 2961 (Kennedy, J., dissenting and concurring).

17. Justices Brennan, Blackmun, and Marshall would have invalidated the law because it infringes upon the minor's right to abortion. Justice Stevens, on the other hand, would have invalidated the statute because it unduly infringed upon the parents' rights. See id. at 295256.

18. Id. at 294950 (O'Connor, J., concurring).

19. See *Roe v. Wade,* 410 U.S. 113 (1973). But cf. *Webster v. Reproductive Health Servs.,* 109 S. Ct. 3040 (1989) (changing the trimester test into a viability standard).

20. 110 S. Ct. 2972 (1990).

21. Id. at 2977. The statute provides for some narrow exceptions to this notification requirement. The physician can notify a close relative other than the parent if the minor and the other relative each file an affidavit in the juvenile court stating that the minor fears physical, sexual, or severe emotional abuse from one of her parents. If the physician is unable to contact the parents after reasonable effort, she or he may perform an abortion forty-eight hours after constructive notice by both ordinary and certified mail. The physician may also perform an abortion if a parent has consented in writing. Id.

22. Id.

23. Before the ninth week of pregnancy the risk of death from an abortion is one in 500,000. Between the ninth and twelfth week the risk is one in 67,000. Between the thirteenth and the fifteenth week of pregnancy the risk of death is one in 23,000. And after the fifteenth week the risk of death is one in 8,700. R. Hatcher, F. Stewart, J. Trussell, D. Kowal, F. Guest, G. Stewart, & W. Cates, *Contraceptive Technology 1990–1992* 146 (1990) hereinafter *Contraceptive Technology*.

24. This is the opinion of Justices Rehnquist, Kennedy, O'Connor, White, Scalia and Stevens. See *Hodgson*, 110 S. Ct. at 2937 (Stevens, J., concurring and dissenting). . . .

25. See, e.g., *Roe v. Wade*, 410 U.S. 113, 17273 (Rehnquist, C.J., dissenting).

26. See, e.g., Id. at 15355.

27. See *Hodgson*, 110 S. Ct. at 2944 (Stevens, J., concurring and dissenting). See also Id. at 2967 (Kennedy, J., concurring and dissenting). Justice O'Connor believes that a statute only receives a higher level of scrutiny if its requirements are unduly burdensome. See, e.g., *City of Akron v. Akron Center for Reproductive Health*, 462 U.S. 416, 46166 (1983) (O'Connor, J., dissenting). The statute in *Hodgson* is the first restriction on abortion that Justice O'Connor held to be unconstitutional.

28. Id. at 2937. In *Webster v. Reproductive Health Servs.*, 109 S. Ct. 3040 (1989), a plurality of the court first suggested applying this lower standard of review —a standard previously unheard of under traditional fundamental rights analysis. This is more evidence that a majority of the Court no longer views abortion as a fundamental right.

29. *Hodgson*, 110 S. Ct. at 294142.

30. See Id. at 2962.

31. Id. at 2942.

32. *Contraceptive Technology, supra* note 23, at 146.

33. The risk of death with an illegal abortion is 1 in 3,000. Id.

34. See *supra* notes 16 and accompanying text.

35. See *Hodgson v. Minnesota*, 110 S. Ct. 2926, 2932 (1990) (citing Minn. Stat. 144.343 (1988)). See also *Ohio v. Akron Center for Reproductive Health*, 110 S. Ct. 2972, 2977 (1990) (citing Ohio Rev. Code Ann. 2919.12 (B)(1)(a)(i) (Anderson Supp. 1988)).

36. *Hodgson*, 110 S. Ct. at 2944 (Stevens, J., concurring and dissenting).

37. See *Contraceptive Technology, supra* note 23, at 146. See also *Hodgson*, 110 S. Ct. at 2954 (Marshall, J., concurring and dissenting). ("A delay of any length in performing an abortion increases the statistical risk of mortality and morbidity.")

38. See *Planned Parenthood of Central Missouri v. Danforth*, 428 U.S. 52 (1976).

39. *Hodgson*, 110 S. Ct. at 2946.

40. Id. at 2938.

41. See *Ohio v. Akron Center for Reproductive Health*, 110 S. Ct. 2972, 299334 (1990) (Stevens, J. concurring). See also *Planned Parenthood v. Danforth*, 428 U.S. 52 (1976), where the majority held that a state cannot constitutionally require parental consent before a minor could obtain an abortion. Justice Stevens, in dissent, however, urged recognition of a state's power to ensure that the pregnant minor consult with her parents before making her decision. Id. at 102. See also *H. L. v. Matheson* 450 U.S. 398 (1981), where the Court held that parental notification is permissible in the case of an unemancipated minor who has not demonstrated her maturity or that the abortion would be in her best interest. Stevens stated that he would have upheld the notification requirement as applied to all minor pregnant women. Id. at 42225.

42. See *Akron Center*, 110 S. Ct. at 297879.

43. Minnesota claimed that the two-parent notification requirement was enacted in order to protect the family unit. See *Hodgson*, 110 S. Ct. at 294142. It is debatable whether protecting the family unit is a legitimate state interest. . . .

44. Justice Stevens's definition of dysfunctional families refers to cases in which there is domestic violence, child abuse or neglect, and sexual molestation. He is also concerned about the divorced, separated, or never-married families where the absent parent does not participate in the child's life in any significant manner. See id. at 293940.

45. See id. at 293839 (citing the district court's findings, 648 F. Supp. 756, 769 (1986)).

46. See e.g., *Ohio v. Akron Center for Reproductive Health*, 110 S. Ct. 2976, 299394 (1990).

47. See *supra* notes 16 and accompanying text.

48. Id.

49. Justices Kennedy, Rehnquist, White, and Scalia held that the two-parent notification requirement is constitutional even without the judicial-bypass procedure. Justices Marshall, Blackmun, Brennan, and Stevens held that the statute was unconstitutional even with the judicial-bypass procedure.

50. *Hodgson v. Minnesota,* 110 S. Ct. 2926, 295051 (1990). Justice O'Connor continued the undue burdens analysis that she articulated most recently in *Webster v. Reproductive Health Servs.,* 109 S. Ct. 3040, 3063 (1989). According to this analysis, heightened scrutiny is only applied to state legislation if it unduly burdens the right to abortion.

51. 110 S. Ct. at 294950.

52. Id. at 2940 (citing 648 F. Supp. 756, 762 (D. Minn. 1986)).

53. Id.

54. Id. (citing 648 F. Supp. at 763).

55. One doctor testified that the minors often dread the court procedure more than the abortion and often have to take a sedative before the bypass procedure. Id. at 2940 n.29.

Maternal-Fetal Conflicts

Maternal-Fetal Relationship:
The Courts and Social Policy

ROBERT H. BLANK, PH.D.

INTRODUCTION

We are in the midst of a revolution in biomedical technology especially in human genetics and reproduction. Rapid advances in prenatal diagnosis and therapy are joined with new reproductive-aiding technologies such as in vitro fertilization and more precise genetic tests. Combined with the burgeoning knowledge of fetal development and the causes of congenital illness, these technologies are altering our perception of the fetus. As a result, prevailing values are being challenged by the new biology, and the courts are being confronted with novel, onerous cases that require a reevaluation of established legal principles.

One critical set of values undergoing reevaluation centers on the relationship between mother and fetus. The technological removal of the fetus

ROBERT H. BLANK, PH.D. is Professor and Chair of Political Science at the University of Canterbury in Christchurch, New Zealand.

from the "secrecy of the womb" through ultrasound and other prenatal procedures gives the fetus social recognition as an individual separate from the mother.[1] The emergence of in utero surgery gives the fetus potential patient status that at times might conflict with that of the pregnant woman who carries it.[2] Moreover, conclusive evidence that certain maternal actions during pregnancy, such as cocaine and alcohol abuse, can have devastating effects on fetal health challenges conventional notions of maternal autonomy.[3] Together, these scientific trends are producing a context in which women's procreative rights achieved only recently after decades of struggle are threatened. In the words of legal scholar George Annas: "Bodies of pregnant women are the battleground on which the campaign to define the right of privacy is fought. The ultimate outcome will likely be shaped at least as much by new medical technologies as by politics or moral persuasion."[4] No applications of medicine promise more acrimonious and intense legal debate in the coming decades than the

The Journal of Legal Medicine, 14 (1993): 73–92. Copyright 1993. Permission granted by The American College of Legal Medicine.

impact of these technologies on the maternal-fetal relationship and on our notions of individual rights.

On the one hand, proponents of fetal rights contend that the health of the unborn fetus must be protected even at the expense of maternal rights.[5] They argue that the state's interest in protecting fetal health must take precedence over the maternal right to privacy. In contrast, proponents of maternal autonomy argue that no one but the pregnant woman can make such intimate decisions.[6] Any attempt at state or third-party intervention, therefore, represents unjustifiable constraints on women and is a return to the days when enslavement of women was justified as biological destiny.

The more we understand about the relationship between the fetus and the mother, the more validity must be ascribed to Aristotle's admonition to pregnant women to "pay attention to your bodies . . . take regular exercise and follow a nourishing diet."[7] It is clear that the well-being of the fetus is inextricably bound to the actions of the mother. Although the courts largely are cognizant of traditional maternal rights and have been hesitant to constrain those rights, recently they have shown a willingness to overrule maternal autonomy and at times her physical integrity when the woman's actions harm or represent probable danger to the life or health of the developing fetus.[8] As scientific evidence corroborates the deleterious effects of maternal behavior, the trend in the courts toward finding a cause of action against a pregnant woman for conduct injurious to her unborn child is bound to heighten.

In the last decade there has been a persistent intensification of policy issues surrounding attempts to define maternal responsibility.[9] Unfortunately, the current policy context and the government response to date have been inconsistent, haphazard, and often contradictory. Considerable interest has focused on the development of case law and the activity of the courts in redefining responsible maternal behavior and the standard of care owed the unborn.[10] It is clear that

the courts are already heavily involved in revising conventional views of maternal autonomy and discretion in procreative matters. Trends in both tort and criminal law appear to be on a collision course with the traditional predominance given maternal autonomy.

An alternative approach to that which emphasizes maternal responsibility is to focus on the social responsibility to provide all pregnant women with access to proper nutrition, counseling, mental health and substance abuse services, and adequate general health care. . . . Programs to provide adequate prenatal care to pregnant women usually return many dollars in benefits for each dollar spent, not to mention the reduction of less tangible social costs.[11] The costs of providing adequate maternal/child health care programs to educate pregnant women is meager compared to the neonatal intensive care costs of treating premature or disabled infants in fully preventable instances. Therefore, before society takes action to coerce responsible maternal behavior, substantial efforts must be made to provide proper education, counseling, and health care to pregnant women, particularly those in high-risk groups such as teenagers and the poor.

I. THE ROLE OF GOVERNMENT IN REDEFINING PROCREATIVE RIGHTS

The progression of Supreme Court decisions on procreative privacy culminating in *Roe v. Wade*[12] and reiterated in *City of Akron v. Akron Center for Reproductive Health, Inc.* and *Thornburgh v. American College of Obstetricians and Gynecologists,*[13] clearly enunciates the right of a woman not to have a child if she so desires. Contraception and abortion in theory at least, are guaranteed for all women, whatever their age and marital status. Although abortion continues to be a volatile issue and recent attention has focused on how tentative the legal context is in light of the new alignment of the Supreme Court,[14] the complementary question of whether all women, whatever their age, marital status, or other characteristics, have a corresponding right to have children is, perhaps, even more problematic. If there is a right to have children, then are there any limits that can be imposed on the number or quality of progeny? Just as the right to abortion is not absolute,[15] it might be that the general right to have children ought to be circumvented under some circumstances. If so, who sets the limits and on what basis and how active a role ought the courts play in shaping these constraints?

What if a woman requires the services of a surrogate mother because she is unable to undergo pregnancy—does she have that right and, if so, who pays?[16] A public furor arose in response to a well-publicized case in which a woman on welfare had a child via artificial insemination by donor.[17] Although the notoriety of this case may not be commonplace, it is a cogent illustration of the dilemmas that arise in interpreting reproduction as a positive entitlement.

Another policy issue regarding the right to have children relates to persons who carry genetic diseases, particularly dominant genetic traits such as Huntington's Disease.[18] Social and legal pressures that will label parents as "irresponsible" who knowingly reproduce children with genetic disorders are likely to intensify. Do chronic alcohol abusers, drug abusers, or women with other high-risk conditions have a constitutional right to procreate without concern for the burden placed on their progeny and society? In the case of young teenagers who are emotionally and physically immature, is it fair to their potential children, others in society, or themselves to guarantee them an unfettered right to reproduce?

If one answers affirmatively that all women have a positive right to reproduce when they desire, then the social policy goals are reasonably straightforward—eliminate to the maximum extent possible any institutional, economic, and political infringements on the free exercise of that right. If one answers negatively, however, the policy context is significantly more troublesome because one must develop a strategy to set constraints without undercutting prevailing social values. Overall, then, in a democratic society, the policy issues in assuming complete reproductive freedom are less troublesome than those surrounding efforts to limit this freedom, because of difficulties in setting the boundaries of legitimate government involvement. . . .

Social policies that focus on the education of high-risk parents to refrain from reproduction or provide other options for having children are likely to enjoy considerably greater support than coercive policies. Voluntary, not mandatory, genetic screening and prenatal diagnostic programs are most compatible with prevailing values concerning procreation in the United States. Although other inducements such as tax incentives might offer the means to supplement educational efforts, they result in inequities based on wealth. In contrast, the elimination or reduction of public support for the indigent, combined with the provision of a full range of family planning services, might encourage some people not to have children, but again at the cost of inequitable impact on various groups. More explicit policies to limit procreative choice historically have depended on sterilization programs.[19] These programs failed to reach even their most modest objectives and continue to personify state intrusion at its extreme for many people. Although new technologies in reversible sterilization and long-term subdermal implant contraceptives promise to ease rationalization of such policies, they will continue to be most controversial.[20] . . .

Despite these caveats, the trends toward legal acknowledgment of fetal rights, torts for wrongful life, torts for prenatal damage, and criminal liability of parents for abuse of their unborn children demonstrate a heightened acceptance by the courts and by the public to place limits on the reproductive choice of individuals.[21] Also, the expanding knowledge of fetal development, in combination with the emergence of intervention technologies, further shifts attention from the idea of reproduction as an unmitigated right to a responsibility to produce healthy children. Those persons who knowingly beget children born unhealthy are increasingly likely to be viewed as acting irresponsibly. They will have to endure mounting social pressure to conform to standards of "responsible" procreative action.[22]

II. THE FETAL ENVIRONMENT: A SUMMARY OF MEDICAL EVIDENCE AND LEGAL TRENDS

A wide range of behavioral patterns and maternal characteristics have been found to be associated with deleterious effects on the fetus. In most cases, it appears that the critical period of development occurs between the third and twelfth weeks of human gestation.[23] However, each organ has its own critical period and for some, such as the brain where cell proliferation does not cease until at least six to eight months after birth, sensitivity to environmental teratogenic agents extends throughout the pregnancy. Although exposure to potential teratogens[24] later in gestation might not result in gross organ system abnormalities, it might still be associated with other serious dysfunctions.

Moreover, research on teratogens indicates that it is probable that most teratogenesis is caused by the combined effects of a number of more subtle agents acting in consort rather than a massive teratogenic action of a single agent. A "simple one-to-one correspondence does not exist for birth defects."[25] The problem is vastly more complex and, thus, the solution depends on unraveling the unique contribution of each of a multitude of intimately related factors. Accordingly, the challenge to the courts in judging

proximate cause is formidable in many of these cases.

Despite the complex nature of the fetal environment and the variation of effects any single stimulus might have on a specific fetus, rapidly expanding medical evidence demonstrates that there are many ways in which maternal behavioral patterns and health status can impair the proper development of the fetus and, in some cases, cause irreparable harm. Although data remain inconclusive in many areas, there is evidence of the importance of providing as risk-free a fetal environment as possible. Maternal smoking, drinking, eating, and general lifestyle can and do have an effect on the fetus.[26]

. . . For law professor Patricia King this "increasing awareness that a mother's activities during pregnancy may affect the health of the offspring creates pressing policy issues that raise possible conflicts among fetuses, mothers and researchers."[27]

Within the context of the growing knowledge of these hazards, the question reemerges as to what right a child has to a safe fetal environment and as normal as possible a start in life? In turn, this demonstrates the potential conflict between the interests of the developing fetus and the mother. It is a tragedy that in an affluent country, such as the United States, children continue to be born with birth defects caused primarily by a lack of proper nutrition or the actions of the mother during pregnancy. However, in a democratic society, the primary responsibility belongs to the woman. She alone is the direct link to the fetus and she alone makes the ultimate decision regarding whether to smoke, use alcohol or other drugs, maintain proper nutrition, and so forth. . . .

As a result of these technological developments, there is a discernible trend in tort law toward recognition of a maternal responsibility for the well-being of the unborn child. Despite many inconsistencies across jurisdictions, there is an unmistakable pattern toward finding a cause of action against third parties for fetal death or prenatal injury even if it occurred at the previable stage.[28] The abrogation of intrafamily immunity and the willingness of some courts to hold parents liable for prenatal injury open the door for increased judicial involvement in defining parental responsibilities.[29] In a short time span, torts against parents for prenatal injury caused either by commission or omission have been recognized by some courts.[30] . . .

III. DEFINING RESPONSIBILITY FOR FETAL HEALTH

. . . The problems in the mother-fetal relationship, then, cannot be separated from the broader social context. Vast socioeconomic inequities and the resulting lack of adequate primary care for a significant minority of the population continue to contribute to the health risks for women and for the fetuses they carry. Although large numbers of women who lack proper health care and education live in isolated rural areas, it is paradoxical that the most vulnerable women are congregated in urban areas, often within sight of the most impressive concentrations of medical technology in the world.

In addition to the macro-social context, one cannot explain an individual pregnant woman's behavior without knowledge of her personal experiences. The emphasis on punishing a pregnant woman diverts attention from the root causes of the woman's often self-destructive behavior that also happens to threaten the fetus. How many of these women were victims of sexual abuse, incest, and other denigration of their self esteem? In the long run, only by understanding why particular women act in ways dangerous to the health of their fetus and ameliorating these base causes can a policy to improve fetal health succeed.

Although no individual can escape ultimate responsibility for personal actions, the social and personal plight of an increasing number of young women makes rational choice problematic and elusive. The birth of addicted, very premature, or otherwise ill babies to these women, however, only extenuates the problem and extends the dreadful cycle into another generation. Despite the expressed concern of policy makers for the health of the children and their right to be born with a sound mind and body, there has been a consistent lack of action. Unless society is willing to expend considerable resources to overcome the problems of poverty, illiteracy, housing, and lack of access to good prenatal care and meaningful employment for women of childbearing age, the future will continue to look bleak for many children.

IV. SOCIETAL RESPONSIBILITY: PREVENTIVE STRATEGIES FOR FETAL HEALTH

Society must place a much higher priority on prevention of health problems.[31] . . .

Coercive governmental action charging a woman who gives birth to a cocaine-addicted baby with a criminal offense or using the tort process to recover damages from a woman for injury to the fetus she is carrying is indicative of a failure of society to address the problem of high-risk behavior before the damage is done. Martha Field is correct when she concludes that if the real goal is not control of women but "protection of the child-to-be and creation of as healthy a newborn population as possible, then appropriate means are education and persuasion, free prenatal care, and good substance abuse rehabilitation programs, available free of charge to pregnant women."[32] Although this approach is more expensive in the short run and requires considerably more effort to implement than ex post facto coercive measures, in the long run it is more fair and cost effective, both monetarily and for the national psyche.

A growing realization of these facts was reflected in the report of many panels in the late 1980s. The Institute of Medicine,[33] the United

States Public Health Service Expert Panel on the Content of Prenatal Care,[34] and the United States Congress Office of Technology Assessment[35] all called for universal access to prenatal care for pregnant women as the critical strategy to improve the health of infants. For instance, the Institute of Medicine concluded that the nation should adopt as a new social norm the principle that all pregnant women should be provided access to prenatal, labor and delivery, and post-partum services appropriate to their need.[36] It is admitted that this will require considerable resources to reorganize the entire maternity care system including the following: removal of all barriers (including personal and cultural) to such care; a vigorous education effort in schools, media, family planning clinics, social service networks, and places of employment; and, research on how to motivate women to seek this care.

The most comprehensive discussion of how to implement prenatal care to deal with these problems is found in the report of the Public Health Service Expert Panel on the Content of Prenatal Care.[37] This report demonstrates that the objectives of prenatal care, instead of pitting mother against fetus, are designed to serve the interests of the woman, the fetus/infant, and the family. Importantly, the panel places considerable emphasis on the need for preconception care to prepare for pregnancy, because it is often too late to ensure a healthy pregnancy once it has begun. In fact, the preconception visit "may be the single most important health care visit when viewed in the context of its effect on the pregnancy."[38] The birth of a healthy baby, then, depends in part on the woman's general health and well-being before conception as well as on the amount and quality of prenatal care. Health care before pregnancy can ameliorate disease, improve risk status, and help prepare the woman for childbearing.[39] . . .

The panel correctly argues that it is "imperative that women who enter pregnancy at risk or develop medical or psychosocial risk during pregnancy receive an augmented program of care,"[40] and the report suggests what this might entail for specific risk factors such as substance abuse.

Society has a responsibility to ensure adequate prenatal care to all pregnant women. Even under the best of circumstances (expanded funding, universal availability, and effective outreach), however, there will be some situations in which a pregnant woman will clearly disregard all attempts to minimize her high-risk behavior and refuse to comply with counseling, referral, and treatment attempts. Reported cases of women who have given birth to two or more addicted babies, despite intensive efforts to encourage responsible behavior,[41] necessitate consideration of policies that encompass coercive intervention strategies. These extreme cases warrant more severe constraints on the woman's capacity to injure additional children.

V. THE RIGHTS CONTEXT: A FORMULA FOR CONFLICT

Although the primacy given individual rights in American political culture has worked to protect the interests of the most vulnerable groups in the past, it creates inexorable dilemmas when strictly applied to the maternal-fetal relationship. The problem is heightened by the fact that proponents both of women's rights and fetal rights often try to optimize their position by insisting that the rights they advocate must be absolute. Often the arguments are framed in either-or terms, emphasizing either the woman's right to privacy or the fetus's right to a sound mind and body. Moreover, the specter of the abortion debate underlies any discussion of this conflict.

. . . The term "fetal rights" is a distortion of the real issue and obscures what ought to be the primary concern—the health of the child when born. It is not the fetus that has rights; rather, it is the child once born that must be protected from avertable harm during gestation. The goal of any policies designed to make the fetal environment as safe as possible should be to maximize the birth of healthy children. The unfortunate, but conscious focus on fetal rights, instead of the rights of the newborn, intensifies opposition without contributing to resolution of the problem. Although the fetus may have interests to be protected that will materialize after birth, it is clear under *Roe v. Wade*[42] that fetuses do not even have a "right" to be born, at least throughout the first two trimesters.

Just as the concept of fetal rights is flawed, so the argument for a pregnant woman's absolute right to privacy is unwarranted in light of current knowledge of fetal development. Unless we are willing to give a woman license to practice infanticide, some constraints will always be imposed. Although in most cases the woman's right to procreative freedom ought to take precedence, in some instances state intervention is not only warranted but also obligatory to protect the interests of the future child by defining the woman's choices more narrowly. One major policy problem, then, is deciding how and where to set these limits. The second is who or what public agent has responsibility for doing so.

VI. THE POLICY PROBLEM: HOW TO BALANCE MATERNAL AND FETAL INTERESTS

Even if there were a consensus that a pregnant woman who chooses to carry her pregnancy to term has a moral responsibility to make reasonable efforts toward preserving fetal health, this would not necessarily translate into a legal duty to do so. By moving from a moral duty to a legal duty, we opt to permit state intervention to force the woman to make a particular moral choice. This may require, in some instances, the creation of a legal duty to accept medical procedures or treatments that benefit the fetus even when it puts the woman at risk and requires invasion of

her bodily integrity. But why should the pregnant woman be singled out for such a duty when other persons are not legally required to undergo medical risk for the benefit of someone other than themselves?[43]

Notwithstanding a hesitancy to move too readily to a legal duty for a pregnant woman, there are instances in which legal intervention is warranted. The problem still remains, however, as to what specific criteria should be used to determine when and how best to constrain maternal action to protect fetal interests. Actions of pregnant women that might affect normal fetal development include the following: abuse of illegal substances; use of alcohol; smoking or breathing secondary smoke; drinking coffee; not eating a balanced diet; use of over-the-counter and prescription drugs; working in a hazardous workplace; living in a high risk environment; exercising too much or too little; travelling late in pregnancy; not obtaining adequate prenatal care; suffering physical harm through accident or illness; not following medical advice to avoid sexual intercourse, stay in bed for duration of pregnancy, agree to cesarean section, agree to stay on life-support system in interests of the fetus, or agree to surgery; being overweight or underweight; not entering a treatment or counseling program, if necessary; not using collaborative conception, if advised; not using prenatal diagnosis, if appropriate; and, not aborting a defective fetus diagnosed by prenatal diagnosis. Certainly, it would be ridiculous to develop a policy that restrains the pregnant woman's behavioral choices for all of the items listed. To do so would make the woman a slave of the fetus. . . .

It is unfortunate that, due to legislative inaction, the courts have been forced to take on the major policy-making role in this area. Although the courts are well-suited for adjudicating specific acts relevant to a particular case, judicial precedents often have broader social implications. The legal penalties that are available to influence the behavior of pregnant women fall into one of several categories. During pregnancy, the courts might order incarceration or detention of the woman to physically constrain her behavior out of concern for fetal health.[44] Legal penalties after birth include various civil tort actions or criminal sanctions.[45] All legal approaches have problems. . . .

Criminal sanctions for maternal behavior also have inherent problems. Although a major argument for legal sanctions is deterrence, there is no evidence, for instance, that prosecution of pregnant drug abusers has any deterrent effect. A report to the American Medical Association concludes that criminal penalties are unlikely to influence behavior because

the use of illegal substances already incurs criminal penalties. Pregnant women who ingest illegal substances are obviously not deterred by existing sanctions; the reasons which prompt them to ignore existing penalties might very well also prompt disregard for any additional penalties. Also, in ordinary instances, concern for fetal health prompts the great majority of women to refrain from potentially harmful behavior. If that concern, generally a strong impetus for avoiding certain actions, is not sufficient to prevent harmful behavior, then it is questionable that criminal sanctions would provide the additional motivation needed to avoid behaviors that may cause fetal harm.[46]

To the contrary, there is some evidence that a major effect of such highly publicized cases is to discourage other pregnant women from obtaining proper prenatal care out of fear of criminal prosecution, thus potentially exacerbating the problem.[47] It seems reasonable that pregnant women who are substance abusers would avoid any medical treatment for fear that their physician's knowledge of their abuse might result in a jail sentence. Moreover, imposing criminal sanctions on pregnant women for potentially harmful behavior could provoke other women to seek abortions in order to avoid legal repercussions. Finally, evidence to date demonstrates that criminal prosecution of pregnant women has a clear bias against minority and low socioeconomic status women.[48] Although criminal sanctions

might be successful in punishing a few women, the lack of deterrence and its likely inequitable application make it unattractive as a policy for assuring the birth of healthy children.

Although judicial intervention is warranted in exceptional cases, particularly when a pregnant woman refuses to undergo, with minimal risk to herself, lifesaving treatment for the fetus she is carrying, any such attempts should require a strict standard of review. Similarly, negligent conduct of a high degree—a conscious and reckless disregard for the welfare of the fetus by the pregnant woman—should be required before holding the woman liable for prenatal injury. Only with clear and convincing evidence, and a presupposition that the pregnant woman is to be given any benefit of doubt, should the case proceed. A closer reading of the trends in case law reviewed here demonstrates that the courts, in their understandable willingness to recognize the interests of those children born with injury, have created precedents that compromise the autonomy and physical integrity of pregnant women by creating increasingly stringent standards of care.

The following statements are meaningful starting points for a vigorous dialogue on how to frame a workable and fair policy to deal with the maternal-fetal relationship that protects the rights of pregnant women in general, but also maximizes societal interest in the birth of healthy children.

1. The well-being of specific unborn children, as well as future generations, demands that pregnant women be educated as to the potential danger of their actions to the developing fetus.

2. The well-being of specific unborn children requires the widespread utilization of emerging technologies for prenatal diagnosis, monitoring, and therapy.

3. The provision of universal prenatal and preconception care for all pregnant women, along with adequate counseling

and substance abuse treatment programs, is essential and would drastically reduce the problems leading to unhealthy maternal behavior.

4. In those instances in which preventive approaches fail and a pregnant woman refuses to modify her behavior, and thus minimize the risk of damage to her offspring, society, primarily through its courts and legislatures, has a duty to intervene to protect the interests of the defenseless fetus.

5. Intervention by the state in the maternal-fetal relationship should always be undertaken in the least intrusive, yet most effective, manner. Healthy children, not punishment of the mother, should be the primary objective of any intervention.

CONCLUSION

The balance between maternal autonomy and the interests of a child to be born with a sound mind and body is a delicate and elusive one, but all efforts must be made to arrive at this balance by fully taking into account these intertwined sets of rights and responsibilities.

NOTES

1. In addition to ultrasound or sonography, other routinely used prenatal diagnostic procedures include amniocentesis, chorionic villus sampling, alpha-fetoprotein screening, and an expanding battery of DNA tests.

2. The first reported surgery on a fetus in utero was performed in April of 1981, on a 31-week-gestation fetus suffering from a life-threatening urinary tract obstruction. See Golbus, Harrison, Filly, Callen, & Katz, In Utero Treatment of Urinary Tract Obstruction, 142 *Am. J. Obstetrics & Gynecology* 383 (1982). Other in utero surgeries have been performed to implant miniature shunting devices in the brains of fetuses diagnosed as having hydrocephalus, a dangerous buildup of fluid in the brain, and heart valve operations. See Rosenfeld, The Patient in the Womb, 82 *Science* 18 (1982). The most dramatic type of fetal surgery involves the removal of the fetus from the uterus with its return upon completion of the surgery. One

recent application of this procedure was conducted to repair a diaphragmatic hernia on a 24-week-gestation fetus. See Harrison, Adzick, Longaker, Goldberg, Rosen, Filly, Evans, & Golbus, Successful Repair In Utero of a Fetal Diaphragmatic Hernia After Removal of Herniated Visera from the Left Thorax, 322 *New Eng. J. Med.* 1582 (1990).

3. For effects of cocaine abuse on the fetus, see Chasnoff, Drug Use in Pregnancy: Parameters of Risk, 35 *Pediatric Clinics N. Am.* 1403 (1988). For effects of alcohol abuse on the fetus, see Wagner, The Alcoholic Beverages Labeling Act of 1988, 12 *J. Legal Med.* 167 (1991).

4. Annas, Predicting the Future of Privacy in Pregnancy: How Medical Technology Affects the Legal Rights of Pregnant Women, 13 *Nova L. Rev.* 329, 329 (1989).

5. See Balisy, Maternal Substance Abuse: The Need to Provide Legal Protection for the Fetus, 60 *So. Cal. L. Rev.* 1209 (1987).

6. See Gallagher, Prenatal Invasions and Interventions: What's Wrong with Fetal Rights, 10 *Harv. Women's L. J.* 9 (1987). See also Johnsen, The Creation of "Fetal Rights": Conflicts with Women's Constitutional Rights to Liberty, Privacy, and Equal Protection, 95 *Yale L.J.* 599 (1986).

7. Aristotle, *Politics*, 7 XVI 14.

8. This can be seen in the willingness of many courts to constrain maternal autonomy in cases involving forced cesarian sections. For a summary of these cases and a discussion of the policy implications, see Kolder, Gallagher, & Parsons, Court-Ordered Obstetrical Interventions, 316 *New Eng. J. Med.* 1192 (1987).

9. See Losco, Fetal Abuse: An Exploration of Emerging Philosophic, Legal, and Policy Issues, 42 *W Pol. Q.* 265 (1989).

10. For a more detailed discussion, see *R. Blank, Mother and Fetus: Changing Notions of Maternal Responsibility* (1992).

11. *The Institute of Medicine, Preventing Low Birthweight* (1985) (concluding that for each dollar spent on prenatal care, $3.38 is saved). See also Nagey, The Content of Prenatal Care, 74 *Obstetrics & Gynecology* 516 (1980) (finding a saving of $3.66 in hospital costs alone for each dollar spent for prenatal care).

12. 410 U.S. 113 (1973).

13. *City of Akron v. Akron Center for Reproductive Health, Inc.,* 462 U.S. 416 (1983); *Thornburgh v. American College of Obstetricians and Gynecologists,* 476 U.S. 747 (1986).

14. Recent shifts in the Court's balance were initially reflected in Webster v. Reproductive Health Servs., 492 U.S. 490 (1989), upholding a Missouri statute affirming that human life begins at conception

and prohibits the use of public funds, employees, and facilities for abortion-related services not necessary to save the life of the mother. The replacement of Justice Thurgood Marshall by Justice Clarence Thomas may have the effect of further undermining *Roe v. Wade.*

15. Even at the height of abortion rights immediately after *Roe v. Wade,* limits could be set by states after the end of the second trimester, or after viability, which is a changing concept due to medical technology.

16. The other side of this question, which is at the center of the surrogate mother controversy, is whether a woman has a right to be a surrogate mother and be paid for her services. See M. Field, *Surrogate Motherhood* (1988).

17. See Case Studies: AID and the Single Welfare Mother, 13 *Hastings Center Rep.* 22 (Feb. 1983).

18. See Purdy, Genetic Diseases: Can Having Children Be Immoral?, in *Genetics Now: Ethical Issues in Genetic Research* 26 (J. Buckley ed. 1978).

19. See P. Reilly, *The Surgical Solution: A History of Involuntary Sterilization* (1991).

20. I have argued elsewhere (R. Blank, *Fertility Control: New Techniques, New Policy Issues* (1991)) that the routine availability of reversible techniques such as NORPLANT will undercut the major assumption of irreversibility that the courts have used to strike down involuntary applications of sterilization since Skinner v. Oklahoma, 316 U.S. 535 (1942).

21. Terms like "wrongful pregnancy," "wrongful life," and "wrongful birth" are constantly being added to the legal lexicon resulting in substantial questioning of previous legal and policy assumptions. It is not surprising that there is wide divergence in the reaction of the courts to these novel cases, both in recognizing a cause of action and determining the appropriate amount of damages, if any, to be awarded. See W. Winborne, *Handling Pregnancy and Birthcases* 5 (1983) (the law in this area is far from being settled; it is just beginning to develop).

22. In some ways, the combination of these more subtle, implicit pressures in the long run are more effective restraints on procreative freedom in a democracy because explicit calls for the same result would be dismissed out of hand.

23. H. Nishimura & T. Tanimura, *Clinical Aspects of the Teratogenicity of Drugs* (1976).

24. Teratogenesis is the development of abnormal structures in an embryo or fetus. Teratogens include any substances or agents that lead to such abnormal development.

25. Melnick, Drugs as Etiological Agents in Mental Retardation, in *Prevention of Mental Retardation and Other Developmental Disabilities* 453 (M. McCormick ed. 1980).

26. R. Blank, *supra* note 10, at ch. 2.

27. King, The Juridical Status of the Fetus: A Proposal for the Protection of the Unborn, in *The Law and Politics of Abortion* 81 (C. Schneider & M. Vinovskis eds. 1980).

28. Increasing numbers of courts have either expressly renounced the viability rule or ignored it. The Georgia Supreme Court, in *Hornbuckle v. Plantation Pipe Line Co.,* 93 S.E.2d 727 (Ga. 1956), held that viability was not the deciding factor in a prenatal personal injury action and that recovery for any injury suffered after the point of conception should be permitted. Similarly, in Wilson v. Kaiser Found. Hosp., 190 Cal. Rptr. 649 (Cal. App. 1983), the California Court of Appeal agreed with this reasoning and concluded that birth is the condition precedent that establishes the beginning of the child's rights. A tort action may be maintained if the child is born alive—whether the injury occurred before viability or after is immaterial once birth takes place. In a further extension of this logic, some courts have recognized a cause of action for personal injuries that occurred prior to conception. In *Renslow v. Mennonite Hosp.,* 367 N.E.2d 1250 (Ill. 1977), a physician was held liable for injuries suffered by an infant girl as a result of a blood transfusion to the mother that occurred nine years before the child's birth. See also Turpin v. Sortini, 643 P.2d 954 (Cal. 1982); *Harbeson v. Parke-Davis,* 656 P.2d 483 (Wash. 1983).

29. Over 40 states have abrogated the immunity doctrine. In the remainder, exceptions to the rule are freely granted such that it seems unlikely that prenatal injury torts against parents would be summarily dismissed. The courts generally agree that the child's personal rights are more worthy than property or contract rights, which are already protected. *Hebel v. Hebel,* 435 P.2d 8 (Alaska 1967). The courts see little family tranquility protected in denying a tort action solely on the basis of the immunity rule. Peterson v. Honolulu, 262 P.2d 1007 (Hawaii 1969). According to the Massachusetts Supreme Court in *Sorenson v. Sorenson,* 339 N.E.2d 907 (Mass. 1975), it is the injury, not the lawsuit, that disrupts harmonious family relations. The child's relationship to the tortfeasor should not result in denial of recovery for a wrong to his or her person. *Briere v. Briere,* 224 A.2d 588 (N.H. 1966).

30. In *Grodin v. Grodin,* 301 N.W.2d 869 (Mich. App. 1980), the Michigan Court of Appeals recognized the possibility of maternal liability for prenatal conduct. The court upheld the right of a child allegedly injured prenatally to present testimony concerning his mother's negligence in failing to take a pregnancy test when her symptoms suggested pregnancy and her failure to inform the physician who diagnosed the pregnancy that she was taking tetracycline, a drug that might be contraindicated for pregnant women. Noting that the Michigan Supreme

Court had determined that a child could bring suit for prenatal injury and that the immunity doctrine had been discarded, the *Grodin* court ruled that the injured child's mother would "bear the same liability as a third person for injurious, negligent conduct that interfered with the child's 'legal right to being life with a sound mind and body.'" In *Stallman v. Youngquist,* 531 N.E.2d 355 (Ill. 1988), however, the Illinois Supreme Court held that no cause of action exists by or on behalf of a fetus, subsequently born alive, against its mother for unintentional infliction of prenatal injuries. In this case, in which action was brought by the infant against the mother for prenatal injuries sustained in an automobile accident, the supreme court reversed the appellate court's finding upholding a cause of action.

31. See R. Blank, *Rationing Medicine* (1988).

32. Field, Controlling the Woman to Protect the Fetus, 17 *Law, Med. & Health Care* 114, 125 (1989).

33. *Institute of Medicine, Prenatal Care* (1988).

34. *Public Health Service, Caring for Our Future: The Content of Prenatal Care* (1989).

35. *Office of Technology Assessment, Healthy Children* (1988).

36. Zylke, Maternal, Child Health Needs Noted by Two Major National Study Groups, 261 *J.A.M.A.* 1687, 1687 (1989).

37. *Public Health Service, supra* note 34.

38. *Id.* at 26.

39. Jack & Culpepper, Preconception Care: Risk Reduction and Health Promotion in Preparation for Pregnancy, 264 *J.A.M.A.* 1147 (1990).

40. *Public Health Service, supra* note 34, at 91.

41. Logli, Drugs in the Womb: the Newest Battlefield in the War on Drugs, 9 *Crim. Justice Ethics* 23 (1990).

42. 410 U.S. 113 (1973).

43. *See* Gallagher, *supra* note 6, at 57. See also Johnsen, *supra* note 6, at 625.

44. One of the most publicized and controversial legal developments in the late 1980s was the increasing number of jurisdictions that tried to impose legal sanctions in an attempt to deter illegal drug use by pregnant women. Women have been prosecuted under statutes against child abuse and neglect, the delivery of a controlled substance to a minor, and involuntary manslaughter. It has been reported that the District Attorney of Butte County, California, announced his intention to prosecute all mothers of newborns with illegal drugs found in their urine; conviction would carry a mandatory minimum sentence of 90 days in jail. Chavkin & Kandall, Between a "Rock" and a Hard Place: Prenatal Drug Use, 85 *Pediatrics* 223 (1990). Likewise, other legal interventions such as civil detention have been sought to control the behavior of pregnant women deemed dangerous to the fetus. See, e.g., *United States v. Vaughn,* 117 Daily Wash. L. Rep. 441 (D.C. Super. Ct. Mar. 7, 1989).

45. Although the details of court cases involving drug abuse by pregnant women vary, several well-publicized cases clearly demonstrate the complex issues facing the courts. In 1989, Jennifer Johnson gave birth to a daughter. At the time, she advised hospital personnel that she was addicted to cocaine and tests confirmed traces of cocaine in her daughter's system. She was subsequently reported to the Florida Department of Health and Rehabilitation and charged with child abuse and delivery of a controlled substance during delivery of her daughter as well as during delivery of a son born in 1987. Although she was acquitted on the child abuse charge due to lack of evidence, she was found guilty on the controlled substance charge and sentenced to 15 years probation, 200 hours of community service, mandatory drug treatment, and participation in an intense prenatal program if she again became pregnant. *Florida v. Johnson,* No. E89-890-CFA (Seminole Cty., Cir. Ct. 1989). The judge reasoned that she had illegally introduced the cocaine into her body and then passed it on to the newborn children in the moments after delivery before the umbilical cord was cut. Children, like all persons, have the right to be born free from having cocaine introduced into their system by others. The Florida Supreme Court later reversed this decision. *Johnson v. State,* 602 So. 2d 1288 (Fla. 1992). For additional details of similar cases, see Janna Merrick's companion article, published as part of this Symposium at pages 57–71.

46. *American Medical Association, Board of Trustees Report: Legal Interventions During Pregnancy* 14 (1990).

47. Johnsen, *supra* note 6.

48. Chavkin & Kandall, *supra* note 44.

Cesareans and Samaritans

NANCY K. RHODEN

UNTIL RECENTLY, if one asked the proverbial person on the street to list maternal–fetal
conflicts, he or she would have mentioned abortion and, when pressed to continue, looked at
the questioner blankly. Now, however, the populace is becoming aware of a host of maternal–
fetal conflicts. Indeed, mother-and-child, long a
somewhat romanticized unity, are increasingly
being created by physicians, courts, and the
media as potential adversaries, locked in battle
on the rather inconvenient battleground of the
woman's belly.

Some of these newly publicized conflicts—
pregnant women abusing drugs or alcohol, or
continuing to work in occupations hazardous to
fetal health—are not all that new: the hazards of
various substances have been known for years.
Other of the conflicts are new, inasmuch as doctors could not recommend Cesareans or other
procedures for the fetus' benefit until they could
detect fetal problems during or before labor. But
probably what is most unprecedented is that
now, suddenly, physicians are seeking court intervention to protect these imperiled fetuses—
intervention that, inevitably, constitutes a significant intrusion into the woman's conduct during
pregnancy or birth.

This essay will discuss just one of the prolifer-
ating array of maternal–fetal conflicts—the question whether courts should have the power to
authorize doctors to perform Cesarean deliveries
against the woman's will. Doctors typically seek
these orders when they believe, based on diagnostic techniques, that vaginal delivery risks
death or neurological damage to the fetus. (In
some cases, vaginal delivery is a risk for the
woman as well.) Women who refuse most commonly do so based on religious beliefs opposed
to surgery, though they may refuse because they
fear surgery, do not believe the doctor's prognoses, or whatever.

I have restricted my focus to this issue for several reasons. First, these cases are more common
than the absence of reported judicial decisions
would make one believe, because many of them
are completely unreported.[1] Some make the local
newspapers,[2] but many don't. For example, during my year as a visiting professor at Albert Einstein College of Medicine, such a case arose at
North Central Bronx, one of the college's affiliated hospitals. It was litigated, and a nonconsensual Cesarean was authorized.[3] But there was no
reported decision, no coverage in local newspapers and, indeed, no way anyone not involved in
the case or present at the hospital would know of
it. Second, these cases are extraordinarily difficult. They pit a woman's rights to privacy and
bodily integrity, normally more than sufficient to
allow a competent adult to refuse major surgery,
against the possibility of a lifetime of devastating

NANCY K. RHODEN, now deceased, co-edited with John D.
Arras the anthology *Ethical Issues in Modern Medicine*.

Journal of Law, Medicine, & Ethics *215, 3 (1987): 118–25. Copyright 1987. This article is a shortened version
of "The Judge in the Delivery Room: The Emergence of Court-Ordered Cesareans," which appeared in the
California Law Review 1987, 74: 1951. Reprinted with the permission of the American Society of Law,
Medicine & Ethics. All rights reserved.*

disability to a being who is within days or even hours of independent existence. Finally, as more and more techniques for diagnosing and treating problems in utero are developed, it is likely that doctors will seek authorization for other nonconsensual treatments.[4] The Cesarean cases, inasmuch as they rest on technology that is standard and routine right now, will constitute important precedents for such future controversies.

The position I will defend is that courts should not order competent women to have Cesareans, despite the potentially tragic consequences to the fetus. This is neither an easy position nor a fully satisfactory one. Indeed, it is the sort of hard line civil libertarian position that I ordinarily find oversimplified in bioethics issues. Yet I believe that it is the morally and legally correct position—albeit merely the "least worst" one—because these orders (1) impose an unparalleled intrusion upon pregnant women; (2) undermine the teachings of the informed consent doctrine that only the individual being subjected to a procedure can assess its risks and benefits; and (3) contain within them the seeds of widespread and pernicious usurpation of women's choices during obstetrical care.

JUSTIFICATIONS FOR NONCONSENSUAL CESAREANS

Abortion Law

In the cases of which I am aware, every judge but one who has ruled on an application for nonconsensual Cesarean delivery has granted the request.[5] Interestingly, *Roe v. Wade,*[6] which has stood firmly for a woman's right to privacy and right to make her own decisions about pregnancy, is the case most commonly invoked by courts to justify these orders.[7] Under *Roe,* women must be allowed to choose abortion prior to fetal viability (subject to state regulation to protect the mother's health in the second

trimester). But once a fetus is capable of independent life outside the womb, albeit with artificial aid, the state's interest in potential life becomes compelling.[8] Then the state can prohibit abortion, unless it is necessary to protect the woman's life or health. Courts invoking *Roe* to support nonconsensual Cesarean delivery reason that since states can prohibit the intentional termination of fetal life after viability, they can likewise protect viable fetuses by preventing vaginal delivery when it will have the same affect as abortion.[9]

At first glance this analysis appears attractive. Attempting a vaginal delivery when responsible medical opinion says that surgical delivery is necessary for the fetus may cause a stillbirth or, perhaps worse, profound neurological damage to the child. These consequences are clearly ones that states have an interest in preventing. But the fact that states have an interest in preventing certain consequences does not mean that any and all action to prevent such consequences is constitutional. For example, states have an interest in preventing use of illicit drugs, and they can make such conduct criminal. But this doesn't mean that they can take any and all other steps to prevent drug use, such as ordering random strip searches at airports (though the way things are going, we may soon see random urine samples). Similarly, the Court in *Roe* said that in the third trimester, the state can even "go so far as to proscribe abortion,"[10] unless the woman's health is at stake. That the state can go this far, prohibiting intentional fetal destruction, doesn't necessarily mean that it can go even farther, and mandate major surgery to protect and preserve the fetus' life. There is a quantum leap in logic between prohibiting destruction and requiring surgical preservation that courts and commentators relying on abortion law have ignored.

In fact, if one reads *Roe* and its progeny more closely, it becomes apparent that court-ordered Cesareans violate *Roe*'s constitutional schema. *Roe* emphasizes that even after the fetus is viable, the woman's life and health come first. If her health is threatened by her pregnancy even after the fetus is viable, she must be allowed to abort.[11] In *Colautti v. Franklin*,[12] the Supreme Court discussed the primacy of maternal health even more specifically. It invalidated a statute that required doctors performing post-viability abortions to use the technique least harmful to the fetus, unless another technique was necessary for the woman's health. Among other infirmities, this statute impermissibly implied that the more hazardous technique had to be *indispensable* to the woman's health, and suggested that doctors could be required to make trade-offs between her health and additional percentage points of the fetus' survival.[13] Abortion law makes clear that such trade-offs cannot be required.

Thus a state could not, under *Colautti*, require that all abortions after viability be done by hysterotomy, a surgical technique that is basically a mini-Cesarean, on the grounds that this is safest for the fetus. A state could not require this because such a technique is less safe for the woman. It may not be immediately apparent that this proscription of compulsory maternal–fetal trade-offs in late abortion applies to the Cesarean dilemma. Yet this becomes quite clear when one realizes that after a fetus is viable, the methods of abortion and of premature delivery simply merge.[14] Although the Supreme Court in *Roe* and subsequent cases has spoken of post-viability abortion, doctors have historically thought of late terminations necessitated by a health problem on the woman's part as premature deliveries — deliveries that may put the fetus at great risk but that are not specifically intended to destroy it. In other words, post-viability terminations of pregnancy are simply inductions of labor, just as might be done at full term.

Once we recognize this, we see that what the Court says about third-trimester abortion should apply to delivery methods as well. When that yardstick is applied, it yields the conclusion that a state clearly could not enact a statute requiring Cesarean over vaginal delivery to protect the fetus. Inasmuch as surgical delivery involves ap-

proximately four times the maternal mortality rate of vaginal delivery,[15] such a statute would impermissibly mandate trade-offs between maternal and fetal health. The state could not statutorily mandate surgical delivery even in those cases where the fetus' health was seriously threatened by vaginal delivery, because the mother's health will still almost always be somewhat threatened by surgical delivery. Likewise, it violates the Constitution for courts to authorize nonconsensual Cesarean delivery in individual cases, since it seems clear that courts should not issue orders in individual cases that, if generalized in the form of a statute, would be unconstitutional.

The Child Neglect/ Fetal Neglect Analogy

Despite the strong argument that nonconsensual Cesareans are at odds with the teachings of *Roe* and other Supreme Court abortion cases, it may be objected that in rejecting maternal–fetal trade-offs, the Supreme Court was thinking only about abortions, not about full-term deliveries. Given the state's strong interest in preservation of life, why, one might ask, must doctors stand by while a baby who could be fine if delivered surgically dies or suffers irreversible brain damage? Whatever abortion law says, should women really have a right to make this potentially lethal choice, when the risk to them is quite minimal?

Courts and commentators have frequently relied on the law of child neglect to argue that harmful choices such as these are not the woman's to make.[16] Parents, of course, cannot refuse needed medical care for their children, even if the provision of such care violates their most cherished religious beliefs.[17] Likewise, it is often argued, pregnant women cannot refuse care necessary for their fetus' well-being. To do so is the prenatal equivalent of child neglect (and, according to this theory, taking substances such as heroin while one is pregnant is the prenatal equivalent of child abuse).

There's a simple charm to this notion that if parents cannot deny care to a child, neither can a pregnant woman deny it to a fetus, at least to a fetus that is fully formed and clearly viable. When analyzed, however, this notion is far from charming. It has far-reaching and very alarming implications, and it is far less simple than it appears. Child neglect is, of course, the failure to perform one's legal duties to one's children. The term "fetal neglect" implies that there are legally enforceable duties to fetuses. But while parents have historically owed a whole panoply of duties to their children, women have not heretofore been held to have legally enforceable duties to fetuses. Of course, we have until recently lacked the technology for visualizing the fetus, diagnosing its problems, and hence recommending procedures for its benefit. Some writers have suggested that the development of such technologies is sufficient to create new maternal duties to the fetus.[18] But before we let technology create entirely new sets of duties, we should at least stop and ask what technology hath wrought.

The technology for treating the fetus as a patient within a patient has transformed the unity of pregnancy into an uneasy duality. Two gestalts are now at work. One sees the pregnant woman as primary and the fetus as secondary; the other reverses the roles. "Fetal neglect" proponents unquestionably see the fetus as primary. They would discern the fetus' needs and then hold the woman responsible for either meeting those needs or justifying her failure to do so. Although they might argue that this is as good a way of reconciling the mother–fetus duality as subordinating the fetus' needs to the mother's, there are good reasons why, under the law, it is not. For one thing, while many women may place the best interests of their fetuses first and foremost, for the law to mandate this approach denies the full import of the fact that the fetus is located inside the woman.

Obviously, "fetal neglect" proponents recognize the *fact* of the fetus' internal location. They then draw the analogy with child neglect by stating that this difference in location is the only difference between a fetus and a child. True, it is (at least for very late-term fetuses). But in terms of what a state must do to end "fetal neglect" as opposed to ending child neglect, this "slight disanalogy" is like the difference between night and day. Children can simply be treated, in opposition to parental demands. But "fetal neglect" cannot be remedied without, as it were, "breaching the maternal barrier"—restraining and physically invading the woman. If one approaches this issue looking to what the fetus needs, there is a tendency to forget the woman is there—or to forget that she is more than, as George Annas puts it, a "fetal container."[19] Instead, one must approach the issue by asking if the woman s privacy can be violated—with the reason for violation being the state's important interest in protecting the life within her.

Giving due weight to the respective locations of mother and fetus debars us from using the simple (and simplistic) child neglect/fetal neglect analogy. It does not, however, answer the question of whether nonconsensual surgery can be imposed. For this, we must consider other cases in which the state's interests may oppose a patient's right to refuse treatment.

The State's Interest in the Well-Being of Third Parties

Competent persons can refuse medical treatment, even when it means their death. Their rights to privacy and bodily integrity are increasingly respected, even though the state has interests, such as in preserving life, that are arrayed against virtually all treatment refusals.[20] In other words, while the state's interests are neither negligible nor forgotten, the patients' privacy rights trump them. But most refusals do not have a direct and devastating effect upon third parties. How do we weigh the individual's right to refuse in these cases against the state's interest in preserving a third party's life—an interest that puts these cases in a class by themselves?

Courts have not taken the interests of third parties lightly, even when the goal was to preserve their emotional welfare rather than to protect them from physical harm. Some courts have overridden treatment refusals by parents of dependent children (usually Jehovah's Witnesses refusing blood transfusions), on the grounds that the parent should not be allowed to orphan his or her child.[21] It can readily be argued that if a parent's privacy right can be overridden to spare his child emotional or financial loss, surely it can be overridden to prevent a stillbirth or a birth injury that may cause profound impairment. The only problem with this argument is that these cases are, in my opinion, clearly wrong.[22] Although the practice is frowned upon, parents can abandon their children by putting them in foster care or even up for adoption; some parents de facto abandon their children by, for example, divorcing and leaving the jurisdiction; and parents take health risks, such as hang gliding, sky diving, or joining the U.S. army, that could potentially result in their children being orphaned. Why, in the one sphere of medical treatment, should they be required to violate their faith and adhere to medical orthodoxy? I see no good reason why here, but not elsewhere, parenthood should obliterate personal autonomy.

Of course, even if one accepted this line of cases, they could still readily be distinguished from the Cesarean dilemma. First, a blood transfusion is a less serious intrusion, involving far less pain, risk, bodily invasion, and recovery time. Second, the imposition of blood transfusions to prevent child abandonment does benefit the parent, in objective or secular terms: it saves his life, even though it does so, according to his faith, at the cost of his future salvation. Except in cases involving conditions such as placenta previa, where vaginal delivery threatens the lives of both woman and fetus, a Cesarean will benefit the fetus but not the woman. Indeed, rather than benefiting, the woman will typically be placed at somewhat greater risk by the proposed surgery. This makes the Cesarean cases truly unusual: one must ask when, if ever, the state can override a

treatment refusal and impose a risk upon one person so as to preserve the life or health of another person.

Having recognized that the true analogue to imposed Cesareans is nonconsensual surgery sought to benefit a third party, we now confront a significant dearth of caselaw. One reason is that there are few fact patterns in which a medical procedure performed on A will save B. Another reason is that compelling A to undergo risks so as to save B has always been considered beyond the reaches of state authority. In setting forth the limits of state authority, philosophers and legal scholars frequently note that the state could not require one citizen to give up a kidney to save another citizen, or to give up an eye so another could see.[23] The idea is outrageous enough to have been burlesqued in a *Monty Python* skit, where a woman minding her own business at home is interrupted by a loud knock on the door. The official-looking man at the door announces, "We've come for your kidney." When she protests, he says, "But you signed a donor card, didn't you?" She stammers that she meant to donate only after she was dead. Looking solemn, he says, unsheathing his surgical tools, "But someone needs it now."

In this country there is no general duty to rescue. There are exceptions, which include a special relationship between the parties such as that of innkeeper and guest, common carrier and passenger, and, most importantly, parent and child.[24] But even when a special relationship gives rise to a duty to rescue, there is still no duty to undertake *risky* rescues.[25] Nor is there such a duty in countries where there is a general duty to rescue.[26] It is easy to see that a demand for someone's kidney falls under the law of rescue (Samaritan law) and goes far beyond what is ever required of potential rescuers. In the one case on point, *McFall v. Shimp,*[27] a man dying of aplastic anemia asked the court to mandate that his cousin donate bone marrow to save him. The court called the relative's refusal to donate morally reprehensible, but held that for the law to "sink its teeth into the jugular vein or neck of one of its members and suck from it sustenance for *another* member, is revolting to our hard-wrought concepts of jurisprudence. Such would raise the spectre of the swastika and the Inquisition, reminiscent of the horrors this portends."[28] Although there are no *McFall*-type cases involving parent–child donation, I think we can say with a fair degree of certainty that the outcome would and should be the same. Parents have a duty to rescue their children—i.e., to be basic Good Samaritans—but they have no duty to be "Splendid Samaritans,"[29] embarking upon rescues that risk their life or health.

THE ILLEGITIMACY OF INTERPERSONAL RISK–BENEFIT COMPARISONS

If what a court does in mandating a Cesarean is no different from mandating a bone marrow transfusion to save a dying relative, it clearly exceeds the state's legitimate authority. While the two seem equivalent to me, they certainly haven't seemed so to most of the courts that have considered requests for nonconsensual Cesareans. For various reasons, court-ordered Cesareans strike many people as legitimate, while court-ordered bone marrow transfusions or kidney donations (a more equivalent intrusion), even from parent to child, seem outrageous. These reasons are important and cannot be ignored—they are what makes this situation so agonizing. However, I will try to show that while these reasons go to the woman's conduct, the appropriate question concerns the nature of the *state's* conduct. When we look to it, all nonconsensual risks imposed on one person to save another are equally illegitimate.

The Cesarean cases unquestionably *feel* different from cases or hypotheticals involving forced intrusions on parents to save children. For one thing, the woman is going to give birth anyway, and if she just does it surgically instead of vagi-

nally the baby will probably be fine. Cesareans are common and relatively safe, and the potential harm from delivering the baby vaginally is very serious. Moreover, it seems to some that women who choose not to abort thereby assume certain obligations to their fetuses, a by no means unreasonable suggestion. Finally, pregnancy simply is a unique situation. A dying relative, even a child, is a separate, independent person. However dire his need, he is not a tiny, helpless, totally dependent creature.

Emotional responses should certainly not be disregarded in bioethics. But neither should they necessarily rule. Physicians understandably become very uncomfortable when a woman appears ready to risk her fetus' life and health for the sake of her religious faith, and they feel even stronger when her reasons appear less weighty. Indeed, trivial reasons for running this risk may justify our casting moral aspersions on the woman's conduct. Despite the uniqueness of pregnancy, however, and despite the strength or weakness of the woman's reason for refusal (assuming she is competent), what the *state* does when it orders a compulsory Cesarean is no different from what it does when it orders compulsory bone marrow or kidney "donation," and what the state does is wrong.

The most significant feature of decisions ordering Cesareans is that the court, explicitly or implicitly, finds that the potential harm to the fetus overrides the woman's rights to privacy, autonomy, and bodily integrity, and justifies imposing a physical harm upon her (because surgery is a harm even if it has no untoward consequences). The court, in other words, takes two people, looks at the potential consequences of a bad situation, and says that the probably severe harm to X warrants imposing a lesser physical harm on Y. The legitimacy of this argument depends upon the assumption that a third party can step in and weigh the risks of surgery for someone who has competently chosen to forego them, and can then order that these risks be run. This is an assumption that has always been rejected in American jurisprudence, and that, if accepted, has far-reaching and extraordinarily frightening implications.

There is something special about the body. In theory, we can all recognize that everyone's body is equally special. But in practice, somehow our own seems far more special than anyone else's. It is very easy for us to say, as objective third parties, that a patient really should have needed surgery, because its risks are minute—perhaps only 1 in 10,000. But when we are thinking about that same surgery for ourselves, the minuteness of that chance may somehow seem less pertinent than the ghastly thought that we might be that one. This different attitude toward low statistical risks when run by a group of strangers and when run by oneself explains the old saying, "Minor surgery is surgery performed on somebody else." Perhaps this difference also explains why even countries with general duties to rescue never require risky rescues. While cowardice may not be admired, it is too human a quality to be formally punished by law.

Needless to say, a court can contemplate surgery for a pregnant woman only as a third-party bystander, albeit a careful and concerned bystander. It can assess the objective risks of surgery to the woman and the corresponding benefits to the fetus. But its ability truly to understand the situation is radically limited. Some limitations are simply due to the impossibility of extrapolating from statistical statements of risks, which apply to groups, to the risks faced by a particular individual. The court cannot know the exact risks it is planning to impose on the individual woman, because statistics don't tell us this. Other limitations relate to the particular, and undoubtedly unusual, circumstance: the risks may be increased if the surgery is done on an emergency basis,[30] and likewise may be magnified by its nonconsensual nature. But perhaps the most significant limitation is that a judge cannot possibly know or take into account the woman's subjective response to these risks, or to the proposed violation of her deeply held religious beliefs. In short, these decisions simply cannot be rendered objective. That is, after all, the whole point of the informed consent doctrine: people should be able to make their own decisions about surgery, even if their choices are idiosyncratic or even harmful.

In ordering surgery, the court is thus rendering objective a determination that cannot rightfully be anything but subjective. Although it is doing so for the best of reasons, its action nonetheless denies to a disturbing extent the woman's uniqueness and individuality. It denies her special fears or her special spiritual reasons for rejecting surgery and "leaving things in the hands of God." When it subjugates her views about having her body invaded (or about interfering with Providence) to its assessment of the "right" action based on potential consequences, it is making an interpersonal risk–benefit comparison and holding that she must run the risk to prevent the greater risk to the baby. Objectively, this may well be the proper assessment. But decisions about major surgery on unconsenting adults simply are not delegated to third parties, and delegating this one is no different from delegating a decision about bone marrow extraction or kidney transplant. I can think of no other instance where a state feels it has the authority to compare the risks faced by one individual to those faced by the other. The court compromises its integrity in making these orders, because whether it realizes it or not, it is treating the woman as a means—a vehicle for rescuing an imperiled fetus—and not as an end in herself.

Two disturbing potential scenarios will help illustrate why a nonconsensual Cesarean is inevitably a wrong against the woman. First, imagine surgery has been authorized, and the woman struggles to try to avoid it. In the case at North Central Bronx, doctors repeatedly asked what they should do if this occurred. Should they hold her down and anesthetize her? Some proponents of intervention would characterize this as merely a practical problem in enforcement—some injunctions being easier to enforce than others. Yet this is much more than a mere enforcement issue. It illustrates the violence lurking here, whether or not it is ever actually committed. The court is at one remove from the violence, because its role is limited to issuing the order. Nonetheless, the court has authorized an act of violence against the woman, even if the violence is obscured by her cowed compliance in the face of judicial power.

Second, imagine that the highly unexpected happens, and the woman is killed or injured by the surgery. Although this is exceedingly unlikely, its possibility raises an interesting moral issue. The court cannot, of course, be held legally responsible for this harm, nor can the doctors, assuming they were not negligent. Yet the court would be, it seems, morally responsible, because it chose to subject the woman to this risk. There is no comparison between the state's responsibility under this scenario and its responsibility if the woman's refusal is upheld and the baby is harmed. If the baby suffers, the woman is causally responsible (assuming surgery would have prevented the harm) and in some cases, at least, will be morally to blame. But the state won't be implicated, because the state does not normally intervene in a person's medical decisions. In other words, a private wrong will have occurred. But if the state has the hubris to intervene in what is ordinarily a private (albeit potentially tragic) choice, it takes on the moral responsibility for the outcome as well. Although the chances of maternal injury are low, the moral risk is great, and this possibility should make courts think twice before mandating surgery.

SOME ADDITIONAL SOCIAL CONCERNS

For purposes of analyzing nonconsensual Cesareans, I have been assuming that the physicians' predictions of harm to the infant are correct. In any individual case, of course, the doctor's alarm is most likely warranted—although it is interesting to note that in *Jefferson, Headley,* and *Jeffries,* the women delivered vaginally and the infants were fine. But when we think of mandatory Cesareans not simply as individual cases but as a social policy, we must recognize that some of the operations will be unnecessary. This is because the tools upon which doctors rely to diagnose problems during pregnancy or labor detect abnormally high risks, but do not necessarily distinguish cases in which the risks will materialize from those in which they will not.

Some tools and diagnoses are better than others. For example, ultrasonography is highly reliable in detecting placenta previa, and diagnosis of complete placenta previa reliably dictates Cesarean delivery. But even here prediction is not 100 percent accurate: both Ms. Jefferson and Ms. Jeffries, who were diagnosed as having complete placenta previa, delivered vaginally. Other tools are as likely to be wrong as right. Electronic fetal monitoring detects abnormal fetal heart patterns during labor that suggest an inadequate flow of oxygen to the fetus. According to the Office of Technology Assessment, the false positive rate of this technology is between 18.5 and almost 80 percent.[31] The rate is around 44 percent even when combined with fetal scalp blood sampling, another test that is believed to be more reliable.[32] A number of controlled studies have shown no difference in perinatal outcome when low-risk women were monitored electronically and when nurses performed intermittent ascultation (listening for heart rate changes).[33]

Physicians should be risk-averse and reluctant to gamble with the lives of babies, and fears of legal liability naturally enhance these traits. However, technological limitations combined with a cautious, risk-averse approach virtually ensure that some of the Cesareans doctors recommend will turn out not to have been required. While the vast majority of women would far rather risk an unnecessary operation than an impaired infant, it is not so clear that, given the technological limitations, it is irrational or immoral to take a different approach to risk. At any rate, mandatory Cesareans will mean that the judicial system requires this risk-averse approach, and forces pregnant women as a group to run some unnecessary risks to ensure healthy babies.

Although it might be suggested that courts can distinguish truly risky situations from only somewhat risky ones, this suggestion unfortunately puts more faith in the judicial system than it deserves, at least in these types of cases. The doctors bringing them will undoubtedly believe that surgery is necessary. The courts will have little choice but to accept the doctor's assessment—especially since in the typical Cesarean case the woman is either not present at all (and of course not represented by counsel) or represented by an attorney appointed only hours or days before and patently incapable of presenting contrary medical evidence even if it could be obtained.[34] These cases have thus far been very one-sided, and given the time constraints will almost surely continue to be so. This may account in part for the fact that most courts have issued the orders. It is interesting to note that in the Pamela Rae Stewart case, where Ms. Stewart was criminally prosecuted for prenatal conduct that allegedly caused her child to be born with brain damage and then to die, there was for once a two-sided debate. Here the American Civil Liberties Union came to Ms. Stewart's defense, and all charges against her were dismissed.[35]

Another social consequence of mandatory Cesareans might well be harm to the babies themselves. When the court authorized nonconsensual surgery for Ms. Jeffries, she went into hiding and could not be found even by a police search. When the court authorized the surgery for Ms. Headley, she avoided the hospital by having a home birth with a lay midwife. If women with unorthodox religious beliefs know that their beliefs will not be honored, they may avoid physicians during delivery or even during their entire pregnancy, thus placing their babies at greatly increased risk. Presumably the informed consent doctrine would dictate that

physicians tell women, early on in prenatal care, that they will not honor their religious beliefs if their fetus is endangered. This disclosure, however, will only serve to make such women avoid prenatal care (much as the reporting of drug abuse will make pregnant drug users avoid doctors and hospitals). Hence as a general social policy, mandatory fetal protection will have questionable success in protecting fetuses.

CONCLUSION

Emotionally compelling cases often make bad law. It is very hard for physicians and judges to resist the urge to save fetuses threatened by what appears to be the irrational conduct of the mother. The benevolence they feel is deeply rooted and deserves our respect. Unfortunately, mandatory rescue of the fetus requires an imposition upon the mother that goes far beyond what our society has imposed, or should impose, on others. Our historical restraint regarding such impositions has strong constitutional and ethical bases. Technology threatens this restraint, by making mandatory intervention possible. But technology cannot change the ethical principles that make mandatory intervention wrong.

REFERENCES

1. Only one of these cases—*Jefferson v. Griffin Spalding County Hospital Authority,* 274 S.E.2d 457 (Ga. 1981)—has been officially reported. Another case —In re Unborn Baby Kenner, No. 79 JN 83 (Colo. Juv. Ct. Mar. 6, 1979)—has been reported in medical literature; see Bowes WA, Selgestad B, Fetal versus maternal rights: Medical and legal perspectives, Obstetrics & Gynecology 1981, 58(2): 209, 211. A recent report of a large-scale survey indicates that courts in eleven states have ordered Cesarean deliveries. Kolder VEB, Gallagher J, Parsons MT, Court-ordered obstetrical interventions, New England Journal of Medicine 1987, 316(19): 1192-96, 1194.

2. See, e.g., *In re Baby Jeffries,* No. 14004 (Mich. P. Ct. May 24, 1982). Developments in the *Jeffries* case

are described in a series of newspaper articles. See Detroit Free Press, May 29, 1982; June 13, 1982; and June 16, 1982.

3. *North Central Bronx Hospital Authority v. Headley,* No. 1992-85 (N.Y. Sup. Ct. Jan. 6, 1986).

4. For discussions of in utero therapy, see, e.g., Robertson JA, The right to procreate and in utero fetal therapy, Journal of Legal Medicine 1982, 3(3): 333–66; Ruddick W, Wilcox W, Operating on the fetus, Hastings Center Report 1982, 12(5): 10–14; Barclay WR, et al., The ethics of in utero surgery, Journal of the American Medical Association 1981, 246(14): 1550–55.

5. *Jefferson v. Griffin Spalding County Hospital Authority,* 274 S.E.2d 457 (Ga. 1981); In re Unborn Baby Kenner, No. 79-JN-83 (Colo. Juv. Ct. Mar. 6, 1979); In re Baby Jeffries, No. 14004 (Mich. P. Ct. May 24, 1982) (order authorizing surgery); *North Central Bronx Hospital Authority v. Headley,* No. 1992-85 (N.Y. Sup. Ct. Jan. 6, 1986) (order authorizing surgery). There is no written decision in the case where the judge refused to authorize surgery. Interview with Judge Margaret Taylor, Family Court, in New York City (Nov. 6, 1985) (describing 1982 case where attorneys for St. Vincent's Hospital sought an order, but she refused to issue one).

6. 410 U.S. 113 (1973).

7. *Jefferson v. Griffin Spalding County Hospital Authority,* 274 S.E.2d 457 (Ga. 1981); *North Central Bronx Hospital Authority v. Headley,* No. 1992–85 (N.Y. Sup. Ct. Jan. 6, 1986), slip op. at 5; In re Unborn Baby Kenner, No. 79-JN-83 (Colo. Juv. Ct. Mar. 6, 1979) slip op. at 6–9.

8. 410 U.S. at 163–64.

9. *North Central Bronx Hospital Authority v. Headley,* No. 1992–85 (N.Y. Sup. Ct. Jan. 6, 1986); In re Unborn Baby Kenner, No. 79-JN-83 (Colo. Juv. Ct. Mar. 6, 1979).

10. 410 U.S. at 163–64.

11. Id.

12. 439 U.S 379 (1979).

13. Id. at 400.

14. Late abortion methods include induction of labor with substances such as prostaglandin or oxytocin — procedures likewise used to induce labor when a live birth is desired (especially oxytocin) — and hysterotomy, a procedure similar to a Cesarean. Pritchard J, Macdonald P, Grant N, Williams' obstetrics, 17th ed., 1985: 428.

15. National Institute of Health, U.S. Dept. of Health and Human Services, Pub. No. 82-2067, Cesarean childbirth: Report of a consensus development conference, Oct. 1981: 268.

16. See, e.g., *Jefferson v. Griffin Spalding County Hospital Authority,* 274, S.E.2d 457 (Ga. 1981); Myers

DBE, Abuse and neglect of the unborn: Can the state intervene?, Duquesne Law Review 1984, 23(1): 1, 26–31; Robertson, supra note 4, at 352, 357–58.

17. For example, in Matter of Jensen, 633 P.2d 1302 (Or. App. 1981), despite the parents' religious objections, the court ordered surgery for a fifteen-month-old child with hydrocephalus (accumulation of fluid in the brain) because her condition, if untreated, could cause major mental and physical disability. Id. at 1305–6. See also *Prince v. Massachusetts,* 321 U.S. 158, 166–67 (1944) (right to practice religion does not include liberty to expose child to communicable disease, ill health, or death).

18. See generally Myers, supra note 16.

19. Annas G, Women as fetal containers, Hastings Center Report 1986 16(6): 13–14.

20. Sec, e.g., Matter of Quackenbush, 383 A.2d 785 (NJ. Super. 1978) (ruling that competent patient with gangrene may refuse recommended leg amputation even though refusal will result in death); *Lane v. Candura,* 376 N.E.2d 1232 (Mass. App. 1978) (holding that irrationality of patient's refusal of amputation does not justify conclusion of incompetence and that surgery cannot be performed against patient's will); In re Melideo, 390 N.Y.S.2d 523 (N.Y. S. Ct. 1976) (Jehovah's Witness' refusal of blood transfusion upheld even though possibly necessary to save her life). These cases illustrate that courts today are likely to hold that the patient's right to privacy overrides that state's interest in preserving life.

21. See In re President and Directors of Georgetown College, Inc., 331 F.2d, 1000, 1008 (D.C. Cir.), *reh. denied en banc,* 331 F.2d 1010, *cert. denied* 377 U.S. 978 (1964); *Powell v. Columbian [sic] Presbyterian Medical Center,* 267 N.Y.S.2d 450 (Misc. 2d 1965). Cf. In re Osborne, 294 A.2d 372 (D.C. 1972) (upholding Jehovah's Witness father's refusal of blood transfusion, noting that even if he died, his children's financial and emotional needs would be met by close relatives and the ongoing family business).

22. At least one court has held that a parent's competent decision to refuse treatment simply supersedes the state's interest in protecting children from the loss of a parent; see In re Pogue, No. M-18-74 (D.C. Nov. 11, 1974). See also In Re Jamaica Hospital (reported in the New York Law Journal, May 17, 1985, at 15) (ordering transfusion for pregnant Jehovah's Witness to save fetus, but noting that if woman, a mother of ten, were the only one whose life were at stake, she could refuse the treatment).

23. See Tribe L, American constitutional law, Mineola, N.Y.: Foundation Press, 1978: 918.

24. Prosser W, Keeton W, The law of torts, 5th ed., St. Paul: West Publishing Co., 1984, §56, 376–77.

25. See, e.g., Vt. Stat. Ann. tit.12, §519(a) (1973); Minn. Stat. Ann. §604.05.01 (West Supp. 1986).

26. European countries, which generally do require rescue, exempt physically hazardous rescues. See, e.g., Code Penal, art. 63 (Fr.).

27. 10 Pa. D. & C. 3d 90 (1978).

28. Id. at 92 (emphasis in original).

29. This terminology is from Judith Jarvis Thomson's famous article defending abortion on the grounds that requiring a woman to continue a pregnancy is requiring her to be a "Splendid Samaritan," a requirement not imposed on anyone else in society. See Thomson JJ, A defense of abortion, Philosophy & Public Affairs 1971, 1(1): 47–66, 48–52.

30. Feldman GB, Freiman JA, Prophylactic Cesarean section at term?, New England Journal of Medicine 1985, 312(19): 1264–67, 1265.

31. Banta HD, Thacker SB, Assessing the costs and benefits of electronic fetal monitoring, Obstetrical and Gynecological Survey 1979, 34(8): 627–42, 628–29.

32. Id. at 629.

33. Leveno KJ et al., A prospective comparison of selective and universal electronic fetal monitoring in 34,995 pregnancies, New England Journal of Medicine 1986, 315(10): 615–19; Haverkamp AD, Orleans M, An assessment of electronic fetal monitoring, Women & Health 1982, 7(3–4): 115–34, 116.

34. In EFM cases, there will seldom be time for more than a hasty phone call to a judge. Even when counsel is appointed for the woman, he or she often has little or no time to prepare the case. In *Jefferson,* Ms. Jefferson's counsel was appointed at 11 a.m. on January 23, 1981; the case was argued at noon that same day. Letter from Hugh Glidewell (July 24, 1981). In *Headley,* North Central Bronx Hospital was represented by Bower and Gardner, a firm specializing in health law, while the woman was not represented at all. Telephone interview with Nancy Gold, of Bower and Gardner, who represented North Central Bronx Hospital (Jan. 13, 1986). According to the survey by Kolder et al., in 88 percent of the cases reported to them, the court order was obtained in six or fewer hours. See Kolder et al., supra note 1, at 1193.

35. *People v. Stewart,* No. M508197 (San Diego Mun. Ct. Feb. 26, 1987). Developments in the *Stewart* case were reported in several newspaper articles. See The New York Times, Oct. 9, 1986; and Feb. 27, 1987.

Compulsory Medical Treatment of Pregnant Women

BONNIE STEINBOCK

COMPULSORY MEDICAL TREATMENT OF PREGNANT WOMEN

. . . Advances in medical technology have enabled doctors to diagnose fetal disorders and sometimes even treat the fetus while still *in utero*. Doctors have treated fetuses with medications, given blood transfusions, implanted shunts, and removed fetuses for minor surgery on their bladders.[1] A dramatic breakthrough occurred in June 1989, when the first successful major surgery on a fetus was performed.[2] The fetus had a diaphragmatic hernia, a fairly common and usually fatal congenital malformation. His stomach, spleen, and large and small intestines had migrated through a hole in the diaphragm, taking up so much space that his lungs could not grow, making it impossible for him to breathe. His parents, Rick and Beth Schultz, were told by a specialist in Detroit that they had three options: end the pregnancy, attempt surgery after birth (which is successful in only about 25 percent of cases), or try experimental fetal surgery. They were referred to Dr. Michael R. Harrison, head of a team of surgeons at the University of California at San Francisco that had successfully performed the operation on baby lambs and fetal monkeys but had never been successful with human fetuses. After talking to Dr. Harrison on the phone and learning of the risks, the Schultzes opted for the prenatal surgery.[3]

With mother and fetus both under anesthesia, Dr. Harrison made an incision in the uterus, drained the amniotic fluid, and exposed the fetus's left arm and side. He cut into the fetus's abdomen and moved the stomach and intestines back into the abdominal cavity. Then he stitched a patch of synthetic Gore-Tex fabric over the hole in the diaphragm. A second patch was placed on the outside of the abdomen to relieve any pressure on the developing organs, and the fetus was returned to the womb. Beth spent the next six weeks in bed, to minimize the danger of a miscarriage. On August 5, 1989, Blake Schultz was delivered by cesarean section, through the same incision made for the surgery. He had to spend three weeks on a respirator in the hospital, but is now at home, growing and developing normally.[4]

The Schultzes are full of gratitude toward Dr. Harrison. Nevertheless, the surgery raises ethical questions. The risks to the mother—two cesarean operations, daily ingestion of a drug to prevent labor, and the danger of uterine rupture—are considerable, while there was no guarantee of a successful outcome for the fetus. Before Dr. Harrison's success with Blake Schultz, he had had six failures.

Less dramatic, but equally ethically problematic, are situations when the lifesaving procedure

BONNIE STEINBOCK is Professor and Chair in the Department of Philosophy at the State University of New York, Albany, with joint appointments in Public Policy and Public Health.

is standard medical practice. Surgeons are unlikely to pressure a patient to consent to experimental surgery; quite the reverse. However, when a commonly performed procedure (such as cesarean section) poses little risk to the woman (or even reduces maternal mortality or morbidity), and may be the only way to secure live birth, physicians may feel an obligation to the fetus to act as its advocate, and to get the woman to consent to lifesaving surgery. Admittedly, refusal in such circumstances is rare. Most women, faced with the possibility of fetal damage or death, readily consent to the treatment their doctors recommend. Nancy Rhoden comments, "The vast majority of women will accept significant risk, pain, and inconvenience to give their babies the best chance possible. One obstetrician who performs innovative fetal surgery stated that most of the women he sees 'would cut off their heads to save their babies.'"[5] Occasionally, however, a woman rejects a physician's recommendation, perhaps on religious grounds, perhaps because she does not think that surgery is necessary, or perhaps because she is afraid of surgery. The courts have long held that competent adults may refuse lifesaving medical treatment. But does the right to refuse treatment for oneself include a right to refuse treatment necessary to save another's life? These cases pose agonizing dilemmas for physicians. Rhoden says, "They pit a woman's right to privacy and bodily integrity . . . against the possibility of a lifetime of devastating disability to a being who is within days or even hours of independent existence."[6]

With a few notable exceptions,[7] most commentators have argued that pregnant women should not be forced to undergo medical treatment for the sake of preserving the life or health of their fetuses.[8] Attitudes among practicing physicians seem to be more split. A study published in 1987 found considerable support among heads of fellowship programs in maternal-fetal medicine for legal intervention of various kinds into the management of pregnancy. Almost half of those surveyed supported involuntary detention of pregnant women whose behavior endangers their fetuses. About the same number thought that the precedents set by the courts for emergency cesareans should be expanded to include other procedures, such as intrauterine transfusion, as these become part of standard medical care.[9]

Sometimes doctors, faced with a refusal, do not resort to the courts, but simply treat without consent. In one case, the placenta of a woman in labor detached prematurely from the inner wall of the uterus (a condition known as abruptio placentae), presenting an imminent threat to fetal survival. The mother repeatedly refused to give consent to a cesarean section, and the attending physicians felt that there was no time to attempt to secure a court order. Despite her refusal of consent, she did not actively resist when given general anesthesia. The physicians then delivered a severely stressed but otherwise healthy infant by cesarean section.[10]

The temptation simply to ignore the mother's refusal is understandable. Doctors are naturally reluctant to stand by and watch a baby who would be fine if delivered surgically die, or perhaps worse, suffer profound neurological damage. If they turn out to be right—the baby's life is saved and it is clear that the baby would have died if they had not operated—it seems harsh to blame them. If the woman herself is later glad that the doctors ignored her refusal, if she is *grateful* to them for having saved her life and that of her child, it does not seem that anyone else can say that they acted wrongly. Nevertheless, I will argue that these conditions cannot be guaranteed in advance, and therefore doctors are not morally justified in ignoring the refusals of competent patients.

It may seem that getting a court order puts doctors in a better ethical and legal position. The rights to privacy and bodily self-determination are not absolute. So it may be argued that doctors who take a patient to court act properly. They do not "take the law into their own hands," but instead give a judge the chance to decide whether there are compelling state interests that

justify forced treatment. This ignores the reality
of emergency decision-making in a medical setting. George Annas comments:

> Physicians should know what most lawyers and
> almost all judges know: When a judge arrives at
> the hospital in response to an emergency call, he
> or she is acting much more like a lay person
> than a jurist. Without time to analyze the is-
> sues, without representation for the pregnant
> woman, without briefing or thoughtful reflec-
> tion on the situation, in almost total ignorance
> of the relevant law, and in an unfamiliar setting
> faced by a relatively calm physician and a
> woman who can easily be labeled "hysterical,"
> the judge will almost always order whatever the
> doctor advises.[11]

A court order gives the misleading impression of
a fair resolution, one that takes seriously the interests of both the woman and the fetus. In reality, the decision to summon a judge simply gives
a legal veneer to the decision the doctors have already made. . . .

MCFALL V. SHIMP AND
THE DUTY TO RESCUE

The principle that pregnant women should not
be compelled to undergo any additional risks for
the sake of the unborn, even after viability, can
be given an equal protection basis. Outside pregnancy, there are virtually no circumstances in
which the body of one person could be required
to save the life of another. One famous case is
McFall v. Shimp,[12] in which Robert McFall, who
was dying of aplastic anemia, asked the court to
order his cousin, David Shimp, the only family
member with potentially compatible bone marrow, to donate bone marrow to him. Bone-
marrow extraction is not an especially risky procedure—far less risky than major surgery—but it
is painful and invasive. Shimp apparently believed that the medical risk to him was greater

than his cousin's doctors assessed it. On a
balancing-interests approach, McFall's interest in
survival might well outweigh Shimp's interests in
avoiding pain and minimal risk. The court rejected this approach. Although the court found
Shimp's behavior to be morally reprehensible, it
refused to order him to donate. The court emphasized that there was no legal duty to rescue
others, and stated that to require this would
change every concept and principle upon which
our society is founded. The court said:

> For a society which respects the rights of *one*
> individual, to sink its teeth into the jugular vein
> or neck of one of its members and suck from it
> sustenance for *another* member, is revolting to
> our hard-wrought concepts of jurisprudence.
> Forcible extraction of living body tissue causes
> revulsion to the judicial mind. Such would raise
> the spectre of the swastika and the Inquisition,
> reminiscent of the horrors this portends.[13]

McFall and Shimp were only cousins, but
there is no doubt that the outcome would have
been the same even had they been father and
child. Angela Holder states, "In no case is an
adult ever ordered to surrender a kidney, bone
marrow, or any other part of his body for donation to his child, to another relative, or to anyone else."[14] In fact, it is doubtful that a parent
could be legally compelled to donate a pint of
blood necessary to save his or her child's life.

The case of minor children is slightly different, since they are often not capable of giving
consent. This is not necessarily a bar to donation, since some courts have allowed parents to
authorize an incompetent sibling to donate a
kidney to a sibling suffering from renal failure,
using a substituted judgment basis.[15] Other
courts have rejected the claim that the test is
whether the incompetent would consent to donate if he could do so, and have simply refused to
authorize the transplant on the grounds that it is
not in the best interest of the incompetent.[16]
While courts have disagreed about whether parents may *authorize* donation on behalf of minor

children, there is agreement that such authorization cannot be *compelled*. In a recent case, Tamas Bosze, a Chicago bar owner, was told that only a marrow transplant could save his son, Jean-Pierre, from dying of leukemia. The boy's only potential donors were twin half-siblings born out of wedlock to the father's former girlfriend. Bosze sued the woman in an attempt to compel her to have the children tested for tissue compatibility. She refused, on the ground that this would not be in the twins' best interest. A court upheld her decision. In so doing, the court upheld the principle that no one is legally required to donate a body part to another, not even when this is needed to save a life. (Shortly thereafter Jean-Pierre Bosze died.[17]) . . . individuals may not be legally compelled to be "good Samaritans." This principle of our legal system must be remembered in assessing compulsory cesareans. To force women to undergo major surgery, even relatively safe major surgery, is to impose an unequal and unjustified burden on pregnant women. Even if we accept—as I do—the premise that women have *moral* obligations to the children they plan to bear, and even if these moral obligations include undergoing risks and making sacrifices to secure the health and well-being of the chldren they have decided to bear, it is quite another matter to think that these moral obligations should be legally coerced. I think we can agree that it would be appallingly selfish for a woman to expose her nearly born baby to the risk of an irreversible handicap simply to avoid an abdominal scar. But even in such a case, the woman should not be legally compelled to undergo surgery.

The above argument is based on the injustice of imposing burdens on pregnant women that are not imposed on other people. But what if the burdens were not unequally imposed? Would the state be justified in legally compelling all citizens, men and women, to undergo bodily risk and invasion where necessary to save a life? The answer to this question depends on one's general political outlook. Those who lean toward a more libertarian perspective will be opposed to "Good Samaritan" laws in general, and find the idea of compulsory donation of bodily parts especially repellent. Those who take a more communitarian approach may argue that all members of a community have a duty to make sacrifices for the good of the whole. For example, requiring healthy adults to make occasional blood donations might be considered justifiable. Communitarians might also argue that women should be legally compelled to undergo cesarean sections, where this is necessary to spare the child lifelong disability or death, given the relatively small objective risk to the woman and the enormous benefit to the child.

I cannot undertake a full-scale treatment of the merits of these opposing political theories. Fortunately, this is not necessary. Even communitarians should oppose compulsory cesareans, because, whether or not they could be justified in theory, there are overwhelming practical objections to them. For example, most doctors, even those who favor legal intervention in some cases, balk at using physical force to perform the surgery.[18] However, the potential for physical compulsion is implicit in legal coercion. Doctors who seek court orders should think about what they are willing to do to ensure that these are carried out. Francis Kenner, a Colorado woman who was told during labor that she needed a cesarean because of fetal distress, became more cooperative after the judge ordered a cesarean section. This was fortunate because, as her physician noted, "had the patient steadfastly refused it might not have been either safe or possible to administer anesthesia to a struggling, resistant woman who weighed in excess of 157.5 kg."[19] George Annas asks, "Do we really want to restrain, forcibly medicate, and operate on a competent, refusing adult? Such a procedure may be 'legal,' especially when viewed from the judicial perspective that the woman is irrational, hysterical, or evil-minded, but it is certainly brutish and not what one generally associates with medical care."[20]

NOTES

1. See Gina Kolata, *The Baby Doctors: Probing the Limits of Fetal Medicine* (New York: Delacorte Press, 1990).

2. Gina Kolata, "Lifesaving Surgery On a Fetus Works For the First Time," *The New York Times,* Thursday, May 31, 1990, A1.

3. "Saving Lives Not Yet Begun," *People,* June 19, 1990, p. 40.

4. Kolata, "Lifesaving Surgery On a Fetus" (see note 2), B8.

5. Nancy K. Rhoden, "The Judge in the Delivery Room: The Emergence of Court-Ordered Cesareans," *California Law Review* 74 (December 1986), p. 1959.

6. Nancy K. Rhoden, "Cesareans and Samaritans," *Law, Medicine & Health Care,* 15:3 (Fall 1987), p. 118.

7. See, for example, Patricia A. King, "The Juridical Status of the Fetus: A Proposal for Legal Protection of the Unborn," *Michigan Law Review* (August 1979), pp. 1647–1687; John Robertson, "The Right to Procreate and In Utero Fetal Therapy," *Journal of Legal Medicine* 3 (1982); and Margery Shaw, "Conditional Prospective Rights of the Fetus," *Journal of Legal Medicine* 5 (1984).

8. See, for example, George Annas, "Forced Cesareans: The Most Unkindest Cut of All," *Hastings Center Report,* June 1982; Janet Gallagher, "Prenatal Invasions & Interventions: What's Wrong with Fetal Rights," *Harvard Women's Law Journal* 10 (1987); Dawn Johnsen, "The Creation of Fetal Rights: Conflicts with Women's Constitutional Rights to Liberty, Privacy, and Equal Protection," *Yale Law Journal* 95 (January 1986); Lawrence J. Nelson and Nancy Milliken, "Compelled Medical Treatment of Pregnant Women," *Journal of the American Medical Association* 259 (Feb. 19, 1988), pp. 1060–1066; and Nancy Rhoden (see notes 5 and 6).

9. Veronika E. D. Kolder, Janet Gallaher, and Michael T. Parsons, "Court-Ordered Obstetrical Interventions," *New England Journal of Medicine* 316 (May 7, 1987), pp. 1192–1196.

10. Jurow and Paul, "Cesarean Delivery for Fetal Distress Without Maternal Consent," *Obstetrics & Gynecology* 63 (1984).

11. George J. Annas, "Protecting the Liberty of Pregnant Patients," *New England Journal of Medicine* 316 (May 7, 1987).

12. *Shimp v. McFall,* 10 Pa. D. & C.3d 90 (1978).

13. Ibid., p. 92 (emphasis in original).

14. Angela Holder, *Legal Issues in Pediatrics and Adolescent Medicine,* 2nd edition (New Haven: Yale University Press, 1985), p. 171.

15. See, e.g., *Hart v. Brown,* 29 Conn. Supp. 368, 289 A.2d 386 (1972); *Strunk v. Strunk,* 445 S.W.2d 145 (Ky 1969).

16. See In re *Richardson,* 284 So 2d 185 (La. Ct. App. 1973); In re *Pescinski,* 67 Wis. 2d. 4, 226 N.W. 2d 180 (1975).

17. Lance Morrow, "Ethics: Sparing Parts," *Time,* June 17, 1991, pp. 54–58.

18. Rhoden, "The Judge in the Delivery Room" (see note 5), footnote 273, p. 2004, citing a statement by Dr. Norman Fost, Presentation on Fetal Therapy at the Hastings Center, Conference on Abortion and Scientific Change, Hastings-on-Hudson, New York (May 24, 1985).

19. W. A. Bowes and B. Selgestad, "Fetal versus Maternal Right: Medical and Legal Perspectives," 58 *American Journal of Obstetrics & Gynecology* (1981), p. 209. The case is In re *Unborn Baby Kenner,* No. 79 JN 83 (Col. Juv. Ct. March 6, 1979).

20. Annas, "Forced Cesareans" (see note 8), p. 45.

Substance-Abusing Women:
False Stereotypes and Real Needs

MARGARET E. GOLDBERG

I DID THE INTAKE for Virginia at a women's shelter. She was a thin, pregnant African American woman of 35 with a tired, narrow face. Although calm, she seemed slightly confused about the dates and details of recent events. . . . Three weeks before she came to the shelter, her husband, angered that the fried chicken was overcooked, attacked her viciously with the cast iron frying pan full of hot grease. (Marks were not apparent because all the injuries were to parts of the body normally covered with clothes.) While Virginia was in the hospital, he told her he would kill her if she ever came back to the house. At discharge she took their seven children, ages one to 13 years, and returned to Providence. . . . At intake, Virginia seemed to be an extreme example of the type of person the shelter was designed to help and an ideal candidate for shelter services in re-establishing her family in a safe location and obtaining legal assistance with regard to her husband. At 9 o'clock that night Virginia disappeared, leaving the oldest daughter in charge of the other children. Around 10 o'clock the next morning she stumbled back, dead drunk but very apologetic. . . . Each of the two subsequent nights she repeated the same behavior. On the fourth day after intake, Virginia and her children were asked to leave. They walked out of the shelter carrying a dozen dark green garbage bags of clothes and personal belongings, headed nowhere. . . .

Dealing with substance-abusing women as an oppressed group is not as easy as dealing with some other groups, because these women are not ideal victims. Unlike the famous "elephant man" described by Treves (1971) who had suffered terrible oppression but had never harmed anyone, substance-abusing women are victims of oppression, but their own behavior frequently puts other innocent people at risk and places a financial burden on society. . . . According to recent estimates published by the Alcohol, Drug Abuse, and Mental Health Administration (Lehman, 1991), about 5 percent of American women abuse or depend on alcohol, and 1.5 percent abuse or depend on nonalcoholic illicit psychoactive drugs. These women come from all races and socioeconomic classes. . . .

Alcohol abuse among women has been known since antiquity. For example, the Old Testament says that when Hannah came into the temple to pray for a son, the priest at first mistook her for a common drunk (Keller, 1970). However, alcohol abuse, to the best of current knowledge, has always been more common among men than women (Fillmore, 1988). Abuse of nonalcoholic drugs has followed a different pattern. Few were known in the United States until the time of the Civil War. After the Civil War opiates and cocaine derivatives became available in unregulated patent medicines until they were outlawed in 1914. Although social

Social Work 40, 6 (1995): 789–798. Copyright 1995, National Association of Social Workers. Used by permission of the National Association of Social Workers.

science surveys as we know them today were not conducted at that time, there is widespread consensus that women were the chief consumers of these products and that many were addicted (Frankel, 1980). Even today, although use of illegal drugs by men exceeds that of women, abuse of prescription medicines such as tranquilizers and diet pills by women exceeds that of men (Lex, 1990) . . . .

Oppression is systematic harm that people with more power do to people with less power. Women . . . are directly discriminated against in hiring, salary, and promotions in the workplace and indirectly discriminated against by employment and educational organizations . . . (Karger & Stoesz, 1990). Women are overrepresented among the poor population because of the financial difficulties faced by single mothers (Karger & Stoesz, 1990). . . . Women are also far more likely than men to be subjected to sexual violence both as children and as adults (Finkelhor, 1986). . . . In fact, domestic violence is believed to be the largest cause of injuries requiring hospitalization among women in the United States (Stark & Flitcraft, 1988). . . . All of these factors affect substance-abusing women, as they do others, but several [childhood sexual abuse and domestic violence] appear to have a special association with the development of substance abuse problems. . . .

But many services developed to help people in these terrible situations are unable to accommodate the needs of substance-abusing women and hence exclude them. . . . Oppression directed at female substance abusers directly reduces the availability of services to promote recovery. Treatment programs are almost all based on methods developed for male substance abusers (Duckert, 1987; Tollett, 1990). . . . Only a few experimental treatment programs provide accommodation for children with their mothers. Mothers receiving public assistance may lose their income if they go into treatment and leave the children with someone else. They then may

be unable to get the benefits back without the children and unable to take the children back without the benefits. . . .

Controversy has arisen about the criminalization of substance abuse during pregnancy: A woman may be charged with drug crimes for using a substance potentially harmful to her unborn baby. Criminalization represents a new level of legal interference with women's rights over their bodies, interference that has no male counterpart (Maher, 1990). Although criminal charges are rare, there is a widespread legal presumption that any woman who abuses substances necessarily is guilty of child neglect or abuse (Maher, 1992). In many states, . . . the infant of a woman known through history or urine testing to have abused a substance during pregnancy automatically comes under the control of the state child protection agency. . . . [W]omen of color are much more likely (according to Chasnoff et al., 1990, 10 times more likely) to be tested than white women, and as a result, criminal charges and child protection interventions are far more often directed at women of color (Maher, 1992). . . .

The need for specific treatment geared toward women is being recognized, and experimental programs are being developed (Brown, 1992; Rahdert & Finnegan, 1993; Tollett, 1990). . . . The federal government is funding a number of innovative research and demonstration projects for treatment of substance-abusing women of childbearing age. . . . Immediate access to treatment without punishment appears to be the best way to alleviate the problems of substance-abusing women who are pregnant (Maher, 1990). Fairer and more widespread testing for drug and alcohol abuse by pregnant women would reveal the problem to be of too large a scope for the state to take over the lives of all affected children. A less intrusive system of monitoring welfare and maternal efforts at regaining sobriety is needed. . . . In addition to greater treatment options, some relatively inexpensive and easy-to-implement modifications of child protective and public assistance policies would reduce barriers to treatment. . . .

Another aspect of improving substance abuse services for women (and men) is better training of primary care physicians to diagnose and treat substance abuse and common emotional symptoms (Lewis, 1992). Better training of primary care physicians could lead to increased early intervention and decreased inappropriate prescription of addictive tranquilizers, such as benzodiazepines, to women who are already struggling to combat chemical dependency or to women who are clinically depressed and vulnerable to chemical dependency. . . .

The most desirable type of remedy is prevention of substance abuse among women. Prevention programs should include not only educational programs in schools, such as programs focused on the dangers of substance abuse to unborn children and special risk factors affecting women, but also real efforts to reduce some major risk factors to women. . . .

REFERENCES

Brown, E., Jay, M., Chaudhury, M., Kayne, H., Zuckerman, B., & Frank, D. (1993, June). Comprehensive day treatment improves outcomes for pregnant drug using women. Poster session presented at the College on Problems of Drug Dependence Meeting, Toronto.

Chasnoff, I., Landress, H., & Barrett, M. (1990). The prevalence of illicit-drug or alcohol use during pregnancy and discrepancies in mandatory reporting in Pinellas County, Florida. New England Journal of Medicine, 322, 1201–1206.

Duckert, F. (1987). Recruitment into treatment and effects of treatment for female problem drinkers. *Addictive Behavior,* 12, 137–150.

Fillmore, K. (1984). "When angels fall": Women's drinking as a cultural preoccupation and as reality. In S. Wilsnack & L. Beckman (Eds.), Alcohol problems in women: Antecedents, consequences, and intervention (pp. 7–36). New York: Guilford Press.

Finkelhor, D. (1986). A sourcebook on child sexual abuse. Beverly Hills, CA: Sage Publications.

Frankel, B. (1980). Human nature, addictions, and the geography of disorder in three cultures. Journal of Drug Issues, 10, 165–202.

Karger, J., & Stoesz, D. (1990). American social welfare policy. New York: Longman.

Keller, M. (1970). The great Jewish drink mystery. *British Journal of the Addictions,* 64, 287–296.

Lehman, M. (1991, July–August). Assessing future research needs: Mental and addictive disorders in women. *ADAMHA News,* pp. 1–7.

Lewis, D. (1992). Medical and behavioral management of alcohol problems in general medical practice. In J. Mendelsohn & N. Mello (Eds.), Medical diagnosis and treatment of alcoholism (pp. 463–500). New York: McGraw-Hill.

Lex, B. (1990). Prevention of substance abuse problems in women. In R. Watson (Ed.), Drug and alcohol abuse prevention (pp. 167–221). Totowa, NJ: Humana Press.

Maher, L. (1990). Criminalizing pregnancy: The downside of a kinder, gentler nation? *Social Justice,* 17(3), 111–135.

Maher, L. (1992). Punishment and welfare: Crack cocaine and the regulation of mothering. *Women and Criminal Justice,* 3(2), 35–70.

Stark, E., & Flitcraft, A. (1988). Violence among intimates: An epidemiological review. In V.

Tollett, E. (1990). Drug abuse and the low-income community. Clearinghouse Review, 24, 495–503.

Treves, F. (1971). The elephant man. In A. Montague (Ed.), The elephant man. New York: Outerbridge & Dientsfrey, pp. 13–38.

Case Study Exercises

CONTRACEPTION AND ABORTION

1. In the case of Darlene Johnson, a Fresno, California, judge offered Johnson the "choice" between Norplant (a long-term contraceptive implant) and jail. Do you think long-term

forced contraception should be a sentencing option for judges in cases such as this one, in which women have been abusive to their own children or have been substance abusers? Share your thoughts on this issue.

2. In 1993 China denied that it had a plan for forced abortions but admitted that a proposed law would require people with diseases that lead to birth defects or mental retardation to either postpone marriage or undergo "long-term contraceptive measures after marriage." (See Rone Tempest, "China Denies Plan for Forced Abortions," *Los Angeles Times,* 30 December 1993.) At least one province already mandates sterilization for people with a history of mental illness or severe mental retardation. In light of these facts, answer the following:
   a. Is this policy just?
   b. What should be our obligations, if any, to ensure that people have healthy children with some minimal level of intelligence?
   c. China's Health Ministry declared that its "better-births policy" is "totally different from the racist 'eugenics' policy pursued by Adolf Hitler during the Third Reich." What are the issues and concerns about any government policy around "better births"?

3. When the FDA was considering whether or not to approve the abortion pill, RU-486, the names of its manufacturer and distributor were kept secret. If the drug is approved for marketing, the distributor's name will be revealed but not the manufacture's. The Population Council says the extreme secrecy is necessary to protect the drug company from threats of boycotts or violence from anti-abortion groups. Marcie Wilder, legal director of the National Abortion Rights Action League in Washington, remarked, "There's never been a drug that's been targeted like this one." (See Gina Kolata, "Abortion Pill Reaches New US Juncture," *New York Times,* 19 July 1996.)
   a. What might be the concerns of anti-abortion groups regarding RU-486?
   b. What might be the concerns of pro-choice groups regarding RU-486?
   c. What are reasons for a boycott of the manufacturer of the abortion pill?
   d. What are reasons against boycotting the manufacturer of the abortion pill?

4 Share your concerns regarding minors seeking an abortion. Should we have a federal policy on this issue, and if so, what should be included in the guidelines?

5. In an open letter to Pope John Paul, professor of Japanese Studies William R. LaFleur called for a reconsideration of the Vatican's position on contraception in light of Buddhist ethics. (See "Dear Pope John Paul," *Tricycle,* Summer 2000.) He writes: ". . . Buddhism— perhaps uniquely among what are sometimes called the 'world religions'—either explicitly or implicitly rejects what I have elsewhere called 'fecundism,' which may be defined most simply as the positing of links between reproductive success and religious value . . . Fecundism has the god or gods as bedside cheerleaders, telling people that the deity's own deep wish is that his or her select people multiply in the greatest possible numbers."
   a. Do you believe LaFleur is right to bring the population explosion before us as an ethical issue?
   b. Along with open letters, what other channels might individuals or religious groups pursue to bring religious and ethical issues before the public eye in trying to effect social change?

6. The Supreme Court, on June 28, 2000, struck down a Nebraska law prohibiting late-term ("partial-birth") abortions. The majority opinion in *Nebraska v. Carhart* (June 28, 2000) held as unconstitutional a Nebraska law prohibiting any "partial-birth abortion" unless that procedure is necessary to save the mother's life. The Nebraska law defines "partial-birth abortion" as a procedure in which the doctor "partially delivers vaginally a living unborn

child before killing the . . . child," and defines the latter phrase to mean "intentionally delivering into the vagina a living unborn child, or a substantial portion thereof, for the purpose of performing a procedure that the [abortionist] knows will kill the . . . child and does kill the . . . child." Violation of the law was a felony, and provided for the automatic revocation of a convicted doctor's state license to practice medicine. Dr. Leroy Carhart, a Nebraska physician, brought the suit that ended up before the U.S. Supreme Court. The Court's ruling was that, "In sum, using this law some present prosecutors and future Attorneys General may choose to pursue physicians who use D & E procedures, the most commonly used method for performing previable second trimester abortions. All those who perform abortion procedures using that method must fear prosecution, conviction, and imprisonment. The result is an undue burden upon a woman's right to make an abortion decision. We must consequently find the statute unconstitutional."

   a. Discuss whether or not you think the Court's reasoning here is justifiable.

   b. If you are able to access pro-life and pro-choice abortion Web sites, how do you see the decision in light of the political climate of the U.S.?

7. Another Supreme Court decision in the year 2000 was *Hill v. Colorado,* which focused on abortion clinics. In their decision, the Court let stand a statute banning protesters from coming within 8 feet of another person, without that person's consent, in order to protest or attempt to counsel a pregnant woman against getting an abortion. Do you agree with the Supreme Court decision to keep protesters at a distance? Does this give proper weight to both the right to freedom of speech and a woman's right to an abortion? Share your thoughts.

8. How do you think we should address abortion clinic violence? After setting out your initial thoughts, answer the following: Given that abortion foes have strong feelings about what they consider to be morally unacceptable, where should we, as a society, draw lines about actions taken because of those beliefs?

9. What ideas or recommendations do you have regarding the following case?

Shelley Shannon, Oregon housewife, admitted on 7 June 95 that she had waged a campaign against abortion clinics and doctors. She was already serving a 10-year prison term for shooting a doctor in Kansas in 1993. She admitted that a year before that shooting she had tried to burn down or disable six abortion clinics on the West Coast. Federal investigators wanted to coax information from her about associates in the anti-abortion movement. But, after disclosing some details and names possibly linked to a conspiracy, she suddenly decided to refuse to cooperate further. Her silence was a setback for the Federal task force trying to determine whether a nation-wide criminal conspiracy exists to inflict violence on abortion doctors and clinics.

   The task force was organized by Janet Reno in Fall 1994, after an abortion doctor and his escort were killed by Paul Hill in Florida. Investigators were seeking to determine whether, in fact, a rumored conspiracy really exists. Thus far, the task force has found evidence that 12 American doctors are targeted for harassment by anti-abortion militants who call the doctors "night crawlers." The most militant members of the anti-abortion movement quote the Bible as a justification to commit murder, arson, and death threats. Shannon said that "Two people convinced me that God is calling them to shoot abortionists," but she refused to name names. (See Timothy Egan, "Conspiracy Is an Elusive Target in Prosecuting Foes of Abortion," *New York Times,* 18 June 1995.)

10. Within the last five years, seven abortion physicians and clinic workers have been killed. In the last several years, the National Abortion Federation alone has been responsible for 39

bombings, 99 acid attacks, and 16 attempted murders. In February 1999, a federal jury ruled that an Internet Web site featuring bloody fetuses and "Wanted" posters targeting doctors and other abortion providers constituted a real threat. They ordered those responsible to pay $107.9 million in damages. The case originated in attempts to stop the rise of abortion-clinic violence and physical harm and/or death threats to those who do abortions. (See Kim Murphy, "Anti-Abortion Web Site Fined $107 Million," *Los Angeles Times,* 3 February 1999.)

Discuss the claims made on behalf of the parties involved, as set out below:

a. "If these posters are threatening, then virtually any document that criticizes an abortionist by name is threatening. I think the effect on political protest will be devastating," said Christopher Ferrara, attorney for the American Catholic Lawyers Association representing several defendants.

b. "Today, my safety and my family's safety depends on the courts upholding this law. . . . Americans are tired of the hassle, and tired of the fear," said Dr. Elizabeth Newhall, Portland physician and one of the plaintiffs.

11. Lisa M. Fleischman, a New York attorney specializing in reproductive issues, has claimed that the question of abortion does not, contrary to the public debate, turn on whether or not the fetus is a life. Rather, the debate exists because we have been unable to face the real moral question at the heart of the abortion debate: namely, "When is killing permitted?" She contends that abortion is killing. It is the taking of a human life. But it is not any more a case of murder than the death penalty is murder or sending soldiers to war is murder. Humanity, she says, "has always believed that, at certain times in certain places, the killing of others is justifiable. The same Catholic Church that so fervently opposes abortion has its doctrine of the 'just war.' Many pro-lifers favor the death penalty." (See Lisa M. Fleischman, "What Abortion Debate Is Really About: When Is Killing Permitted?" *Los Angeles Times,* 18 March 1990.)

a. Discuss the strengths and weaknesses of either of Fleischman's analogies (between abortion and the death penalty and abortion and sending soldiers to war) to see if the analogy holds.

b. Fleischman claims the abortion debate centers on the question, "When is killing permitted?" One argument favoring the use of fetal tissue (e.g., in transplants or research) is that it is a way for something good to come out of an evil (an abortion). Respond to this position.

12. To what extent should we put pressure on or pass laws to require prostitutes and sex workers to use condoms as an attempt to address the explosion of sexually transmitted diseases (STDs) and AIDS? Set out your view in light of the following:

Sex trade workers in Eastern Europe and Asia are enslaved to international crime syndicates. Clients demand unprotected sex and prostitutes must accept these "workplace" conditions if they hope to make a living. For anatomical reasons, women are four times more vulnerable to contracting HIV. They get it and they give it while repressive laws discourage them from seeking treatment because their profession is a crime. . . . In the East and the South . . . HIV infection has exploded into pandemic proportions. What was once primarily a disease of gay men, certainly in North America, HIV/AIDS has been transformed into an affliction that threatens millions upon millions of women and children. Globally, 10.3 million young people (between the ages of 15 and 24) have contracted HIV, about a third of all those infected, with girls and young women 50 percent more likely to get it now than boys and young men . . .

"The condom is to the sex worker what a hard hat is to a construction worker," said Cheryl Overs, former coordinator of the International Network of Sex Workers

Projects. . . . "At the most, we find we can reach women for a maximum of three months before they disappear again," said Licia Brussa, who administers an Amsterdam-based humanitarian agency that works with prostitutes in 47 European and North African countries. "These women are extremely limited in being able to access health care services. They're afraid of being deported. They're under the control of international crime syndicates. They have no autonomy about where they live and work, about whether they can marry. . . . This can no longer be viewed as a local or national problem, but as an international one." (See "'Morality' still clouds the debate over prevention," *The Toronto Star,* 13 July 2000.)

MATERNAL-FETAL CONFLICTS

1. In an unprecedented action, South Carolina's Supreme Court ruled that a woman could be prosecuted for child abuse if she takes drugs during pregnancy. Pregnant women are the only people who can be arrested for using a drug—i.e., for prior drug use. Arguing that a viable fetus can be considered a "child" or "person" under state law, the Court then gave a fetus legal protection. Consequently, the ruling reinstated an eight-year sentence given to Cornelia Whitner, whose son (now a healthy eight-year-old boy) tested positive for cocaine after he was born. (See Robert Tanner, "Mom Abused Drugs," *Chattanooga Free Press,* 17 July 1996; see also Matt Owen, "Advocate for Pregnant Woman Wants to Bring Changes in Law," *The Post and Courier* (Charleston, SC, 25 July 1999.)

   a. Some argue that this ruling would discourage pregnant drug abusers from seeking medical help. Do you think this concern is sufficient grounds to consider the South Carolina Supreme Court ruling misguided?

   b. In his dissent, Justice James E. Moore commented on the ruling, "Is a pregnant woman's failure to obtain prenatal care unlawful? Failure to take vitamins and eat properly? Failure to quit smoking or drinking?" He said that, under this decision, a woman would be better off to illegally abort a third-trimester fetus and face a two-year sentence than give birth to a baby after taking drugs and then face a ten-year sentence for child abuse. What would you reply to Judge Moore?

2. Two researchers in Boston produced startling numbers to support the long-held belief that smoking during pregnancy can prove fatal to fetuses and infants. They found that expectant mothers who smoke cause the deaths of about 5,600 babies and cause between 19,000 and 141,000 miscarriages in America every year. Furthermore, as many as 26,000 newborn infants are put in intensive care units each year because of smoking-related low birth weight. (See "Study on Smoking Tallies Baby Deaths," *Los Angeles Times,* 13 April 1995.)

   a. Given the statistical data about the dangers of smoking to infants, what should be done? It may help to look at distinctly different perspectives (e.g., of the fetus, the pregnant woman, the medical profession, societal interests).

   b. How might you defend or attack the claim, "Pregnant women who smoke should be prosecuted for child abuse"?

3. In a report on dioxin, scientists at the EPA claimed that the most serious health hazard of exposure to dioxin is not cancer—it is harm to the fetus. Dioxin and its related toxic compounds, PCBs and furans, are by-products of heating or burning chlorine-based chemicals (e.g., in manufacturing or in waste incinerators). As a consequence of the burning, minute particles fall to the earth and enter the food chain. The report pointed out that "the human embryo may be very susceptible to long-term impairment of immune function from in-utero effects." (See Keith Schneider, "Fetal Harm, Not Cancer, Is Cited as Primary Threat from Dioxin," *New York Times,* 11 May 1994.)

a. If a couple planning to have a family read the report, what issues and concerns would arise? What would be the key recommendations from this perspective?
b. If an obstetrician or other health care giver read the report, what issues and concerns would arise? What would be the key recommendations from this perspective?
c. If EPA personnel or members of an environmental watch-dog group read the report, what issues and concerns would arise? What would be the key recommendations from this perspective?

4. Share your thoughts on the following claim: "Given evidence that AZT can cut the risk of transmission of HIV between a pregnant woman and her fetus from 8 percent to 25 percent, mandatory AIDS testing of all pregnant women is justified."

5. How do we find a balance of competing interests in maternal-fetal conflicts? Set out your suggestions for finding a balance between the interests of the pregnant woman (patient autonomy) and those of her fetus (fetal rights), taking into consideration the following: occupational concerns, environmental concerns, and lifestyle concerns (such as consumption of alcohol, smoking, and drug abuse).

6. Studies done in 1994 found there might be a link between silicone breast implants and damage to the esophagus in breast-feeding implants. In a study of eleven infants whose mothers had silicone implants, it was found that six of the eight breast-fed babies had damage to the esophagus that made it difficult to swallow, caused vomiting, and weakened the esophagus. Also, most of them were underweight. The bottle-fed infants showed no such abnormalities (see Philip J. Hilts, "Risks Found in Nursing Infants of Implant Recipients," *New York Times,* 19 January 1994). Assuming further studies confirm this problem, should the risks to the babies outweigh the woman's right to decide whether or not to get breast implants, particularly when the implants are for cosmetic (versus reconstructive) reasons? Share your reflections on this dilemma.

7. In what sort of situation might a forced caesarian be justifiable? What sorts of issues arise regarding the woman's right to privacy and/or bodily integrity? When, if ever, are those rights trumped by the fetus's right to life?

8. Contrary to widely held perceptions about "crack babies," a key study indicated the fears of long-term aftereffects are overblown. The Maternal Lifestyle Study is said to be the largest research project to date on drug-exposed infants. According to Charles Bauer, professor of pediatrics at the University of Miami,

People were worried [in the 1980s] that the school system would be flooded with retarded, uncontrollable children. That just didn't happen. The recent studies show that prenatal drug exposure has a greater impact on children's social development than on their medical condition, and its effects are subtle and not always detrimental." (See Megan Twohey, "The Crack-Baby Myth," *National Journal,* 13 Nov 1999.)

Evidently, the foster care environment can be just as damaging as the biological mother's drug environment. Barry Lester, director of the Infant Development Center at Brown University, recommends putting money into intervention right after birth, rather than taking the baby away from her mother. Clearly, treating drug-addicted mothers is not easy, and lack of drug treatment for women just exacerbates the situation. However, since taking babies away from cocaine-abusing mothers has not resulted in a better situation for the child, offer your recommendations for addressing this difficult social problem.

InfoTrac College Edition

1. Tu Ping; Qiu Shuhua; Fang Huimin; Herbert L. Smith, "Acceptance, Efficacy, and Side Effects of Norplant Implants in Four Counties in North China"
2. Deborah Haas-Wilson, "The Impact of State Abortion Restrictions on Minors' Demand for Abortions"
3. John Ellis, "It's OK to Kill Babies? And That's Fit to Print? [Response to an Article by Steven Pinker, *New York Times Magazine*, Nov 2, 1997]"
4. Yvette R. Harris, " Adolescent Abortion"
5. Mike Hoyt, " Abortion: Partial Truths. [Interview]"
6. Susan E. Wills, "BACK TO THE ALLEY CLINICAL PSYCHOSIS: Unsafe Abortions Are Not a Thing of the Past"
7. James Ciment, "Most Deaths Related to Abortion Occur in The Developing World"
8. Carolyn Egan, "How We Won Abortion Rights. [Canada]"
9. *The Christian Century,* "Responsibility Claimed for Abortion Clinic Bomb"
10. Melanie Conklin, "Lights out on Abortion. [Punitive, Broad Wisconsin 'Partial Birth' Abortion Law Provokes Strike by All Abortion Providers]"
11. Henry Morgentaler, "A Letter to Pope John Paul II. [About Hate Speech and Violence Committed by Anti-Abortion Activists]"
12. *The Christian Century,* "Postabortion Counseling"
13. *Pediatrics,* "Neonatal Drug Withdrawal. [American Academy of Pediatrics Committee on Drugs]"
14. Francis M. Donnelly, Joy L. Mowery, D. Gail McCarver, "Knowledge and Misconceptions among Inner-City African-American Mothers Regarding Alcohol and Drug Use"

Web Connections

For links to Contraception, Abortion, and Maternal Fetal Conflicts Web sites, articles, cases, and more exercises go to our abortion page at philosophy.wadsworth.com/teays.purdy/ abortion

Chapter 7

Reproductive Technology and Surrogacy

ONE OF THE MOST controversial topics in reproductive ethics is the use of new technologies and new social arrangements to facilitate childbearing. Reproduction is an especially sensitive issue because of the ways it intersects with traditional views, especially religious views, about the moral status of the fetus, women's social roles, and the family. At one end of the spectrum are those who believe that reproduction should take place only in a traditional marriage as a result of sexual intercourse between a woman and man. At the other end are those who condone any attempts to reproduce that result from informed choices; only the high probability of serious harm justifies limits on such choices. In between lie a vast array of possible ethical positions, expanding in number as new options become available.

Reproductive technology offers a veritable panoply of opportunities. First, it can make childbearing possible in cases where it would otherwise be virtually impossible. Also, it can make childbearing easier or safer than it would otherwise be. Moreover, it can help us shape the nature of the resulting child; e.g., by allowing us to intervene at very early stages in the development of the fetus in order to address medical problems. It also allows for the selection of eggs, sperm, and even embryos in order to obtain the best candidate for creating a healthy (or genetically engineered) child.

One key technology here is in vitro fertilization, or IVF. In IVF, eggs are obtained from a fertile woman (either the intended mother or a donor egg) and fertilized in a petri dish with sperm obtained from the intended father or a donor. The eggs are then implanted in either the donating woman or another woman who has been hormonally prepared to receive them. The success rate is low, the process is expensive, and the long-term effects on the women and the children produced are unknown.

There are objections to all of the aims of reproductive technologies, as well as to the means, such as IVF, used to achieve them. One objection is that we have no business meddling in these matters: They are for God or nature to decide, and we ought not tamper with the hand that nature has dealt us. Those who believe that embryos and fetuses have moral status also tend to object on the grounds that the experimentation involved in these new approaches fails to respect human life, especially when "damaged" or "excess" embryos are destroyed. They similarly raise objections to sex selection, which entails the abortion of a fetus rejected because of gender.

Among the critics are feminists who are wary of changes in reproductive practices. On the one hand, the use of new reproductive technology could promote pronatalism and a kind of biological determinism that finds women's chief value in reproduction and nurturing. On the other hand, it could exploit women, financially and in other ways, all in the name of promoting individual choice. One of the claims in this regard is that women and children are demeaned by such practices; that, for example, a surrogate pregnancy is a form of "alienated labor": A woman is contracted to deliver a product, the child, by going through a process of creation in which she is supposed to separate herself emotionally from the child developing inside of her, hand it over upon birth, and have no other relationship with it the rest of her life. Some contend that this arrangement brings about the commodification of both women and children.

The most enthusiastic supporters of nontraditional reproduction are those who see science as liberating us from oppressive social traditions and who thus consider reproductive technology just one more tool at our disposal. By this view, we have every right to use these means, particularly since the benefits, they contend, clearly outweigh the risks. Such concerns as potential exploitation of women and children thus get dismissed by arguments about informed consent and the right of self-determination on the part of participating individuals. Proponents of this view believe that we need to honor women's right to make choices, even if we find the decision morally repugnant; that autonomous individuals are entitled to make even bad decisions with respect to their own affairs and to what happens in their own bodies. For some thinkers, such as John Robertson, people have a right to procreative liberty, and this right entails the use of reproductive technology, including surrogate parenting.

Nevertheless, the matter is not so clearly resolved. We therefore need to look closely at the issues and concerns resulting from the new reproductive technologies. It is especially important to engage in the kind of critical thinking that neither rejects all new developments out of hand, ignoring their potential benefits, nor indiscriminately embraces them all. Such thinking attempts to ferret out the assumptions underlying the opposing positions and seek out evidence (theoretical, empirical, historical, social) for the claims inherent in them.

So-called "surrogacy" is perhaps the most controversial of all the new developments in reproduction. The simplest sort of surrogacy requires no complex technology at all: a woman gestates a baby to be handed over to others, and fertilization is done either by artificial insemination (AI) or sexual intercourse. Because the resulting child is genetically as much the gestating woman's as the fertilizing man's, some object to seeing her role as mere "surrogacy," suggesting instead we call it "contract pregnancy."

Surrogacy brings to the forefront the questions:

- What is it to be a mother?

- Should surrogate contracts be enforceable?

- How much value should be placed on genetics in decisions over custody arrangements?

- Can human life be a subject for a contract?

- How can we arrive at what's in the best interest of the child in disputes over surrogate arrangements?

- What sorts of safeguards could minimize the potential for abuse and exploitation?

- Is surrogacy demeaning to women and children?

All of these questions deserve our attention as we set forth public policy guidelines.

As recognized in the "Baby M" (*Stern v. Whitehead*) case, the biological surrogate is legally the mother of the child and thus has enforceable rights which she can exercise. For Mary Beth Whitehead, mother of Melissa (Baby M), that meant she got broad visitation rights when she sued for custody of the child. Because of this precedent, couples seeking surrogates have sought a less risky legal path, such as gestational surrogacy.

Newer, higher-tech forms of surrogacy involve a gestating woman, as the fertilized egg is provided by others. In this case, the surrogate mother has no genetic relationship to the child she bears. Not only does this seem appealing biologically to the contracting couple (as they can then be the genetic parents of the child), but it lifts a significant legal burden.

Gestational surrogates who want to sue for custody have considerably less legal standing than those who are biological surrogates (i.e., the genetic mothers)—as the Anna Johnson case showed. Because she had no genetic relation to the baby she gave birth to under contract to the Calverts, Anna Johnson's maternal standing was dismissed by the California Supreme Court. She was seen as having no right to raise, or be part of raising, the child she bore. In addition, the fact that Johnson was African-American and the contracting woman, Crispina, was Filipina and her husband, Mark, white, raised questions about race and the possible bias in the ruling itself and the handling of the case by the media. Furthermore, the case of *Calvert v. Johnson* fueled the debate about the potential for exploitation of third world women by wealthy members of the dominant society. We need to look at the wide range of issues so that we can arrive at policies that are rooted in justice.

Many of the same questions arise with contract pregnancy as with genetic and reproductive technologies in general. Should we be "playing God"? Should we be "meddling with nature"? Does it harm the family? Does it harm the children thus produced, either physically or psychologically? Does it exploit women—especially disempowered, poor, and minority women? Both supporters and opponents of these methods admit that there is potential for new and difficult problems; such as custody decisions in litigious cases or in cases in which nobody wants the child because it was born with health problems or the baby was the "wrong" gender.

These questions deserve serious scrutiny. Their answers may help us fashion public policy, although attempting to construct a morally tenable public policy raises still more questions. On balance, is contract pregnancy immoral? In all forms? Should it be made illegal? Or should any form be legal? Should it be highly regulated to protect the competing interests at stake in it? Should contracts be considered unenforceable?

Should commercial pregnancies (those undertaken for pay) be banned, retaining only those undertaken for love, so-called "altruistic" surrogacy?

These questions have no easy answers, and thus far the law has addressed them only on the state level. Some states ban surrogacy, some allow it with restrictions, some have given it a virtual green light. We are still in the process of arriving at some semblance of public policy on the issue of reproductive technology. Because of this, it is important for us to look at these issues and try to arrive at some resolution in order for us to shape future decision making on the issue.

The readings in this chapter will help clarify and advance our thinking about this difficult issue. This chapter is divided into two sections. The first considers both general issues raised by assisted reproduction and considers some specific practices; the second focuses on the vexed issue of surrogacy.

In the first section, that of reproductive technology, the readings are as follows:

1. Susan Sherwin argues that there are good reasons for a cautious attitude toward in vitro fertilization and the new technologies generally.

2. John A. Robertson argues for a permissive approach to assisted reproduction, positing a wide-ranging right to procreative liberty.

3. Michelle Stanworth comments that concern about women's (and children's) welfare must be multifaceted and that it doesn't necessarily support the conclusion that assisted reproduction should be prohibited.

4. Hilde Lindemann Nelson examines the issue of personhood of the fetus arising from the use of new reproductive technology.

5. An editorial from *The Globe and Mail* (Toronto) asserts that reproductive technology is creating a "morass" of multiple births and suggests that we need to give more thought to how we are proceeding.

The readings in the second section look at surrogacy and the ethical dilemmas it raises.

1. Herbert Krimmel argues that surrogacy commodifies children and raises other serious moral problems.

2. Anita L. Allen provides a historically based objection to the view that surrogacy involves slavery, and argues that privacy arguments are inappropriate for judging the moral permissibility of surrogacy.

3. Christine Sistare applies the concepts of freedom and choice to make the case for women's right to engage in contract pregnancy.

4. Alexander Morgan Capron considers what should be done to prevent or remedy one risk of surrogacy: the existence of too many parents.

Reproductive Technology

Feminist Ethics and In Vitro Fertilization

SUSAN SHERWIN

. . . LET ME BEGIN with a quick description of IVF for the uninitiated. In vitro fertilization is the technology responsible for what the media likes to call "test tube babies." It circumvents, rather than cures, a variety of barriers to conception, primarily those of blocked fallopian tubes and low sperm counts. In vitro fertilization involves removing ova from the woman's body, collecting sperm from the man's, combining them to achieve conception in the laboratory, and, a few days later, implanting some number of the newly fertilized eggs directly into the woman's womb with the hope that pregnancy will continue normally from this point on. This process requires that a variety of hormones be administered to the woman—which involve profound emotional and physical changes—that her blood and urine be monitored daily, and then at 3 hour intervals, that ultrasound be used to determine when ovulation occurs. In some clinics, implantation requires that she remain immobile

SUSAN SHERWIN is Professor of Philosophy and Women's Studies, Dalhousie University.

for 48 hours (including 24 hours in the head down position). IVF is successful in about 10–15% of the cases selected as suitable, and commonly involves multiple efforts at implantation. . . .

. . . IVF is a difficult issue for feminists.

On the one hand, most feminists share the concern for autonomy held by most moral theorists, and they are interested in allowing women freedom of choice in reproductive matters. This freedom is most widely discussed in connection with access to safe and effective contraception and, when necessary, to abortion services. For women who are unable to conceive because of blocked fallopian tubes, or certain fertility problems of their partners, IVF provides the technology to permit pregnancy which is otherwise impossible. Certainly most of the women seeking IVF perceive it to be technology that increases their reproductive freedom of choice. So, it would seem that feminists should support this sort of technology as part of our general concern to foster the degree of reproductive control women may have over their own bodies. Some

From Science, Morality, and Feminist Theory, *Marsha Hansen and Kai Nielsen, eds. (Calgary, Alberta, Canada: University of Calgary Press, 1987), 265–284. Copyright 1987. Reprinted by permission of University of Calgary Press.*

feminists have chosen this route. But feminists must also note that IVF as practiced does not altogether satisfy the motivation of fostering individual autonomy.

It is, after all, the sort of technology that requires medical intervention, and hence it is not really controlled by the women seeking it, but rather by the medical staff providing this "service." IVF is not available to every woman who is medically suitable, but only to those who are judged to be worthy by the medical specialists concerned. To be a candidate for this procedure, a woman must have a husband and an apparently stable marriage. She must satisfy those specialists that she and her husband have appropriate resources to support any children produced by this arrangement (in addition, of course, to the funds required to purchase the treatment in the first place), and that they generally "deserve" this support. IVF is not available to single women, lesbian women, or women not securely placed in the middle class or beyond. Nor is it available to women whom the controlling medical practitioners judge to be deviant with respect to their norms of who makes a good mother. The supposed freedom of choice, then, is provided only to selected women who have been screened by the personal values of those administering the technology.

Further, even for these women, the record on their degree of choice is unclear. Consider, for instance, that this treatment has always been very experimental: it was introduced without the prior primate studies which are required for most new forms of medical technology, and it continues to be carried out under constantly shifting protocols, with little empirical testing, as clinics try to raise their very poor success rates. Moreover, consent forms are perceived by patients to be quite restrictive procedures and women seeking this technology are not in a particularly strong position to bargain to revise the terms; there is no alternate clinic down the street to choose if a woman dislikes her treatment at some clinic, but there are usually many other

women waiting for access to her place in the clinic should she choose to withdraw.

Some recent studies indicate that few of the women participating in current programs really know how low the success rates are.[1] And it is not apparent that participants are encouraged to ponder the medical unknowns associated with various aspects of the technique, such as the long term consequences of superovulation and the use of hormones chemically similar to DES. Nor is it the case that the consent procedure involves consultation on how to handle the disposal of "surplus" zygotes. It is doubtful that the women concerned have much real choice about which procedure is followed with the eggs they will not need. These policy decisions are usually made at the level of the clinic. It should be noted here that at least one feminist argues that neither the woman, nor the doctors have the right to choose to destroy these embryos: ". . . because no one, not even its parents, owns the embryo/fetus, no one has the *right* to destroy it, even at a very early developmental stage . . . to destroy an embryo is not an automatic entitlement held by anyone, including its genetic parents."[2]

Moreover, some participants reflect deep seated ambivalence on the part of many women about the procedure—they indicate that their marriage and status depends on a determination to do "whatever is possible" in pursuit of their "natural" childbearing function—and they are not helped to work through the seeming imponderables associated with their long term well-being. Thus, IVF as practiced involves significant limits on the degree of autonomy deontologists insist on in other medical contexts, though the nonfeminist literature is insensitive to this anomaly.

From the perspective of consequentialism, feminists take a long view and try to see IVF in the context of the burgeoning range of techniques in the area of human reproductive technology. While some of this technology seems to hold the potential of benefitting women generally—by leading to better understanding of conception and contraception, for instance—there is a wary suspicion that this research will help foster new techniques and products such as human cloning and the development of artificial wombs which can, in principle, make the majority of women superfluous. (This is not a wholly paranoid fear in a woman-hating culture: we can anticipate that there will be great pressure for such techniques in subsequent generations, since one of the "successes" of reproductive technology to date has been to allow parents to control the sex of their offspring; the "choice" now made possible clearly threatens to result in significant imbalances in the ratio of boy to girl infants. Thus, it appears, there will likely be significant shortages of women to bear children in the future, and we can anticipate pressures for further technological solutions to the "new" problem of reproduction that will follow.)

We must look at the sort of social arrangements and cultural values that underlie the drive to assume such risks for the sake of biological parenthood. We find that the capitalism, racism, sexism, and elitism of our culture have combined to create a set of attitudes which views children as commodities whose value is derived from their possession of parental chromosomes. Children are valued as privatized commodities, reflecting the virility and heredity of their parents. They are also viewed as the responsibility of their parents and are not seen as the social treasure and burden that they are. Parents must tend their needs on pain of prosecution, and, in return, they get to keep complete control over them. Other adults are inhibited from having warm, stable interactions with the children of others—it is as suspect to try to hug and talk regularly with a child who is not one's own as it is to fondle and hang longingly about a car or a bicycle which belongs to someone else—so those who wish to know children well often find they must have their own.

Women are persuaded that their most important purpose in life is to bear and raise children; they are told repeatedly that their life is incomplete, that they are lacking in fulfillment if they do not have children. And, in fact, many women do face a barren existence without children. Few women have access to meaningful, satisfying jobs. Most do not find themselves in the centre of the romantic personal relationships which the culture pretends is the norm for heterosexual couples. And they have been socialized to be fearful of close friendships with others—they are taught to distrust other women, and to avoid the danger of friendship with men other than their husbands. Children remain the one hope for real intimacy and for the sense of accomplishment which comes from doing work one judges to be valuable.

To be sure, children can provide that sense of self worth, although for many women (and probably for all mothers at some times) motherhood is not the romanticized satisfaction they are led to expect. But there is something very wrong with a culture where childrearing is the only outlet available to most women in which to pursue fulfillment. Moreover, there is something wrong with the ownership theory of children that keeps other adults at a distance from children. There ought to be a variety of close relationships possible between children and adults so that we all recognize that we have a stake in the well-being of the young, and we all benefit from contact with their view of the world.

In such a world, it would not be necessary to spend the huge sums on designer children which IVF requires while millions of other children starve to death each year. Adults who enjoyed children could be involved in caring for them whether or not they produced them biologically. And, if the institution of marriage survives, women and men would marry because they wished to share their lives together, not because the men needed someone to produce heirs for them and women needed financial support for their children. That would be a world in which we might have reproductive freedom of choice. The world we now live in has so limited women's options and self-esteem, it is legitimate to question the freedom behind women's demand for this technology, for it may well be largely a reflection of constraining social perspectives.

Nonetheless, I must acknowledge that some couples today genuinely mourn their incapacity to produce children without IVF and there are very significant and unique joys which can be found in producing and raising one's own children which are not accessible to persons in infertile relationships. We must sympathize with these people. None of us shall live to see the implementation of the ideal cultural values outlined above which would make the demand for IVF less severe. It is with real concern that some feminists suggest that the personal wishes of couples with fertility difficulties may not be compatible with the overall interests of women and children.

Feminist thought, then, helps us to focus on different dimensions of the problem then do other sorts of approaches. But, with this perspective, we still have difficulty in reaching a final conclusion on whether to encourage, tolerate, modify, or restrict this sort of reproductive technology. I suggest that we turn to the developing theories of feminist ethics for guidance in resolving this question.[3]

In my view, a feminist ethics is a moral theory that focusses on relations among persons as well as on individuals. It has as a model an interconnected social fabric, rather than the familiar one of isolated, independent atoms; and it gives primacy to bonds among people rather than to rights to independence. It is a theory that focusses on concrete situations and persons and not on free-floating abstract actions.[4] Although many details have yet to be worked out, we can see some of its implications in particular problem areas such as this.

It is a theory that is explicitly conscious of the social, political, and economic relations that exist among persons; in particular, as a feminist theory, it attends to the implications of actions or policies on the status of women. Hence, it is necessary to ask questions from the perspective of feminist ethics in addition to those which are normally asked from the perspective of mainstream ethical theories. We must view issues such as this one in the context of the social and political realities in which they arise, and resist the attempt to evaluate actions or practices in isolation (as traditional responses in biomedical ethics often do). Thus, we cannot just address the question of IVF per se without asking how IVF contributes to general patterns of women's oppression. As Kathryn Payne Addelson has argued about abortion,[5] a feminist perspective raises questions that are inadmissable within the traditional ethical frameworks, and yet, for women in a patriarchal society, they are value questions of greater urgency. In particular, a feminist ethics, in contrast to other approaches in biomedical ethics, would take seriously the concerns just reviewed which are part of the debate in the feminist literature.

Feminist concerns cited earlier made clear the difficulties we have with some of our traditional ethical concepts; hence, feminist ethics directs us to rethink our basic ethical notions. Autonomy, or freedom of choice, is not a matter to be determined in isolated instances, as is commonly assumed in many approaches to applied ethics. Rather it is a matter that involves reflection on one's whole life situation. The freedom of choice feminists appeal to in the abortion situation is freedom to define one's status as childbearer, given the social, economic, and political significance of reproduction for women. A feminist perspective permits us to understand that reproductive freedom includes control of one's sexuality, protection against coerced sterilization (or iatrogenic sterilization, e.g. as caused by the Dalkon Shield), and the existence of a social and economic network of support for the children we may choose to bear. It is the freedom to redefine our roles in society according to our concerns and needs as women.

In contrast, the consumer freedom to purchase technology, allowed only to a few couples of the privileged classes (in traditionally approved relationships), seems to entrench further the patriarchal notions of woman's role as child-bearer and of heterosexual monogamy as the only acceptable intimate relationship. In other words, this sort of choice does not seem to foster autonomy for women on the broad scale. IVF is a practice which seems to reinforce sexist, classist, and often racist assumptions of our culture; therefore, on our revised understanding of freedom, the contribution of this technology to the general autonomy of women is largely negative.

We can now see the advantage of a feminist ethics over mainstream ethical theories, for a feminist analysis explicitly accepts the need for a political component to our understanding of ethical issues. In this, it differs from traditional ethical theories and it also differs from a simply feminine ethics approach, such as the one Noddings offers, for Noddings seems to rely on individual relations exclusively and is deeply suspicious of political alliances as potential threats to the pure relation of caring. Yet, a full understanding of both the threat of IVF, and the alternative action necessary should we decide to reject IVF, is possible only if it includes a political dimension reflecting on the role of women in society.

From the point of view of feminist ethics, the primary question to consider is whether this and other forms of reproductive technology threaten to reinforce the lack of autonomy which women now experience in our culture—even as they appear, in the short run, to be increasing freedom. We must recognize that the interconnections among the social forces oppressive to women underlie feminists' mistrust of this technology which advertises itself as increasing women's autonomy.[6] The political perspective which directs us to look at how this technology fits in with general patterns of treatment for women is not readily accessible to traditional moral theories, for it involves categories of concern not accounted for in those theories—e.g. the complexity of issues which makes it inappropriate to study them in isolation from one another, the

role of oppression in shaping individual desires, and potential differences in moral status which are connected with differences in treatment.

It is the set of connections constituting women's continued oppression in our society which inspires feminists to resurrect the old slippery slope arguments to warn against IVF. We must recognize that women's existing lack of control in reproductive matters begins the debate on a pretty steep incline. Technology with the potential to further remove control of reproduction from women makes the slope very slippery indeed. This new technology, though offered under the guise of increasing reproductive freedom, threatens to result, in fact, in a significant decrease in freedom, especially since it is a technology that will always include the active involvement of designated specialists and will not ever be a private matter for the couple or women concerned.

Ethics ought not to direct us to evaluate individual cases without also looking at the implications of our decisions from a wide perspective. My argument is that a theory of feminist ethics provides that wider perspective, for its different sort of methodology is sensitive to both the personal and the social dimensions of issues. For that reason, I believe it is the only ethical perspective suitable for evaluating issues of this sort.

NOTES

1. Michael Soules, "The In Vitro Fertilization Pregnancy Rate: Let's Be Honest with One Another," *Fertility and Sterility* 43, 4 (1985) 511–13.

2. Christine Overall, *Ethics and Human Reproduction: A Feminist Analysis* (Allen and Unwin, forthcoming), 104 ms.

3. Many authors are now working on an understanding of what feminist ethics entail. Among the Canadian papers I am familiar with, are Kathryn Morgan's "Women and Moral Madness," Sheila Mullett's "Only Connect: The Place of Self-Knowledge in Ethics," both in this volume, and Leslie Wilson's "Is a Feminine Ethics Enough?" *Atlantis* (forthcoming).

4. Sherwin, "A Feminist Approach to Ethics."

5. Kathryn Payne Addelson, "Moral Revolution," in Marilyn Pearsall, ed., *Women and Values* (Belmont, CA: Wadsworth 1986), 291–309.

6. Marilyn Frye vividly describes the phenomenon of inter-relatedness which supports sexist oppression by appeal to the metaphor of a bird cage composed of thin wires, each relatively harmless in itself, but, collectively, the wires constitute an overwhelming barrier to the inhabitant of the cage. Marilyn Frye, *The Politics of Reality: Essays in Feminist Theory* (Trumansburg, NY: The Crossing Press 1983), 4–7.

The Presumptive Primacy of Procreative Liberty

JOHN ROBERTSON

PROCREATIVE LIBERTY has wide appeal but its scope has never been fully elaborated and often is contested. The concept has several meanings that must be clarified if it is to serve as a reliable guide for moral debate and public policy regarding new reproductive technologies.

WHAT IS PROCREATIVE LIBERTY?

At the most general level, procreative liberty is the freedom either to have children or to avoid having them. Although often expressed or realized in the context of a couple, it is first and foremost an individual interest. It is to be distinguished from freedom in the ancillary aspects of reproduction, such as liberty in the conduct of pregnancy or choice of place or mode of childbirth.

JOHN A. ROBERTSON is Thomas Watt Gregory Professor, School of Law at the University of Texas at Austin.

The concept of reproduction, however, has a certain ambiguity contained within it. In a strict sense, reproduction is always genetic. It occurs by provision of one's gametes to a new person, and thus includes having or producing offspring. While female reproduction has traditionally included gestation, in vitro fertilization (IVF) now allows female genetic and gestational reproduction to be separated. Thus a woman who has provided the egg that is carried by another has reproduced, even if she has not gestated and does not rear resulting offspring. Because of the close link between gestation and female reproduction, a woman who gestates the embryo of another may also reasonably be viewed as having a reproductive experience, even though she does not reproduce genetically.[1]

In any case, reproduction in the genetic or gestational sense is to be distinguished from child rearing. Although reproduction is highly valued in part because it usually leads to child rearing, one can produce offspring without rearing them and rear children without reproduction. One who rears an adopted child has not reproduced, while one who has genetic progeny but does not rear them has.

In this book the terms "procreative liberty" and "reproductive freedom" will mean the freedom to reproduce or not to reproduce in the genetic sense, which may also include rearing or not, as intended by the parties. Those terms will also include female gestation whether or nor there is a genetic connection to the resulting child.

Often the reproduction at issue will be important because it is intended to lead to child rearing. In cases where rearing is not intended, the value to be assigned to reproduction *tout court* will have to be determined. Similarly, when there is rearing without genetic or gestational involvement, the value of nonreproductive child rearing will also have to be assessed. In both cases the value assigned may depend on the proximity to reproduction where rearing is intended.

Two further qualifications on the meaning of procreative liberty should be noted. One is that "liberty" as used in procreative liberty is a negative right. It means that a person violates no moral duty in making a procreative choice, and that other persons have a duty not to interfere with that choice.[2] However, the negative right to procreate or not does not imply the duty of others to provide the resources or services necessary to exercise one's procreative liberty despite plausible moral arguments for governmental assistance.

As a matter of constitutional law, procreative liberty is a negative right against state interference with choices to procreate or to avoid procreation. It is not a right against private interference, though other laws might provide that protection. Nor is it a positive right to have the state or particular persons provide the means or resources necessary to have or avoid having children.[3] The exercise of procreative liberty may be severely constrained by social and economic circumstances. Access to medical care, child care, employment, housing, and other services may significantly affect whether one is able to exercise

procreative liberty. However, the state presently has no constitutional obligation to provide those services. Whether the state should alleviate those conditions is a separate issue of social justice.[4]

The second qualification is that not everything that occurs in and around procreation falls within liberty interests that are distinctively procreative. Thus whether the father may be present during childbirth, whether midwives may assist birth, or whether childbirth may occur at home rather than in a hospital may be important for the parties involved, but they do not implicate the freedom to reproduce (unless one could show that the place or mode of birth would determine whether birth occurs at all). Similarly, questions about a pregnant woman's drug use or other conduct during pregnancy, a controversial topic . . . implicates liberty in the course of reproduction but not procreative liberty in the basic sense.

THE IMPORTANCE OF PROCREATIVE LIBERTY

Procreative liberty should enjoy presumptive primacy when conflicts about its exercise arise because control over whether one reproduces or not is central to personal identity, to dignity, and to the meaning of one's life. For example, deprivation of the ability to avoid reproduction determines one's self-definition in the most basic sense. It affects women's bodies in a direct and substantial way. It also centrally affects one's psychological and social identity and one's social and moral responsibilities. The resulting burdens are especially onerous for women, but they affect men in significant ways as well.

On the other hand, being deprived of the ability to reproduce prevents one from an experience that is central to individual identity and meaning in life. Although the desire to reproduce is in part socially constructed, at the most basic level transmission of one's genes through reproduction is an animal or species urge closely linked to the sex drive. In connecting us with nature and future generations, reproduction gives solace in the face of death. As Shakespeare noted, "nothing 'gainst Time's scythe can make defense/save breed."[5] For many people "breed"—reproduction and the parenting that usually accompanies it—is a central part of their life plan, and the most satisfying and meaningful experience they have. It also has primary importance as an expression of a couple's love or unity. For many persons, reproduction also has religious significance and is experienced as a "gift from God." Its denial—through infertility or governmental restriction—is experienced as a great loss, even if one has already had children or will have little or no rearing role with them.

Decisions to have or to avoid having children are thus personal decisions of great import that determine the shape and meaning of one's life. The person directly involved is best situated to determine whether that meaning should or should not occur. An ethic of personal autonomy as well as ethics of community or family should then recognize a presumption in favor of most personal reproductive choices. Such a presumption does not mean that reproductive choices are without consequence to others, nor that they should never be limited. Rather, it means that those who would limit procreative choice have the burden of showing that the reproductive actions at issue would create such substantial harm that they could justifiably be limited. Of course, what counts as the "substantial harm" that justifies interference with procreative choice may often be contested, as the discussion of reproductive technologies in this book will show.

A closely related reason for protecting reproductive choice is to avoid the highly intrusive measures that governmental control of reproduction usually entails. State interference with reproductive choice may extend beyond exhortation and penalties to gestapo and police state tactics. Margaret Atwood's powerful futuristic novel *The Handmaid's Tale* expresses this danger by creating a world where fertile women are forcibly impregnated by the ruling powers and their pregnancies monitored to replenish a decimated population.[6]

Equally frightening scenarios have occurred in recent years when repressive governments have interfered with reproductive choice. In Romania and China, men and women have had their most private activities scrutinized in the service of state reproductive goals. In Ceauşescu's Romania, where contraception and abortion were strictly forbidden, women's menstrual cycles were routinely monitored to see if they were pregnant.[7] Women who did not become pregnant or who had abortions were severely punished. Many women nevertheless sought illegal abortions and died, leaving their children orphaned and subject to sale to Westerners seeking children for adoption.[8]

In China, forcible abortion and sterilization have occurred in the service of a one-child-per-family population policy. Village cadres have seized pregnant women in their homes and forced them to have abortions.[9] A campaign of forcible sterilization in India in 1977 was seen as an "attack on women and children" and brought Indira Ghandi's government down.[10] In the United States, state-imposed sterilization of "mental defectives," sanctioned in 1927 by the United States Supreme Court in *Buck v. Bell,* resulted in 60,000 sterilizations over a forty-year period.[11] Many mentally normal people were sterilized by mistake, and mentally retarded persons who posed little risk of harm to others were subjected to surgery.[12] It is no surprise that current proposals for compulsory use of contraceptives such as Norplant are viewed with great suspicion.

TWO TYPES OF PROCREATIVE LIBERTY

To see how values of procreative liberty affect the ethical and public policy evaluation of new reproductive technologies, we must determine whether the interests that underlie the high value accorded procreative liberty are implicated in their use. This is not a simple task because procreative liberty is not unitary, but consists of strands of varying interests in the conception and gestation of offspring. The different strands implicate different interests, have different legal and constitutional status, and are differently affected by technology.

An essential distinction is between the freedom to avoid reproduction and the freedom to reproduce. When people talk of reproductive rights, they usually have one or the other aspect in mind. Because different interests and justifications underlie each and countervailing interests for limiting each aspect vary, recognition of one aspect does not necessarily mean that the other will also be respected; nor does limitation of one mean that the other can also be denied.

However, there is a mirroring or reciprocal relationship here. Denial of one type of reproductive liberty necessarily implicates the other. If a woman is not able to avoid reproduction through contraception or abortion, she may end up reproducing, with all the burdens that unwanted reproduction entails. Similarly, if one is denied the liberty to reproduce through forcible sterilization, one is forced to avoid reproduction, thus experiencing the loss that absence of progeny brings. By extending reproductive options, new reproductive technologies present challenges to both aspects of procreative choice. . . .

THE FREEDOM TO PROCREATE

In addition to freedom to avoid procreation, procreative liberty also includes the freedom to procreate—the freedom to beget and bear children if one chooses. As with avoiding reproduction, the right to reproduce is a negative right against public or private interference, not a positive right to the services or the resources needed to reproduce. It is an important freedom that is widely accepted as a basic, human right.[13] But its various components and dimensions have never been fully analyzed, as technologies of conception and selection now force us to do.

As with avoiding reproduction, the freedom to procreate involves the freedom to engage in a series of actions that eventuate in reproduction and usually in child rearing. One must be free to marry or find a willing partner, engage in sexual intercourse, achieve conception and pregnancy, carry a pregnancy to term, and rear offspring. Social and natural barriers to reproduction would involve the unavailability of willing or suitable partners, impotence or infertility, and lack of medical and child-care resources. State barriers to marriage, to sexual intercourse, to conception, to infertility treatment, to carrying pregnancies to term, and to certain child-rearing arrangements would also limit the freedom to procreate. The most commonly asserted reasons for limiting coital reproduction are overpopulation, unfitness of parents, harm to offspring, and costs to the state or others. Technologies that treat infertility raise additional concerns that are discussed below.

The moral right to reproduce is respected because of the centrality of reproduction to personal identity, meaning, and dignity. This importance makes the liberty to procreate an important moral right, both for an ethic of individual autonomy and for ethics of community or family that view the purpose of marriage and sexual union as the reproduction and rearing of offspring. Because of this importance, the right to reproduce is widely recognized as a prima facie moral right that cannot be limited except for very good reason.

Recognition of the primacy of procreation does not mean that all reproduction is morally blameless, much less that reproduction is always responsible and praiseworthy and can never be limited. However, the presumptive primacy of procreative liberty sets a very high standard for limiting those rights, tilting the balance in favor of reproducing but not totally determining its acceptability. A two-step process of analysis is envisaged here. The first question is whether a distinctively procreative interest is involved. If so, the question then is whether the harm threatened by reproduction satisfies the strict standard for overriding this liberty interest.

The personal importance of procreation helps answer questions about who holds procreative rights and about the circumstances under which the right to reproduce may be limited. A person's capacity to find signficance in reproduction should determine whether one holds the presumptive right, though this question is often discussed in terms of whether persons with such a capacity are fit parents. To have a liberty interest in procreating, one should at a minimum have the mental capacity to understand or appreciate the meanings associated with reproduction. This minimum would exclude severely retarded persons from having reproductive interests, though it would not remove their right to bodily integrity. However, being unmarried, homosexual, physically disabled, infected with HIV, or imprisoned would not disqualify one from having reproductive interests, though they might affect one's ability to rear offspring. Whether those characteristics justify limitations on reproduction is discussed later.[14] Nor would already having reproduced negate a person's interest in reproducing again, though at a certain point the marginal value to a person of additional offspring diminishes.[15]

What kinds of interests or harms make reproduction unduly selfish or irresponsible and thus could justifiably limit the presumptive right to procreate? To answer this question, we must distinguish coital and noncoital reproduction. Surprisingly, there is a widespread reluctance to speak of coital reproduction as irresponsible, much less to urge public action to prevent irresponsible coital reproduction from occurring. If such a conversation did occur, reasons for limiting coital reproduction would involve the heavy costs that it imposed on others — costs that out-weighed whatever personal meaning or satisfaction the person(s) reproducing experienced. With coital reproduction, such costs might arise if there were severe overpopulation, if the persons reproducing were unfit parents, if reproduction would harm offspring, or if significant medical or social costs were imposed on others.

Because the United States does not face the severe overpopulation of some countries, the main grounds for claiming that reproduction is irresponsible is where the person(s) reproducing lack the financial means to raise offspring or will otherwise harm their children. As later discussions will show, both grounds are seriously inadequate as justifications for interfering with procreative choice. Imposing rearing costs on others may not rise to the level of harm that justifies depriving a person of a fundamental moral right. Moreover, protection of offspring from unfit parenting requires that unfit parents not rear, not that they not reproduce. Offspring could be protected by having others rear them without interfering with parental reproduction.

A further problem, if coital reproduction were found to be unjustified, concerns what action should then be taken. Exhortation or moral condemnation might be acceptable, but more stringent or coercive measures would act on the body of the person deemed irresponsible. Past experience with forced sterilization of retarded persons and the inevitable focus on the poor and minorities as targets of coercive policies make such proposals highly unappealing. Because of these doubts, there have been surprisingly few attempts to restrict coital reproduction in the United States since the era of eugenic sterilization, even though some instances of reproduction — for example, teenage pregnancy, inability to care for offspring — appear to be socially irresponsible.

An entirely different set of concerns arises with noncoital reproductive techniques. Charges that noncoital reproduction is unethical or irresponsible arise because of its expense, its highly technological character, its decomposition of parenthood into genetic, gestational, and social components, and its potential effects on women and offspring. To assess whether these effects justify moral condemnation or public limitation, we must first determine whether noncoital reproduction implicates important aspects of procreative liberty.

The Right to Reproduce and Noncoital Technology

If the moral right to reproduce presumptively protects coital reproduction, then it should protect noncoital reproduction as well. The moral right of the coitally infertile to reproduce is based on the same desire for offspring that the coitally fertile have. They too wish to replicate themselves, transmit genes, gestate, and rear children biologically related to them. Their infertility should no more disqualify them from reproductive experiences than physical disability should disqualify persons from walking with mechanical assistance. The unique risks posed by noncoital reproduction may provide independent justifications for limiting its use, but neither the noncoital nature of the means used nor the infertility of their beneficiaries mean that the presumptively protected moral interest in reproduction is not present.

Are Noncoital Technologies Unethical?

Judgment about the reproductive importance of noncoital technologies is crucial because many people have serious ethical reservations about them, and are more than willing to restrict their use. The concerns here are not the fears of overpopulation, parental unfitness, and societal costs that arise with allegedly irresponsible coital reproduction. Instead, they include reduction of demand for hard-to-adopt children, the coercive or exploitive bargains that will be offered to poor women, the commodification of both children and reproductive collaborators, the objectification of women as reproductive vessels, and the undermining of the nuclear family.

However, often the harms feared are deontological in character. In some cases they stem from a religious or moral conception of the unity of sex and reproduction or the definition of family. Such a view characterizes the Vatican's strong opposition to IVF, donor sperm, and other noncoital and collaborative techniques.[16] Other deontological concerns derive from a particular conception of the proper reproductive role of women. Many persons, for example, oppose paid surrogate motherhood because of a judgment about the wrongness of a woman's willingness to sever the mother-child bond for the sake of money.[17] They also insist that the gestational mother is always morally entitled to rear, despite her preconception promise to the contrary. Closely related are dignitary objections to allowing any reproductive factors to be purchased, or to having offspring selected on the basis of their genes.

Finally, there is a broader concern that noncoital reproduction will undermine the deeper community interest in having a clear social framework to define boundaries of families, sexuality, and reproduction. The traditional family provides a container for the narcissism and irrationality that often drives human reproduction. This container assures commitments to the identifications and taboos that protect children from various types of abuse. The technical ability to disaggregate and recombine genetic, gestational, and rearing connections and to control the genes of offspring may thus undermine essential protections for offspring, couples, families, and society.

These criticisms are powerful ones that explain much of the ambivalence that surrounds the use of certain reproductive technologies. They call into question the wisdom of individual decisions to use them, and the willingness of society to promote or facilitate their use. Unless one is operating out of a specific religious or deontological ethic, however, they do not show that all individual uses of these techniques are immoral, much less that public policy should restrict or discourage their use.

. . . [T]hese criticisms seldom meet the high standard necessary to limit procreative choice.

Many of them are mere hypothetical or speculative possibilities. Others reflect moralisms concerning a "right" view of reproduction, which individuals in a pluralistic society hold or reject to varying degrees. In any event, without a clear showing of substantial harm to the tangible interests of others, speculation or mere moral objections alone should not override the moral right of infertile couples to use those techniques to form families. Given the primacy of procreative liberty, the use of these techniques should be accorded the same high protection granted to coital reproduction.

NOTES

1. Whether labeled reproductive or not, gestation is a central experience for women and should enjoy the special respect or protected status accorded reproductive activities. On this view, a woman who receives an embryo donation or who serves as a gestational surrogate is having a reproductive experience, whether or not she also rears.

2. The distinction between liberty and claim right follows Joel Feinberg's account of those terms in his "Voluntary Euthanasia and the Inalienable Right to Life," *Philosophy and Public Affairs* 7(1978):93–95.

3. Constitutional rights are generally negative rather than positive. With the exception of counsel in criminal trials, there is no obligation on the government to provide the means necessary to exercise constitutional rights.

4. Dan Brock has argued that contraceptive services are so cheap and their lack has such a substantial impact on persons that the state has a moral obligation to provide contraceptives to poor persons. Dan Brock, "Reproductive Freedom: Its Nature, Bases, and Limits" (unpublished paper, 1992).

5. Sonnet 12 ("When I do count the clock that tells the time/And see the brave day sunk in hideous night"). Sonnet 2 ("When forty winters shall besiege thy brow/And dig deep trenches in thy beauty's field")

also sings the praises of reproduction as an answer to death and old age.

6. Margaret Atwood, *The Handmaid's Tale* (Boston: Houghton Mifflin, 1986).

7. "Where Death and Fear Went Forth and Multiplied," *New York Times,* 14 January 1990.

8. B. Meredith Burke, "Ceaucescu's Main Victims: Women and Children," *New York Times,* 25 January 1990.

9. Sheryl WuDunn, "China, with Ever More to Feed, Pushes Anew for Small Families," *New York Times,* 2 June 1991.

10. The 1977 sterilization campaign plays a key role in the denouement of Salmon Rushdie's *Midnight's Children: A Novel* (New York: Knopf, 1981). The narrator cries, just before he too is sterilized: "They are doing nashendi — sterilization is being performed. Save our women and children. And a riot is beginning" (p. 414).

11. Phillip Reilly, *The Surgical Solution* (Baltimore: Johns Hopkins University Press, 1991).

12. Paul A. Lombardo, "Three Generations, No Imbeciles: New Light on *Buck v. Bell,*" *New York University Law Review* 60(1985):30.

13. This right has received explicit recognition in the United Nations' 1978 Universal Declaration of Human Rights ("men and women of full age . . . [have the right] to marry and found a family"), the International Covenant of Civil and Political Rights (Art. 23, 1976), and the European Convention on Human Rights (Art. 12, 1953).

14. See chapters 4 and 7 [of *Children of Choice*] for further discussion.

15. The low marginal value of additional reproduction would ordinarily be relevant only when one has already had a large number of children, and thus may not be important for many of the issues discussed in this book [i.e., *Children of Choice*].

16. Catholic Church, Congregation for the Doctrine of the Faith, "Instruction on Respect for Human Life in Its Origin and on the Dignity of Procreation," *Origins* 16(1987):698–711.

17. They are also concerned that women will be exploited or pressured by circumstances into arrangements that turn out to harm their interests.

Birth Pangs: Conceptive Technologies and the Threat to Motherhood

MICHELLE STANWORTH

. . . ONE BASIS FOR feminist hostility to the conceptive technologies is a powerful theoretical critique which sees in these new techniques a means for men to wrest "not only control of reproduction, but reproduction itself" from women.[1] It has been suggested that men's alienation from reproduction—men's sense of disconnection from their seed during the process of conception, pregnancy, and birth—has underpinned through the ages a relentless male desire to master nature, and to construct social institutions and cultural patterns that will not only subdue the waywardness of women but also give men an illusion of procreative power. New reproductive technologies are the vehicle that will turn men's illusions of reproductive control into a reality. By manipulating eggs and embryos, scientists will determine the sort of children who are born—will make themselves the fathers of humankind. By removing eggs and embryos from some women and implanting them in others, medical practitioners will gain unprecedented control over motherhood itself. Motherhood as a unified biological process will be effectively deconstructed: in place of "mother," there will be ovarian mothers who supply eggs, uterine mothers who give birth to children, and, presumably, social mothers who raise them. Through the eventual development of artificial

MICHELLE STANWORTH is an author on bioethics issues and the editor of *Reproductive Technologies: Gender, Motherhood, and Medicine* (University of Minnesota Press).

wombs, the capacity may arise to make biological motherhood redundant. Whether or not women are reduced by this process to the level of "reproductive prostitutes," the object and the effect of the emergent technologies is to deconstruct motherhood and to destroy the claim to reproduction that is the foundation of women's identity.

While this theoretical account of the new technologies may be in some ways extremely radical, in other respects it ironically tends to echo positions that feminists have been keen to challenge. In the first place, this analysis entails an exaggerated view of the power of science and medicine, a mirror image of that which scientists and medical practitioners often try themselves to promote. Science may well be, as Emily Martin argues, a hegemonic system; but as she shows, that system does not go unchallenged.[2] The vigorous critique of science in this account needs to be tempered with a deeper understanding of the constraints within which science and medicine operate, and of the way these can be shaped for the greater protection of women and men. Second, in the urgent concern to protect infertile women from the sometimes unscrupulous attentions of medical science, infertile women are all too often portrayed as "desperate people," rendered incapable by pronatal pressures of making rational and ethical decisions.[3] This view of infertile women (and by implication, of all women) comes uncomfortably close to that espoused by some members of the medical profession. Third,

From Conflicts In Feminism, *Marianne Hirsch and Evelyn Fox Keller, eds. New York: Routledge, 1990.*
Reprinted by permission of Michelle Stanworth and Evelyn Fox Keller.

this theoretical account sometimes seems to suggest that anything "less" than a natural process, from conception through to birth, represents the degradation of motherhood itself. But motherhood means different things to different women, and to identify motherhood so exclusively with nature, with the absence of technology, and indeed, with pregnancy and childbirth runs the risk of blunting the cutting edge of feminist critique. . . .

Conceptive technologies are accused of being:

Unsuccessful: Whatever the image of in vitro fertilization with embryo transfer, or of GIFT, as miracle cures for infertility, the miracle works in remarkably few cases.[4]

Unsafe: Risks are associated with the hormonal drugs used to stimulate ovulation for ivf patients, and those used to regulate cycles in some types of surrogacy. Where several embryos are transferred, infant and maternal health may suffer because of the frequency of multiple births. Women undergoing conceptive treatments are subject even more frequently than other women to procedures (e.g., ultrasound, caesarian deliveries) the routine use of which has been challenged by the women's health movement.[5]

Unkind: Whether treatment is "successful" or not, the pressure, emotional upheaval, disruption, and indignities involved do incommensurable damage to a woman's quality of life. The very existence of conceptive technologies makes it difficult for women to reconcile themselves to childlessness.[6]

Unnecessary: Infertility is a social condition, the seriousness of which depends entirely on the social evaluations attached to childlessness. Infertility does not require in vitro fertilization, or surrogacy, or any medical solution at all. If there were less hype about conceptive technologies, and if infertile people were less obsessed with securing their own biological child, then infertility might be resolved by the more satisfactory strategy of adoption.[7]

Unwanted: Women who expose their bodies to conceptive technologies or submit themselves as "surrogate" mothers have been coerced (1) by pressure from male partners, (2) by the limited economic opportunities for women and restricted avenues of self-esteem, which mean (especially in the case of "surrogate" mothers) that the "choice" isn't really a choice, (3) by pronatalist values and practices, which ensure that women who fail to bear children face constant reminders of the extent to which they fall short of hegemonic ideals. As Grundberg and Dowrick so clearly put it, none of us is free in our choices until it is possible to say aloud without fear of censure, "I don't wish to have children," (4) by unscrupulous and authoritarian doctors, who mislead them about the risks, intimidate them into "consent," or whose clinics offer "counseling into treatment" rather than counseling about treatment.[8]

Unsisterly: Women who use conceptive technologies harm other women, including women who don't (1) by seeking medical solutions to infertility, and thereby reinforcing the illusion that childbearing is a necessary component of femininity, (2) by providing doctors with experimental data and material to further their knowledge of the reproductive process and thus, by contributing to the expansion of a medical empire, the power of which is inimicable to women, (3) by taking advantage of a "surrogate" mother's poverty and powerlessness (or altruism) for their own benefit; this exploitation is potentially racist or imperialist, since women from subordinate ethnic communities and from poorer countries might be extensively used as "surrogate" mothers by privileged Western women in the future.[9]

Unwise: The low success rate of conceptive technologies as well as their many disadvantages make them an unwise focus for resources. Greater benefits would be derived if the resources currently being absorbed by in vitro fertilization and associated techniques were redeployed to fund research into the causes of infertility, or into preventative measures.[10]

The above charges constitute a powerful analysis of the impact of conceptive technologies, an analysis that goes beyond the unacceptably narrow terms of conventional medical assessment. But the strength of the feminist position we ultimately evolve depends upon the care with which these accusations are deployed and upon the implications for action that are drawn from them. Take, for example, the accusations that conceptive technologies are both *unwanted and unsisterly.* Underlying these charges is a telling critique of coercive pronatalism and of the place of medical practice in relation to it. But even this extremely useful analysis raises a number of questions.

While challenging the ways that coercive pronatalism shapes women's motivations to mother, we must be very clear that "shaped" is not the same as "determined." The battery of sanctions and rewards designed to entice women into motherhood indicates, not that conformity is guaranteed, but that childlessness is a genuine option, which efforts are made to contain. The most effective analyses of pronatalism are scrupulous about recognizing that even the pain of infertility does not prevent infertile women from making rational decisions about motherhood, and that the rejection of childbearing, while a difficult option for many women, is not necessarily a more authentic one.

As well as exposing pronatalist ideologies, we need also to articulate more convincing rationales for childlessness. For instance, in recent critiques of pronatalism (perhaps reacting against the fragile compromise involved in "having it all"?) it sometimes seems as if eschewing motherhood depends upon the compensation provided by a career. As one article says about protagonists in the Baby M surrogacy case:[11]

the Sterns are not free either. . . . The Sterns, two people deeply committed to challenging professional careers, still feel the cultural imperative to "have" a child.

But why is it relevant to such a compulsion that people are committed to challenging professional careers? If it is assumed that a career can

and should displace the wish for a child, then what type of economism does that bespeak? And what are we to make of the implied contrast: that professional women might be expected to have their minds on higher things, but that motherhood is the sensible course for women without rewarding careers? These interpretations may well not be what the authors of the above remarks on the Sterns had in mind, but they do signal how difficult it is for us to deal with the question of voluntary childlessness in a theoretically adequate way. To the extent that our discussions of pronatalism inadvertently justify childlessness in terms of career commitment, we run the risk of leaving no justification for childlessness—no refuge against pronatalist pressures—for the majority of women.

Finally, indignation at coercive pronatalism needs to be matched by an equally resolute opposition to the invidious distinctions that target some women as mothers and label others, on grounds that have little to do with their capacity to nurture a child, as unfit. As all participants in the debate are aware, pro-motherhood propaganda is not uniformly disseminated;[12] it coexists with disincentives and obstacles to motherhood for women from disempowered groups. According to ideologies of motherhood, all women want children; but single women and teenagers, women from ethnic minorities and those on state support, lesbian women and women with disabilities are often urged to forgo mothering "in the interests of the child." Do some feminists unintentionally endorse a similar pattern of invidious distinctions when it seems to be suggested that infertile women should not be mothers, or that their desire for children (and only theirs) is selfish, misguided, and potentially dangerous? . . .

One of the most politically sensitive elements of the case against conceptive technologies is the claim that these are *"unnecessary"*—that infertility does not dictate a medical solution, and that the condition of involuntary childlessness can be resolved satisfactorily by adoption. For some infertile women (and I count myself among them) this happy ending is indeed possible. But it is a long and implausible leap from there to the conclusion that conceptive technologies are in general unnecessary.

For one thing, the description of infertility as a social condition of involuntary childlessness doesn't hold for all women. For some women, pregnancy and childbirth are not only a route to a child, but a desired end in itself.[13] Our passionate concern as feminists to defend the integrity of the experience of childbirth (against intrusive obstetricians, for example) would sit uneasily with the view that the attachment to giving birth of some infertile women reflects a misguided commitment to biological motherhood.

For another, it would be naive to regard the adoption process as necessarily free of the drawbacks and risks that characterize medically assisted conception. Adoption and fostering are often subject to strict surveillance and regulation and that surveillance and regulation is not necessarily benign to women. Adoption agencies in many countries are (rightly) rigorous about who may exercise parental rights: but their policies and criteria of assessment are framed against a conventional notion of parenting—and particularly, of motherhood—which will deter many would-be mothers. Adoption agencies in Britain may (and often do) refuse single women or those aged over thirty; may (and usually do) refuse those who are not heterosexual, whether married or not; may (and sometimes do) refuse women who have jobs, women who have had psychiatric referrals, women with disabilities, women whose unconventional life-styles cast doubt—for the social workers at least—on their suitability as mothers. They are also likely to refuse, in spite of the long and uncertain waiting period for adoption, women who intend to continue trying to achieve a pregnancy. For many would-be mothers, particularly those who want their relationship with a child to begin while it is still in infancy or toddlerhood, the conceptive technologies are not so much about biological motherhood as about having a child at all. The tensions surrounding the adoption process, the

raising and dashing of hopes, the rejection by adoption agencies of prospective mothers who would have endured no questions about their fitness had they been fertile—all of these mean that adoption may, like the conceptive technologies, sometimes be "unsuccessful," sometimes "unsafe" and often "unkind."

And there is, of course, another complication when we consider the adoption process from the point of view of the birthmother. To the same extent that surrogacy can be seen as *"unsisterly"*—as involving the exploitation of birthmothers by infertile women—adoption can be seen as unsisterly too. The pressures that lead some women to surrender their babies for adoption are very like those condemned in the case of surrogate mothers, right down to the possibility of exploitation of women from subordinate ethnic communities or from poorer nations. Indeed, in Britain, the potential for exploitation has been an element in a largely successful campaign to eliminate "trans-racial" adoptions of black children by white parents. It is ironic that while adoption is often presented in a positive light as a solution to infertility, the sometimes painful experiences of women who have surrendered their children to adoption are also invoked to demonstrate the dangers of surrogacy.[14]

In highlighting the difficulties of adoption, I am not arguing for an end to adoption, nor am I identifying it as an unsatisfactory practice. On the contrary, I think adoption is to be encouraged; it is often the basis for strong and joyful mother-child relationships, and it enables many birthmothers to find a secure and loving home for children whom they decide not to mother.[15] What I would like to emphasize is that the impact of adoption on women (like that of surrogacy or other conceptive technologies) depends upon the conditions we create for these practices. We cannot ensure that a birthmother s decision to surrender her child for adoption will be painless (any more than we can make abortion decisions easy). But what we can and must do is to try to create conditions—crucially, about freedom from restriction during pregnancy and about custody—that will preserve her autonomy and help to ensure that the decision is hers;[16] and we can commit ourselves with renewed vigor to efforts to secure forms of economic and social support for all mothers so that fewer such decisions are coerced by poverty and need.

. . . Before setting our minds against conceptive technologies, we have to consider whether this is really the best way to protect women who have sought (and will continue to seek) their use. An implacable opposition to conceptive technologies could mean that any chance of exerting pressure on those who organize infertility services—for example, pressure for better research and for disclosure of information; for more stringent conditions of consent; for means of access for poorer women, who are likely to be the majority of those with infertility problems—would be lost. Would it be wise to abandon infertile women to the untender mercies of infertility specialists, when a campaign, say, to limit the number of embryos that may be implanted (and thereby to reduce multiple pregnancies, pressures for selective reduction, and so forth), or to regulate the use of hormonal stimulation, might do a great deal to reduce the possible risks to women and to their infants?[17]

Perhaps in the light of these reflections, we might reconsider the claim that these technologies are *"unwise"*—that it would be better to divert resources to fund research into causes of infertility. Better for whom? Infertility services are often the poor cousin of health services—poorly funded, badly organized, extremely unequally distributed, and run in an authoritarian and insensitive fashion.[18] Do we really want to argue that resources be removed from the already inadequate provision for infertile people, and redeployed for the protection of those who are currently fertile? Surely this kind of divisive strategy runs counter to the feminist concern to improve health care provisions for all women, and to be sensitive to the needs of the infertile. On the other hand, a feminist campaign for a better range of services around infertility (research into causes, independent woman-staffed counseling services, and a range of treatments, high-tech and low) would make common cause with infertile women and men, who are often themselves very critical of the quality of help they are offered and the terms on which it is available. . . .

NOTES

1. Janice Raymond, "Preface," p. 12, in Gena Corea et al., ed., *Man-Made Women* (London, Hutchinson, 1986). This critique is associated with FINRRAGE, the Feminist International Network of Resistance to Genetic and Reproductive Engineering, whose views are elaborated in a number of books, including Jocelynne Scutt, ed., *The Baby Machine: the Commercialisation of Motherhood* (Carlton, Australia: McCulloch Publishing, 1988).

2. Emily Martin, *The Woman in the Body* (Milton Keynes: Open U. Press, 1989). Feminists have been responsible for broadcasting alternative views of women and health, while the women's health movement has campaigned vigorously for the extension of health services and for their transformation, to make them more accountable to women and more responsive to women's needs.

3. Infertile women are far from being passive victims of medical technology, not only in the sense that they actively seek out infertility treatments (as Gerson rightly points out) but also (as Pfeffer argues) in the sense that they question those treatments, stop them, reject them in favor of others, or never present for treatment at all. Deborah Gerson, "Infertility and the construction of desperation," *Socialist Review*, vol. 19, no. 3 (July–September 1989) and Naomi Pfeffer, "Artificial insemination, in-vitro fertilisation and the stigma of infertility," in Michelle Stanworth, ed., *Reproductive Technologies: Gender, Motherhood, and Medicine* (Minneapolis: U. Of Minnesota Press, 1988).

4. E.g., Gena Corea and Susan Ince, "Report of a survey of IVF clinics in the USA," in Patricia Spallone and Deborah Steinberg, eds., *Made to Order: the Myth of Reproductive and Genetic Progress* (Oxford: Pergamon Press, 1987).

5. E.g., Renate Duelli Klein and Robyn Rowland, "Women as test-sites for fertility drugs," *Reproductive and Genetic Engineering* vol. 1, no. 3 (1988), pp. 251–73.

6. E.g., Christine Crowe, "Bearing the consequences—women experiencing IVF," in Jocelynne Scutt, ed., *The Baby Machine*.

7. This has been argued most elegantly by Deborah Gerson, "Infertility and the construction of desperation"; also Mary Sue Henifin, "Introduction" to Elaine Hoffman Baruch et al. eds., *Embryos, Ethics and*

Women's Rights (New York and London: Harrington Park Press, 1988).

8. E.g., Judith Lorber, "In vitro fertilization and gender politics," in Elaine Hoffman Baruch et al., eds., *Embryos, Ethics and Women's Rights,* for a very thoughtful analysis of the dominance of male partners in reproductive decisions. The restricted "choice" of women with regard to reproductive technologies is argued eloquently by Andrea Dworkin, *Right-Wing Women* (London: The Women's Press, 1983), pp. 181–82; and by various contributors to Renate Duelli Klein, ed., *Infertility: Women Speak Out* (London: Pandora Press, 1989), who also offer vivid illustration of the power of pronatalism. For the way that clinics may manipulate women into treatment, see e.g. Gena Corea, *The Mother Machine* (New York: Harper and Row, 1985). Stephanie Dowrick and Sibyl Grundberg's sensitive discussion of pronatalism is in their edited collection, *Why Children?* (London: The Women's Press, 1980).

9. E.g., Sultana Kamal, "Seizure of reproductive rights? A discussion on population control in the third world and the emergence of new reproductive technologies in the west," in Patricia Spallone and Deborah Steinberg, eds., *Made to Order.* In her extended discussion of surrogacy contracts, Carole Pateman makes the pertinent observation that the view of surrogacy as involving women in helping or exploiting other women conveniently obscures the part of men in surrogacy arrangements; Carole Pateman, *The Sexual Contract* (Cambridge: Polity Press, 1988).

10. E.g., Mary Sue Henifin, "Introduction: women's health and the new reproductive technologies," in Elaine Hoffman Baruch et al., eds., *Embryos, Ethics and Women's Rights;* or Marion Brown, Kay Fielden, and Jocelynne Scutt, "New frontiers or old recycled?" in Jocelynne Scutt, ed., *The Baby Machine.*

11. Janice Doane and Devon Hodges, "Risky business: familial ideology and the case of Baby M," *differences,* vol. 1, no. 1 (Winter 1989), pp. 67–81.

12. Linda Singer, "Bodies—pleasures—powers," *diferences,* vol. 1. no. I (Winter 1989), pp. 45–65, writes tellingly of the "differential strategies" by which motherhood is currently marketed to particular segments of the female population.

13. Naomi Pfeffer and Anne Woollett, *The Experience of Infertility* (London: Virago, 1983).

14. Betty Jean Lifton urges us to consider also the psychological effects of surrogacy on children, in the light of the experiences of some adopted children; "Brave new baby in the brave new world," in Elaine Hoffman Baruch et al., eds., *Embryos, Ethics and Women's Rights.*

15. Feminist support for adoption rests, among other things, on the recognition that motherhood is not a unitary experience, to which all women have the same relationship (or to which any woman necessarily has the same relationship throughout her life). Different orientations to pregnancy and childbirth are discussed in, for example, Emily Martin, *The Woman in the Body,* pp. 104–5; Kristin Luker, *Abortion and the Politics of Motherhood* (Berkeley and London: U. of California Press, 1984); see esp. Sara Ruddick, *Maternal Thinking: Toward a Politics of Peace* (Boston: Beacon Press, 1989).

16. There have been encouraging calls in recent articles for the risks to be shared more equally by all parties to a surrogacy contract, rather than being all taken by the mother; this might entail no restrictions on behavior, diet, health, or even abortion during pregnancy, and full rights to change her mind for a period of time after the birth. Janice Doane and Devon Hodges, "Risky business: familial ideology and the case of Baby M," pp. 77–79; and Linda Singer, "Bodies—pleasures—powers," p. 63.

17. These are merely off-the-cuff examples of campaigns that might benefit women using infertility services; but it is the principle of feminist intervention to improve safety standards that interests me, and I am by no means committed to these particular campaigns.

18. Lesley Doyal, "Infertility—a life sentence? Women and the National Health Service," in Michelle Stanworth, ed., *Reproductive Technologies;* Naomi Pfeffer and Alison Quick, *Infertility Services: A Desperate Case* (London: GLACH, 1988); David Mathieson, *Infertility Services in the NHS—What's Going On?* Report prepared for Frank Dobson, M.P., Shadow Minister of Health, 1986.

Dethroning Choice: Analogy, Personhood, and the New Reproductive Technologies

HILDE LINDEMANN NELSON

THERE IS SOMETHING about the debate over reproductive technologies of all kinds—from coerced use of Norplant to trait-selection technologies, to issues surrounding in vitro fertilization (IVF), to fetal tissue transplantation—that seems to invite dubious analogies. A Tennessee trial court termed Mary Sue and Junior Davis's frozen embryos "in vitro children" and applied a best-interests standard in awarding "custody" to Mary Sue Davis;[1] the Warnock Committee drew an implicit analogy between human gametes and transplantable organs in its recommendation of a voluntary, nonprofit system for collecting and distributing gametes in the United Kingdom;[2] Owen Jones compares the right to trait-selection to the right to abortion;[3] Robert Veatch once claimed that if a woman had signed an organ donation card and then died while pregnant, she had in effect given consent to the attempt to sustain the pregnancy after her death;[4] John Robertson has argued that contract pregnancy poses no problems we have not already encountered with adoption;[5] and Andrea Bonnicksen has compared the wonders of preembryonic genetic screening to the riches housed in the gold museum in Bogota, Colombia.[6]

The second noteworthy feature of the debate over the new reproductive technologies is the rather widespread assumption that the permissibility of employing them rests on the quality of the contract between the person seeking the services and the provider. A private agreement made for the purpose of satisfying one's self-regarding preferences is, on this view, permissible so long as no fraud or force is used; government oversight ensures that the choice is free. In this way of framing the question, procreative liberty is given presumptive priority in all conflicts over the use of a procreative technology, and the burden of proof falls on its opponents, who must show that sufficient harm results from its use to justify limiting procreative choice.[7] At the same time, the sole source of obligation is the explicit or implicit consent to arrangements designed to satisfy those choices. This is such a common method of proceeding that it excites little attention. It participates fully in the dominant bioethical paradigm.

These two features of much of the reproductive ethics discussion—dubious analogy and the emphasis on choice—are, I think, connected by a rather impoverished but widely shared account of what it is to be a person. The idea is that a person is a private chooser, and, like other concepts of personhood, this one invites the use of certain analogies and repels the use of others. In this essay, I shall argue that a careful look at the analogies and disanalogies used in the debates over reproductive technologies tells you something about the model of personhood that has been tacitly or deliberately adopted; and that this

HILDE LINDEMANN NELSON is Director, Center for Applied and Professional Ethics, University of Tennessee, Knoxville.

Journal of Law, Medicine & Ethics, 23, 2 (1995): 129–35. Copyright 1995. Reprinted by permission of Hilde Nelson and the American Society of Law, Medicine & Ethics. All rights reserved.

in turn provides some insight into the moral assumptions that are likely to underlie the discussion, and the sources of moral goodness that are likely to be invoked. I want to argue further that the idea of the self as private chooser is an inherently contradictory concept, as privileging private choice over all other sources of value ultimately permits our *technologies*—not our personal selves—to determine what persons shall be, and the technological concept of personhood (which elicits its own analogies) is very different indeed from the private preference-maximizer the reproductive ethics literature so frequently promotes. At the same time, I shall argue, the person constructed by the technological imperative is heavily *dependent* on the person-as-chooser. As I think both notions of personhood are ultimately unsatisfactory, I shall close by offering a third alternative—one that might make it easier for us to pick our way through the ethical thicket that surrounds the use of the reproductive technologies.

ANALOGIES AS WEATHERVANES

Case law proceeds by analogy, as does a fair amount of bioethics, where one of its uses is to test the consistency of one's principles. To return to one of the analogies with which I began: if contract pregnancy really is morally equivalent to adoption, and adoption is socially acceptable, then consistency demands that contract pregnancy be accepted by society as well. Whether the analogy will seem convincing depends on the kind of normative light in which one is standing. If one's primary source of moral illumination is personal choice, then one will find a certain intuitive plausibility in looking at contract pregnancy from the choosers' point of view: as the contracting parents see it, this child, like the adopted child, did not arrive by accident but was chosen lovingly and willingly to be a new member of the family. If, however, one's moral light emanates

from a belief that those who put a child into the world (whether they chose to or not) are obliged to weave a relationship of love and care around that child, the analogy between contract pregnancy and adoption will seem less convincing: from this point of view, when that relationship never forms or ceases to exist, something of great value is lost—something too valuable to be handed off casually or deliberately to others.

The moral force of the analogy between adoption and contract pregnancy will very much depend on the web of beliefs about persons, families, causality, and so on that informs one's outlook. For this reason, careful scrutiny of an analogy might reveal a great deal about the assumptions and beliefs that underlie it. Analogies, if you will, serve as weathervanes that indicate which way the moral wind is blowing.

I want to use this observation about analogies as a tool for investigating the social meaning of various reproductive technologies. It seems to me that if an analogy between a new development and an established social practice can tell you something about the moral commitments underlying the arguments for or against the new development, then a look at the disanalogies ought to show up other moral saliencies that have, from the first perspective, been hidden from view.

DISANALOGIES AS TIP-OFFS

Let me begin with a disanalogy between contract pregnancy and adoption—the one I hinted at earlier. Adoption is ordinarily a response to misfortune: a child's parents are either unable to care for it, which is sad, or they are unwilling to care for it, which is reprehensible. Inability to care for one's child is sad because the child is uniquely one's own, of one's body, a part of one's self; and when this connection must be severed, something of value to both parent and child is lost. Accounts of what exactly is lost may differ, but that the loss is significant is attested to by the many adopted children who, even though lovingly cared for by attentive adoptive parents, nevertheless feel that something is missing in their lives.[8] Contract pregnancy, by contrast, deliberately engineers the loss: one of the parents undertakes the pregnancy with the intent of severing her connection with the child after it is born.

When this disanalogy is noted, *consent* as a basis for obligation can be complemented by the notion of obligation based on *causality*. I have directly caused this particular child to exist. Because she is a human child, she enters the world with enormous bodily, emotional, and interpersonal needs, and, as I have put her in this needy state, I am obliged to help get her out of it. Because what is at stake here is nothing less than another person's life and happiness, my responsibility is too great to be performed by proxy. I cannot be sure the rearing parents are discharging my duty as I ought to do it, especially if I have removed myself from any contact with them. I therefore must, if I can, meet this obligation myself.[9]

In his classic *Methods of Ethics*, Sidgwick sounds this causal theme: "For the parent, being the cause of the child's existing in a helpless condition, would be indirectly the cause of the suffering and death that would result to it if neglected."[10] From the standpoint of causality, the analogy to contract pregnancy is not adoption, but rather something more like disownment. Here the conception of personhood is social and narrative: persons have histories and connections to other people, and these connecting threads are not only temporal, social, and contractual, but sometimes also causal. In the act of relinquishing the child at birth, as in the act of disowning, the contract birthgiver refuses to honor the causal and personal relationships that bind her to the child.

The argument using disownment as its analogy is based in causality *in contradistinction to* choice, but there have been attempts to create causal accounts that proceed *by way of* choice.

These attempts are, I think, ultimately unsuccessful because the choice motif crowds out other sources of value: the concept of the person is once again the independent contractor, bound not by her relationships to others, but by the choices she has made. Kant's account of personhood is considerably more sophisticated than the current notion of the private preference-maximizer, but it is still at bottom an image of the self as autonomous chooser, and choice will out in the end. Here is Kant's attempt to incorporate causality into the paradigm of contract:

> It is a quite correct and even necessary Idea to regard the act of procreation as one by which we have brought a person into the world without his consent and on our own initiative, for which deed the parents incur an obligation to make the child content with his condition so far as they can. They cannot destroy their child as if he were something they had *made* (since a being endowed with freedom cannot be a product of this kind) or as if he were their property, nor can they even just abandon him to chance, since they have brought not merely a worldly being but a citizen of the world into a condition which cannot now be indifferent to them even just according to concepts of Right.[11]

It looks as if Kant is arguing that the parents owe the child because they caused him to be born, but then we note that the parents did this on their "own initiative"—that is, they agreed to have sexual intercourse. For Kant, then, the causal line originates in consent. The man and woman freely chose to engage in behavior that caused a person's existence, and so they must take responsibility for that choice.

Would the obligation to the child still hold if they had not chosen freely to have sex? To answer this question, we have to think about the context in which the act of procreation takes place. Kant makes it clear in this section of *The Doctrine of Right* that he is talking about intercourse within marriage. He is discussing the begetting and bearing of children not as it proceeds from a given act of procreation, but as it proceeds from marriage—the state in which intercourse can and should take place. And marriage, for Kant, is a state which both parties consent to enter.

To engage in sex outside of marriage, on the other hand, is to be in the state of nature. A woman giving birth in this state may have caused her child to be born, but the birth is so shameful, Kant argues, that even if she murders the child, she should not be punished for murder.[12] One's duties to the child would therefore seem to have less to do with *whether* one caused its existence than with *where* one did so—within the social contract or in the state of nature. Kant's use of the language of the social contract—itself an analogy between living in a well-ordered society and freely entering into a legally binding exchange of goods or services with someone—underscores his view of persons as rational agents who, for a consideration, give up some of their autonomy to other rational agents. It is a view that creates only surface-room for causality as a source of obligation. The causal account is quickly elbowed out, leaving the contract alone to do the moral work. For this reason, the Kantian analysis of parental obligation is incomplete.

TWO OTHER DISANALOGIES

I have been pursuing merely one example of how disanalogies can point to unnoticed or underexplored avenues of ethical investigation. Now I propose to broaden my focus by noting two disanalogies between assisted procreation in general and ordinary coitus. By using the term *assisted procreation* rather than *reproductive technology,* I mean to exclude, for the moment, contraceptive technologies, but to include prenatal screening, trait selection, and genetic enhancement of existing traits. The first disanalogy between assisted procreation and coitus, then, as Marjorie Schultz has pointed out, is that the intent to have a child is more readily apparent in assisted procreation.[13]

If, for example, you are going to the trouble of undergoing IVF, you are clearly trying to get pregnant rather than to have a good time in bed. No child resulting from the procedure can be considered an accident. There is, of course, still the problem of invisible pressure (say, from the rest of the family) to have a baby, or false consciousness—perhaps the woman mistakenly believes she cannot be fulfilled as a woman unless she gives birth. Considerations of this kind blur the question of intent even here, but, in separating procreation from sexual intimacy, it is considerably easier to see which is which. Disentangling the strand of intent from those of passion, coercion, or mishap permits a more personal sense of reproductive agency. The baby is now not something that happened to us, but what you and I, severally rather than jointly, have willed. This value of the exercise of personal will sits just below the surface of assisted procreation in a way that it cannot for ordinary coitus.

The second disanalogy between assisted procreation and coitus is that the activity of adding a new generation to one's family becomes a more public activity. It is no longer simply a private act, intended or unintended, between a man and a woman, but rather enlists the help of other moral agents. For that reason it may be argued that it is quite right to hold those seeking assistance to a somewhat higher standard of accountability than we ordinarily hold prospective parents. By this I do not mean that the reasons for *having* a child have to pass a more rigorous moral muster. These reasons are often frivolous or nonexistent, but the child is none the worse for this so long as she receives loving care once she arrives on the familial scene. The higher standard of accountability I am arguing for has less to do with why one has a child than with how one intends to treat her when she comes into existence. It is that intention and whether the prospective parent is in a position to fulfill her or his responsibilities to the child that become the business of those who are asked to help bring about the child's existence. When medical responses to subfertility move the decision to have a child from a private choice to a more broadly shared cooperative activity, we can see more clearly that notions of the common good—particularly, of what is conducive to children's flourishing—and not just personal preferences are at play in human procreation.

of a live birth) is on national average only a rather depressing 16 percent and its cost in most clinics is over $10,000 per attempt, leads some women to undergo the procedure upward of eight or even ten times; they feel that because the option is there, they ought to avail themselves of it. And so forth.

FROM PERSON-AS-CHOOSER TO PERSON AS TECHNOLOGICAL CONSTRUCT

In exploring the disanalogies between assisted procreation and ordinary coitus, I have so far found at least two important differences—namely, intention and number of persons involved—that can be overlooked if one focuses exclusively on the similarities between the practices. Disanalogies between technologies of contraception and organic infertility could doubtless also be identified, but these would require a separate analysis. Rather than perform it here, I move on to another sort of difference—this time between using reproductive technologies in general, whether conceptive or contraceptive, on the one hand, and letting nature take its course, on the other. The difference is that technology multiplies choices. This is hardly a novel observation, but its consequences have not always been well understood.

An accumulation of choices can be a burden as well as a blessing, as Barbara Katz Rothman[14] and others have remarked. In the circles where safe, legal abortion is readily available, for example, not exercising this option, even though prenatal screening has revealed the likelihood of a serious defect in the fetus, may invite censure. Similar censure may arise from the failure to choose among birth control options, even within a monogamous marriage. The possibility that IVF could provide a remedy for subfertility, even though its success rate (measured in terms

THE TECHNOLOGICAL SELF

In this way, medical technologies exert power over persons and not the other way around. Technologies create their own culture of practices, institutions, and discourses, and these become a powerful force that inscribes individual bodies to its own specifications. In a kind of mirror image of the person as free chooser, the person created by technology is shaped by outside forces to particular cultural norms. This concept of personhood, described (but arguably not endorsed) by Michel Foucault, is I think at least as disturbing and morally inadequate as its mirror image. Let me describe it briefly; say how it mirrors the free chooser, and offer a third alternative.

Bodily inscription might be considered a metaphorical flight of fantasy, but it can also be taken literally. Consider, for example, how the culture created by the technologies of television, capitalism, personal computers, and private automobiles has contributed to obesity in the United States. Market forces favor cars over public transportation, so people drive their cars to work and deny themselves even the walk from the bus stop or train station. Then they sit for many hours each day typing words and numbers into a computer, and return home by car to an evening of television, sponsored by companies that advertise heavily processed foods designed to be consumed while watching television. In the way of life these technologies have spawned, there are insufficient natural opportunities for exercise and far too many opportunities to overeat. We are of course free to set aside time for exercise and to pass up the fatty snacks, but to do this we have to resist the forces created by widespread use of the technologies in question. Left to themselves, these forces exert pressure on the body that increases its size.

The power of technological culture, however, is not merely an unthinking force that makes us gain weight; it is often *disciplinary* power. This can be distinguished from the power of the state, which imposes the sovereign will on its citizens through such sanctions as fines or prison terms; it is also different from the power of individual persons, who may have the wealth, publicity, social stature, or moral suasion to force others to do their will. The disciplinary power of technological culture, as Foucault conceives of it, is a grid of everyday practices, people, tools, techniques, market forces, social arrangements, sciences, and patterns of thought that imposes itself on individuals and molds them according to its dictates. It is power from the bottom up.

"Power," Foucault explains, "is employed and exercised through a net-like organisation. . . . [It] reaches into the very grain of individuals, touches their bodies and inserts itself into their actions and attitudes, their discourses, learning processes and everyday lives."[15] Foucault was particularly interested in the way this net-like organization functions as a social discipline, imposing taboos against masturbation or homosexuality, for example, or forcing behavioral norms in the army or in orphanages.

In our own time, he believed, power is exercised simultaneously through force of law ("sovereignty") and through the cultural practices, institutions, economic arrangements, collectivities, scientific techniques, social attitudes, and ideologies (collectively, "technologies") that compel us to conform to the social norms this disciplinary grid itself creates. But the two systems of power are incompatible, Foucault argues, and because their incompatibility is increasingly more apparent, it was necessary that a mediating discourse be found that would allow them to interact continually. This mediating discourse, Foucault

claims, is medicine. "The developments of medicine, the general medicalisation of behaviours, conducts, discourses, desires etc., take place at the point of intersection between the two heterogeneous levels of discipline and sovereignty."[16]

Medicine mediates between discipline and sovereignty when, for example, people who pose a political threat to the state are declared insane and shut up in mental institutions. But the mediation of medicine and power we want to look at here is that involving the technologies medicine has created—particularly those aimed at subfertility and procreation. Medicalizing subfertility with the help of procreative technologies sets up norms: bodily norms, behavioral norms, ethical norms. A subfertile woman who wants to have a child is not merely unlucky—she is abnormal. She should go to an infertility clinic, where various technologies will normalize her into pregnancy. Simply accepting whatever child will be produced by IVF is abnormal; the embryo should undergo genetic screening for quality control of the resulting child. The refusal to sacrifice greatly to bring a fetus to term is abnormal; the mother should have consented to fetal surgery to repair a neural tube defect, or to a caesarean section because a perinatologist has predicted fetal distress. In these and other ways, medicine—a kindly, benevolent knowledge aimed at our good—becomes a technology that disciplines and standardizes individual bodies.

Foucault takes this insight one step farther. His claim is that, far from being the rational, free agents of the Kantian paradigm (or the autonomous preference-satisfiers that abound in the bioethics literature), the individual is *constructed* by these disciplinary technologies. "The individual is not a pre-given entity which is seized on by the exercise of power. The individual, with his identity and characteristics, is the product of a relation of power exercised over bodies, multiplicities, movements, desires, forces."[17] There is, as Foucault sees it, no interior self that constitutes one's personhood. "Nothing in man—not even his body—is sufficiently stable to serve as the basis for self-recognition or for understanding other men."[18] This does not mean there is no self, but rather that the self is *exterior* to the person: "it is produced permanently around, on, within the body" by the net-like organization of disciplinary power.[19]

This exterior self, created by the disciplinary grid as mediated by medicine, is utterly dependent, I suggest, on a conception of persons as natural entities who choose freely. The illusion of an autonomous, unencumbered agent, who independently enters into agreements or seeks the goods he prefers, conceals the coercive power of the reproductive technologies as they produce persons according to their own specifications of what is normal or desirable. The concealment of this coercive aspect of technology is essential if technology's use is to be justified by free choice; the concept of person as technologically constructed requires the ideology of choice to drive the technologies. Autonomy becomes one piece of the net-like organization that inscribes itself forcefully on the body and so perpetuates this disciplinary form of power. We *are* persons-as-choosers, but not because we choose to be. We are persons-as-choosers because the disciplinary grid forces us to be. Choice is normal. Choice is required.

The concept of person as free choice maker could not, I believe, have arisen outside the vast proliferation of technologies that has given the self the options from which it may choose. It is no accident that the Kantian Enlightenment Man came into being at the same time as the Industrial Revolution. Until the technologies were available that made alternative ways of living possible, until people had practical means for realizing private notions of the good life, a concept of the person that laid great emphasis on the faculty of choice would have been deeply puzzling, to say the least. A liberal society, in which it is left to the individual to determine his or her own conception of the good, cannot exist without the technologies that permit one to put one's conceptions into practice. In this way, the Kantian

person-as-chooser and Foucault's technologically constructed and normalized self take in each others' washing: diametrically opposed, each is necessary to the other.

AN ALTERNATIVE ACCOUNT OF THE SELF

When personal preference is taken to be the most appropriate or even the only appropriate standard of conduct for the use of reproductive technologies, the public understanding of motherhood, paternity, family, and the like rests uneasily on an incoherent conception of persons as autonomous contractors who are simultaneously technological constructs. The ideology of choice, it seems, gives us a conception of the self that is at once too much at the mercy of social and cultural forces and too isolated from them. Persons both become mere functions of their place in the net-like disciplinary grid and stand self-contained, seeking to maximize their preferences in unattached Cartesian solitude. Neither conception of the self is very satisfactory; taken together, they self-destruct.

When choice sounds the dominant note in a culture, it is likely to silence other notes. Or, to change the metaphor, the intense emphasis on choice drives society in certain directions and leaves other avenues invisible. Our society has become so used to the Kantian account of persons that we sometimes fail to notice how badly it fits the realities of human procreation. It cuts against the very kinds of persons reproductive technologies are designed to produce — dependent, vulnerable babies with deep connections to other human selves, rather than independent, mature, unattached, free agents. The Kantian self leaves out too much of what it is to be human: the socialization that we receive from our families, friendships, and formal schooling; the webs of interpersonal relationships that encumber us with responsibilities at the same time as they provide us with identity and meaning; and the very languages we learn, which determine what categories of perception and understanding will be open to us. Yet the technologically constructed self seems so completely a function of one's position in the disciplinary grid as to deny the possibility of personal freedom, and hence any moral or legal or political agency. On this model, there is no real possibility of rational reflection or ethical suasion, only the assertion of one's desires, and the exercise of such power as is available to achieve them. And, if I am right about the way in which the Kantian and Foucauldian selves rely on one another, and the incoherence of that relationship, then both accounts of personhood are inadequate.

We need another model — one that lets us stop vacillating wildly between unfettered choice and no choice. The alternative I have in mind (and others may be put forward) is an account not of the person, but of *persons* — some of whom are helpless, unformed, and inexperienced; others of whom are capable of independent action, however constricted by the practices and institutions of their society; still others whose powers of independence as well as of interaction with others are now waning. This account of personhood is that of selves through time in community, most of whom will, during some significant part of their lives, engage in collaborative reflection and action with others — reflection and action aimed toward some notion of their common good. Collaborative work of this kind requires at least a minimum of ethical and epistemic elbow-room for each person involved — a modest amount of rational free agency that allows the person to take some responsibility for her commitments and the actions that flow from them. It also requires, I think, not a thick conception of the common good, but a rather more slender notion — one that is respectful of the wide variety of persons who are entitled to share in it.

What I am advocating is a concept of selves in dialogue with others. Recognizing our common good requires a public discourse in which we self-consciously examine the analogies we use, paying careful attention to the conceptions of personhood at which they hint. To what extent, for example, should the common good of refusing to perpetuate images of women as maternal backgrounds or flowerpots constrain a prospective father's preference for sustaining a postmortem pregnancy for more than a few days? To what extent ought the common good of affirming the worth of people with short stature act as a side constraint on a private choice, in the not-too-distant-future, to screen one's pre-embryo for height?

In the absence of sustained and thoughtful public debate over these and related questions, there is reason to argue that we are not justified in passing laws that forbid the use of any reproductive technology — at least, not unless the technology can clearly be shown to cause personal harm. Nor, on my own showing, are we justified in leaving these matters to the market and to other social and disciplinary forces that wield a power over us which we neither fully understand nor fully control. If we can neither look to the law nor count on market forces to see us through — if, in Foucault's language, neither sovereign nor disciplinary power will answer here — our best alternative appears to be a reliance on moral suasion. But to achieve a shared moral understanding of these reproductive questions, the debate will have to be framed in a way that lets us see what we are passing up if we decide that personal preference needs more vigorous legal and ethical protection than any other value. When the framework rests heavily on personal choice, we cannot even see what is missing, let alone whether it is worth having. And we have no publicly accessible means of deciding, rationally and reflectively, whether to ratify or resist the normalizing powers of the technologies in question.

IN ADDITION TO CHOICE: A FINAL ANALOGY

What this all comes down to, to return to the example of contract pregnancy one final time, is that the analogy to adoption and the ethical orientation that underlies it is ultimately unsuccessful: its dominant call of personal choice has, as it were, drowned out the baby's cry. I have already tried to show how causality complements choice as a source of morality, but what other moral notions might allow us to hear that baby better? There are a number of excellent answers to this question,[20] but I want to close by reflecting briefly on just one: the goodness of solidarity with the disenfranchised.

Consider a lesbian couple in a long-term and loving relationship, who want, like other couples, to have children, and who want, like other couples, to have them as children of their own bodies. Transvaginal oocyte retrieval permits Carla, as we will call her, to give eggs that will be fertilized in vitro by sperm from her partner Charlotte's brother; a resulting embryo will be implanted in Charlotte's uterus. Later, when they want a second child, it will be Carla's cousin whose sperm fertilizes Charlotte's eggs and Carla who will be the birthgiver.

People in Carla and Charlotte's situation will almost certainly have experienced pervasive, invidious, and destructive discrimination. They will be stigmatized as immoral, unnatural, perverted. If their sexual orientation is known, they may be fired from their jobs, or not offered jobs for which they are well qualified. They may be denied housing, or become the target of a hate group. They may be harassed and intimidated. Or, more subtly, they may be thought unfit to rear children. None of these forms of discrimination can be justified. Considerations of sexuality per se are entirely irrelevant to one's ability to be a good tenant, a productive worker, a loving parent. Procreative technology, then, can be a benefit to Carla and Charlotte not simply because it advances a conception of the good they have chosen personally, but also because it advances a conception of the common good: namely, to make the world a better place for disenfranchised people capable of rearing children in a loving household, and for the children so reared.

Carla and Charlotte's children will have two mothers as well as a father, but while this may

strike many of us as exotic, it is not likely to harm the children, who seem to do rather well under these arrangements.[21] What is needed as we set policy for the new reproductive technologies is a greater openness to unexpected results of this kind and better judgment about what is and is not worth protecting. We can begin by noting the model of personhood that is at work in our deliberations. When we do this, we are likely to end up with a richer notion not only of what it is to be a human being, but also of what is involved in living a good life.

REFERENCES

1. *Davis v. Davis v. King,* E-14496 (5th Jud. Ct., Tenn. 1989).

2. Great Britain, Department of Health and Social Security (chairman Mary Warnock), *Report of the Committee of Inquiry into Human Fertilisation and Embryology* (London: Her Majesty's Stationery Office, 1984).

3. Owen D. Jones, "Reproductive Autonomy and Evolutionary Biology: A Regulatory Framework for Trait-Selection Technologies," *American Journal of Law & Medicine,* XIX (1993): at 601.

4. Robert Veatch, "Maternal Brain Death: An Ethicist's Thoughts," *JAMA,* 248 (1982): 1102–03.

5. John A. Robertson, "Surrogate Mothers: Not So Novel After All," *Hastings Center Report,* 13, no. 5 (1983): 28–34.

6. Andrea Bonnicksen, "Genetic Diagnosis of Human Embryos," *Hastings Center Report,* 22, no. 4, Supp. (1992): at S5.

7. John Robertson, *Children of Choice: Freedom and the New Reproductive Technologies* (Princeton: Princeton University Press, 1994): at 16.

8. When it comes to familial connections, it seems that people are not readily replaceable. That is why we laugh at W.C. Field's encounter with a distraught mother whose baby has just died. "No matter, Madam," he leers, "I will gladly get you with another."

9. For a more detailed account of this kind of argument, see Hilde Lindemann Nelson and James Lindemann Nelson, *The Patient in the Family* (New York: Routledge, 1955): at ch. 5.

10. Henry Sidgwick, *The Methods of Ethics* (Chicago: University of Chicago Press, 1962): at 249. Sidgwick's argument is discussed in Jeffrey Blustein, "Child Rearing and Family Interests," in Onoral O'Neill and William Ruddick, eds., *Having Children* (Oxford: Oxford University Press, 1979); discussion of Blustein on Sidgwick is found in James Lindemann

Nelson, "Parental Obligations and the Ethics of Surrogacy: A Causal Perspective," *Public Affairs Quarterly,* 5 (1991): at 51.

11. Immanuel Kant, *Metaphysical First Principles of the Doctrine of Right,* trans. Mary Gregor (Cambridge: Cambridge University Press, 1991): at PA 281.

12. *Id.* at PA 336.

13. Marjorie Maguire Schultz, "Reproductive Technology and Intent-Based Parenthood: An Opportunity for Gender Neutrality," *Wisconsin Law Review,* 1990 (1990): at 308–09.

14. Barbara Katz Rothman, *The Tentative Pregnancy: Prenatal Diagnosis and the Future of Motherhood* (New York: Viking, 1986).

15. Michel Foucault, *Power/Knowledge: Selected Interviews & Other Writings, 1972–1977,* ed. Colin Gordon (New York: Pantheon, 1980): at 98, 39.

16. *Id.* at 107.

17. *Id.* at 73–74.

18. Michel Foucault, "Nietzsche, Genealogy, History," in *Language, Counter-Memory, Practice: Selected Essays and Interviews by Michel Foucault,* trans. Donald F. Bouchard and Sherry Simon (Ithaca: Cornell University Press, 1977): at 153.

19. Michel Foucault, *Discipline and Punish: The Birth of the Prison,* trans. Alan Sheridan (New York: Vintage, 1979): at 29.

20. For excellent answers from the feminist ethics of care alone, see Virginia Held, "Non-Contractual Society," in Marsha Hanen and Kai Nielsen, eds., *Science, Morality and Feminist Theory* (Calgary: University of Calgary Press, 1987): 111–37; Sara Ruddick, *Maternal Thinking: Toward a Politics of Peace* (Boston: Beacon Press, 1989); Rita Manning, *Speaking from the Heart: A Feminist Perspective on Ethics* (Lanham: Rowman & Littlefield, 1992); and Joan C. Tronto, *Moral Boundaries: A Political Argument for an Ethic of Care* (New York: Routledge, 1993).

21. See Michael B. King and Pat Pattison, "Homosexuality and Parenthood," *British Medical Journal,* 303, 3 Aug. (1991): 295–97.

A Multiple-Birth Morass

WE LIVE IN AN AGE in which many people keep mistaking the Guinness Book of Records for the Bible as life's Good Book.

Consider Nkem Chukwu's remarks on the reason why her recent, fertility-drug enhanced pregnancy resulted in a new world record—eight live-born children. "I wanted to have as many as God gave me so I'm really glad I had eight," she told a news conference in Houston this week.

God, in this view, has added fertility drugs to the arsenal of strange ways in which He works.

We don't think so. It is infertility technology and parents' wills—and not the Lord's—that produce octuplets; it is fertility drugs and parents' obsessions—and not God's fault—if such multi-birth events produce children who are blind, have cerebral palsy, or are afflicted with various immune system and neurological disorders.

The question is what to do about what is a growing problem. Statistics in the United States suggest the number of births involving three or more babies have leaped by 178 percent in the past decade. The vast majority of these births are

From The Globe and Mail, *January 4, 1999. Copyright 1999. Reprinted with permission from* The Globe and Mail.

related to infertility treatments. It is not the sheer numbers that are important, but the ills that befall the children. Statistics out of Europe indicate that 43 percent of twins are born prematurely and 8 percent require intensive care; the number jumps to 92 percent and 34 percent in triplets.

And the above does not take into account the added risk of long-term, life-debilitating illnesses that plagued the lives of many multiple-birth children. It is easy to see there is a problem, but more difficult to know what to do about it. We don't want laws that tell parents they can't have multiple children. If Pierre Trudeau once argued that there was no place for the state in the bedrooms of this country, it is even more true that the state should stay out of this country's wombs.

Therefore, all pressures should be extralegal. A logical first step is to stop Guiness Book beatification of these events. A part of us would like the media, including this newspaper, to take a vow to stop reporting on multiple births. This is probably unworkable, but at the very least we should report these events with a hard, reportorial eye. A suitably cold headline for the Chukwu births might have read: "A potential tragedy in Texas — Octuplets."

As well, it is probably true that those outside the media should stop making multiple births a kind of life jackpot. About three thousand people have already made contributions to the Chukwu family; the McCaughey septuplets in Iowa resulted in a new custom-designed house and van for the family.

We know it sounds Draconian, but there are better and more socially responsible uses for your money. Give it to abandoned single mothers, families with children with birth defects and adoptive parents of AIDS babies. Don't reward risk-taking, multiple birth parents. If the Chukwus truly believe what happened is God's will, then let God look after them.

Surrogacy

Surrogate Mother Arrangements from the Perspective of the Child

HERBERT T. KRIMMEL

A DOZEN OR SO YEARS from now, when the children already born from surrogate mother arrangements start to ask questions about the way in which they were brought into this world, what will we tell them? What can we expect their feelings to be?[1]

They will learn that they were different from other babies; that they were the product of what some call "collaborative reproduction."[2] They will discover that what this means in their cases is that their biological mothers decided to conceive them, not because their biological mothers wanted to raise, know, and love them, but for some other reasons. That, for these other reasons, their biological mothers entered into contracts to transfer custody of them to their biological fathers and their biological fathers' wives,[3] in order to fulfill a need that those couples had: the desire to experience the joys of having a baby.

If the emotional experiences of adopted children are a guide,[4] the children born under surro-

HERBERT KRIMMEL is a Law Professor at Southwestern University School of Law, Los Angeles.

gate mother arrangements will want to know why their mothers gave them up. How will these children feel about the various reasons surrogate mothers[5] are giving today for why they enter into surrogate mother arrangements? And, if the experiences of adopted children are a guide, the children born under surrogate mother arrangements will want to know more than just the why of it. They will also want to know *how* it was possible for their biological mothers to have given them up. Will these children find complete solace for the fact that their mothers were able to part with them in the love of the parents who raised them?

And how will these children feel about the parents who raised them? What will they think about their parents' arranging for their existence with contracts, terms, conditions, and warranties? How will they feel that they had to meet specifications before their intended parents had to accept them?[6]

How will these children feel about the language that surrogate mothers use to describe themselves and them?

From LOGOS, *Vol. 9 (1988): 97–112. Reprinted with permission of Herbert T. Krimmel and* LOGOS.

The purpose of this article is to address the practice of surrogate parenting from the perspective of the children who will be born under these arrangements; in order, I hope, to convince you that surrogate mother arrangements are both unethical and inimical to the interests of children and of society.

THE ETHICAL PROBLEM WITH SURROGATE MOTHER ARRANGEMENTS

What is fundamentally unethical about surrogate mother arrangements is that they, of necessity, treat the creation of a person as the means to the gratification of the interests of others, rather than respect the child as an end in himself.[7] They treat a person (the child) as though he were a thing, a commodity.

Essential and indispensible to the operation of each and every surrogate mother arrangement is the shared and common intention of the parties to transfer the baby at birth from his biological mother to his adopting parents.[8] But surrogate mother arrangements are more than just contracts about the custody of children vis-à-vis their biological parents. They are also contracts for the creation of children;[9] the irreducible core of which is that the surrogate mother must be willing to create a child with the premeditated intention to transfer him at birth. By the very nature of the transaction, the surrogate mother cannot desire to keep the child. Nor can she make a pretense to valuing the child in and for himself, since she would not otherwise be creating the child but for the monetary and other emotional consideration she receives under the surrogate mother contract.[10] Indeed, the very purpose and design of the surrogate mother arrangement is to separate in the mind of the surrogate mother her decision to create the child from the decision to have and raise that child. Her desire to create the child must necessarily be the result of some motive other than the desire

to be a parent. The child is conceived, not because he is wanted by his biological mother, but because he can be useful to her and others. He is conceived in order to be given away.

THE MOTIVATIONS OF SURROGATE MOTHERS

Why do the women who sign up to be surrogate mothers enter into surrogate mother arrangements? According to the reasons thus far advanced by surrogate mothers themselves and those who have studied them:[11]

1. Most do it for the money. Ninety percent of surrogate mothers say they would not be surrogates if they were only reimbursed for their expenses.[12]

2. Many do it in order to deal with some past emotional trauma. About one-third of the surrogate mothers in the Parker study[13] say that an important reason for them is to work through guilt, or other negative feelings, associated with a past abortion or with the giving up of a child for adoption.

3. Some of them do it, at least in part, because they enjoy being pregnant. These women cite as reasons both enjoyment of the physical sensations of being pregnant and of receiving the cultural deference and attention accorded pregnant women.[14]

4. Many cite the so-called "altruistic" motive. They want to do something nice for someone else, often expressed as wanting to give an infertile couple "the gift of life."[15]

5. The vast majority normally give some combination of the above as their motivation.

What is clearly absent from this list of reasons for procreating a child, and what *must* be absent for surrogate mother arrangements to work, is the motive of wanting the child. For, if the desire to have and raise the child were more important to surrogate mothers than the motives listed above, they could never enter into a surrogate mother arrangement.

However one may feel about the relative merits of the surrogate mothers various motives, common to them all is the use of the child as a means to the surrogate mother's happiness. Each of the motives given above clearly indicates that the child is being *valued* by the surrogate mother, primarily, if not exclusively, for his utility as a means to her economic or psychological well-being. The child is a source of income, therapy, self-esteem, or good feelings. That, is his raison d'être. Implicitly, if not explicitly, the child has a price.

Even the so-called "altruistic" motive is not altruistic at all when viewed from the perspective of the child. Children should not be given away as elegant gifts to make others happy for the same reason one does not give one's spouse to a lonely friend. To do so is to treat them as things and not as persons. Moreover, it quite clearly communicates to the person being given away that he is of lesser importance to you than the happiness of the third party.

REGARDING THE MOTIVES OF PARENTS IN NATURAL PROCREATION

But, it has been asked,[16] How are the motives of surrogate mothers really all that different from those of parents who use natural means of procreation? Professor Robertson argues that with natural parents "ends and means intertwine. Children are instruments for parental meaning and satisfaction, at the same time that they are loved for themselves."[17] He goes on to argue that "[p]ersons making this charge [that surrogate mother arrangements are ethically wrong because they use children as a means] usually overlook how traditional reproductive practices could also be condemned on this basis."[18] Professor Robertson's comparison is erroneous for two

reasons: first, because one evil does not justify another; and second, because it overlooks a very important distinction.

For any parent to treat his child, however conceived or acquired, solely as a means,[19] seems to me to be a pretty good theoretical definition of child abuse. We readily perceive and condemn this type of behavior in the case of overly ambitious parents; for example, those more interested in having a famous child actress, Olympian, pianist, and so on, than they are in their child's welfare. Surrogate mother arrangements, however, are not justified because parents using natural means of procreation *could* commit equal evils.[20] They are condemned because they cannot, by their very nature, rise to an ethical treatment of children that is possible for natural parents. Which leads to the second fallacy in Professor Robertsons comparison.

Interestingly enough though, Professor Robertson has unwittingly suggested the answer to his own argument. The distinction that he fails to recognize is that for the surrogate mother the ends and means *cannot* intertwine. She cannot treat the child as an end valued for himself alone if she is going to enter into a surrogate mother contract;[21] while, conversely, with natural procreation it is *possible*[22] for the parents to treat their child as an end.

Furthermore, that natural parents commonly do have mixed motives for having children, valuing them for themselves, while at the same time expecting to derive pleasure from them, is not ethically impermissible, so long as the latter does not preclude the former. To use Kantian ideology, the pursuit of one's happiness and the performance of one's moral duty (to treat persons as ends) may coincide.[23] For example, one may enter into a marriage expecting to enjoy conjugal relations, but to value one's husband solely as a means of sexual gratification is to turn him, in your mind, into a prostitute. One may enter into marriage expecting to receive financial support, aid, and succor; but to view one's wife solely as a means of support is to treat her, in your mind, as though she were a slave.

What is this treatment of the child as an end, that natural parents are capable of, but surrogate mothers cannot attain and still be surrogate mothers? It is to love the child simply for who he is, selflessly and unconditionally. It is not possible for the surrogate mother even to make a pretense of loving the child in this manner[24] when she would not have created him but for the dual assurances that someone else would take him off her hands at birth *and* make it worth her while.

WHY SURROGATE MOTHER ARRANGEMENTS AND ADOPTION ARE DIFFERENT

If this is true, how is it possible for adoption to be ethical?[25] How is it possible to voluntarily part with someone you truly love? You cannot, by definition,[26] if it is in exchange for something else; no, not even for good feelings.[27] You can only do so if it is solely for the good of the one you love. In other words, only if it is a selfless act. The distinction between surrogate mother arrangements and adoption is that the latter can be a selfless act of love, while the former cannot be.[27a]

The typical situations that give rise to the placement of a child for adoption are (1) the child was unintentionally conceived and his mother decides to bring him to term, or (2) the parents desired to have a child, but because of some serious and unfortunate circumstances arising after conception decide that they cannot keep him. What is important for our discussion, however, is what does not happen in adoption. There, the child's mother does not conceive him for the purpose of giving him up. Adoption is an emergency: What will we do with the baby if the mother cannot keep him? Surrogate mother arrangements, on the other hand, are premeditated.

This results in a distinction of ethical importance. In adoption, the mother can make her decision on whether to keep the child or to place him for adoption on the basis of what is in the best interests of the child, regardless of her own preferences. What she cannot legally do is sell the child.[28] The surrogate mother, on the other hand, does not, and cannot, decide the question of the child's custody on the basis of what is in the child's best interests. That is what is expressly precluded by the very idea of surrogate parenting. She must have decided this issue on the basis of contract even before the child was conceived, and for reasons that suited her purposes.[28a]

WHY THE LOVE OF THE ADOPTING PARENTS IS NOT ENOUGH

But, it might be asked, why should it matter what the motivation of the surrogate mother is, when according to the surrogate mother arrangement it has been prearranged that the child will be taken by an adopting couple? Why isn't the love of the adopting couple a complete and adequate substitute for that of the surrogate mother?[29]

Parental love is not fungible. One wouldn't expect a child who is unloved by his father to find complete solace in his mother's devotion. To demur to a child's question of why his mother didn't love him enough to keep him, by saying that he needn't trouble himself seeking an answer to that question because someone else loves him, is not an emotionally adequate answer. If anything, our experience with adopted children should have taught us this: that children suffer terribly about the question why they were given away.[30] (And we are starting to see a similar manifestation of this phenomenon with children conceived through artificial insemination by donor.[31]) Parental love is not fungible any more than romantic love is. One does not comfort a person who has just lost his spouse with the thought that the "woods are full" of eligible persons of the opposite gender.

An adopted child deeply appreciates the love of his adopting family, but he feels the loss of his biological parents nevertheless.[32] At least the adopted child—although still feeling the loss—can perhaps find some consolation in the explanation, if true, that his parents loved him but couldn't keep him.[33] This explanation cannot be used to comfort the child conceived through a surrogate mother arrangement for the simple reason that the surrogate mother never wanted the child for herself.[34]

In surrogate mother arrangements it is only a deflection, not an answer, to tell a child that because some other people love him, it is unimportant that his mother did not love him enough to keep him. Such a response willfully misses the emotional point of the child's question. This inquiry is made all the more poignant because the surrogate mother's giving up of her baby was not unavoidable, which the child might otherwise eventually come to understand and forgive. Rather, it was the very essence of the deal, without which the child would never have been conceived. The child will come to learn that it was *only because* his mother had the assurance of a binding contract that she could give him up for the money for which she conceived him in the first place. That is, this child came into existence on order, as a custom-made commodity for a guaranteed purchaser. Can any child be expected to understand, much less forgive, that?

THE MOTIVATIONS OF ADOPTING PARENTS

Why do the adopting parents enter into surrogate mother arrangements? Typically,[35] those who are currently[36] seeking to utilize surrogate mother arrangements are, for the most part, infertile couples. They generally have gone to great lengths to remedy their infertility, and when that proved to be of no avail, they sought to adopt infants. Their attempts to adopt children proved unsatisfactory or frustrating to them either because they were turned down, or they were able to adopt children but were discouraged by the long wait (for white infants), or they were dissatisfied with the type of children available for im-

mediate adoption (that is, older, "wrong race," handicapped, retarded).[37] A few couples utilizing surrogate mother arrangements never sought to adopt. They are particularly attracted to the surrogate mother arrangement because it results in a child with a biological link to one of the adopting parents, which they find to be a highly desirable advantage in comparison with adoption.[38] These couples would choose surrogate mother arrangements in preference to adoption.

What motivates the adopting parents is, for the most part, the desire to raise a child. So, what can be wrong with this desire? And, what can be wrong with the desire to procreate and raise a child of one's own blood in preference to adopting a child? Isn't that what almost all of us desire? Nothing is wrong with these desires per se. What is wrong is what is being done in utilizing surrogate mother arrangements in order to satisfy these desires. Surrogate mother arrangements are wrong because you should not purchase[39] people;[40] because a child should not be an item of manufacture, which you create to specifications as you would a car; and because persons do not *exist* for your pleasure or in order to fulfill your needs. And yet, this is precisely the type of thinking that surrogate mother arrangements necessarily encourage and inevitably entail.[41] The evil that surrogate mother arrangements do is to deprive the child of the dignity to which he is entitled as a person, by treating him as a means. It matters not that the adopting parents' objective is worthy if their method of obtaining it is corrupt.[42]

COMMODIFICATION: THE RESULT OF TREATING AND PERCEIVING THE CHILD AS A MEANS RATHER THAN AS AN END

It is when children are thought of as existing in order to fulfill needs that they become, in our minds, commodities. Surrogate mother arrangements entail and embody this type of thinking in two related ways: first, simply by virtue of the fact that they are, in essence, contracts for the creation and custody of children; second, because they encourage and tempt the adopting parents to view children as items of manufacture.

The surrogate mother and the adopting couple enter into the surrogate mother contract for the same reason that any person contracts: because the subject matter of the contract is more highly valued by one party than its quid pro quo, and vice versa. A contract is thereby designed to maximize the satisfaction of the contracting parties, and the subject matter of the contract is seen as a means to this end. The interests of the thing traded (if such a notion has any meaning at all) is unimportant.[43]

One hundred years ago, if an expecting couple were asked whether they wanted a boy or a girl, it was largely an idle question. They took what they got. If they had a preference, which they very well might, there was very little they could do about it. It was not a preference about which they expected to be able to exercise control. Today, with the techniques of amniocentesis, ultrasound, and sperm centrifuge, one can choose the sex of one's children.[44] And, as our knowledge of genetics, and equally important, our ability to manipulate and engineer results, increases, the proponents of collaborative reproduction invite us in earnest to consider what type of baby we would like—even arguing that the parents have a "right" to so decide.[45] What they do not seem to consider is that what is being invited is also a change in our attitude toward children. Their viewpoint would move us away from a simple, loving, and grateful acceptance of the child we in fact receive, and toward a critical consumerism of the "perfect" child we're entitled to, can afford, and therefore must have.[46]

The proffered *ability* to pick and choose builds expectations. It does with products. It will, and already has, with children.[47] Why does one buy a product? Because it fulfills a real or perceived need. How does one value a product? By how well it performs in fulfilling one's expectations. Defective and inferior products are those that disappoint us. What implications does this have for the child? If the parents have a right to a perfect baby of their own design, who has the correlative duty? Does it not become the baby's duty to please his parents and to meet their expectations?[48] Is it any surprise that a recent study of 8,000 abortions performed at clinics in Bombay, India, reveals that 7,997 of them were of female fetuses?[49]

That surrogate mother arrangements do encourage and tempt the adopting parents to think of the child born through that process as a means to their happiness is quite evident from the not so subtle language used by them and the proponents of surrogate mothering.[50] One magazine article quotes an adopting couple as referring to their "right to have a normal newborn infant."[51] To speak as though your need and desire to have a child give rise to a "right" to a child is wrong for the same reason it would be wrong to argue that your loneliness entitles you to a spouse. It is neither your needs nor your desires that provide the justification for another's existence. It is wrong to act and talk as though another person's reason for being were to satisfy your needs, to be the means to your happiness.[52]

DOES THE CHILD HAVE GROUNDS TO COMPLAIN?

Professor Robertson has argued that "[e]ven if there is a higher degree of confusion, unhappiness, or maladjustment in donor-assisted reproduction, a child would seem better off under this collaborative structure than not to exist at all."[53] Be that as it may, one may agree that no human life is without value and still find the practice of surrogate parenting to be unethical. By analogy, although it might be both objectively true, and subjectively felt, that a life without the use of one's legs is preferable to no life at all, that does not mean that a person would not be wronged by someone intentionally setting forth to manufacture him without legs in order to serve another's purposes.[54] By Professor Robertson's logic, no black American could object that his ancestors were brought to this country as slaves, since otherwise he most probably would not be living here today. That an evil act may have good consequences as well as bad ones does not justify the act, allow the actor to take credit for them, or erase the stain of their origin.[55]

The fundamental mistake underlying Professor Robertson's argument is that he addresses the wrong question. Even if the children born under surrogate mother arrangements are objectively "better off" in comparison with nonexistence, and even if we presume hypothetically that subjectively they would prefer life with these impairments in preference to no life at all, this does not mean that they were not wronged. The ethical issue is not resolved simply by knowing that the impairments imposed by surrogate parenting have not succeeded in depriving the child's life of all value, or even by knowing whether the child would have consented if presented with the limited choice of having either an impaired existence or no existence at all. Rather, we must also address the question of why, in the first place, the parents should have a right to premeditatedly create a child with planned and intended impairments.[56]

Viewed from this perspective the answer becomes clear. It is unethical for parents to treat their children as things even if such acts do not succeed in depriving their children's lives of all meaning. And, furthermore, it is not right to treat persons as means, and not as ends, even if they grudgingly[57] consent to being so treated. For example, I suppose one could also say that sweatshop laborers are objectively "better off" than having no jobs at all, but this would not make taking advantage of their plight by paying them less than a fair wage ethically justifiable. Neither are blackmail nor armed robbery justified because the victim chooses the subjectively

less loathsome alternative presented to him. Indeed, we do not even hold the consent of the victim to be valid in such instances, and not because it didn't reflect the victim's true preference on the occasion of his choice, but rather, because we don't consider the person who forced the choice upon him as entitled to make the victim choose from such a limited menu. Simply stated, one is not entitled to purposely stack the deck with Hobson's choices and then plead consent as a justification for one's evil act.

Professor Robertson has discovered that children are largely at the mercy of their parents. This, however, should be a cause for heightened responsibility, not for exploitation. People do not have an obligation to create children. The choice is theirs; but that choice does not encompass the right to abuse them.[58]

CONCLUSION

Surrogate mother arrangements are unethical. They preclude the surrogate mother from treating the child as an end in himself, and they strongly encourage and tempt the adopting couple to do the same. What is at stake here, however, is more than some persnickety concern over moral tidiness. The children born from these surrogate mother arrangements are going to hurt for the same reasons you and I would hurt. The ethical concerns I have raised in this article are those born of a concern for their feelings.[59]

CODA

It is reported that following the birth of a baby girl in April 1986, twenty-three-year-old Shannon Boff of Redford Township, Michigan, having twice been a surrogate mother, announced her retirement with these words: "Any more babies coming from me are going to be keepers."[60] The fundamental question the advocates of surrogate mother arrangements must answer is why any child should have to grow up with the knowledge that he was created in order to be "given" away, that *he* was not a keeper.

NOTES

1. Many perhaps will dismiss this questioning as hypothetical and speculative. After all, who can know how anyone will feel in the future, and can't we expect that there will be a broad range of feelings on the part of these children? Generalization? Certainly. It is the general case that we want to inquire about: What will the typical child born of these surrogate mother arrangements feel? Yes, we can expect that different persons might exhibit a range of reactions to being orphaned, for example, but no one doubts that for the average orphan it must be a thoroughly miserable feeling—a feeling that anyone who was once three years old and "lost" his mommy in the department store can relate to. (But see note 54, *infra*.) Speculation? Perhaps. But if so, it is one for which there is a strong basis in fact arising from the known experiences of adopted children, a schooled speculation based on what we have learned from past analogous experiences. The same rule that teaches me that if I wouldn't like something done to me that probably you won't like it done to you either. Perhaps we are engaging in speculation, but if so, it is what we had better do for the sake of these children.

2. J. Robertson, *Embryos, Families, and Procreative Liberty: The Legal Structure of the New Reproduction*, 59 S. Cal. L. Rev. 939, 1001 (1986) [hereinafter cited as Robertson (1986)] .

3. For simplicity, I will refer hereafter in this article to the biological father and his wife as the "adopting parents."

4. See generally, A. Sorosky, et al., *The Adoption Triangle* (1978); and see Testimony of Suzanne Rubin before the California Assembly Committee on Judiciary, Surrogate Parenting Contracts, Assembly Publication No. 962, pp. 72–75 (Nov. 19, 1982) (hereinafter cited as Rubin); C. Gorney, *For Love and Money*, California Magazine p. 88, at 151 (Oct. 1983) (hereinafter cited as Gorney).

5. Although I am in complete accord with Katha Pollitt's point that we should refer to the surrogate mother simply as the mother, since the term mother "describes the relationship of a woman to a child, not to the father of that child and his wife" (K. Pollitt, *The Strange Case of Baby M*, 244 The Nation 667, at 682–83 (May 23, 1987) (hereinafter cited as Pollitt)): nevertheless, the term "surrogate mother" unfortunately has caught hold, and I have decided to continue to use it for the sake of clarity. But see *In re Baby M.*, 537 A. 2d 1227, 1234 (N.J., 1988) (hereinafter cited as *In re Baby M.*—Sup. Ct. Opn.).

6. See, e.g., B. Kantrowitz, et al., *Who Keeps Baby M'?* Newsweek p. 44, at 47, 49 (Jan. 19, 1987) (hereinafter cited as Kantrowitz); Gorney, *supra* note 4, at 90 (box); *In re Baby M.*—Sup. Ct. Opn., *supra* note 5, at 1268 (Appendix A).

7. See I. Kant, *Metaphysical Foundations of Morals* (1785) in C. Fredrich (ed.), The Philosophy of Kant, 176–78 (1949) (hereinafter cited as Kant).

8. See *supra* note 3.

9. There has been a lot of loose talk that surrogate mother arrangements are not baby bartering because the adopting parents are merely renting the services of the surrogate mother. See, e.g., *In re Baby M.*, 525 A. 2d 1128, 1160 (N.J. Super. Ch., 1987), rev'd, 537 A. 2d 1227 (N.J., 1988) (hereinafter cited as *In re Baby M.* —Ch. Ct. Opn.). The argument is a red herring. Surrogate mother arrangements are about procuring babies. The adopting couple want the end product, and would dearly love to dispense with the services of the surrogate if they could. In general they have tried, having only come to surrogacy after attempting to acquire a baby by adoption. As has been pointed out by Professor Capron (L.A. Times, April 7, 1987, Sec. II, p. 5, col. 7), and others, most surrogate mother contracts only provide for compensation to the surrogate mother on delivery of a baby, no payment being made if the surrogate miscarries (i.e., renders the service but fails to deliver the product). But even the more sophisticated contracts currently being drafted, which provide for some compensation to the surrogate mother if she miscarries, do not change what these contracts are about. Surrogate mother contracts are not pure, or even primarily, service contracts. They are mixed contracts for both services and a product. If anything, the service portion is incidental to the expectations, and in the minds, of the adopting parents. For example, if I contract to have a masseur give me a back rub, it is to the service alone that my expectations lie. But if I contract to have my portrait painted, I am not satisfied that the artist performs all the necessary services well. The essence of the contract was that I wanted a picture of myself. Until that is delivered I am not satisfied. So it is with the adopting couple in surrogate mother arrangements. If the surrogate mother miscarries, through no fault of her own—i.e., she performs the service—the adopting parents will be disappointed, and their disappointment will not relate to the service, but to the failure to get the product. See, e.g., Gorney, *supra* note 4, at 150. An example of a mixed contract where the sale of a product is incidental to the service would be where you employ a doctor to sew up a wound that entails the sale of the stitches. Quite a different case. And see *In re Baby M.*—Sup. Ct. Opn., *supra* note 5, at 1240–41, 1248.

10. In point of fact, surrogate mothers do not create these children merely for the sake of bringing them into existence. Were we to find such a person, however, would her actions be ethical? No, for the same reason that it is not ethical for the proverbial sailor, acting solely of course in the interest of adding to human existence, to cheerfully bestow the "gift of life" on all naive females he can talk into it. To desire something to exist requires one to desire all those things that are necessary for its existence, and all those things that are essential elements of it or are inseparably connected with it. To desire a child is to desire the responsibilities that come with a child, for that is what a child is, a package. Separating the decision to procreate a child from the desire to have and raise that child fails to respect that child as an end in himself because that act is incompatible with loving him. See notes 21–34 and accompanying text *infra.*

11. See, e.g., P. Parker, *Motivations of Surrogate Mothers: Initial Findings,* 140 Am. J. Psych. p. 117–18 (Jan. 1983); Kantrowitz, *supra* note 6, at 47; M. Gladwell, *Surrogate Parenting Industry Goes into Legal Labor Pains,* Insight p. 20, at 21 (Sept. 22, 1986) (hereinafter cited as Gladwell); Gorney, *supra* note 4.

12. *Id.* and see, e.g., *Womb for Rent,* Los Angeles Herald Examiner, Sept. 21, 1981, A3, col. 1; S. Lewis, *Baby Bartering?* Los Angeles Daily Journal, April 20, 1981; B. Krier, *The Moral and Legal Problems of Surrogate Parenting,* L.A. Times, Nov. 10, 1981, Sec. V, p. 1, col. 1; E. Markoutsas, *Women Who Have Babies for Other Women,* Good Housekeeping p. 96, at 99 (Apr. 1981).

13. See Kantrowitz, *supra* note 6, at 47; Gladwell, *supra* note 11, at 21; P. Avery, *Surrogate Mothers: Center of a New Storm,* U.S. News & World Report p. 76 (June 6, 1983).

14. See, e.g., Gorney, *supra* note 4, at 94–95.

15. See, e.g., *In re Baby M.*—Sup. Ct. Opn., *supra* note 5, at 1236; Kantrowitz, *supra* note 6, at 44, 47; Gorney, *supra* note 4, at 95.

16. Robertson (1986), *supra* note 2, at 1025.

17. *Id.*

18. *Id.* at 1025 n. 296.

19. A mere means, to use Kantian parlance. Kant, *supra* note 7, at 176–78.

20. See L.A. Times, April 17, 1979, Sec. I, p. 2, col. 1, reporting the case of parents who conceived a child for the purpose of having him serve as a bone marrow donor for his sister.

21. See text accompanying notes 7–16 *supra.*

22. Kant did not say that it was easy to be good or to be free, only that it was possible. Kant, *supra* note 7, at 199.

23. Kant, *supra* note 7, at 144–45.

24. I am not speaking here of love in the sense of an emotion (i.e., affection: *philia*), but rather in the sense of an act of will (*agapē*). And see Kant, *supra* note 7, at 147. For example, an antebellum slave owner might have had affection for some of his slaves, but his actions prove that he did not love them in the sense in which I am using the word.

25. I am not implying that all offerings of children for adoption are necessarily ethical. In order to be so they must be done in the best interests of the child. See H. Krimmel, *The Case Against Surrogate Parenting,* 13 Hastings Center Report 35, at 36 (Oct. 1983) (hereinafter cited as Krimmel).

26. See *supra* note 24. The fact remains that man is incapable of giving a non-religious justification for his existence and essential worth. It is precisely for this reason that a secular society must treat persons as ends in themselves. No man is required to justify his existence, because no man can. To violate this "taboo" and challenge another's right to exist is to challenge one's own. To require a reason for a person's being is to treat him as a means, which makes his worth to depend both upon his ability to satisfy some end, and also upon the value of that end itself, and *that* is a pit from which no man can escape.

27. See Kant, *supra* note 7, at 145.

27a. Surrogate mother arrangements and adoption also differ in their essential purposes and functions. The purpose of adoption is to provide good homes for existing children who need them. The purpose of surrogate mother arrangements is to create "desirable" children for people who want to be parents.

28. See, e.g., Cal. Penal Code Sec. 273; L. Andrews, *The Stork Market,* 70 A.B.A.J. 50, at 54–55 (Aug. 1984).

28a. See *In re Baby M.*—Sup. Ct. Opn., *supra* note 5, at 1238, 1242, 1246, 1248.

29. Using the term "surrogate mother" here, rather than mother, especially brings home the truth of Katha Pollitt's point to which I have previously alluded. See *supra* note 5.

30. See *supra* note 4; and see, e.g., Gorney, *supra* note 4, at 151; B. Lifton, *Twice Born: Memoirs of an Adopted Daughter* (1975).

31. See Rubin, *supra* note 4, at 72–75; L. Dusky, *Brave New Babies?* Newsweek p. 30 (Dec. 6, 1982); J. Hollinger, *From Coitus to Commerce: Legal and Social Consequences of Noncoital Reproduction,* 18 J. L. Reform 865, at 922–23 (1985).

32. See Rubin, *supra* note 4, at 72–75.

33. See, e.g., E. Keerdoja, et al., *Adoption: New Frustration, New Hope,* Newsweek p. 80, at 83 (Feb. 13, 1984).

34. Katha Pollitt's discussion of this point in her critique of the trial court's opinion in the *Baby M* case compels quotation:

> To be sure, there are worse ways of coming into the world, but not many, and none that are elaborately prearranged by sane people. Much is made of the so-called trauma of adoption, but adoption is a piece of cake compared with contracting. Adoptive parents can tell their child, Your mother loved you so much she gave you up, even though it made her sad, because that was best for you. What can the father and adoptive mother of a contract baby say? Your mother needed $10,000? Your mother wanted to do something nice for us, so she made you? (Pollitt, *supra* note 5, at 688.)

35. See, e.g., D. Gelman and D. Shapiro, *Infertility: Babies by Contract,* Newsweek p. 74 (Nov. 4, 1985) (hereinafter cited as Gelman and Shapiro); Gorney, *supra* note 4.

36. There is nothing, however, inherent in the technology of surrogate parenting that limits its use to infertile couples. See Krimmel, *supra* note 25, at 35. It has been suggested that surrogate parenting might be used by single men, by homosexual couples, by career women too busy to be pregnant, and even by models who want a baby but no stretch marks. See, e. g., Gorney, *supra* note 4, at 92, 94 (box); B. Beyette, *Bar's Family Law 'Think Tank' Tackles Surrogate Motherhood Issue,* L.A. Times, Jan. 21, 1987, Sec. V, p. 2, col. 3; J. Robertson, *Procreative Liberty and the Control of Conception, Pregnancy, and Childbirth,* 69 Vir. L. Rev. 405, at 430 n. 68 (1983) [hereinafter cited as Robertson (1983)].

37. See, e.g., "Adoption in America," *Hearing before the Subcommittee on Aging, Family and Human Services of the Senate Committee on Labor and Human Resources,* 97th Congress, 1st session (1981), p. 3 (comments of Sen. Denton) and pp. 16–17 (statement of Warren Master, Acting Commissioner of Administration for Children, Youth and Families, HHS); Gorney, *supra* note 4, at 91.

38. See, e.g., Gelman and Shapiro, *supra* note 35, at 77; cf. Gorney, *supra* note 4, at 150.

39. No one doubts that the adopting parents truly want a child. But in surrogate mother arrangements, as with the more traditional forms of baby bartering, paying for the child corrupts their good intentions. In this sense surrogate mother arrangements are like the sin of simony: attempting to purchase, and thereby corrupting, that which is given as a matter of grace.

40. See *supra* note 9. In the Baby M case, the trial court judge, Harvey Sorkow, made quite a point of arguing that surrogate mother arrangements couldn't be baby buying because a father couldn't buy what was already his. *In re Baby M.*—Ch. Ct. Opn., *supra* note 9, at 1157. I believe that Judge Sorkow made a factual error, which led him into making a legal one. First, what is it that makes a baby yours? If it is the biological link, the surrogate mother's claim is equal, if not superior, to the father's. See Pollitt, *supra* note 5, at 686. And indeed, if you are only claiming what is yours already, what is the need of paying anyone anything? What the adopting parents are paying for is the termination of the biological mother's custody rights in the child, and that is no different than paying off the co-owner of a piece of land because you want undisputed ownership of the whole. Second, parental agreements concerning custody rights are subject to court approval. See 15 S. Williston, *A Treatise on the Law of Contracts* Sec. 1744A (3rd ed. 1972). If, in a divorce case, one spouse attempted to trade custody rights in children as a pawn in the marital property settlement, one wonders how Judge Sorkow would react, and how he would distinguish that from what happens in surrogate mother agreements. And, while we are on the subject, how would we expect a child to feel when he finds out his mother traded him for the house?

41. See, e.g., Robertson (1983), *supra* note 36, esp. at 408–09, 412, 424, 429–430.

42. See *supra* note 39.

43. Cf. E. Landes and R. Posner, *The Economics of the Baby Shortage,* 7 J. L. Stud. 323 (1978); J. Prichard, *A Market for Babies?* 34 Toronto L. J. 341 (1984).

44. See M. Shapiro and R. Spece, *Bioethics and Law* 448 (1981).

45. See Robertson (1983), *supra* note 36, at 429–30.

46. The following exchange of letters in the Hastings Center Report is illustrative of the point:

> [I]f the happiness of the infertile couple is genuine, what good reason is there to suppose that the child will not benefit by being loved, cared for, and provided with suitable surroundings for growth and happiness? [M. Goodman, *Correspondence,* 14 Hastings Center Report at 43 (June 1984).]

> Goodman . . . asks rhetorically what good reason there would be to suppose that a couple made happy by the newborn would not reciprocate. There would be many, if the analysis begins, as does Goodman's, with the implicit assumption that it is somehow the infant's duty to make the *parents* happy, or even that there is some sort of mutual or equal measure of responsibility and expectations on that score. And yet, as Goodman unconsciously suggests to us, in the surrogate arrangement, there certainly will be. Those par-

ents have contracted, at substantial fee, for that infant. Who among us willingly purchases damaged goods? Will a child with birth defects be as willingly and lovingly received from the surrogate as a "perfect" child? Will it? [Krimmel, *Correspondence*, 14 Hastings Center Report at 44 (June 1984).]

47. See, e.g., *No Other Hope for Having a Baby*, Newsweek p. 50 (Jan. 19, 1987); Gorney, *supra* note 4, at 94; cf. K. Lowry, *The Designer Babies Are Growing Up*, L.A. Times (Magazine) p. 7 (Nov. 1, 1987); Robertson (1983), *supra* note 36, at 429–30, 430 n. 66.

48. See *supra* note 46; cf. F. Pizzulli, *Asexual Reproduction and Genetic Engineering: A Constitutional Assessment of the Technology of Cloning*, 47 S. Cal. L. Rev. 476, esp. 507–544 (1974) (hereinafter cited as Pizzulli).

49. C. Campbell, *A Homeric Constraint on Sex Selection*, 17 Hastings Center Report 2 (Oct. 1987); and see also, M. Stenchever, *An Abuse of Prenatal Diagnosis*, 221 J.A.M.A. 408 (1972); C. Westoff and R. Rindfus, *Sex Preselection in the United States: Some Implications*, 184 Science 633, 636 (1974).

50. See, e.g., Robertson (1983), *supra* note 36, esp. at 408–10, 412, 424, 429–436.

51. Gorney, *supra* note 4, at 155.

52. See *supra* notes 20 and 46.

53. Robertson (1986), *supra* note 2, at 1000; and see *Surrogate Parenthood*, A.B.A.J. p. 39 (June 1, 1987).

54. See Pizzulli, *supra* note 48, at 520. Professor Robertson apparently would agree that his proposed right of procreational autonomy would not extend to "harming" the child. Robertson (1983), *supra* note 36, at 432. He believes, however, that "fabrication or manipulation alone is not harmful, or at least not harmful enough." *Id.* at 432 n. 76. Elsewhere (Robertson (1986), *supra* note 2, at 995–97) he suggests that posthumous conception of children even "fifty or one hundred years after the genetic source's death, would not necessarily subject offspring to a life worse than death." *Id.* at 996. And to ban such a practice "might . . . interfere with the procreative liberty of the deceased person, who contemplated posthumous reproduction." *Id.* at 997. If planning an orphan doesn't count as harm, one must wonder how Professor Robertson defines the word.

55. See A. Lincoln, Second Inaugural Address, reprinted in II *The Collected Works of Abraham Lincoln 1848–1858*, at 333 (Brasler, ed., 1953).

56. It is precisely at this point that surrogate mother arrangements are distinguished from the problem posed by "wrongful life" cases such as *Gleitman v. Cosgrove*, 49 N.J. 22, 227 A. 2d 689 (1967).

Although both surrogate mother arrangements and "wrongful life" cases involve the situation where the cause that results in a person's existence is inseparably connected to that cause that results in an injury to the person as well; they differ due to the dissimilar characters of their causal elements; i.e., the reasons why existence and damage are inseparably connected. Stated otherwise, "wrongful life" cases and surrogate mother arrangements are similar in that, in both, existence and injury *are* inseparably connected, but they differ from one another in *why* this is so. In a majority of jurisdictions, in "wrongful life" cases the child has not been allowed to sue for being born deformed because his deformity and existence are inseparably connected, and the courts, for the most part, are unwilling to say that there is such a thing as a life without value. Hence, the large majority of courts have concluded, the child was not wronged by being born deformed because he could not otherwise have been. See G. Tedeschi, *On Tort Liability for "Wrongful Life,"* 1 Israel L. Rev. 513 (1966). In "wrongful life" cases the injured child could not have been other than he was and still be. In this respect "wrongful life" cases and surrogate mother arrangements are indistinguishable. However, when we inquire in each of these situations into the *reason* for why there is a connection between existence and damage we see the distinction. In the case of "wrongful life," the reason for the connection between the child's existence and his deformity is not due to any choice his parents made, but rather, is the result of some natural or accidental cause beyond human control. In surrogate parenting, however, the parents are only willing to create the child if he has the impairment (of being born under a surrogate other arrangement). It is the parents' choice that forges the link between existence and impairment. The connection between these elements is due not to nature, but to human will. The child still is not damaged by being brought into existence, per se, but the premeditated planning of his parents to give him a substandard or limited existence is evil.

57. I am not implying that a freely given consent would alleviate the ethical difficulty here. For, neither is one entitled to treat one's self as a means, and not as an end. See Kant, *supra* note 7, at 178. The criminal law provides an interesting illustration of this point. Both the common law and modern authorities concur in the principle that consent is not a defense to the crime of mayhem. See *Wright's Case*, Co. Lit. 127a (1604) (defendant complying with a beggar's request, cut off the beggar's hand in order to give him more "colour to begge."); *State v. Bass*, 255 N.C. 42, 120 S.E. 2d 580 (1961) (defendant assisted in his accomplice's scheme

to cut off the latter's fingers in order to obtain insurance money).

58. Furthermore, Professor Robertson's argument proves too much. The implications of his logic go far beyond the situation posed by surrogate parenting. For if a child has no ethical complaint about the manner of his conception or the specifications of his manufacture, so long as these do not make his life "worthless," why couldn't parents using traditional methods of procreation strike similar deals? What, for example, would prevent them from saying: "We will conceive a child only on the condition that he serve as a serf on our farm until he reaches the age of 35"? Or, once the technology of cloning becomes available to humans, how could it then be ethically objectionable

to clone a replicant only on the condition that he serve as your organ donor if needed. (Cf. *supra* note 20.) When it comes time to take the replicant's kidneys, might one say to him: "You didn't get such a bad deal. You got to live up until now, and besides, had I not wanted an organ donor, I never would have made you"? This argument, when coupled with the belief that human existence is of incomparable worth, becomes a variation on the theme: I created you; therefore, I own you, and you owe me everything. Under such a view, child abuse would be a theoretical impossibility.

59. See *supra* note 1.

60. N. Blodgett, *Who is Mother?* 72 A.B.A.J. p. 18 (June 1, 1986).

Surrogacy, Slavery, and the Ownership of Life

ANITA L. ALLEN

SURROGATE PARENTING[1] is one of the most discussed solutions to the problems of female sterility, infertility,[2] and disability.[3] Surrogacy is also discussed as a possible option for fertile, able-bodied women who would like to raise children but do not wish to undergo pregnancy. It is uncertain how many couples or individuals seriously consider surrogacy. In recent years, however, hundreds of women have signed contracts to become surrogate mothers,[4] giving up

ANITA ALLEN, now Anita Allen-Castellitto, is a Professor of Law at the University of Pennsylvania, with an expertise in privacy law, legal philosophy, constitutional law, torts, race relations, gender studies, and law and literature.

their parental rights in exchange for rewards such as money or the joy of altruism.

The practice of surrogacy has raised a complex web of legal issues. Among the most important are whether surrogacy is best characterized as selling babies or providing personal services; whether participants should undergo mandatory screening; whether legal paternity is affected by surrogacy; whether surrogacy contracts are enforceable in whole or in part; whether surrogacy fosters the exploitation of women, children, and the poor, thereby undermining public policy; and finally, whether state and federal governments may legally interfere with an individual's private procreative choices.[5] Courts have already

Harvard Journal of Law and Public Policy, *Vol. 13, 139 (1990). Permission granted by the* Harvard Journal of Law and Public Policy.

faced a number of difficult cases concerning the validity and enforceability of surrogacy contracts,[6] and legislatures of at least six states have enacted laws that tightly regulate or prohibit commercial surrogacy.[7] In the meantime, ethical and constitutional debate regarding the practice of surrogacy continues in both the academic and family service communities.

Opposition to surrogacy often stems from a sense that it violates general notions of human morality. Notably, this kind of opposition is sometimes premised on the claim that surrogacy is tantamount to the unlawful and immoral institution of slavery.[8] To equate surrogacy with slavery, however, distorts both practices. It is therefore not helpful to think of the two as simply different examples of the same immoral principle. Nevertheless, while surrogacy is certainly not the same thing as slavery, American slavery had the effect of causing black women to become surrogate mothers on behalf of slave owners.[9] Thus, although slavery and surrogacy are not coterminous, this particular aspect of American slavery may be instructive for present efforts to determine rationally surrogacy's legal and moral status.

Support for surrogacy is sometimes premised on privacy-related constitutional rights and liberties.[10] Professor John A. Robertson has argued that the constitutional right of privacy regarding procreation, as evidenced by Supreme Court cases ranging from *Meyer v. Nebraska*[11] to *Eisenstadt v. Baird*,[12] limits state regulation of noncoital reproduction to cases of serious harm.[13] He argues that "moral condemnation, commercialism, and slippery slopes" should not justify interference with fundamental decisions about family function.[14] But surrogacy arguments based on the right of privacy are not without their difficulties. As I have argued in detail elsewhere,[15] it is doubtful that women or childless couples have privacy rights entitling them to engage in commercial surrogacy. On the other hand, the proposition that States may not regulate surrogacy, but must enforce all surrogacy

agreements like other commercial contracts, is even more doubtful.[16]

My comments here, then, are intended to take issue with two very seductive and often-used arguments in the surrogacy debate: one cited in *opposition* to surrogacy — the slavery equation argument, and the other cited *in favor* of surrogacy — the privacy argument.

I. SLAVERY

In a different way or to a different degree than adoption,[17] surrogacy has been characterized as "baby selling,"[18] that is, as commercial trafficking in human beings. Accordingly, contemporary surrogate parenting has been dubbed by some as a form of slavery.[19] In addition to "baby selling," the "womb renting" and "autonomy sharing"[20] aspects of surrogacy contracts also make the surrogate mother, like the child she bears, a victim, a kind of slave.

The characteristic feature of slaves is that they lack self-ownership. Slave owners sell, use, and dominate. Although there are a few who would argue that slavery is not inherently immoral, ethicists commonly use slavery as the paradigm case of a socio-economic practice that is profoundly and patently immoral.[21] According to ethicists, slavery is plainly wrong, and thus anything that closely resembles slavery must also be wrong. Legal scholars also use slavery as a paradigm, but as a paradigm of practices that are illegal under the Constitution and unacceptable to public policy. Hence the normative advice given to policymakers by both ethicists and jurists is the same: Avoid practices that have too many traits in common with slavery.

Labelling surrogacy as "slavery" is thus both a moral and a policy condemnation. This kind of condemnation implies that well-meaning surrogates, as well as their consumers and facilitators, are immoral or complicitous in immorality. When taken to an extreme, this logic implies that well-meaning lawyers and judges, like Noel Keane[22] and Judge Sorkow of the *Baby M* case,[23] who help draft and enforce surrogacy agreements, are parties to immorality.

Surrogacy, however, is not slavery, and equating the two does not prove surrogacy immoral. By treating the two practices as moral equivalents, one ignores the enormous scope of control the slave owner exerts over the slave, a feature quite lacking in surrogacy arrangements. Nevertheless, the following little-known, true story illustrates how one aspect of slavery can shed light on the moral and legal policy debates regarding surrogacy today.[24]

In the early 1800s, a happy little girl by the name of Polly Crocket was living in Illinois. One dismal autumn night, Polly was kidnapped and sold into slavery in Missouri. Her first owner was a poor farmer; the second, a wealthy gentleman named Taylor Berry whose wife trained Polly as a seamstress. Polly grew up and was permitted to marry another of Berry's slaves. Polly managed to have two children, Lucy and Nancy, before her husband was sold to a distant owner "way down South."[25]

The years passed. With deaths and marriages, the ownership of Polly and her daughter was passed in and out of the Berry family. Encouraged by Polly, daughter Nancy escaped to freedom in Canada. Desperate to join her, Polly attempted to escape and made it all the way to Chicago. Because the Fugitive Slaves Laws were in effect, however, "negro-catchers" were permitted to arrest her and return her to her owner in Missouri.[26]

Upon return to Missouri, Polly took the bold step of finding a good lawyer. She successfully sued for her freedom on the theory that she was not a slave, but legally a free woman who had been wrongfully sold into slavery.

Now a free woman and anxious to have her family together again, Polly decided to buy her daughter Lucy out of slavery. But Lucy was not for sale. Lucy was "legitimately" owned by a Mr. Mitchell, who wanted to keep Lucy to please his wife. Polly filed a lawsuit against Mr. Mitchell on September 8, 1842, for the possession of her daughter, Lucy.[27] During the seventeen-month pendency of her mother's civil suit, poor Lucy was locked away in jail.

Polly's suit finally ended in victory, and she was awarded possession of Lucy. On the final day of the trial, Polly's lawyer, the slave-holding jurist Edward Bates, summed up his case to the jury:

> Gentleman of the jury, I am a slave-holder myself, but thanks to Almighty God I am above the base principle of holding anybody a slave that has a right to her freedom as this girl has been proven to have; she was free before she was born; her mother was free but kidnapped in her youth, and sacrificed to the greed of negro-traders, and no free woman can give birth to a slave child, as it is in direct violation of the laws of God and man.[28]

This poignant story vividly illustrates the sense in which the legal concept of ownership completely lacks inherent moral content. It can work like a two-edged sword. Polly legally owned herself, yet she lived most of her life as a slave. Once she proved in court that the master who possessed her did not lawfully own her, she gained standing to sue for the recovery of her own daughter, Lucy. But Lucy was also the precious putative property of another owner, who had acquired her through a "legitimate" commercial transaction and was not willing to sell her to Polly. Extant property law favored Mr. Mitchell; it certainly could not compel him to sell. Thus, Polly resorted to slave law to prove unlawful possession. By proving that she was not in fact a slave at the time of her daughter's birth, Polly was able to persuade the court that she was the rightful owner of her daughter. In the end, mother and daughter owned themselves. But the institution of slavery remained intact, and Mr. Mitchell was out the price of a housemaid.

This story is a stark reminder that as a result of the American slave laws, all black mothers were de facto surrogates. Children born to slaves were owned by Master X or Mistress Y and could be sold at any time to another owner. Slave women gave birth to children with the understanding that those children would be owned by others.

The story of Polly also teaches us several other important lessons. First, Polly's case reminds us that well-meaning people, including business people, lawyers, and judges sometimes participate in unjust, immoral practices. Most people would agree with this proposition in the abstract but are reluctant to confront it in concrete cases. To declare that a controversial practice, engaged in by well-meaning citizens, is immoral is to appear presumptuous, intolerant, and self-righteous. These kinds of attitudes are often thought of as threatening to the philosophical underpinnings of modern liberal government, as manifest by the often asked questions: Who are you to judge? What gives you the right to say? Liberalism is sometimes interpreted to treat all moral judgment as moralism and all public moral inquiry as an invasion of privacy. As a result, notions of morality are rarely invoked in public discourse and are thus relegated to secrecy. This is not good. Sometimes we have to be willing to criticize public officials and even our friends and neighbors in light of our own moral intuitions. That is, after all, how we eventually abolished slavery.

Polly's case also brings to mind a subtler point. The fact that the law is receptive to the claims of some individuals wronged by a practice does not necessarily vindicate the practice. Polly's daughter was returned to her because of an earlier injustice. But the practice of slavery—with its resulting surrogacy—continued. The fact that Polly was able to get judicial redress within the legal framework of slavery did not legitimate slavery. Analogously, the fact that Mary Beth Whitehead Gould of the *Baby M* case also got her day in court when things went wrong does not necessarily mean we should condone the practice of surrogacy. A corollary to this is that just because child custody arrangements are judi-

cially obtainable when surrogacy agreements are breached does not mean we should support the practice.

Polly's case suggests a third point. Even in social contexts where the expectations of motherhood do not exist—where one understands that one is a member of an enslaved race without meaningful claims to one's own children—the desire to parent and to enjoy the companionship of one's children can be very strong. We can imagine that Mary Beth Whitehead Gould's anguish at losing her daughter was not unlike Polly's.[29] Both women's sense of security—responsibility and identity—were very connected to the children to whom they had given birth but supposedly had no right to parent.[30]

A fourth and final message to be drawn from Polly's case is that the law can easily accommodate the commercialization of human life. We must therefore be careful. As the legal positivists John Chipman Gray and Hans Kelsen made plain, in principle, anything can have a right to anything.[31] In our jurisprudence, the conceptual vocabulary is in place to make alienable property[32] of women, of children, of kidneys, of hearts, of spleens, and even an individual's cell line.[33] The concepts of property and ownership are elastic enough to let us buy and sell anything we want. We cannot simply look to the language of law to know where to draw the lines. We must first draw the lines where we want them to go and then make those lines into law.

II. PRIVACY

Under the modern jurisprudence of constitutional privacy, the Constitution embodies protection for certain privacy rights regarding human reproduction. These include the right to procreate,[34] to use contraception,[35] and, under *Roe v. Wade*,[36] to obtain medically safe abortions. Courts and commentators have appealed to constitutional privacy rights as a basis for concluding that surrogacy agreements must be validated and specifically enforced.[37]

Privacy and equal protection arguments favoring surrogacy, and against state prohibitions, are not convincing. To be sure, surrogacy involves the intimate decision to bear a child, which courts have repeatedly held to be an appropriately private decision.[38] But the pre-planned, commercial, third-party, and burdensome nature of surrogacy makes it strikingly unlike ordinary child-bearing and adoption. The argument is often made that since sperm donation and artificial insemination are available to women, surrogacy must be available to men.[39] There is a relevant difference between the burdens imposed upon a man, who in an hour of time can make a sperm donation, and the burdens imposed upon a woman, who must endure a nine-month pregnancy and all the emotional and physical health risks associated with pregnancy.

"The right to privacy" is ill-suited as a principle of adjudication in custody suits between natural fathers and natural, surrogate mothers. The procreative privacy interests of both mothers and fathers would seem to argue for access to their natural children, even where one parent originally intended to be only a surrogate mother. Contract principles seem inapposite in the child custody context as well. Surely, procreative privacy rights — rights of constitutional dimensions — and the best interest of the child dwarf mere contractual rights. The New Jersey Supreme Court was convinced of this point. It unanimously rejected the argument that childless couples have constitutional privacy rights demanding state validation and enforcement of surrogacy agreements.[40]

Surrogacy agreements are best viewed as unenforceable personal commitments or vows between unmarried individuals. When disputes over child custody arise, courts should decide the cases as child custody disputes are always decided, without regard to the principles of commercial contract law. Any prenatal agreement to waive or terminate parental rights should be

deemed void as a matter of public policy. Would-be surrogate mothers should be deemed to have constitutional privacy rights so strong as to limit their own capacities for alienating their procreative and traditional parental prerogatives. This approach is permissive, in the sense that it does not criminalize surrogacy agreements. It is restrictive, in that it is likely to discourage the practice, certainly the business, of surrogacy.

Some feminists have a more welcoming view of surrogacy than mine.[41] They say surrogacy is a source of liberation for women. It frees them from traditional roles which limit childbirth to marriage. Yet the motives and values actual surrogates emphasize are the motives and values of Nineteenth-Century "true womanhood."[42] One strains to see female liberation in a practice that pays so little, capitalizes on the traditionally female virtues of self-sacrifice and caretaking, and enables men to have biologically related children without the burden of marriage.

Finally, one of the more compelling arguments for surrogacy focuses on its potential to aid disabled women.[43] It is argued that disabled women should be able to parent, but they often cannot because of physical infirmity or confinement to wheelchairs that makes gestation risky or impractical. This argument for surrogacy has considerable force, but less so when one considers that it requires sacrifices by one disadvantaged group to help another.

It is often speculated that in the long-run it is poor women and women of color who will stand to suffer most by uses of surrogate mothers and surrogate gestators.[44] Some fear that minority women will become the "surrogate class." This outcome would be ironic in the case of black women because, as a class, black women have a higher rate of infertility than white women[45] and are less able to pay for surrogacy services on their own behalf. Although religious and political beliefs could constrain participation, opportunities to earn money through surrogate gestation may be difficult to refuse for the poor women of the future.

III. CONCLUSION

I suspect Professor Peter Schuck would denigrate these objections to surrogacy as "natural law."[46] He has argued that surrogacy can be seen as a "praiseworthy act of generosity and commitment to the creation of a wanted life."[47] He believes surrogacy "will generate very large, widely distributed private and social benefits."[48] Unless its costs outweigh its benefits, he argues, "the law should uphold surrogacy contracts, not categorically condemn them."[49] Because my sense of the relevance and strength of non-consequentialist concerns differs from his, I disagree that the burden of proof is on opponents of surrogacy.

An ample basis for viewing the burden of proof on the side of surrogacy proponents is suggested by the socially retrogressive character of surrogacy and the equal, competing "privacy" interests of biological parents in the companionship of their offspring. As previously urged, the practice of surrogacy depends upon Nineteenth-Century conceptions of female self-sacrifice and self-denial. It depends as well on our willingness to yield to additional pressures to commercialize certain aspects of human life. Although privacy rights are cited in an effort to explain why surrogacy contracts must be validated, the privacy principle is simply not dispositive. Privacy rights do not dictate that parental rights must be deemed commercially alienable, nor that surrogacy contracts must be treated as more than unenforceable personal commitments. More importantly, privacy rights do not dictate which one of two competing natural parents should have custody of a child that both want to rear.

NOTES

1. Surrogate parenting can be characterized as a practice whereby a women ("surrogate mother") bears a child for another woman, man, or couple. In the highly publicized cases of the past decade, a surrogate mother has agreed prior to conception to be artificially inseminated and to surrender custody of the resulting child in exchange for a fee.

2. See, e.g., *New Approaches to Human Reproduction: Social and Ethical Dimensions* 117–216 (L. Whiteford and M. Poland eds. 1988) (social science and ethical perspectives); Colloquy: In Re *Baby M,* 76 *Geo. L.J.* 1717 (1988) (legal and ethical perspectives); Ethical Considerations of the New Reproductive Technologies, 46 *Fertility and Sterility* 62S (Supp. 1 1986) (biomedical and ethical perspectives); M. Warnock, *A Question of Life: The Warnock Report on Human Fertilization and Embryology* 42–47 (1985) (ethical perspectives).

3. See, e.g., Asch, Reproductive Technology and Disability, in *Reproductive Laws for the 1990s* 69 (N. Taub & S. Cohen eds. 1989).

4. See Torry, Wrestling with Surrogate Motherhood, *Wash. Post,* Feb. 12. 1989, at A31, col. 4.

5. See *New Approaches to Human Reproduction: Social and Ethical Dimensions, supra* note 2, at 162.

6. See *Surrogate Parenting Associates, Inc. v. Kentucky ex rel. Armstrong,* 704 S.W.2d 209 (Ky. 1986) (surrogacy held not to violate Kentucky statute prohibiting buying and selling of babies); In re *Adoption of Baby Girl L.J.,* 132 Misc.2d 972, 505 N.Y.S.2d 813 (Sur. Ct. 1986) (surrogacy agreement not expressly prohibited by legislature and therefore allowed despite court's strong reservations); *Doe v. Kelley,* 106 Mich. App. 169, 307 N.W.2d 438 (1981) (state statute subjecting to court scrutiny any exchange of consideration in adoption proceedings, other than court costs, held not to violate constitutional right to privacy, and Michigan statutes prohibiting payment to surrogate mothers held constitutionally permissible), cert. denied, 459 U.S. 1183 (1983); see also Allen, Privacy, Surrogacy and the *Baby M.* Case, 76 *Geo. L.J.* 1759, 1760 n. 7 (1988); In re *Baby M,* 217 N.J. Super. 313, 525 A.2d 1128 (Ch. Div. 1987), aff'd in part, rev'd in part, remanded, 109 N.J. 396, 537, A.2d 1227 (1988).

7. See Torry, *supra* note 4.

8. See, e.g., Schneider, Mothers Urge Ban on Surrogacy as Form of Slavery, *The New York Times,* Sept. 1, 1987, at A13, col. 1.

9. Slave mothers had no legal claim of right or ownership over their natural children they had given birth to. Slave owners not only had ownership over the slaves but owned their children too, and could buy and sell them to third parties without regard to the wishes of the natural mother. This phenomenon of American slavery thus resembled a de facto system of certain elements of surrogacy. See *infra* note 24 and accompanying text.

10. See Robertson, Embryos, Families, and Procreative Liberty: The Legal Structure of the New Reproduction, 59 *S. Cal. L. Rev.* 939, 954–66 (1986).

11. 262 U.S. 390 (1923) (invalidating a state law prohibiting elementary schools from teaching subjects in and language other than English).

12. 405 U.S. 438 (1972) (invalidating Massachusetts law prohibiting contraceptive distribution to non-married persons).

13. See Robertson, Procreative Liberty and the State's Burden of Proof in Regulating Noncoital Reproduction, 16 *Law, Medicine & Health Care* 18 (1988).

14. *Id.* at 19–20.

15. See Allen, Privacy, Surrogacy, and the *Baby M* Case, 76 *Geo. L.J.* 1759 (1988).

16. See *id.* at 1771–74.

17. Often the fact that surrogacy agreements precede the child's conception is pointed to as the feature distinguishing it from adoption.

18. Schuck, Some Reflections on the *Baby M* Case, 76 *Geo. L.J.* 1793, 1794 (1988).

19. See Schneider, *supra* note 8.

20. Schuck, *supra* note 18, at 1794 n.3.

21. Cf. Feinberg, Autonomy, Sovereignty, and Privacy: Moral Ideals in the Constitution?, 58 *Notre Dame L. Rev.* 445 (1983) (considering morality of voluntary slavery). *But see G. Dworkin, The Theory and Practice of Autonomy* 127–29 (1988) (presumption against slave as involuntary bondage may be rebutted in particular cases).

22. Noel Keane is the foremost legal expert on surrogacy arrangements, having arranged many surrogate contracts, including the one involved in the *Baby M* case. See Torry, *supra* note 4. Mr. Keane is also the author of a book on surrogacy. See N. Keane, *The Surrogate Mother* (1981).

23. In re *Baby M,* 217 N.J. Super. 313, 525 A.2d 1128 (Ch. Div. 1987), aff'd in part, rev'd in part, remanded, 109 N.J. 396, 537 A.2d 1227 (1988).

24. See Delaney, Struggles for Freedom, in *Six Women's Slave Narratives* 9 (1988) (woman held wrongly in slavery sues to have her daughter Lucy delivered out of slavery and returned to her; court awards the mother "the right to own her own child").

25. *Id.* at 14.

26. *Id.* at 23.

27. See *id.* at 33.

28. *Id.* at 42.

29. Mary Beth Whitehead had entered into a surrogate-parenting agreement with William Stern in which she agreed to be artificially inseminated with Mr. Stern's sperm, to carry the child to term, and to turn over the child to the Sterns. In return for this and Ms. Whitehead's renouncement of parental rights to the child, Mr. Stern agreed to pay her $10,000 and all medical and related expenses. After the birth of "Baby M," Ms. Whitehead decided not to give up the child. Her intense desire to keep Baby M led Ms. Whitehead to defy a court order granting the Sterns temporary custody and to take the child away with her to Florida. A court awarded the Sterns permanent custody of Baby M but allowed Ms. Whitehead to retain her parental rights and to have some visitation rights. See In re *Baby M,* 217 N.J. Super. 313, 525 A.2d 1128 (Ch. Div. 1987), aff'd in part, rev'd in part, remanded, 109 N.J. 396, 537 A.2d 1227 (1988).

30. A woman's security may be linked to her children by the responsibility she feels for bringing them into the world and providing them with the psychological and financial care they need. In addition, a woman's sense of identity is tied to her children by virtue of the strong physical connection with them experienced during the final stages of pregnancy and a belief that the children's genetic and biological makeup creates a link with her past, and her stake in the future. See Allen, *supra* note 6, at 1790.

31. See J. Gray, *The Nature and Sources of Law* 28–63 (1909) (rights can be ascribed to human beings, supernatural beings, animals, inanimate objects, and juristic persons such as corporations); H. Kelsen, *General Theory of Law and State* 93–109 (1945) (rights can be ascribed to anything).

32. See Radin, Market-Inalienability, 100 *Harv. L. Rev.* 1849 (1987); see also D. Meyers, *Inalienable Rights* (1985) (philosophical discussion of inalienable rights).

33. See *Moore v. Regents of Univ. of California,* 202 Cal. App. 3d 1230, 249 Cal. Rptr. 494 (1988).

34. See *Skinner v. Oklahoma,* 316 U.S. 535 (1942).

35. See *Griswold v. Connecticut,* 381 U.S. 479 (1965).

36. 410 U.S. 113 (1973).

37. See e.g., Doe v. Kelley, 106 Mich. App. 169, 174, 307 N.W.2d 438, 441 (1981); *Surrogate Parenting Associates, Inc. v. Kentucky ex rel. Armstrong,* 704 S.W.2d 209, 212 (Ky. 1986); Bitner, *Womb for Rent: A Call for Pennsylvania Legislation Legalizing and Regulating Surrogate Parenting Agreements,* 90 *Dick. L. Rev.,* 227, 236–37 (1985); Coleman, *Surrogate Motherhood: Analysis of the Problems and Suggestions for Solutions,* 50 *Tenn. L. Rev.* 71, 82 (1982).

38. See, e.g., *Thornburgh v. American College of Obstetricians and Gynecologists,* 476 U.S. 747, 772 (1986).

39. See Schuck, *supra* note 18, at 1798.

40. See In re *Baby M,* 109 N.J. 396, 537 A.2d 1227 (1988).

41. See, e.g., Davis, Commentary: Alternative Modes of Reproduction: The Locus and Determinants of Choice, in *Reproductive Laws for the 1990s, supra* note 3, at 421. But see Chavkin, Rothman &

Rapp, Alternative Modes of Reproduction, in *id.* at 405.

42. See Welter, The Cult of True Womanhood: 1820–1860, 18 *Am. Q.* 151 (Summer 1966) (characteristics of Nineteenth-Century womanhood were domesticity, self-denial, submission to male domination, and a willingness to fulfill the needs of others).

43. See Asch, *supra* note 3.

44. See Nsiah-Jefferson, Reproductive Laws, Women of Color, and Low-Income Women, in *Reproductive Laws for the 1990s, supra* note 3, at 23.

45. See *id.* at 49.

46. See Schuck, *supra* note 18, at 1798–1801.

47. *Id.* at 1793.

48. *Id.*

49. *Id.* at 1793–94.

Reproductive Freedom and Women's Freedom: Surrogacy and Autonomy

CHRISTINE T. SISTARE

. . .

WOMEN'S FREEDOM

I believe that a fundamental moral issue in the surrogacy debate is the nature and extent of women's freedom: their freedom to control their bodies, their lives, their reproductive powers, and to determine the social use of those reproductive capacities. This issue is fundamental both normatively and descriptively. That is, respect for woman's personal freedom ought to be a guiding moral concern in resolving the debate, and

CHRISTINE T. SISTARE is Associate Professor of Philosophy, Director of the Center for Ethics, and Co-Director of Philosophy/Political Thought Program at Muhlenberg College, PA.

recognition of the centrality of this issue is, I think, a basic source of the controversy and of much of its intensity.

I accept, as a premise, that women have often been manipulated and oppressed because of and through their reproductive capacities. The bearing of children is a biologically and socially important role, one which makes women valuable even when they seem least valued. The limitations which pregnancy itself imposes and the limitations which can be imposed through the mystification of reproduction, generally, and of maternity, in particular, have proven highly useful in the control of women. Such control has been enhanced insofar as women have internalized these limitations. Motherhood has been both pedestal and prison.

Now, however, there are social and technological contexts which provide a way for women to benefit through the free use of their reproduc-

The Philosophical Forum, *Vol. XIX, No. 4, Summer 1988; pp. 228–236. Reprinted with permission of Christine T. Sistare and Blackwell Publishers.*

tive powers. The social context, itself, is the result of the increased freedom of women in this society: the acceptance of childbearing and rearing by single mothers, the availability of contraception and abortion, independence from men through access to jobs and fulfillment without matrimony, the real possibility of life without husbands or children. The effect has been to place childbearing at a premium.[1]

The technological context arises in the possibilities of impregnation without intercourse, of gestation with or without genetic contribution, and of related medical novelties. These technologies are such that any person can become a parent—even a genetically related parent—if only he or she can find a person of the other gender willing to make the necessary biological contribution to complete the process. The relevant effect, *vis à vis* surrogate maternity, is that women can contract with other persons for the use of their wombs. In fact, for a simple surrogate pregnancy, little by way of technology is required; the new technological background mostly acts, in this case, to reinforce the social context.

When the social and technological contexts are combined, of course, the result is that people who want a [genetically related] child but who cannot or will not provide for gestation can achieve their goal by arranging for a surrogate. Thus, women can demand payment for their service, their reproductive labors, and can do so in a way—really for the first time in our history—which greatly relieves them of the control of men and of traditional social constraints. Women need not accept marriage or some other promise of support without control as their payment. They need not provide access to their reproductive capacities on demand. They may make the arrangements they like and take their payment in unencumbered money. And that, I contend, is the deep source of the present controversy.

I take it to be a fundamental, if sometimes forgotten, principle of our common political morality that adults have a presumptive right to conduct their private lives and make important personal decisions without unwarranted interference by other individuals or by the law. This is the general liberal tendency of American thought. Surely, some right to primary control over one's body must be the necessary correlate.[2] The question which ought primarily to occupy us, therefore, is this: is there sufficient justification for society to deny to adult women the disposition of their reproductive capacities according to their own desires? Is there, perhaps, some weighty reason for refusing women the right to bear children under circumstances chosen or created by them [some person which would not, similarly, license society either to prohibit or require sterilization of women who choose otherwise]?

Freedom and the Body as Property

No doubt there are cogent arguments for social control over the disposition of individuals' bodies and their functions in some cases. One reason for overriding women's right to reproductive freedom which is pertinent to surrogacy might be that surrogacy amounts to no more than selling one's body and to treating the human body as property. This apparently reasonable concern seems to feature in the prohibition of slavery and has prompted recent restrictions on organ donation.

However, this is hardly sufficient as a general condemnation of surrogacy, since we do acknowledge the individual's right to primary control over her body, and since we certainly allow people to treat their bodies as property in a variety of ways: *e.g.,* the selling of blood, of antibodies, and (most apropos) of *sperm. A fortiori,* in our society, we permit people to sell their labor and even think well of them for it. In fact, the surrogate is more a laborer than a seller of body parts, since she really only sells her services while renting out her body. Moreover, surrogacy is not analogous to conduct which clearly endangers the life, health, or liberty of the agent; so, unlike organ selling or self-enslavement, surrogacy does not pose a hard case for liberal anti-paternalism.

Of course, we might consider limiting the total number or frequency of surrogate pregnancies undertaken by any woman, especially by those who really are at peril from pregnancy. Such paternalistic regulations *must be justified,* of course. And, in justifying them, we must ask ourselves this: would we ever consider protecting women from themselves by limiting their reproductive choices in these ways if they were not being paid for the pregnancies? Would we legislate the number or frequency of pregnancies of any woman (healthy or not) who became pregnant as a result of any circumstances other than a surrogacy contract? I expect the answer to these questions will be a quiet "No." What is most objected to about the labor-for-hire character of surrogacy contracts is not the potential for harm to women; on the contrary, it is the potential for gain.

Freedom and Consent

We might argue that women must be treated paternalistically in a legitimate sense because, with respect to surrogacy, there can be no truly informed or voluntary consent. Thus, in the current public debate we hear comments to the effect that "a woman can never consent to giving up a child because she can never know how she will feel after it is born." Of course, an obvious objection to this claim is that many people [men and women] seem to have given voluntary and informed consent to having their children adopted or to giving custody of their children to others. If such choices are said to be not really free, we must ask for the model of free choice, of consent, being promoted.

We can never know what it will feel like to do anything before the time of actual performance —certainly nothing likely to be fraught with strong emotions. Indeed, even if I have engaged in some type of conduct in the past, I cannot be *certain* as to how I will feel about a different instance of the same type of conduct in the future. If knowing how one will feel is a criterion of in-

formed consent, there can never be such consent to any choice for the future. Thus, if we take this model of choice seriously, we will have to refuse people the right to determine their own fates in most personally significant or weighty situations. We will have to conclude that the persons most immediately concerned are incompetent to decide about their wills, their medical treatments, their marriages, even about the decision to become parents or not become parents. I submit that no one will embrace this conception of free choice, not even those who have specific doubts concerning the reliability of consent in certain types of cases.[3]

The operant but unavowed notion, here, is that maternity (or, perhaps, the feeling of Being-a-Mother) is such a primal, mystical experience that no one can appreciate its power to transport in advance of the moment. In the face of this notion, the genuine mystery is how we are to understand women who act as surrogates and do not regret doing so or women who choose to forfeit custody of their offspring.[4] Are all such women *monsters*? Surely it is not necessarily the case that to recognize the wonderful power of reproduction is to desire to keep all the products of it. We can and should value reproduction as both a capacity and an experience without mystifying it; what is naturally beautiful need not be regarded as preternatural to ensure appreciation.

We have many devices at hand in the law for the protection of those individuals who really are not capable of protecting themselves or of making their own choices competently. We recognize that there are such special cases. But neither a model of consent which precludes the possibility of consent nor the mystifying representation of maternal feeling as a primal urge too potent to admit of rational control can provide adequate grounds on which to *violate the right of all women* to be the dispositors of their own reproductive capacities. Women are not and should not be treated as a special subclass of adults by virtue of their reproductive capacities or their parental feelings. Such an interpretation is grossly insulting to women as well as *to men,* who are depicted as detached bystanders to an essentially female enterprise.

Reproductive Freedom and Other Interests

Naturally, we must take account of interests other than the surrogate's interest in renting her reproductive services. Some critics of surrogacy argue that children born of surrogates may be disturbed when, in later life, they learn of the arrangement which brought them into the world. Now here is a curious argument. We know that such problems may arise in custody or adoption cases, as well, but I have never heard it suggested that children should not be adopted or that parents should be forced to retain custody of their offspring. There is something odd about the idea that it is better to not be born than to be born from one woman's body but raised by someone else. This is only plausible against a social background which depicts surrogacy as abnormal. Besides, children might equally be impressed with the devotion of persons so determined to become parents. Furthermore, the present distress of those who want but cannot have children should count for something in our weighing of interests. But, most importantly, that some children may have trouble dealing with their origins is not sufficient warrant for preemptive denial of freedom to all women. The probable harm just does not outweigh the fundamental interest of women in the control of their reproductive lives and the social use of their reproductive powers.

"Well then," we are told, "this fundamental interest will actually be impaired by surrogacy." Women will be enslaved by impossible contracts — forced to undergo unimagined indignities by ruthless baby-seeking males or heartless women unwilling to bear children themselves. Of course, the contractual worries are easily dealt with. The surrogate and the contractors agree upon her obligations, including prenatal care, on their obli-

gations to her, and on stipulations for default according to a plan which is acceptable to all the parties. (We might borrow from the model of contracts in professional athletics in designing standard surrogacy arrangements.) At any rate, the surrogate will not become a birthing-machine without rights. A good surrogate contract could protect a woman from that fate more surely than most traditional maternal roles afforded to women past or present. Once again, we see that simple social intelligence and careful forethought will preclude most of the envisioned horrors of social change.

What of the *other woman?* Shouldn't she carry her own child? On the other hand, if she can't, isn't it better that she do without than that she be subjected to a humiliating inquiry into her inability to bear a child? I believe that, if there is another woman involved, her freedom must also be respected. Her decision to employ a surrogate must be entirely free and private. Her fertility, her health, her personal situation — these are no more our business than the fertility, etc., of her male partner. Society cannot force on any woman any standard of reasonable risks and sacrifices for parenting. It certainly has no grounds to demand that women set their desire to be parents above all other values or interests. It makes no such demand of men; and any man informed that he must subject himself to a legal determination of his health, must abandon his work, and must prove that he could become a parent by no other means would be rightfully outraged.

People choose to have children, and have always done so, for a variety of reasons — some frivolous, some even perverse. Perhaps social inattention to the fitness of future parents discloses the moral poverty of our culture, but there it is. Social discussion of appropriate reasons for undertaking parenting is almost nonexistent: we just assume that most people will become parents. It is a cruel irony of the debate over surrogacy that, now, women who want to become parents by contracting with a surrogate are said to be selfish. It used to be said that anyone who did not want children was selfish. And, of course, any *woman* who did not want to raise children was branded as unnatural.

We cannot have it all ways. Women must not be held to expectations or standards so radically divergent from the social norm and, in fact, so self-contradictory. Until we require social approval of every individual's decision to become a parent, we cannot require approval of the way in which any woman does become one. To claim otherwise is to embrace the view that a woman's reproductive role renders her very much a second-class person. The new technologies and social milieu enable some women to capitalize on their gestational capacity. That gestation is a reproductive role exclusive to women should not, now, be used as grounds for invading the privacy or limiting the choices of women who wish to become parents through different means.

EXPLOITATION OF WOMEN

Much is made, in very loose terms, of the inevitable exploitation of women which will follow from socially and/or legally sanctioned surrogacy arrangements. The projected exploitation is framed, primarily, in class terms: poor women will be used as baby-gestators by the rich and sterile—or, worse yet, by the rich and vacuous whose obsessive concern for physical preservation and uninterrupted jet-setting will outweigh any inclination to become parents through more direct traditional means. So, we are told, "It will always be poor women who have babies and rich women who get them." Yet, if we inspect this farrago of complaints, we will see that the expected massive exploitation is neither very likely nor very different from a host of ways in which women [and men] are presently exploited with little or no legal interference.

To begin with, such trepidations fly in the face of what appears to be a deep cultural fixation

with genetic or blood relationships. Indeed, the cross-cultural ubiquity of attention to biological links between parents and children suggests that there is some natural origin of our genetic narcissism. Innate or not, an obsessive determination to reproduce with as much genetic input as possible seems to be shared by persons of all classes. Even if the heartless, body-conscious women of the upper class have escaped this emotional investment in biologically exclusive reproduction, I suspect their male partners have not.

A surrogate could be employed, of course, only for gestation, with no genetic contribution. But, given the real class prejudices which can be expected to influence surrogate hirings, it hardly seems probable that wealthy persons will eagerly seek the services of women from impoverished or seriously disadvantaged backgrounds. Even the most inanely self-absorbed contractors will avoid the perceived risks of unhealthy or deficient children.[5] The reality of racial and ethnic prejudices must also be confronted in assessing the threat of exploitation: racially or ethnically privileged groups will not rush to have their children borne by members of despised minorities. These are ugly truths, but they must be acknowledged. Contractors will want their babies borne by surrogates with whom they themselves feel comfortable, and people typically feel most comfortable with others like themselves.

More to the point, the nature of the projected exploitation is obscure. This is a capitalist society. We do not, as a society, bemoan the fate of women who work as domestics or in truly degrading service and industrial jobs for minimum wages. Nor have we, as a society, evinced much concern with emotional strains on individuals when those strains were freely undertaken. Should awareness of the powerful emotions evoked by pregnancy and childbearing suddenly induce us to renounce our historical indifference to the emotional well-being of our fellows, we can simply stipulate that surrogate contracts will only be legally enforceable if the surrogate undergoes psychological screening, or has previously experienced pregnancy, etc.

It is just too difficult to see how being a self-employed surrogate, renting out one's reproductive capacity according to one's own determination, can be anything but an improvement on the opportunities presently available to many women. A surrogate may live in her own home, raise her own children, and be assured of good medical care. She can protect herself from the personal abuse and indignities which attend much of women's work in our society. She might pursue education or a career. Moreover, to guard against real rather than fantasized exploitation, we can impose legal minimum and maximum fees for surrogacy and apply the usual legal requirements to surrogate contracts. Ensuring that surrogates are paid well and treated well is the way to prevent their misuse, and this can be done through thoughtful regulation which both respects and protects all parties. We could start by limiting the role of lawyers and medical technicians so as to distribute payments in favor of the surrogates and away from these inessential third parties [typically white men].[7]

But what should we make of the complaint that rich women will somehow gain the benefits of parenting at the expense of poor women? Children are not, after all, a limited resource; presumably, poor people can get children, too. In fact, any woman who can serve as a surrogate can bear children of her own. I suppose we might consider public fertility services for those who can't afford current private rates. The prospect that the lure of payment will keep poor women too busy incubating babies for the rich to reproduce for themselves is implausible and easily debarred by maximum fees or other regulations. I do not believe, however, that many opponents of surrogacy are genuinely concerned about the reproductive futures of economically disadvantaged women or classes. After all, to the extent that we are worried about any possible effects on the social fabric, our preferred course should be the intelligent use of regulations to control social consequences.

No, I fear that the animating thrust of comments like this lies elsewhere. Perhaps some opponents of surrogacy make such claims out of anger and envy inspired by the class system and directed at those who benefit most from it. These *feelings* are suspect, at best, as moral or legal considerations. More to the point, if we do not like capitalism, we should do something about capitalism, as a system. Our dislike for the system or its beneficiaries ought not to be a reason for restricting the *freedom of women, both rich and poor.* To deny women their basic rights on such grounds is to penalize those who have traditionally *not* benefited from the present system. It would be morally wrong and politically wrong-headed to force women to live according to a standard higher than and quite disparate from that presently actualized in this society. To do so by means of the coercive power of the law of the present social system in honor of a cultural ideal which does not even figure in the foreseeable future of our society would be, in my opinion, morally and politically perverse.

Other critics of surrogacy may express qualms about relations between classes because of a newly discovered aversion to capitalism as the culture of money. How ironic that those long-satisfied with our system and our culture should choose to refuse women an opportunity to enjoy the benefits of capitalism just when technology and social change have opened access to those benefits through women's special reproductive capacities. It is the sort of irony which ought to make us curious. We should wonder why there is this new fear of capitalist exploitation just when women have attained special access to the capitalist game—access not open to men and largely independent of traditional social controls.

The fact of the matter is that we, as a society, do not believe the best things in life are free. Cost is value and money is power. Unless and until our society and culture are radically altered, assuring women who act as surrogates full legal standing can only serve to prevent exploitation. We certainly do not want to drive surrogacy into a legal underground where exploitation can flourish. Nor should we forget that pinchbeck veneration of an idealized maternal role has always been a primary device for the very real exploitation and oppression of women. Women will best be protected when they are recognized as autonomous adults with full rights. That recognition cannot be won through either the mystification of Motherhood or a false idealization of our social values. . . .

CONCLUSION

I do not want to suggest that the surrogacy issue — or any of the social conundra arising from the new birth technologies — is a simple one. I doubt that the complex of issues and concerns involved can be perspicuously or fruitfully *reduced to* matters of the freedom of surrogates. I do not even think this complex can be reduced to a question of individual freedom, generally: the freedom of women and men playing any of the pertinent parts in surrogate arrangements or in society at large.

I do, however, believe that freedom — particularly the freedom of women to be the dispositors of their reproductive capacities and to control their lives — is a central consideration in this controversy. It is central normatively in that it ought to be taken account of and respected. I believe it is also central in the present waging of the debate, though it remains — as a consideration — very well hidden. I have tried to evince, here, the ways in which our fear of women's reproductive freedom informs much of the current opposition to surrogacy. I have attempted, as well, to disclose the way in which genuine concern for women and women's rights should inform our response to other social interests, values and aims. . . .

ENDNOTE

. . . I wish to clarify certain points. 1) It is not my view that anyone who wishes to renege on a contractual agreement, is behaving irrationally. I claim, rather, that women can rationally choose to become surrogates and that women's reproductive role does not render them irresponsible [to make legal contracts]. 2) Nor is it my view that it is better to be born, *simpliciter,* than to not be born. It is my view that the claim "to not be born is better, *simpliciter,* than to be born through surrogacy" is, at least, odd. (In fact, I find both claims odd in much the same way.) 3) Finally, it is certainly not my view that everyone who opposes surrogacy does so simply from sympathy with patriarchy or from aversion to women's freedom; I hope I am neither that narrow-minded nor that pessimistic. Rather, I believe that much of the current debate is informed by patriarchy and indifferent to issues of women's freedom.

NOTES

1. Unfortunately, an increase in the incidence of infertility and other childbearing problems has augmented the rarity and value of woman able to bear children.

2. Note that the right to control over one's body claimed here is not to be regarded as an absolute right. It is also not to be pasted onto the abortion issue insofar as that involves any conflict of rights.

3. *E.g.,* cases of suicide, voluntary euthanasia, or drug abuse, in which the verity and reliability of consent are placed in doubt by the typical extremity of the surrounding situation.

4. The majority of those who have served as surrogates appear to be happy with their role, describing it in terms of personal fulfillment and of contributing to the happiness of others. This is a fact which is curiously under-reported in the present debate. The little attention given to the perspective of the surrogate focuses on those few women who have been unhappy with the arrangement.

5. I suspect that it is just the inanely self-absorbed who will be most insistent on obtaining quality surrogates to bear their children.

6. My impression is that most of the calls for privatization — or, rather, continued non-regulation — of

surrogacy come from those who presently benefit from the absence of legal control: *i.e.,* lawyers and fertility counselors. Surrogates and contractors must share roughly half the money earned and spent with these middlemen and are left with no recourse should the intermediary resources be unsatisfactory. Lack of legal standing for surrogates is an immediate boon to these third parties who are typically remunerated at least as well as the surrogate but who carry no liability should matters go awry. The suggestion that market competition and the desire to maintain a good record of service obviate need for regulation of their roles strikes me as unpersuasive.

Too Many Parents

ALEXANDER MORGAN CAPRON

BIOMEDICAL DEVELOPMENTS have generated countless challenges for the law. While the legal system's response is not always awe-inspiring, its confused and faltering reaction to medically assisted reproduction is in a class by itself. Perhaps this is not surprising, since of late virtually every bizarre possibility hypothesized in the early days of artificial baby-making has materialized, first in the fertility clinics and then in the courthouses.[1]

Yet even courts that have responded with some semblance of ad hoc justice have failed to respect the central interests at stake, which are not those of the warring adults but of the children who are and will be produced using the new reproductive methods. Two recent cases from opposite coasts demonstrate the limitations of the contract law model on which the courts

have relied with increasing frequency and make clear the need to read present legislation wisely and to craft new legislation that is astute as well as comprehensive.

IN RE MARRIAGE OF BUZZANCA

Orange County, California, which has given rise to the most widely discussed surrogate motherhood cases — occasionally involving facts so weird the cases have gone straight to the talk-show circuit without first being litigated — recently outdid itself: On 10 June 1998, the state's highest court declined to review a Court of Appeal decision reversing a trial court holding that a little girl with eight people who could arguably be called her parents was actually parentless.

Behind the birth of that little girl, Jaycee Buzzanca, lies a convoluted tale. About five years

ALEXANDER CAPRON is the University Professor Henry W. Bruce Professor of Law at the University of Southern California.

The Hastings Center Report, *Sept–Oct 1998: pp. 22–24. Reprinted with permission of Alexander M. Capron and The Hastings Center. Copyright 1998 The Hastings Center.*

ago, Erin Davidson agreed to become an egg donor, on the condition that she and her husband, who have four children, would approve who got her eggs. Once Mr. and Mrs. X (who remain anonymous) passed muster, seventeen eggs harvested from Mrs. Davidson were fertilized with Mr. X's sperm. Four were implanted in Mrs. X, who then gave birth to twins; the remaining embryos were kept in frozen storage. After the twins' birth, the fertility center offered the Xs three choices: destroy the embryos, donate them for research, or donate them for other couples. Mr. and Mrs. X checked off the third option. The Davidsons seem to have been unaware any further donation might occur.

Meanwhile, John and Luanne Buzzanca had failed to produce a child with five different surrogate mothers. On 13 August 1994, one of the Xs' frozen embryos was implanted in the uterus of "professional surrogate" Pamela Snell, who had served that role in the birth of three previous babies. Twelve days later, John and Luanne Buzzanca and Pamela and her husband Randy Snell signed a written surrogacy agreement, which—in what proved an understatement—warned that the peculiar circumstances of the case made parenthood legally unpredictable. The delay in formalizing the agreement was eventually found by the appellate court to be without legal significance, but its psychological meaning shortly emerged when John separated from Luanne. Eight months later, just weeks before Jaycee's birth on 26 April 1995, he filed for divorce.

In that filing, John alleged the marriage had produced no children, which Luanne denied in her response. Her attempt to get temporary child support was initially rebuffed by the family court because John was not Jaycee's biological father nor was she born to Luanne during the course of the marriage (the two ways the law typically establishes fatherhood). In February 1996, however, an appellate panel ruled that Luanne had made sufficient showing that she would prevail at trial to entitle her to child support pending the litigation.

In March 1997 the lower court heard John's petition for divorce as well as a petition Luanne had filed in September 1996 to establish herself as Jaycee's legal mother. Based only on oral arguments, the court ruled that John was not the legal father because he had not contributed the sperm, that Luanne was not the legal mother because she had neither contributed the egg nor borne Jaycee, and that the surrogate was not the legal mother because the parties had so stipulated. The gamete donors and their spouses were unknown to the court and not parties to the case.

In reversing these conclusions, the appellate panel looked to the Uniform Parentage Act as enacted in California. The act does not directly address the tangled circumstances of the case, but the court extrapolated a basic principle from the act: people should be held responsible for the reproductive outcomes of their actions. In addition to the two bases for establishing fatherhood that John Buzzanca failed to meet, the act provides that if a man consents to his wife's artificial insemination by donor (AID), he is deemed the father, and the donor of the semen "is treated in law as if he were not the natural father of a child thereby conceived."[2] While John's wife was not the one who bore Jaycee, Presiding Justice David Sills concluded that John fit within the act's assignment of fatherhood to one "who intends to raise [a] child but who otherwise does not have any biological tie" to the child whose procreation he "contemplate[d] by [his] consent to a medical procedure."[3]

The appellate court faced a bigger hurdle when it turned to Luanne's relationship with Jaycee because the act does not address the female equivalent of AID. Furthermore, in the leading California case on surrogate motherhood, *Johnson v. Calvert*,[4] the state supreme court had set forth only two ways to establish maternity: giving birth to a child or following the procedures (blood tests) used to determine paternity, neither of which applied to Luanne. Yet as the *Buzzanca* panel noted, the *Johnson* court had reached its conclusions about maternity through reasoning by parity from "statutes which, on their face, referred only to paternity." Having decided that an unrelated man could be deemed the father of a child because he intended the child to be born, the panel by a parity of reasoning ruled the same was true of a woman. Hence Luanne is Jaycee's mother.

MAKING POLICY, NOT READING STATUTES

This would be a sensible result, were the sole question whether John and Luanne could be held to have financial obligations to support Jaycee, but much more is actually at stake, especially as regards the assignment of maternity. Although presented as statutory interpretation, the opinion not merely makes up law out of whole cloth but actually goes against the policies embodied in the parentage and adoption laws.

First, the California Supreme Court itself stretched the parentage act beyond recognition in *Johnson* when it treated the law's two ways of identifying the natural mother as though they were separate "definitions" of motherhood that could yield two separate mothers, when in fact they are simply two ways of establishing that a woman is the "natural mother" because she gave birth to the child. The identity of a birth mother is not usually in doubt, but when it is, it may be resolved through genetic tests.[5]

Although the act's drafters did not contemplate that biological motherhood could have two facets, genetic and gestational, that has come to be the reality in many assisted reproduction cases. A policy decision must now be made about when if ever to rely on genetics over gestation. While the act does not address this issue directly, the only hint of the weight the legislature would give to these competing considerations favors the birth mother, since under the act genetic testing was in service of establishing birth, not the other way around. To reach the opposite conclusion, as the *Johnson* court did, and to premise the result on treating men and women "in parity,"

fails to recognize that women make a different contribution to reproduction than men and profoundly devalues the gestational aspect of that contribution.

Second, the *Buzzanca* court carried this illogic one step further by generalizing a narrow statutory provision. It interpreted the AID provision to embody the principle that obligation follows intention, whereas in fact the act simply bars a husband who has consented to AID performed by a physician from using a paternity test to defeat the presumption that a child born to his wife during the marriage is his legal issue. The act does not, however, govern the relationship of a man to a child not borne by his wife, much less the relationship of the wife to a child who is not the product of her womb and to whom neither she nor her husband are genetically related.

During gestation and at the moment of birth, the only mother-child relationship that is beyond question is that of child and birth mother, and the interests of the child will be best served if all concerned, including "professional surrogates," keep that mother-child relationship in mind. Recognizing this recognizes the need for responsible *maternal* behavior during pregnancy and for having someone clearly authorized to make *maternal* decisions about the newborn, without having first to sort through contracts or genetic relationships with the child that others claim to hold, on the basis of which they claim entitlement to make decisions about the pregnancy or the newborn child.

This is the issue that *Buzzanca* elides by going beyond assigning financial responsibility to imply parental status. Not surprisingly, the panel read the AID provision of the parentage act as expressing the age-old doctrine of estoppel, that a person who consents to an act should not be able to disclaim responsibility when others act accordingly. But it is one thing to say that a husband who consents to his wife's AID shoulders the responsibility of fatherhood, and quite another to say that the woman who commissions a surrogate contract is more entitled to be the mother of the resulting child than either the surrogate who bears the child or the woman whose egg is used.

The appellate panel in *Buzzanca* did not have to tackle this issue directly because the gamete donors remained out of the picture, and because Pamela Snell, who had filed for custody of Jaycee around the same time that Luanne petitioned to be named Jaycee's mother, apparently withdrew, and because by February 1997 the trial court had accepted the parties' stipulation that the Snells were not Jaycee's "biological parents." But had Pamela not relented—indeed, had she refused to turn over Jaycee at birth to a divorcing couple (as Luanne apparently feared, since she forged a "forwarding" order on Pamela's mail to keep her from receiving notice of the divorce action)—it goes well beyond any existing statute to conclude that Luanne's intent to be a mother should necessarily outweigh Pamela's undeniable biological relationship with Jaycee.

BROADENING RESPONSIBILITY

A further difficulty with the "intent" model of parenthood[6] is that its reliance on contract law not only turns children into commodities (in a marketplace where fertility centers charge ever higher prices for "elite" gametes and surrogates[7]) but treats public decisions as private, especially by evading adoption laws. People wishing to become parents of unrelated children can now sidestep the child-protective regimen established by the adoption laws simply by contracting for adoption prenatally.

Of course, draconian prohibitions on all forms of surrogacy may simply lead to ingenious evasions, as illustrated by *Doe v. Doe,* a divorce case decided in April by the Connecticut Supreme Court.[8] Though that case involved fewer participants, it was also very peculiar and

actually began before the Does got married. Plaintiff "Jane Doe," who had several children from a first marriage, had become infertile, so defendant "John Doe" advertised in the local paper for a surrogate, who was then inseminated with the defendant's semen, using a syringe but not under medical supervision. When the surrogate was four months' pregnant, Jane and John Doe married, and the surrogate assumed Jane's identity for purposes of receiving prenatal care and delivery.

The child was twelve years old by the time the superior and probate courts came to rule on John Doe's divorce complaint and his petitions to be declared the child's lawful father and to terminate the parental rights of the surrogate mother and her by-then ex-husband. Therefore, both in the interests of the child and in recognition of the maternal role long played by Mrs. Doe, the Connecticut court was right to accept a probate court ruling that John was the child's father and to utilize a state statute under which Jane could enjoy the status of an interested third party with "a powerful, albeit nonparental, claim to custody." In determining child custody issues, a "court's paramount consideration," as Justice David M. Borden noted, "is the child's welfare."[9]

Like many cases in which the new reproductive technologies have been examined legally, *Doe* is a divorce case; in such cases, children's status and needs are often pawns in the divorcing couple's battles over money, power, and revenge for hurt feelings. Given these circumstances, the steps needed to protect the interests of children in the context of a divorce action may not be the steps that best protect the children of the new reproductive technology at or before birth or even before conception. Furthermore, the claims of the other germinal and gestational participants in assisted reproduction are not best worked out in the context of a divorce case, which directly involves only the "social" parents. Indeed, the surrogate mother in *Doe* had apparently not sought to establish her legal parentage earlier, despite her dissatisfaction. Shortly after the child's birth, the surrogate wrote to the Does expressing deep "hurt" over their failure to live up to assurances that the relationship was more than a "business deal" and would involve their providing pictures of, and visits with, the baby. Seven years later, after the surrogate's own daughter had died, she asked John Doe's help in traveling to conceive a child with a Florida man; she also stated that she still considered the child to be hers and his (and not Jane Doe's) and that she desired to see "our daughter" but did not want a visit with Jane, who "is not a part of this as far as I am concerned. . . . My feelings towards our daughter concern you and I, and no one else."[10]

If society really wants to hold all the parties involved responsible for the consequences of their intentional acts, at least three steps are needed. First, it should make it clear to all those involved that they are at risk of financial and other responsibilities, while the benefits they gain will always be tempered by the goal of achieving what is best for the innocent third parties involved, namely, the children.

Second, the incentives to carry out artificial reproduction under medical supervision could then be increased by minimizing the financial and other risks of certain parties (particularly gamete donors) who participate in assisted reproduction run by legitimate fertility centers operated under supervision both by physicians and by adoption authorities or other agencies concerned with child welfare.

Third, the law should make the fertility centers that arrange for gamete donation, in vitro fertilization, and surrogate gestation responsible for the consequences. Of course, a center could insist that "intended" parents agree to indemnify the center for the child-support payments and other expenses that arise when death, divorce, or disagreement complicates the outcomes sought. But the effect of an indemnity agreement would still be to leave the first obligation on the centers' shoulders, giving them an incentive to screen all participants well and to structure arrangements

in the way that would be most protective of the children produced. Any inability or unwillingness of the adults involved to make good on their responsibilities would be at the expense of the fertility center, not the innocent victims. Fertility centers, as the "repeat players" in assisted reproduction, are easier to supervise than the individuals involved; moreover, it would be much easier and more cost-effective for centers to obtain the necessary liability coverage. More even than the "intended" parents, the fertility centers are responsible for bringing these children into existence since they assemble the necessary participants and carry out the key laboratory and clinical procedures. Thus, it is not only fair to hold the centers ultimately responsible should the children's interests be placed at risk, but it would be most protective of the children, since it would induce greater caution and care on the part of the leading actors. Success has many parents, disaster only one: in the case of assisted reproduction, protecting the well-being of those most at risk from disasters means that the role of "the one parent" should be placed on the fertility centers, which will be most able—and available—to pay the piper.

REFERENCES

1. Alexander M. Capron, "The New Reproductive Possibilities: Seeking a Moral Basis for Concerted Action in a Pluralistic Society," *Law Medicine & Health Care* 12 (1984): 192–98.
2. Uniform Parentage Act § 5.
3. In re Marriage of Buzzanca, 61 Cal. App. 4th 1410, 1418 (1998).
4. 5 Cal.4th 84, 851 P.2d 776 (1993).
5. Alexander Morgan Capron, "Whose Child Is This?" *Hastings Center Report* 21, no. 6 (1991): 37–38.
6. John A. Robertson, "Meaning What You Sign," *Hastings Center Report* 28, no. 4 (1998): 22–23.
7. Gina Kolata, "Clinics Selling Embryos Made For 'Adoption'," *New York Times,* 23 November 1997.
8. 244 Conn. 403, 710 A.2d 1297 (1998).
9. 244 Conn. at 441, citing *Manter v. Manter,* 185 Conn. 502, 441 A.2d 146 (1981).
10. 244 Conn. at 445, n. 47.

Case Study Exercises

REPRODUCTIVE TECHNOLOGIES

1. In 1995, it was charged that three physicians at a fertility clinic associated with University of California at Irvine stole or misused eggs of couples trying to have children and implanted them in infertile women who came to the clinic for help. A number of children were born to the women who were not genetically related to them. The women who gave birth consider the babies they bore to be *their* children. The couples who had stored eggs for their own use contend that they never intended or authorized that they be used by anyone else and, thus, they (the genetic parents) are the parents of the children who were born. Federal prosecutors filed charges against two of the UCI fertility clinic doctors, including accusing Dr. Ricardo Asch, the scandal's key figure, of misappropriating the eggs of some former patients at the center. The total settlements thus far in the 113 civil lawsuits are nearly $20 million. The biggest settlements went to women who never conceived a baby but whose eggs were implanted in other women who then had children. On May 12, 2000 a woman filed a lawsuit claiming physicians from the UCI clinic secretly took an embryo stored by her and her husband and implanted it into another woman for profit. The suit claims that the embryos of as many as 500 couples may have been sold to other women, adding a new twist to what is already a moral quagmire. (See H. G. Reza, "Largest Settlements Okd in Fertility Scandal," *Los Angeles Times*, 6 November 1997, and Hector Becerra, "Lawsuit Claims Defunct Clinic Stole Embryo," *Los Angeles Times*, 13 May 2000.)

   a. Discuss what might be said in support of the couple who stored eggs or embryos at the UCI clinic, intending to use them to produce their own genetic children.

   b. Discuss what might be said in support of the couple who went to the clinic and used what they thought were "donated" eggs or embryos.

   c. Two of the physicians involved (Drs. Asch and Balmaceda) fled the country. What responsibility do you think the clinic bears in a case such as this one?

2. In the case of William E. Kane, the California Supreme Court ruled that he had the right to bequeath his frozen sperm. Kane committed suicide in 1991, but had designated in his will that his sperm would go to his girlfriend, Deborah E. Hecht, so that she could be impregnated. Was this a wise decision? Should people be allowed to will eggs, sperm, or frozen embryos for use after they die? Discuss what we ought to do if such cases arise.

3. Share your thoughts on the following case:

   In 1995, a woman in Italy gave birth to a baby conceived from the egg of her sister-in-law, Elena, and the sperm of her brother. To complicate matters further, the sister-in-law, Elisabetta, had been killed two years previously (in December 1992). Dr. Pasquale Bilotta had attempted to implant in Elisabetta four of the eight embryos conceived through IVF, but each pregnancy failed and the four other embryos were frozen for future use. After the woman died, her husband asked the doctor to implant one of the remaining embryos in his sister. The baby is legally parented by the sister-in-law and her husband, though the man (Elena's brother and the biological father of the baby) intends to adopt the infant. Condemned by the Vatican, the matter has also raised questions whether this represents a kind of incest. A majority of Italians polled found it "morally unacceptable." At least one member of the Italian Parliament called the birth "immoral and incestuous." Some Italians have urged new Italian laws to curb some forms of artificial fertilization. (See John Tagliabue, "In Italy a Child is Born, and so is a Lively Debate," *The New York Times*, 13 Jan 1995.)

   a. Do you think it wise for the frozen embryo to be implanted in the sister-in-law, Elena? Note what sorts of issues and obstacles there are.

   b. Speaking from the point of view of those who find it morally unacceptable, what would the strongest argument be that such methods be banned?

4. Tony Randall became a father at age 77, as did Anthony Quinn and Saul Bellow at 84, and George Plimptom became the father of twins at age 69. Few, if any, voices were raised in opposition to such elderly men becoming parents—even though it is highly unlikely they'll live to see their child or children graduate from college. However, when a 63-year old woman gave birth with the help of fertility doctors, there was an outpouring of negative sentiment and derisive comments about the woman herself. This Susan Sherwin referred to as "cultural horror" (that a postmenopausal woman should move back into the role of a fertile woman). (See Gina Kolata, "Old Mother Hubbard Was Never a Sex Pot," *New York Times,* 27 April 1997.)

   a. Set out your position on men who are over 60 becoming fathers.

   b. Set out your position on women who are over 60 becoming mothers.

5. In December 1993 a 59-year-old postmenopausal British woman gave birth to twins after having fertilized eggs implanted in her uterus by a clinic in Rome. The same clinic gave a similar treatment to a 62-year-old woman. As a result of the criticism of allowing postmenopausal women to be artificially impregnated (presumably the central concern is the age of the woman), France's conservative government moved to impose strict controls on artificial impregnation—including requiring the consent of the sperm donor and a judge's permission before receiving an embryo implant. (See Alan Riding, "French Government Proposes Ban on Pregnancies After Menopause," *The New York Times,* 5 Jan 1994.)

   a. How would you respond to French Health Minister Philippe Douste-Blazy, who said artificial late pregnancies were immoral and women seeking such methods were egoistic?

   b. How would you respond to Elizabeth Badinter, who challenged the ban, saying, "Nobody has ever banned a 20-year-old girl who is deeply neurotic, addicted to drugs or has AIDS from having a baby—why should a woman of 60, who could be a good mother, not have the right to have a child?"?

   c. How would you respond to Claude Sureau, president of the ethics committee of the International Federation of Gynecology and Obstetrics, who said, "I don't think a law forbidding such things is good. How does one define the normal age of menopause? And if one allows the law to interfere in such a private domain, one is in a dangerous ethical situation of genetic totalitarianism."?

6. The number of children born from donated eggs has increased more than tenfold since 1989 and continues to grow. This has spawned a new business—egg brokerages—with fees that range up to $6,000 and beyond for matching recipients with donors. However its perceived benefits for the various parties, there are a number of ethical issues, such as: Should recipients tell their children about the circumstances of their birth? Who should be allowed to donate or sell eggs? How should donors be screened, if at all? Do children of such arrangements suffer long-term psychological problems? Will disclosure stigmatize the child? What are the potential problems with the asymmetry brought about by introducing a third party into the process of procreation? No one yet knows if donation can have lasting emotional effects, and there are few long-term studies of donors. (See Traci Watson, "Sister, can you Spare an Egg?," *U.S. News and World Report,* 23 June 1997). Share your thoughts on the following:

   a. Do you think egg donation or sale necessarily gives rise to the commodification of human beings?

   b. Are women as a group harmed by the use (some say exploitation) of women whose eggs are donated or sold?

   c. Should individuals or brokers be allowed to place ads in college newspapers in order to recruit college-age women to donate or sell eggs?

    d. Should there be any restrictions (such as warning signs as to physical risks) placed on the ads?

7. In March 1999 *The New York Times* reported on an advertisement soliciting "smart" egg donors (i.e., college students who had SAT scores over 1400) who were also tall. Evidently the contracting couple sought an egg donor that would "resemble" themselves. Is it morally distasteful to allow such targeted ads? Set out your argument as to whether a couple should advertise for the egg donor of their dreams.

8. Through an embryologist's mistake, a New York woman, Donna Fasano, who used in vitro fertilization (IVF) to get pregnant, gave birth to twins. One twin, however, was not genetically related to either her or her husband. Evidently the embryologist knew another couple's embryos had been implanted in the first batch, and corrected his mistake in the second batch, but told no one about his error. The woman of the other couple failed to get pregnant. Mrs. Fasano, who is white, suspected something went astray when she saw the babies —one is white and one is black.

    a. Do you think the Fasanos are morally obligated to give up the child that they are not biologically related to? If they refused to run DNA tests on the baby, claiming he is theirs regardless of genetics, do you think they ought to be forced to test the baby? Set out your views on this case.

    b. What do you think of the resolution of the case, as noted below:

    The baby's birth parents, Richard and Donna Fasano, had filed suit to force the Rogerses to live up to a visiting agreement. Mrs. Fasano gave birth to the boy and to her own biological son last December after a Manhattan fertility clinic mistakenly placed fertilized embryos from both couples in her womb. The Fasanos said they wanted the two boys to know each other as brothers, and they had reached a visiting agreement with the Rogerses before they turned the boy over in May. Mrs. Fasano and her lawyers contended in court that the boy should be considered both her son and Mrs. Perry-Rogers's son. But Justice Lebedeff ruled yesterday that the Rogerses were the sole parents. Lawyers for the Fasanos said they would not contest the judge's decision. (See David Rohde, "Biological Parents Win in Implant Case," *The New York Times,* 17 July 1999.)

SURROGACY

1. Should there be any restrictions on family members being either gestational or traditional surrogate mothers? Discuss the issues and concerns raised by the following case for both the individuals involved and the society as a whole:

    In 1991 a South Dakota woman, Arlette Schweitzer, 42 years old, was the gestational surrogate mother of twins for her daughter, who was born without a uterus. The eggs came from her daughter and the sperm from her son-in-law. The embryos that resulted from IVF were then implanted in Schweitzer's womb. This was the first time in the U.S. that a woman gave birth to her own grandchildren. Schweitzer did not receive any payment for serving as a surrogate mother and said she bore the children out of love for her daughter. In 1991, according to the American Fertility Society, there were 198 attempts at gestational surrogacy, with 33 deliveries. In July 1991, San Francisco Giants pitcher, Dave Righetti, and his wife became the parents of triplets because of Dave's sister who served as a gestational surrogate. (See Gina Kolata, "When Grandmother Is the Mother, Until Birth," *The New York Times,* 5 August 1991.)

2. The most celebrated surrogacy case involved a couple, William and Elizabeth Stern, and a woman, Mary Beth Whitehead, who was contracted to be the surrogate for the Sterns. This

was a case of traditional surrogacy, with William Stern providing the sperm and Mary Beth Whitehead providing the egg and bearing the child. Elizabeth Stern was not infertile. Stern, a pediatrician, diagnosed herself as having a mild case of multiple sclerosis and decided that pregnancy could worsen her condition.

   a. Should women who are not infertile be allowed to use a surrogate to bear them a child?

   b. What sorts of precautions, if any, should be taken to prevent possible abuse in the event that the contracting woman in a surrogacy arrangement was not infertile?

   c. If surrogacy is permitted at all, is there any good reason, so long as the surrogate is willing, to set down restrictions about the contracting woman who intends to raise the child the surrogate will bear?

3. Virtually all surrogacy contracts require the potential surrogate be subjected to psychological testing to determine her stability and whether, in fact, she would be able to part with the baby she bears.

   a. Critics argue that this stipulation is in itself suspect, claiming that the goal is to find women who see the infant they give birth to as a commodity that can be given away (or sold). How would you reply to the critics' concern?

   b. Should the couple that contract a surrogate and who intend to raise the child the surrogate bears also be subjected to psychological tests to determine their emotional stability?

4. If we as a society allow surrogacy, why shouldn't we consider surrogacy a potential occupation for women and pay women a respectable salary to bear children for infertile couples? Share your thoughts on this idea.

5. In the case of gestational surrogate Anna Johnson who was contracted by the Calverts to bear the child of which they were the genetic parents, the specter of racism was raised. It seems that Johnson was African-American, Crispina Calvert was Filipina and Mark, her husband, was white. Some worried that this would open the door to rich, white couples seeking out poor minority women to be the gestational surrogate of "their" children.

   a. Should there be a prohibition or restrictions on using a surrogate of a different race from the contracting couple?

   b. Would paying the gestational surrogate of another race from the contracting couple a generous salary be a way to ensure that poor minority women are not exploited as part of a baby-bearing underclass?

6. The contract with the Sterns that surrogate Mary Beth Whitehead signed stated that William Stern could order her to abort (e.g., if the fetus had severe medical problems). Although this stipulation, as one of Stern's lawyers conceded, was not legally enforceable, it may have had a coercive effect on Whitehead. Discuss the concerns about the addition of such an "abortion clause" in a surrogacy contract.

7. How much control should a contracting couple have over the actions of a surrogate? Offer some guidelines, taking the following into consideration: use of legal (controlled) substances such as over-the-counter drugs; use of legal substances such as alcohol and cigarettes; use of illegal substances such as marijuana, cocaine, and heroin; exercise and other physical activity; and diet and nutrition.

8. Surrogate "brokers" (lawyers who help couples find surrogates and make up the resulting surrogacy contracts) receive a hefty sum for their services. Indeed, such lawyer-brokers net much more money than the surrogate herself.

   a. What would be the strongest case for "Let the buyer beware" with respect to the use of surrogate "brokers"?

   b. What would be the strongest case for strict regulations limiting how much money a broker-lawyer can make in arranging a surrogacy contract?

    c. What would be the strongest case for eliminating any exchange of money from surrogacy arrangements (whether it be at the lawyer's gain or payment for the surrogate's services or medical fees)?

9. A woman who (with or without her husband) seeks a surrogate arrangement assumes much greater legal risks if she uses a biological surrogate, rather than a gestational surrogate. That is, her genetic connection to the child carries much more legal weight than any intentions to rear a child to whom she is not biologically related. Thus, it would be less risky to employ a gestational surrogate. Do you think this is ethically preferable?

10. Some critics of surrogacy argue that all forms of commercial surrogacy should be prohibited — that it commodifies women and children. Furthermore, some contend that commercial surrogacy is a form of alienated labor on the part of the surrogate. Do you think prohibiting any money exchange would address such problems of surrogacy?

11. Uma Narayan, among others who comment on surrogacy, argues that "gift" (or altruistic) surrogacy, in which no money changes hands, has the potential for abuse. Do you think she is right to oppose this form of surrogacy?

12. A new specialty service consists of surrogates who are willing to bear children for gay men. This raises the question of whether surrogacy could be seen as a means for nontraditional marriages or couples to have families — something that has not normally been available to them. Discuss the advantages and disadvantages of gays, lesbians, or single men and women using surrogacy as a way to have children. Is there any reason to see this method as problematic?

13. Ought we to change surrogacy arrangements to allow surrogate mothers to change their mind about relinquishing the child (so it is similar to birth mothers having a few months before adoptions are finalized)? State the strongest claims for or against establishing a three-month waiting period after the birth of a child conceived under a surrogate arrangement in which the surrogate mother has the right to change her mind about relinquishing the child.

14. Share your thoughts on this case:

> A couple who used a surrogate but provided neither the egg nor the sperm were found to be the legal parents of the child by the California appeals court in March of 1998. The court ruled that intent outweighed the biological relationship and, thus, declared Jaycee Louise Buzzanca the legal daughter of John and Luanne Buzzanca. The couple broke up after the surrogate mother was implanted with the embryo and the father wanted no responsibility for the child. The court, however, in finding him the legal father, also ruled that John Buzzanca must pay child support until the girl is 18. In responding to Buzzanca's statement that he was not responsible because technology made it possible using a sperm and egg donation from other people, [an] ACLU attorney noted that biological ties are not the exclusive definition of a family. (See Greg Hernandez and Davan Maharaj, "Couple Who Used Surrogate Ruled Parents," *Los Angeles Times,* 11 March 1998.)

15. In an article in *The Washington Post,* in May 1999, lawyer Lori B. Andrews wrote,

> Four years ago, I got a call from an infertility specialist who was in the midst of a procedure. He was just about to transfer an embryo created by a childless couple's egg and sperm to the woman who had volunteered to carry the baby for them. But he suddenly had second thoughts. "I've got an embryo from a couple in a catheter," he told me hurriedly. I pictured him, catheter in one hand, telephone receiver in the other. "I'm about to implant it in the surrogate, who is the husband's sister," he explained, and wanted to know if it would

violate his state's ban on incest. If he decided not to go through with the implantation and the embryo died, he asked, could he be found guilty of murder?

As a lawyer specializing in reproductive technologies for the past two decades, I've become used to such calls, and I shared this doctor's frustration about how little law there was to guide him. No, I told him, this probably wouldn't be incest. But the question of murder was more complicated. In some states, such as Louisiana, embryos that are created in vitro are viewed as people and cannot be destroyed. The incident reminded me once again that the United States lacks a national policy for dealing with reproductive technology—and is the only technologically sophisticated nation without one. (See Lori B. Andrews, "Embryonic Confusion," in *The Washington Post*, 2 May 1999.)

a. Do you think it would be murder if the embryo died?
b. What sorts of policy guidelines do you think should there be to address cases such as these?
c. Later in the article, Andrews says of the gap between medicine and the law, "Nowhere is the lack of precedents more complicated than in dealing with frozen embryos." Assuming this is the case, how should we look at frozen embryos when drawing up laws?

InfoTrac College Edition

1. Thomas A. Shannon, "Eggs No Longer Cheaper by the Dozen"
2. Rebecca Dresser, "And Baby Makes Three . . . or Four . . . or Five: Assisted Reproduction"
3. Monica Konrad, "Ova Donation and Symbols of Substance: Some Variations on the Theme of Sex, Gender and the Partible Body"
4. Traci Watson, "Sister, Can You Spare an Egg? Donors Get Money. Couples Get Babies"
5. Ian Craft, "An 'Inconvenience Allowance' Would Solve the Egg Shortage"
6. Kathryn Jean Lopez, "Egg Heads. [In vitro fertilization]"
7. *The Christian Century*, "Bishop Responds to Embryo, Abortion Cases. [Cardinal Basil Hume; Destruction of Frozen Embryos in the United Kingdom]"
8. *Jet*, "Couple Claims Wrong Sperm Used During Fertilization"
9. John Travis, "Brave New Egg. [New Technologies to Produce Human Oocytes]"
10. Ziba Kashef, "Miracle Babies: One in Ten Black Women Will Face the Anguish of Being Unable to Conceive, But Today's Fertility Treatments Are Improving the Odds"
11. Alexis Jetter, "Could You Kiss This Baby Good-Bye? [Trials of One Surrogate Mother]"
12. Hugh V. Mclachlan and J.K. Swales," Commercial Surrogate Motherhood"
13. *The Ecologist* "The Baby Brokers"
14. Caroline White, "Banking on Interest. [Medicine and the Media]"

Web Connections

For links to Contraception, Abortion, and Maternal-Fetal Conflicts Web sites, articles, cases, and more exercises go to our abortion page at philosophy.wadsworth.com/teays.purdy/abortion

Chapter 8

Genetics and Cloning

GENETICS IS ONE of the most exciting new areas in bioethics. In the last 40 years or so, our understanding of genetics has grown enormously, opening up the potential for powerful new technologies. Some people are wary of this new knowledge because they believe that some things are better left unknown — we shouldn't be "playing God." Many others are concerned about its practical potential for harm. And with the mapping of the human genetic code, we will likely see significant changes and new directions in medicine in the next few years and in decades to come.

The possible benefits of new DNA-based treatments may make it seem unduly negative to be concerned about its dangers. Yet the human track record in using new discoveries is checkered. Often pioneers have plunged ahead with new projects on the basis of incomplete or inadequate knowledge; often, too, people have focused on their own goals, failing to consider the consequences of their acts for others, and over the long-term.

The history of medicine provides us with many examples of practices intended as therapies being adopted without sufficient evidence of their safety and efficacy, therapies that caused suffering and even death. Purging and bleeding were two common practices in earlier days; surgery, radiation, and electricity have also been used in a variety of harmful ways as they became available. Often, members of relatively disempowered groups have borne the brunt of such experimentation (although white middle-class men have not been immune, either). Notorious in the annals of medicine, as Diana Axelsen noted in Chapter 3, are Marion Sims' experiments involving gynecological surgery on black women slaves without their consent.

Another disastrous chapter in medical history has been the indiscriminate use of estrogens. Even though it has been known since the 1940s that estrogens encourage the proliferation of cancer cells, they have been prescribed for many women. In the 1940s and 1950s, for example, a form of estrogen, diethylstilbestrol (DES), was given to pregnant women, in the belief that it would help protect their pregnancies. Although it did not do so, it did lead to an epidemic of cancer in their children.

More recently, minority women have been used as research subjects in the development of hormonal contraceptives. Sometimes unsafe devices, like the IUD (the Dalkon Shield), are rushed to market. In this case, one poorly designed component led to infection, infertility, and even death for some users. For all these reasons, new applications in medicine cry out for careful scientific and moral assessment. Nobody can promise that they will prevent future harms, but such ongoing scrutiny is surely essential for minimizing them.

This realistic perspective on medical history might lead one to conclude that we should reject new possibilities out of hand. But that would be to ignore the real benefits scientific knowledge has brought us. Advances in prevention and treatment have taken place because society has acted on scientific knowledge about the prerequisites for health (like clean water and safer food supplies). Also critical has been biological research about diseases like puerperal fever, pneumonia, and polio, as well as progress in pain relief and rehabilitation.

Many of us now take these benefits for granted and have no conception of the suffering that once plagued human life, and that still plagues the millions for whom they are currently inaccessible. Moreover, there are plenty of other health conditions that continue to burden more affluent individuals, and if reducing suffering is a morally urgent goal, further health progress is needed. Human suffering can also be alleviated by the use of biological and medical knowledge to control reproduction. Thus concern for suffering requires us to pursue and use new knowledge, but to do so cautiously.

Genetics, like any important new source of knowledge, could eventually show us how to prevent suffering; its very power also means that it could be used in ways that threaten well-being. It promises to help us prevent or cure some diseases; it might also provide the means to change or enhance our biologically based characteristics. But genetic research may itself pose serious risks, and even if we can use genetics to achieve our intended goals, it may enable us to undertake projects that are themselves unwise — say by removing certain genes from the gene pool because of their apparently deleterious nature.

Even where such projects may not be intrinsically unwise, the fact that they will unfold in capitalist, racist, or sexist societies may render them harmful. For example, if individuals know of their genetic weak links, that knowledge might help them prevent disease. However, if such knowledge leads to discrimination by employers or insurance companies, it may well do more harm than good.

More subtle dangers may also await us. Because of the apparent power of genetic explanation, we may attempt to extend it beyond its appropriate sphere. For example, a tendency to try to trace human behavior to genetic causes emerges during certain periods in human society. An important source off this bent is hierarchical political philosophies with an interest in persuading us that social inequality is inevitable (because biologically based) and therefore morally defensible.

These theories generally try to show, for example, that it is right and proper for women to confine their activities to the domestic sphere and that members of other disadvantaged classes such as the poor, minorities, the disabled, and homosexuals deserve their subordinate status. This point of view is currently popular, and is one of the major motivators for huge biological projects like the Human Genome Project, which is attempting to map the whole genome of a particular individual—and, as we saw in July 2000, this goal has become a reality. This genetic determinist perspective also tends to squelch inquiry into alternative explanations for difference and inequality.

An equally serious matter is that this perspective funnels resources into attempts to find genetic remedies for problems that result from, or could more easily be solved by, social or political changes. These approaches delay or prevent progress in alleviating suffering from disease and disability. Thus, for example, if we really want to prevent the excess disease, disability, and death suffered by African-American babies, it would be sensible to make sure their mothers enjoy the same health-related amenities as populations with better outcomes. Among them would be high-quality prenatal care, good food, and protection from toxic substances. Only then might one reasonably pursue the hypothesis that any remaining differences might be genetic. Even where problems are genetic in origin, it doesn't follow that genetic treatment is the best solution. Suppose it turns out, for example, that some women's breast cancers are a consequence of genetic susceptibility to exposure to certain pesticides. It's likely that it would be preferable to reduce human exposure to pesticides than to attempt to alter these women's genetic structure.

Is genetic inquiry "too hot to handle"? Even if this conclusion were warranted, it looks as if it is now too late to stuff the genie back into the bottle. And the potential benefits from progress in genetics are substantial. If, for example, it were possible to prevent or cure such horrid diseases as Huntington's disease, that would contribute enormously to human welfare. The crucial point here is that society must control the development of biological science to ensure that it does not violate our consciously chosen moral, political, and social goals—without undermining good science. We must find a way to avoid both "state" science, as exemplified by the Soviet Union's politically motivated adoption of the view that acquired characteristics are inherited (Lysenkoism), and an individualistically driven pursuit of "progress" heedless of consequences.

Given that genetics in medicine will not go away, and that it can be a force for good as well as for evil, we as a society are faced with a variety of moral problems about how to proceed. Space limitations in a text of this sort preclude anything but a taste of the myriad of fascinating issues that have already begun to face society. One set of questions is associated with the interface between genetic knowledge and particular individuals who might want to use it. What, for example, are appropriate forms of screening? What counts as good genetic counseling?

Another set of questions is raised at the broader social level. Should there be limits on the kinds of research acceptable to society? And, how can such judgments be enforced? When the potential uses of DNA research were becoming evident in the 1970s, some scientists—and lay people as well—were alarmed by its potential misuse and the harm that could ensue. Those who were in favor of continued research carried the day, arguing that the elaborate safeguards they proposed would ensure public safety. Concern about such research seems to have been forgotten, and accounts of the controversy have tended to disappear from texts on the subject. Whether this outcome is warranted remains to be seen.

One major issue is whether genetic manipulation should be limited to somatic (or body) cells in particular persons, or whether it could be justifiable to alter germ cells (which pass traits on to offspring) as well. After all, individuals might be able to give informed consent to risky experimentation or therapy on their own bodies, but the situation is entirely different when future persons might be harmed.

GENETICS AND REPRODUCTION

Our growing understanding of genetics poses numerous questions about parental rights and duties in the context of reproduction. For example, can it ever be wrong to knowingly take the risk of passing on a serious disease by having children? Or does an affirmative answer open up too many difficult issues, such as where to draw the line, the justification of selective abortion, and quality-of-life concerns for those currently living with the disease or disability? A common reaction to these questions is that the matter should be left to fate.

Another controversial question is whether anything is wrong with sex selection. Sex selection is currently possible after conception via ultrasound and abortion; it can also be achieved before conception by using pre-implantation genetic diagnosis. In the future, it may be possible to select the sex of the fetus far more easily and cheaply.

Sex selection could be used to choose either girls or boys. Some people believe that wanting a child of a given sex is sexist, no matter what the motive. Furthermore, most human societies are undeniably sexist, preferring boys to girls, and female fetuses are aborted far more often than male ones. Of course, women living in the most sexist societies might have feminist reasons—wanting to spare girls oppressed lives—for aborting females. So the moral status of such abortions is by no means clear.

Would a just society ban abortions aimed at producing a child of a preferred sex? The moral indeterminacy of sex selection would argue against that view, and such abortions would be difficult to prevent, in any case. Moreover, banning such abortions undermines women's legal right to abortion. Yet sex selection, by any means, may lead to potentially disastrous sex imbalances in the human population. In China, for example, where population concerns have led the state to develop a "one-child per family" goal, so many families have opted for boys that there is likely to be a serious shortage of women in the next generation. In India, selective abortion and the neglect of girls is leading to similar results. Perhaps education can prevent such individual choices from undermining the common good.

The readings in this chapter are divided into two sections: genetics and cloning. The first considers the broader issues raised by progress in genetics.

1. The A.M.A. Council on Ethical and Judicial Affairs considers issues raised by the imminent availability of multiple genetic tests.

2. Sherman Elias and George J. Annas discuss the pros and cons of somatic and germ-line genetic therapies.

3. James D. Watson argues in favor of germ-line genetic engineering.

4. Laura M. Purdy argues that it can sometimes be wrong to have genetically related children.

5. Abby Lippman provides a wide-ranging critique of the increasing geneticization of health and reproductive discourse.

In the second section we look at cloning.

1. Jacque Cohen and Giles Tomkin look at embryo cloning and attempt to separate fact from fiction.

2. Responding to the National Bioethics Advisory Commission's statement in favor of banning human cloning is Susan M. Wolf, who opposes the decision, which is discussed here. She argues that the policy necessary to enforce a ban will be too intrusive and may lead to the banning of other technologies that have health benefits.

3. In "Human Cloning and the Constitution," Clarke D. Forsythe looks at the issues raised by use of the terms "person" and "human," and examines the embryo's constitutional status. He argues that the only way to protect a human embryo is to avoid cloning.

4. Lee M. Silver examines some of the religious arguments used against cloning, attempts to defuse the rhetoric he sees being employed, and criticizes some of the assumptions held by opponents of cloning.

5. Lisa Sowle Cahill considers some of the issues raised by the new technologies, such as cloning, showing how issues around global justice are brought to the foreground (e.g., by stem cell research).

Issues in Genetics

Multiplex Genetic Testing

THE COUNCIL ON ETHICAL AND JUDICIAL AFFAIRS, AMERICAN MEDICAL ASSOCIATION

AMONG THE MOST SIGNIFICANT advances in the development of genetic medicine is the ability to test for genetic origins of specific conditions. In previous reports, the American Medical Association's Council on Ethical and Judicial Affairs has addressed many ethical issues associated with the application of the growing body of genetic information and accompanying technologies.[1]

Here, analysis is offered regarding testing for multiple genetic conditions simultaneously, or "multiplex genetic testing."

The term *multiplex genetic testing* can mean different things. It commonly refers to testing for multiple mutations that give rise to a single disorder, such as cystic fibrosis or phenylketonuria. This report deals instead with multiplex genetic testing where tests for completely different conditions are offered in a single session. As the mapping of the human genome progresses and tests for newly discovered genes are developed, the possibility has arisen that many differ-

ent testing "packages" could be administered simultaneously. This latter kind of multiplex testing creates a new level of complexity because the modes of heredity, social implications, and availability of treatment can differ greatly among the conditions tested.

Existing tests can be divided into three broad categories: first, tests can be performed to find genetic conditions that will lead to future inevitable disease onset as in the case of Huntington disease. Second, tests can be designed to find specific genetic information that indicates a heightened risk to possible disease onset. Often referred to as "susceptibility testing," this type of test can be used to provide information about the possibility of contracting specific cancers, such as colon or breast cancer. Finally, genetic tests can be used to determine a patient's carrier status, providing information about the existence of a gene or gene mutation that is not necessarily manifested in an individual's phenotype, but that may be passed to children. The implications of the in-

Permission granted by the American Medical Association.

formation conveyed by each test are different and are best addressed in separate ethical analyses.

The implications of genetic tests also differ depending on the population targeted for testing. For instance, genetic information provided to couples in the process of making reproductive decisions will likely have a different impact from information provided to an individual who has no intentions of having children. Similarly, providing genetic tests to children at the request of their parents may have different ramifications from providing the same tests to consenting adults.[2] These differences are crucial to any analysis of genetic testing and must be given careful consideration as the availability of genetic medicine continues to grow.

Multiplex testing may compound the ethical complexities associated with single genetic tests rather than simply combining them. It should not be concluded that safeguards designed to limit the ethical risks associated with single genetic tests will be sufficient to meet the challenges that arise when tests are offered in combination. While this may be true in limited circumstances, in general the clinical application of multiplex testing should not proceed without a careful examination of the associated regulatory and ethical issues. Marketing of multiplex testing, both directly to consumers and through physicians' offices, could provide appealing financial returns to the biotechnology industry as well as to genetic testing centers.[3] In the face of these incentives encouraging rapid development and distribution of multiplex tests, it is critical to confront the relevant ethical issues before these tests are widely conducted without necessary safeguards. As a response to this need and as a part of its continued efforts to address the ethical implications of genetic medicine, the Council presents the following analysis of multiplex genetic testing.

SENSITIVITY, SPECIFICITY, AND PREDICTIVE VALUE

Among the variety of genetic tests, some yield high rates of false-positive and false-negative results, while others are characterized by findings that are precise but of uncertain clinical or predictive value.[4] These problems with current genetic testing technology are complicated rather than reduced when single tests are combined to form a multiplex test.

Any single test's clinical validity is determined by three factors: the test's sensitivity, its specificity, and its positive predictive value. Sensitivity measures the test's ability to register true-positive results, while specificity measures its ability to provide true-negative results. The positive predictive value of a test is the probability that a person with a true positive will get the disease. A key determinant of the total number of false positive results is the frequency of the trait in the tested population. As an example, if a test that yields false positives 10 percent of the time is used to screen a population of 100 people in which 90 people actually have the disease, then of the ten people who are actually negative we can expect that one of them will test positive. In this case, the number of false positives would be one in 100. Thus, when high-risk groups are tested, positive results can be interpreted with greater confidence than when general populations of unknown risk are tested. Conversely, if low-risk groups are tested, the likelihood of false-positive results is correspondingly higher.

Consider the BRCA1 mutation and its relative predominance among Ashkenazi Jews. It is estimated that approximately 1 percent of all women of Ashkenazi Jewish descent carry the mutation, while approximately 0.1 percent of women in the population at large carry a mutated gene.[5] If only Ashkenazi Jewish women were tested for the trait, the rate and number of false-positives would be much lower than if all women were tested for the BRCA1 mutation. If, on the other hand, BRCA1 were tested as part of a multiplex test that targeted populations without an elevated risk for the BRCA1 mutation, the rate of false-positives would be high.

Multiplex testing contributes to the problem of false results by combining several tests, each of which carries its own risk of producing a false result. The chance that the multiplex test will yield a false positive result increases as the number of tests included in the panel increases. For example, consider a single test that produces accurate results in 90 percent of cases. If five tests with similar rates of accuracy are conducted at once, the laws of probability suggest that the chance that they will all yield accurate results falls just below 60 percent.

The real clinical value or utility of a panel is also questionable in multiplex genetic testing. Even when tests are accurate, providing a meaningful interpretation of the results is often complicated.[6] Genetic tests can only provide information about the state of genetic material (genotype) without saying much about physical manifestations (phenotype). In some cases where the gene mutation is manifested phenotypically in all patients who inherit the gene, a genetic test can provide results that are entirely predictive, as in the case of Huntington disease. In many cases, however, genetic tests attempt to assess presymptomatic risk for developing a disease. With these susceptibility tests, a positive result does not ensure that the individual will develop the disease, and a negative result does not preclude one from risk. Tests for the BRCA1 mutation are helpful in illustrating this point. By age seventy, the risk of breast cancer among carriers of the BRCA1 mutation has been shown to be 56 percent and the risk of ovarian cancer, 16 percent.[7] It is important to recognize, however, that those identified as having the BRCA1 mutation may not actually develop either form of cancer. Furthermore, it has been shown that only 7 percent of women with a family history of breast cancer had this specific genetic mutation. Thus even individuals with supposed risk over 90 percent would gain no predictive advantage from being

tested for BRCA1.[8] In fact, obtaining the negative results of a BRCA1 test might provide false reassurance and discourage the use of important screening techniques such as breast self-examination and mammography.

INFORMED CONSENT AND COUNSELING

It is critical to assess the degree to which the nature of current genetic tests could affect the ability of patients to give informed consent. Patient autonomy is given its clearest voice in the process of consent, and the medical community has established conditions that must be met to ensure that patients' freedom to make decisions is protected. One of the most crucial of these conditions is disclosure by the physician of all relevant information. Without such disclosure, the patient cannot reasonably be expected to make a decision that represents a clear analysis of available options and possible outcomes. The nature of genetic information, however, provides several challenges to this requirement.

As with many laboratory tests, results from genetic testing are typically assumed by patients to be correct. Many genetic tests do not validate these assumptions of near-perfect performance.[9] Communicating the problems of sensitivity and predictive value—and the need for caution when interpreting test results—to patients (who may believe that tests are by their very nature conclusive) is a difficult task. This difficulty is amplified when factors such as specificity vary for each of the different tests of the multiplex package.

Moreover, tests conducted for diagnostic purposes, susceptibility, and carrier status have different implications and counseling needs. While tests for diagnosis are associated with near-certain predictions of disease development, susceptibility tests provide information only about illness risk. Counseling in the latter cases must, for instance, include interpretation of the risks associated with particular mutations. Carrier screening is designed to provide information to potential parents about the possibility of passing a gene mutation to children. Although a carrier test itself may be fairly straightforward, assessing the implications of the test requires, for instance, an understanding of reproductive genetics. In cases involving a single genetic mutation that is either dominant or recessive, a basic discussion of Mendelian inheritance may be sufficient. However, in more complicated cases of polygenic traits or linked genes, a substantially more sophisticated understanding of biology may be required. If tests for all three purposes were combined to form a single multiplex test, substantially more counseling would be required in order to convey all the information relevant to a patient's final decision.

Not only does each type of test require different, unique information backgrounds, the tests trigger different social or personal contextual concerns. For instance, different susceptibility tests have different implications for patients, and the information required for meaningful interpretation of the results may vary substantially.[10] As a result, grouping tests by general category will not necessarily alleviate the problems associated with counseling for multiplex tests.

The third principal challenge to obtaining informed consent lies in the nature of the information resulting from many genetic tests, particularly those designed to determine susceptibility. In many cases, receiving a positive test result for a genetic mutation does not provide any conclusive predictive evidence that one will eventually develop the disease. There may also be instances in which test results can provide insight into actual future disease onset, but in which no preventive measures or treatments exist with which to stave off or mitigate the inevitable condition. In still other cases, such as tests for cystic fibrosis, patients may be asked to consider that certain tests may predict disease onset but cannot distinguish between the often vastly disparate levels of severity. When these uncertainties are coupled with the possibilities of false results, providing

patients with the information necessary to consider a multiplex test appears difficult at best.

Some will argue that clinicians can overcome these difficulties by carefully counseling patients and working through the complexities with those considering testing. Behind this position is the view that physicians should not assume that there is anything their patients cannot understand and consider in the process of giving informed consent. Furthermore, it would be paternalistic to deny patients access to tests simply because the profession recognizes the possibility that appropriate information might be lost in the process of disclosure. These are certainly compelling points; however, it is also important to examine how closely our current medical system can approximate the conditions under which adequate counseling could occur. A Human Genome Project survey found that only 54 percent of the physicians surveyed had even one course in basic genetics.[11] Experts in medical genetics concur with this finding, arguing that there currently exists a shortage of clinicians trained in genetic counseling and interpreting genetic tests. In sum, many physicians who will be asked to provide patients with tests and information about genetics will not have the background necessary to meet the challenges of that task.

Another possible solution is to refer patients to genetic counselors. Again, however, the feasibility of this solution must be evaluated in terms of currently available resources. Counseling a patient about a genetic condition is a time-consuming process consisting of pre-test information sessions, informed consent sessions, and post-test counseling sessions. Many of these sessions last over three hours, and as a result some counselors see as few as 300 new patients a year.[12] Even without the availability of the multiplex test, trained genetic counselors are under strain to meet the increasing demand for genetic services. The time demanded of these professionals will only increase with the combination of several tests conveying different information and implications with varying levels of accuracy. This poses a problem. Despite the fact that multiplex testing will require genetic clinicians to spend significantly more time with each patient, no systemic change has been proposed to handle this potentially overwhelming shift in practice. This raises profound questions about the profession's ability realistically to meet the information needs of patients attempting to make decisions about multiplex tests.

It should also be noted that the increase in time demanded of counseling physicians by multiplex testing would come at a time when physicians are often under considerable pressure to economize their interactions with patients. Incentives currently in place often have the intended or secondary effect of requiring physicians to see more patients in the course of their practice rather than fewer. In this environment, it is unlikely that physicians will be able to meet the counseling requirements presented by multiplex testing. Even if the burden of conveying strictly genetic information is shifted to nonphysicians, the process of counseling must include the consideration of clinical implications that can only be conveyed by physicians.

Such concerns are only compounded by questions of whether insurers will reimburse for appropriate — and expensive — counseling services.

PHYSICIAN RESPONSIBILITY TO INDIVIDUAL PATIENTS

Past council opinions on genetic testing have assumed a link between testing and risk, addressing those circumstances in which individuals considered "at risk" for a specific condition are offered testing for genetic status. Yet as more conditions are included in a multiplex test, a wider group of the general population becomes at-risk for at least one of the included genetic traits. It is likely that these patients would be offered the entire panel of tests rather than the single, clinically relevant test. As genome research continues, the genetic root of an increasing number of conditions will be established, thereby expanding the pool of patients considered eligible for genetic tests. It seems safe to predict that eventually virtually all patients will be shown to have a genetic disposition for some trait, and that might encourage a trend toward a large proportion of the population seeking evaluative genetic testing. If these tests are grouped in multiplex packages without concern for the relevant risks of the individual, a substantial number of patients would receive results from evaluations that are not clinically indicated.

Experience with laboratory test panels (often referred to as "chem 7," "chem 12," etc.) supports the assertion that multiplex testing would lead to a breakdown in the link between clinical indication and genetic evaluation. In daily practice, it is often less expensive and equally convenient to order a fixed battery of laboratory tests rather than each individual test suggested by the patient's condition. It may not be readily apparent, especially to a busy practitioner, why genetic tests should be treated differently, particularly if multiplex tests could provide a less expensive alternative to single trait testing.

This prospect is cause for some concern. Abnormal results from specific tests in laboratory panels are routinely provided to patients even if the test in question was not clinically indicated. In some instances, the information may be benign, or there may be treatments available that can be of material benefit to the patient. In other cases, however, information provided by nonindicated testing may result in unnecessary psychological distress, lifestyle modifications that negatively affect quality of life with no resulting benefit, or requests for treatment that are founded on misconceptions rather than medical science. While these problems may be resolved in cases where communication of information is unimpeded and straightforward, they are significantly more serious when associated with those tests, including genetic tests, that convey information that is difficult to explain and to understand.

The challenges facing physicians who attempt to help patients deal with fears and to clarify misconceptions by providing sufficient information about many genetic tests are not limited to scientific and personal contextual uncertainties, however. Current popular conceptions regarding the information contained in a genetic test also complicate significantly the task of patient communication. There is a substantial body of misleading information relayed to the public almost daily about the implications of genetics. Stories in the media repeatedly claim that science has uncovered an inheritable gene responsible for a wide variety of conditions and behaviors, often implying that a cure is not far behind. The response among many members of the general public is to believe that genetic information is the key to understanding future disease onset and to establishing the immutability of certain traits and characteristics. In short, genes are often portrayed as the source of inevitable outcomes and predetermined conditions. To many, genes are even thought to represent the essence of human beings. Providing accurate information in the face of these powerful assumptions is extremely difficult.

In general terms, many patients perceive genetic information to be an indicator of their fundamental health. Despite the fact that diseases and traits cannot be reduced solely to their genetic components and that environmental and behavioral influences are critical components to the development of most conditions, current social conceptions of self place tremendous significance on genetic composition. Physicians have a responsibility to appreciate the power of genetic information and to exercise appropriate caution when providing access to tests that may be interpreted by patients as evaluations of their basic "wellness."

The far-reaching, conceptual impact genetic information may have on patients strengthens the claim that only those tests that are clinically indicated should be offered. Providing general access to testing in the clinical setting validates misconceptions that genetic information is inherently valuable and that surveying genes is a legitimate assessment of overall health. Furthermore, even seemingly benign tests that provide information about genetic status but that have no bearing on phenotypic expression or reproductive decisions may have a psychological impact on the patient who interprets the presence of a mutation as a deep-seated flaw.

Given the significance of genetic information, it is also critical to ensure that test results are accurate. It has already been established that providing access to tests that are not justified by the clinical evidence may substantially compromise the clinical validity of a multiplex test. The increased risk of false-positive results inherent in expanding the pool of tested patients beyond those with a personal or family history outweighs the benefits gained by those patients who seek genetic tests to provide a survey of their genes, even if there is a small chance the test could provide information valuable to the patient. It is critical to recognize the limitations of testing as well as the potential impacts of affording access to genetic information that may be incorrect.

POPULATION TARGETING AND MULTIPLEX TESTS

Targeting of genetic testing to individuals who have an elevated risk for a specific condition has many merits. The challenge is to define and find those patients who are eligible for a given test according to this approach. One possibility is to design multiplex packages based on patterns of risk found in different populations. These populations could be identified by rates of disease incidence, and multiplex tests could be constructed that target the conditions found in a particular population. This method has been explored by a group of practitioners within the Department of Human Genetics at the Mount Sinai School of Medicine, who developed a multi-disease carrier screening program consisting of a multiplex test designed to target diseases found in an Ashkenazi Jewish population.[13] Their multiplex test encompassed individual tests for Tay-Sachs disease, cystic fibrosis, and Type I Gaucher disease.

But there are a number of potential problems with designing multiplex tests on the basis of incidence patterns in defined populations. The assumption of such testing is that elevated rates of risk are distributed throughout the selected population, such that every individual within the population presents a history that supports the need for testing. However, this assumption relies upon a history of reproductive isolation that is not evident in many socially defined populations. Individuals tend to associate according to cultural features: these may not be representative of gene pools that track with targeted mutations. The reproductive overlap between populations may be extensive. Programs that rely upon the patient's self-identification with a population to determine eligibility for testing risk targeting cultural features rather than appropriate genetic inheritance. If tests are provided to those who are not in fact members of high-risk groups, the number of false-positive results will increase and possible harm could result. These problems, both with defining a broad population that actually represents a pool of patients each having elevated risk and with selecting patients whose membership in that group is established biologically, present compelling arguments against designing multiplex tests on the basis of populations.

Proceeding with programs to test socially defined populations for multiple genetic mutations using specifically designed multiplex tests could result in different forms of discrimination. Because of the problems in defining "at risk" populations that should in fact be eligible for multiplex testing, it is likely that any such testing programs will disproportionately subject one group of patients to the negative impacts either of false results or forms of generic discrimination. Patients who are tested according to actual risk based on clinical evaluation will benefit from more accurate test results than those given tests because of their membership in an inevitably ill-defined genetic population.

Moreover, multiplex tests that attempt to group individuals into broader populations could disrupt the patient-physician relationship by introducing an element of perceived discrimination into the clinical setting. One of the primary duties of physicians is to treat each patient according to his or her individual medical needs. To the extent that ethnic heritage may contribute to particular health concerns, it is clinically relevant and should be considered. Offering multiplex tests that are bundled according to race or ethnicity, however, serves to categorize patients rather than to address their distinct needs. Furthermore, the criteria upon which this categorization is based are the genetic mutations and diseases prevalent in a population. The profession can ill afford the perception that science is being used to bring attention to the genetic flaws present in lines of inheritance.

Perhaps the most troubling potential application of multiplex tests would be the construction of test panels explicitly designed to discriminate against specific ethnic groups. For instance, a multiplex test could be built around a single test for which elevated risk exists in a particular population. The other tests in the multiplex bundle could be any tests for which reasonable risk exists in the general population. By using the one race-related trait to target the population, the remainder of the tests could point to mutations that exist in other populations but which go unnoticed for lack of testing. The insidious implication of such testing would be that one ethnic group had an abundance of mutations and must therefore be considered inferior. While this possibility might seem improbable, history provides many examples of such discrimination in other contexts, and society must not discount the possibility of such unprincipled actions.

POTENTIAL FOR DISCRIMINATION

In any discussion of genetic tests, one of the fears most commonly expressed by patients and society is the possibility that this private information might be used in discriminatory practices. Safeguards and regulations must be put in place to prevent insurers and health care service organizations from denying coverage for or discriminating against people who have tested positive for a genetic trait.[14] This basic premise should also be extended to employers, especially self-insured employers, who could use genetic information in their hiring and promotion decisions.

Potential discrimination by insurance companies and employers could be further complicated by multiplex tests designed to target specific groups. For example, a test that coupled BRCA1 and Tay-Sachs could be used to discriminate disproportionately against Ashkenazi Jews. A similar test coupling sickle-cell anemia and prostate cancer could discriminate against African-American males. The formulation of the test itself and the determination by society, industry, and health care providers of conditions to be tested could become a powerful means of social control.

USING MULTIPLEX TESTS WISELY

Increasingly, genetic science is helping to characterize the etiology of illnesses. Genes are inherited and passed on to future generations. Viewed by many as fundamental to conceptions of self, knowledge of their genes may influence many important decisions and options in peoples' lives. However, the impact of environmental factors and behaviors on health should not be ignored, and diseases should not be reduced to their genetic components only.

Multiplex testing presents a series of challenges to adequate communication between the patient and the physician. It increases the total number of marginally indicated or non-indicated tests, thereby bolstering the rate of false results. These results may lead to psychological stress and misinformed life-altering decisions, and may also affect the ability of a physician to obtain informed consent. The inherently uncertain nature of genetic information as well as the lack of clinical geneticists and counselors available to provide adequate information also suggest that standards of disclosure will be difficult if not impossible to maintain.

Finally, multiplex testing and its resultant information may have widespread societal implications. When coupled with society's emphasis on the primary role of genetics in pathology and suffering, expanded provision of genetic tests might lead to varied forms of discrimination against those with genetic conditions. Furthermore, multiplex tests could be constructed specifically to target defined populations, which could lead to selective discrimination against particular populations.

Although multiplex tests have not reached the general health care market, the potential for their widespread application is readily apparent. Before such tests reach health care providers, clinics, and drugstores, the ethical and social implications of these tests must be well understood, and careful restrictions and regulations must be established.

The Council offers the following recommendations on the future possibilities of multiplex genetic testing:

1. Physicians should not routinely order tests for multiple genetic conditions.
2. Tests for more than one genetic condition should be ordered only when clinically relevant and after the patient has had full counseling and has given informed consent for each test included in the panel.

3. Efforts should be made to educate clinicians and society about the uncertainty surrounding genetic testing.

ACKNOWLEDGMENTS

Members of the Council on Ethical and Judicial Affairs include the following: Charles W. Plows, MD, Santa Ana, Calif. (chair); Robert M. Tenery, Jr., MD, Dallas, Tex. (vice chair); Alan Hartford, MD, PhD, Boston, Mass.; Dwight Miller, University Park, Md.; Leonard J. Morse, MD, Worcester, Mass.; Herbert Rakatansky, MD, Providence, R.I.; Frank A. Riddick, Jr., MD, New Orleans, La.; Victoria Ruff, MD, Columbus, Ohio; George T. Wilkins, Jr., MD, Culver, Ind.; Linda L. Emanuel, MD, PhD, Chicago, Ill. (vice president, ethics standards); Michael Ile, JD, Chicago, Ill. (council secretary); Stephen R. Latham, JD, PhD, Chicago, Ill. (director, ethics division); Jeffrey C. Munson, Chicago, Ill. (senior staff associate and staff author); Jessica Berg, JD, Chicago, Ill. (staff consultant); Eric Nadler, Chicago, Ill. (intern and staff author).

The Council on Ethical and Judicial Affairs acknowledges the helpful comments of Pilar Ossorio, section leader for genetics at the Institute for Ethics at the American Medical Association, and anonymous editorial reviewers.

This report was adopted by the House of Delegates of the American Medical Association in December 1996 and has been subsequently revised in response to comments from peer reviewers.

REFERENCES

1. Council on Ethical and Judicial Affairs, American Medical Association, "Prenatal Genetic Screening," *Archives of Family Medicine* 3 (1994): 633–42; "Genetic Testing by Employers," *JAMA* 266 (1991): 1827–30; *Physician Participation in Genetic Testing by Health Insurance Companies Reports of the Council on Ethical and Judicial Affairs* (Chicago: American Medical Association, 1993); *Ethical Issues in Carrier Screening of Cystic Fibrosis and other Genetic Disorders. Reports of the Council on Ethical and Judicial Affairs* (Chicago: American Medical Association 1991); *Testing Children for Genetic Status Reports of the Council on Ethical and Judicial Affairs* (Chicago: American Medical Association, 1996).

2. Council on Ethical and Judicial Affairs, *Testing Children.*

3. Committee on Assessing Genetic Risks, Institute of Medicine, *Assessing Genetic Risks: Implications for Health and Social Policy, Executive Summary* (Washington, D.C.: National Academy Press, 1994), p. 2.

4. Committee on Assessing Genetic Risks, *Assessing Genetic Risks.*

5. Frances Collins, "BRCA1—Lots of Mutations, Lots of Dilemmas," *NEJM* 334(1995): 186–88.

6. Philip Kitcher, *The Lives to Come* (New York: Simon and Schuster, 1996). See in general pages 65–86.

7. Jeffrey P. Struewing, Patricia Hartge, Sholom Wacholder et al., "The Risk of Cancer Associated with Specific Mutations of BRCA1 and BRCA2 among Ashkenazi Jews," *NEJM* 336 (1997): 1401–8.

8. Fergus J. Couch, Michelle L. DeShano, M. Anne Blackwood et al., "BRCA1 Mutations in Women Attending Clinics That Evaluate the Risk of Breast Cancer," *NEJM* 336 (1997): 1409–15.

9. Kitcher, *The Lives To Come.*

10. See, for example, Sherman Elias and George Annas "Generic Consent for Genetic Screening" [Sounding Board], *NEJM* 330 (1994): 1611–13.

11. Ethical, Legal and Social Implication of the Human Genome Project: Education of Interdisciplinary Profession. Funded by: Office of Health and Environmental Research at the Department of Energy and National Institute of Health (ELSI), Georgetown University, 10 June 1996.

12. Neil A. Holtzman, *Proceed with Caution: Predicting Genetic Risks in the Recombinant DNA Era* (Baltimore, Md.: Johns Hopkins University Press, 1989).

13. Christine M. Eng, Brynn Levy, Tania S. Burgert et al., "Evaluation of a Model Program for Multi-Disease Carrier Screening in a Target Population" [Abstract], *Pediatric Research* 35 (1994): 151A.

14. Over half of the states have enacted laws prohibiting insurers and employers from the adverse use of information derived from genetic testing.

Somatic and Germline Gene Therapy

SHERMAN ELIAS AND GEORGE J. ANNAS

RECENT REPORTS of human gene therapy experiments have been heralded worldwide with praise from the medical and scientific communities as well as the general public. A new medical journal, *Human Gene Therapy,* devoted entirely to this topic, has also been introduced. The stage is now set for more experiments involving human somatic cell genes, with the objective of ameliorating or correcting genetic defects.[1] In mid-1990 Steven Rosenberg and colleagues reported the use of retroviral-mediated gene transduction to introduce the gene coding for resistance to neomycin into human tumor-infiltrating lymphocytes before their infusion into five patients with metastatic melanoma.[2] The distribution and survival of these "gene-marked" lymphocytes were then studied, and for the first time, the feasibility and safety of introducing new genes into humans were demonstrated. We are now witnessing the transition from theoretical possibility to practical reality of the "dawn of a new age of cancer treatment" based on novel gene therapy strategies.[3] In September 1990, Michael Blaese and colleagues at the National Institutes of Health (NIH) announced the first human gene experiment in a young girl with adenosine deaminase (ADA) deficiency, a very rare autosomal recessive genetic disorder resulting in severe combined immune deficiency.[4] Affected individuals usually die during childhood

from chronic infections. The investigators obtained circulating lymphocytes from the patient, expanded the number of cells in culture, infected the cells with a recombinant retrovirus carrying the ADA gene, and then reinfused the cells into the patient.

SOMATIC CELL THERAPY

Some believe that somatic cell gene therapy is an unwise pursuit. Their underlying concern is that it will inevitably lead to the insertion of genes to change the character of people, reduce the human species to a technologically designed product, or even "change the meaning of being human."[5] These fears rest on the presupposition that somatic cell gene therapy differs in a significant way from accepted forms of treatment.[6] This has not, however, been the consensus of panels of experts who have analyzed the issues. Both the President's Commission for the Study of Ethical Problems in Medicine and Biomedical and Behavioral Research[7] and the European Medical Research Councils[8] concluded that somatic cell gene therapy is not fundamentally different from other therapeutic procedures, such as organ transplantation or blood transfusion. The only important differences between somatic cell gene therapy and other treatments are the issues of safety and the possibility that viral vectors may also infect germ cells.

At present, among the various methods for introducing genetic material into cells, retroviral-based vectors appear to be the most promising

SHERMAN ELIAS is Professor and Head of Obstetrics & Gynecology at the University of Illinois at Chicago. GEORGE ANNAS is a Professor of Medical Ethics at the Boston University School of Public Health.

approach for gene transfer in humans.[9] Concern has been raised that despite elaborate "built-in safety features" with redesigned mouse retroviral vectors, there is a finite risk that these vectors could recombine with undetected viruses or endogenous DNA sequences in the cell and so become infectious. This risk of "viral escape," as well as other potential risks that would be limited to the patient, such as activation of a protooncogene or disruption of an essential functioning gene, has resulted in society demanding very critical review and participation in any decisions to embark on human gene therapy.[10]

In the United States, recombinant DNA research funded by the NIH must first be reviewed by the local Institutional Review Board and local Institutional Biosafety Committee. In addition, the NIH has established the Recombinant DNA Advisory Committee (RAC) to review proposals to be funded by the NIH. An interdisciplinary subcommittee of RAC, called the Working Group on Human Gene Therapy, was formed that consisted of three laboratory scientists, three clinicians, three ethicists, three attorneys, two public-policy specialists, and one lay member. Based on a draft from this subcommittee, the RAC composed a document called "Points to Consider in the Design and Submission of Human Somatic-Cell Gene Therapy Protocols."[11] This document is intended to provide guidance in preparing proposals for NIH consideration, and focuses on: (1) objectives and rationale of the research, (2) research design, anticipated risks and benefits, (3) selection of subjects, (4) informed consent, and (5) privacy and confidentiality. The RAC has deliberately limited its purview to somatic cell gene therapy, emphasizing that the "recombinant DNA is expected to be confined to the human subject" to be treated.[12]

W. French Anderson, a leading NIH investigator in the field of gene therapy, contends that "somatic cell gene therapy for the treatment of severe disease is considered ethical because it can be supported by the fundamental moral principle of beneficence: It would relieve human suffer-

ing."[13] He also argues that after the appropriate approval of therapeutic protocols by Institutional Review Boards and the NIH,

> it would be unethical to delay human trials. . . . Patients with serious genetic disease have little other hope at present for alleviation of their medical problems. Arguments that genetic engineering might someday be misused do not justify the needless perpetuation of human suffering that would result from unethical delay in the clinical application of this potentially powerful therapeutic procedure.[14]

And more recently, Anderson has insisted that it is time to be less tentative about somatic cell therapy, saying "What's the rush? The rush is the daily necessity to help sick people. Their (our) illnesses will not wait for a more convenient time."[15] A large majority of Americans seem to agree. According to a survey reported by the Office of Technology Assessment, 83 percent of the public say they approve of human cell manipulation to cure usually fatal genetic diseases.[16]

It should be emphasized, however, that human experimentation regulation has a long history, and it is easy to forget even its basic lessons in the rush to research. We are unlikely to repeat Martin Cline's unapproved beta-thalassemia experiments [see note 4], but we do continue to concentrate early experiments on children (who cannot consent for themselves) and the terminally ill (who are especially vulnerable to coercion), repeating many of the same ethical mistakes made with artificial heart and xenograft transplants in the 1980s. The point is that just because somatic cell experiments are not fundamentally different than transplant experiments, it does not mean that there are no ethical or legal problems of consequence involving these experiments, or that we have reached a consensus on how to resolve them.

GERMLINE CELL THERAPY

In contrast to somatic cell gene therapy, which is limited to the individual patient, germline gene therapy entails insertion of a gene into the reproductive cells of the patient in such a way that the disorder in his or her offspring would also be corrected. This can be interpreted either as the corrective genetic modification of gametes (sperm or ova) or their precursor cells, or insertion of genetic material into the totipotential cells of a human conceptus in refined variations of the techniques used for germline modification in the creation of transgenic animals.[17] As such, germline gene therapy constitutes a definitive qualitative departure from any previous medical interventions because the changes would not only affect the individual, but also would be deliberately passed on to future generations.[18]

Should human germline gene therapy be permitted? Until now there has been some comfort in the fact that technical difficulties would preclude consideration of such genetic engineering in human beings for many years to come. However, one need only look at the scientific advances presented at the First International Symposium on Preimplantation Genetics, held in Chicago in September 1990, to realize that the pace of technology in this area has become much faster than previously predicted. Although in the past it may have seemed politically prudent to avoid the subject, we must now begin to seriously discuss the ethical issues before germline gene experiments in humans are technically possible, in order to assist future policymakers in their deliberations.[19]

At the Workshop on International Cooperation for the Human Genome Project, in Valencia in October 1988, French researcher Jean Dausset suggested that the Genome Project posed such great potential hazards that it could open the door to Nazi-like atrocities. In an attempt to avoid such consequences, he suggested that the conferees agree on a moratorium on genetic manipulation of germline cells and a ban on gene transfer experiments on early embryos. The proposal won widespread agreement among the participants at the meeting and was only defeated after a watered-down resolution using "international cooperation" was suggested by

Norton Zinder, who successfully argued that the group had no authority to enforce such a resolution. Leaving the question of authority for later debate, should we take Dausset's proposal for a moratorium on germline cell experimentation seriously?

ARGUMENTS AGAINST HUMAN GERMLINE GENE THERAPY

The ethical arguments against the use of a human germline gene therapy fall into three categories: (1) its potential clinical risks, (2) the broader concern of changing the gene pool, the genetic inheritance of the human population, and (3) social dangers.[20]

Potential Clinical Risks

Major advances in knowledge must be made to overcome the significant technical obstacles for human germline gene therapy. Methods would have to be developed to stably integrate the new DNA precisely into the right chromosomal site in the appropriate tissues for adequate expression and proper regulation. The possibilities for dangerous mistakes are formidable: examples would include insertional mutagenesis, in which a normally functioning gene is disrupted or a proto-oncogene activated by the newly integrated gene, or the regulatory signals of the nonfunctional or dysfunctional gene could adversely affect the regulation of the new exogenous gene.[21] These safety concerns are compounded by practical problems, including loss of gametes or embryos by instrument manipulation and the inherent limitations and inefficiency of reproductive technologies such as in vitro fertilization (IVF). Of course, many medical experiments have significant risks, and in this respect, germline research is not unique. IVF itself was opposed on similar grounds in the late 1960s and early 1970s.

On the other hand, unless there is overwhelming evidence that the procedure will be successful and not cause harm to the resulting child, there is no justification for doing genetic experiments on an early embryo and then reimplanting it. The more reasonable position would be not to reimplant the genetically defective embryo in the first place. The same logic applies to gamete manipulation. This argument suggests that except in the vanishingly rare case in which both parents are homozygous, and thus all embryos produced will be affected with their condition, and this condition is seen as unacceptable by them, *and* they refuse to use either donor ovum or donor sperm, there will be no clinical role for genetic therapy to replace or substitute for defective genes in embryos. Even in this case, of course, such research may never be justifiable because of the significant risks of introducing even worse problems for the resulting child.

Changing the Gene Pool

In germline gene therapy the objective would be to correct a genetic defect for future generations and hence restore the individual's lineage to the "normal" state. But what may be considered a harmful genetic trait today could be neutral in the future or could even conceivably serve a beneficial function, depending on environmental pressures in which the trait operates. Arno Motulsky has used the example of wearing eyeglasses. For primitive humans, genetically controlled myopia could prove fatal if one could not keep a sharp eye out for predators. The relatively high frequency of myopia and the need for some to wear eyeglasses represents loss of an adaptive biological trait in modern civilization. Nonetheless, myopia is never fatal, and some people, particularly ophthalmologists, optometrists, and eyeglass makers, might even say that the existence of myopia and other refractory deficits has been of benefit by creating a livelihood for them.[22] One danger is that we may wrongly eliminate a characteristic, such as sickle-cell trait, that by protecting against malaria has advantages

for the carrier. On the other hand, much of medicine has the potential for altering the next generation by helping the current one survive to reproductive age. As Alexander Capron has noted:

> The major reasons for drawing a line between somatic-cell and germ-line interventions . . . are that germ-line changes not only run the risk of perpetuating any errors made into future generations of nonconsenting "subjects" but also go beyond ordinary medicine and interfere with human evolution. Again, it must be admitted that all of medicine obstructs evolution. But that is inadvertent, whereas with human germline genetic engineering, the interference is intentional.[23]

Capron continues the argument by noting that "the results produced by evolution at any points in time are hardly sacrosanct," producing, as they do, genetic diseases, and he concludes that intentionally interfering "in humankind's genetic inheritance is not a sufficient reason to foreswear the technique forever, though it is reason enough to distinguish it from somatic-cell interventions."[24] Robert Morison's warning is an appropriate note on which to close our gene pool discussion:

> The nominalist biological position is that there can be no such thing as an ideal man. Men are brothers simply because they all draw their assortment of genes from a common pool. Each individual owes his survival and general wellbeing partly to his own limited assortment of characters and partly to the benefits received through cultural interchange with other individuals representing other assortments. It follows that the brothers in such a human family have a sacred obligation to maintain the richness and variety of their heritage—their human gene pool and their common culture. Every man in a sense must become his brother's keeper, but the emphasis is on keeping and expanding what both hold in common, not on converting one brother to the ideal image held by the other.[25]

Social Dangers

The intentional alteration of germline genes seems to be the real reason that some condemn it as presumptuously "playing God" and crossing a symbolic barrier beyond which medicine and mankind become involved not in treating disease, but in recreating ourselves. It is feared that we may begin to lose our footing on the slippery slope when we extend our notions of gene therapy toward "enhancement genetic engineering." This would involve insertion of a gene to enhance a specific characteristic: for example, adding an extra gene that codes for growth hormone into a normal child in an attempt to achieve a taller individual or, in the context of germline manipulation, to create taller future generations. From the medical perspective, French Anderson points out that adding a normal gene to correct the harmful effects of a nonfunctional or dysfunctional gene is different from inserting a gene to make more of an existing product. Selectively altering a characteristic might endanger the overall metabolic balance of individual cells or the body as a whole.[26] He has also warned:

> I fear that we might be like the young boy who loves to take things apart. He is bright enough to be able to disassemble a watch, and maybe even bright enough to get it back together again so that it works. But what if he tries to "improve" it? Maybe put on bigger hands so that the watch is "better" for viewing. But if the hands are too heavy for the mechanism, the watch will run slowly, erratically, or not at all. The boy can understand what he can see, but he cannot comprehend the precise engineering calculation that determined exactly how strong each spring should be, why the gears interact in the ways that they do, etc. Attempts on his part to improve the watch will probably only harm it. We will soon be able to provide a new gene so that a given property involved in a human life would be changed—e.g., a growth hormone gene. If we were to do so simply because we could, I feel that we would be like that young boy who changed the watch hands. We, like him, do not really understand what makes the object we are tinkering with tick. Since we do not understand, we should avoid meddling. Medicine is still so inexact that any modification

(except perhaps one which returns towards normal a defective property) might cause severe short-term or long-term problems.[27]

The issues raised by such enhancement efforts are similar to those of athletes taking steroids, but with the added complication of perpetuating the effects to unborn generations. But assuming that all the medical concerns can be addressed, and even if such issues as scarcity of resources and equal access to care are resolved, one major ethical problem remains—the likelihood of genetic discrimination. Using the example of inserting the gene for growth hormone, if being tall were considered a social virtue, say for basketball players, it would only be an advantage if "opponents" could be kept relatively shorter by selectively limiting their access to the "treatment." What if a gene could be inserted to prevent a certain type of cancer in susceptible, yet otherwise normal, individuals? Could they lose their children's health insurance if they refused to have their gametes or embryos "treated"?[28] Will we be able to resist "encouraging" parents to decrease the "genetic burden" and thus not undermine individual autonomy and dignity?

The most troublesome of all forms of genetic engineering is "positive" eugenics. Human beings seem to have an urge to "improve" our own species by genetic manipulations. Throughout history men and women have practiced assortive mating based on physical characteristics, intelligence, artistic talent, disposition, and many other traits. It was the English aristocrat and mathematician Francis Galton, a cousin of Charles Darwin, who in 1883 coined the term "eugenics" from the Latin word meaning "wellborn." In his writings, Galton defined eugenics as the science of improving human condition through "judicious matings . . . to give the more suitable races or strains of blood a better chance of prevailing speedily over the less suitable."[29] Eugenic genetic engineering includes attempts to alter or "improve" complex human traits that are at least in part genetically determined—for example, intelligence, personality, or athletic ability. Because such traits are polygenic, purging the genome of undesirable genes and replacing them with an array of desirable genes would require technological advances that we cannot even foresee. Moreover, even if such replacement could be achieved, the interplay between the newly introduced genetic material and the recipient genome would result in entirely unpredictable results. Nonetheless, the scenario remains in the realm of remote possibility.

We need not envision a return to the "racial hygiene" totalitarianism of National Socialism under the Nazis to see that the genetic screening of preimplantation embryos might become popular, or even standard. As the U.S. Congress's Office of Technology Assessment (OTA) put the case in 1988, such screening need not be mandated by government at all, since individuals can be made to *want* it (as they are now made to want all sorts of things by advertising), even to insist on it as their right. In the words of the OTA report, "New technologies for identifying traits and altering genes make it possible for eugenic goals to be achieved through technological as opposed to social control."[30]

Sheldon Krimsky has persuasively argued that there are two potential moral boundaries for gene therapy: the boundary between somatic cells and germline cells, and the boundary between the amelioration of disease and the enhancement of traits. But as he has noted also, the first involves a clear distinction, but a dubious rule, whereas the second involves a desirable rule, but a fuzzy distinction. The problem is that the distinction between disease and enhancement has no objective, scientific basis; disease is constantly being redefined. Krimsky asks, for example, "is chemical hypersensitivity a disease? Any trait that has a higher association with the onset of a disease may itself be typed as a proto-disease, such as fibrocystic breasts."[31]

Thus the problem is that we want to use germline gene therapy only to correct devastating diseases to avoid, among other things, the creation of a "super class" of privileged and gene-

enhanced individuals who have the advantage of both wealth and enhanced genetic endowment. But the solution is unlikely to be drawing a line between disease and enhancement, both because that line is inherently fuzzy and because once "treatment" techniques are established, it may be impossible, as a practical matter, to prevent these same techniques from being used for enhancement. Because many traits one might want to enhance, such as intelligence or beauty, are polygenic, we may also comfort ourselves that they may never actually be susceptible to predictable genetic manipulation.[32]

ARGUMENTS FOR HUMAN GERMLINE THERAPY

Efficiency

Leroy Walters suggested two rationales for which human germline therapy is ethically defensible.[33] The first rationale is efficiency. Assuming that somatic cell gene therapy became a successful cure for disorders caused by single-gene abnormalities, such as cystic fibrosis or sickle-cell disease, treated patients would constitute a new group of phenotypically normal, homozygous "carriers" who could then transmit abnormal genes to their offspring. If a partner of such an individual had one normal copy for the gene and one abnormal one, there would be a 50 percent likelihood of an affected offspring. If two treated patients with the same genetic abnormality reproduced, all of the offspring would be affected. Each succeeding generation could be treated by means of somatic cell gene therapy; however, if available, some phenotypically cured patients would consider it more efficient, and in the long run less costly, to prevent transmission of the abnormal gene to their offspring via germline gene therapy. Andreas Gutierrez and colleagues appear to have accepted this efficiency rationale as well by suggesting that germline gene therapy might be used to *prevent* cancers in individuals carrying defective tumor suppressor genes (for example, the retinoblastoma gene in retinoblastoma and p53 in Li-Fraumeni syndrome).[34]

It has also been suggested that germline therapy would be needed to treat genetically defective embryos of couples who believe it is immoral to discard embryos (because they are human life) regardless of their genetic condition.[35] This argument, however, is not persuasive. First, individuals with this belief might not be able to justify putting their embryos at risk of extracorporeal existence in the first place, and even if they could, would find it even more difficult to justify manipulations of the embryos with germline gene therapy that may cause their demise. Further, even those who adamantly oppose abortion do not equate the failure to implant an extracorporeal human embryo with the termination of a pregnancy. Thus, germline gene therapy cannot be justified solely on the basis of the religious beliefs of those who hold that protectable human life begins at conception. Moreover, as has been argued previously, it cannot be justified solely on the basis of treating the embryos of homozygous parents, since alternatives, such as ovum and sperm donation, exist that put the potential child at no risk.

Unique Diseases

The second rationale for the germline approach would arise if some genetic diseases could only be treated by this method. For example, in hereditary diseases of the central nervous system, somatic cell gene therapy may be impossible because genes could not be introduced into nerve cells due to the blood-brain barrier. Early intervention that did not distinguish between somatic cells and germ cells may be the only means available for treating cells or tissues that are not amenable to genetic repair at a later stage of development or after birth.

On the surface, the efficiency argument seems reasonable if one is dealing with a genetic characteristic in all sperm and one could remove it from all sperm by manipulating testicular cells.

On the other hand, if, as seems most likely, screening will be done on preimplantation embryos, and those with genetic "defects" identified, then the *most efficient* method of dealing with the defective embryos is to simply discard them, implanting only the "healthy" ones.

For now at least, it seems that the second rationale is the stronger one, but since we have no coherent theory for treating such diseases by germline therapy, actual experimentation is at best premature.

SHOULD GERMLINE THERAPY BE PERMITTED?

Even though Jean Dausset's moratorium proposal did not pass at Valencia, there is currently a de facto moratorium on germline therapy because it is unclear both how to do it and for what conditions it might be appropriate. Consequently, a formal moratorium seems unnecessary. It also seems unwise. A review of the literature and this summary of it make it clear that the issues have not been well thought-out or well debated. The arguments against germline gene therapy tend to be basically the same as those previously used against somatic cell therapy: work with genes seems to arouse greater concern primarily because of the "genetic theories" of the Nazis and their horrible acts to put them into practice, and the early work on recombinant DNA in the United States and the concern that it might create a dangerous strain of virus or an uncontrollable pathogen. The "future generation" argument is actually no different than the original arguments raised against IVF and any extracorporeal manipulation of the human embryo.

What seems most reasonable now is to continue the public debate on whether, and under what conditions, germline experimentation should be attempted. As a way to better focus this debate, we recommend the following prerequisites be met prior to attempting any human germline gene therapy:

1. Germline gene experimentation should only be undertaken to correct serious genetic disorders (for example, Tay-Sachs disease).

2. There should be considerable prior experience with human somatic cell gene therapy, which has clearly established its safety and efficacy.

3. There should be reasonable scientific evidence using appropriate animal models that germline gene therapy will cure or prevent the disease in question and not cause any harm.

4. Interventions should be undertaken only with the informed, voluntary, competent, and understanding consent of all individuals involved.

5. In addition to approval by expert panels such as the NIH's Working Group on Gene Therapy and local Institutional Review Boards, all proposals should have prior public discussion.

An international consensus is desirable, because germline gene manipulation is the area in which there is the most international concern. This presents us with the first real opportunity to develop an international forum for policy debate and perhaps even resolution. Since we are dealing with the future of the species, this does not seem like too much to expect.

NOTES

1. D. J. Weatherall, "Gene Therapy in Perspective," *Nature* 349:275–6, 1991; B. J. Culliton, "Gene Therapy on the Move," *Nature* 354–429, 1991; and M. Hoffman, "Putting New Muscle into Gene Therapy," *Science* 254:1455–6, 1991.

2. S. A. Rosenberg, P. Aebersold, K. Cornetta, A. Kasid, R. A. Morgan, R. Moen, E. M. Karson, M. T. Lotze, J. C. Yang, S. L. Topalian, M. J. Merino, K. Culver, A. D. Miller, R. M. Blaese, and W. F. Anderson, "Gene Transfer into Humans—Immunotherapy of Patients with Advanced Melanomas, Using Tumor-Infiltrating Lymphocytes Modified by Retroviral Gene Transduction," *New England Journal of Medicine* 323:570–8, 1990.

3. A. A. Gutierrez, N. R. Lemoine, and K. Sikora, "Gene Therapy for Cancer," *Lancet* 339:715–21, 1992; and A. Abbott, "Italians First to Use Stem Cells," *Nature* 356:465, 1992.

4. L. Thompson, "Human Gene Therapy Debuts at NIH," *Washington Post*, September 15, 1990, p. A1. Other researchers may claim to have conducted the first human gene transfer experiments. In the early 1970s, German researchers conducted an experiment on German sisters who suffered from a rare metabolic error that caused them to develop high blood levels of arginine. Left uncorrected, this genetic defect leads to metabolic abnormalities and mental retardation. Using Shope virus (which induces a low level of arginine in exposed humans), the researchers infected the girls in the hope that the virus would transfer its gene for the enzyme that the body needs to metabolize arginine. The attempt failed. The next experiments took place in 1980 in Italy and Israel. Turned down by the UCLA Institutional Review Board for an experiment to introduce the globin gene (by mixing the patient's bone marrow with cells with DNA coding for hemoglobin in the hope that a normal hemoglobin gene would stably incorporate into the bone marrow cells) in a patient with beta-thalassemia, Dr. Martin Cline later unsuccessfully performed this experiment on two children, one in Italy and one in Israel. He was sanctioned by the NIH for failure to obtain IRB approval and his case became notorious. See President's Commission for the Study of Ethical Problems in Medicine and Biomedical and Behavioral Research, *Splicing Life,* U.S. Government Printing Office, Stock no. 83-600500, Washington, D.C., 1982, pp. 44–5; and materials in J. Areen, P. King, S. Goldberg, and A. M. Capron, *Law, Science and Medicine,* Foundation Press, Mineola, NY, 1984, pp. 165–70.

5. For example, "Gene Therapy (Editorial)," *Lancet* 1:193–4, 1989; G. Kolata, "Why Gene Therapy Is Considered Scary but Cell Therapy Isn't," *New York Times,* September 16, 1990, p. E5.

6. E. K. Nichols, *Human Gene Therapy,* Institute of Medicine, National Academy of Science, Harvard Press, Cambridge, MA, 1988, p. 163.

7. President's Commission for the Study of Ethical Problems in Medicine and Biomedical and Behavioral Research, *Splicing Life.*

8. "Gene Therapy in Man. Recommendations of European Research Councils," *Lancet* 1:1271–2, 1988.

9. W. F. Anderson, "Human Gene Therapy: Scientific and Ethical Considerations," *Journal of Medical Philosophy* 10:275–91, 1985.

10. B. Culliton, "Gene Therapy: Into the Home Stretch," *Science* 249:974–6, 1990.

11. Department of Health and Human Services, "National Institutes of Health Points to Consider in

the Design and Submission of Human Somatic-Cell Gene Therapy Protocols," *Recombinant DNA Technical Bulletin* 9:221–42, 1986.

12. Ibid.

13. W. F. Anderson, "Human Gene Therapy: Why Draw a Line?" *Journal of Medical Philosophy* 14:681, 1989.

14. Ibid.

15. W. F. Anderson, "What's the Rush?" *Human Gene Therapy* 1:109–10, 1990.

16. U.S. Congress, Office of Technology Assessment, "New Developments in Biotechnology—Background Paper," *Public Perceptions of Biotechnology,* OTA-BBP-BA-45, U.S. Government Printing Office, Washington, D.C., May 1987.

17. G. Fowler, E. T. Juengst, and B. K. Zimmerman, "Germ-Line Gene Therapy and the Clinical Ethos of Medical Genetics," *Theoretical Medicine* 10:151–65, 1989.

18. S. Elias and G. J. Annas, *Reproductive Genetics and the Law,* Year Book, New York, 1987.

19. L. Walters, "The Ethics of Human Gene Therapy," *Nature* 320:225–7, 1986.

20. Fowler et al., 1989, and Nichols, 1988. And see generally, on human embryo experiments, P. Singer and H. Kuhse, "The Ethics of Embryo Research," and G. J. Annas, "The Ethics of Embryo Research: Not as Easy as It Sounds," *Law, Medicine & Health Care* 14:133–40, 1987.

21. Anderson, 1985.

22. A. G. Motulsky, "Impact of Genetic Manipulation on Society and Medicine," *Science* 219:135–40, 1983.

23. A. Capron, "Which Ills to Bear: Reevaluating the 'Threat' of Modern Genetics," *Emory Law Journal* 29:665–96, 1990.

24. Ibid.

25. R. Morison, "Darwinism: Foundation for an Ethical System?" *Zygon* 1:352, 1966.

26. Anderson, 1985, 1989.

27. W. F. Anderson, "Human Gene Therapy: Where to Draw the Line," unpublished draft, 1986, p. 607. Reprinted in 1987 supplement to Areen et al., 1984, p. 27.

28. Anderson, 1985, 1989.

29. D. Suzuki and P. Knudtson, *Genetics: The Clash between the New Genetics and Human Values,* Harvard Press, Cambridge, MA, 1989.

30. U.S. Congress, Office of Technology Assessment, *Mapping Our Genes,* OTA-BA-373, U.S. Government Printing Office, Washington, D.C., April 1988.

31. S. Krimsky, "Human Gene Therapy: Must We Know Where to Stop before We Start?" *Human Gene Therapy* 1:171–3, 1990.

32. B. Davis, "Limits to Genetic Intervention in Humans: Somatic and Germline," in *Human Genetic Information: Science, Law and Ethics,* Ciba Foundation Symposium 149, John Wiley and Sons, New York, 1990.

33. Walters, 1986.

34. Gutierrez et al., 1992.

35. R. M. Cook-Deegan, "Human Gene Therapy and Congress," *Human Gene Therapy* 1:163–70, 1990.

All for the Good:
Why Genetic Engineering Must Soldier On

JAMES D. WATSON

THERE IS LOTS OF ZIP in DNA-based biology today. With each passing year it incorporates

DR. JAMES WATSON is President of Cold Spring Harbor Laboratory, New York, and winner of the 1992 Nobel Prize in medicine.

an ever increasing fraction of the life sciences, ranging from single-cell organisms, like bacteria and yeast, to the complexities of the human brain. All this wonderful biological frenzy was unimaginable when I first entered the world of

From Time *magazine, January 11, 1999. Reprinted by permission of James D. Watson.*

genetics. In 1948, biology was an all too descriptive discipline near the bottom of science's totem pole, with physics at its top. By then Einstein's turn-of-the-century ideas about the interconversion of matter and energy had been transformed into the powers of the atom. If not held in check, the weapons they made possible might well destroy the very fabric of civilized human life. So physicists of the late 1940s were simultaneously revered for making atoms relevant to society and feared for what their toys could do if they were to fall into the hands of evil.

Such ambivalent feelings are now widely held toward biology. The double-helical structure of DNA, initially admired for its intellectual simplicity, today represents to many a double-edged sword that can be used for evil as well as good. No sooner had scientists at Stanford University in 1973 begun rearranging DNA molecules in test tubes (and, equally important, reinserting the novel DNA segments back into living cells) than critics began likening these "recombinant" DNA procedures to the physicist's power to break apart atoms. Might not some of the test-tube-rearranged DNA molecules impart to their host cells disease-causing capacities that, like nuclear weapons, are capable of seriously disrupting human civilization? Soon there were cries from both scientists and nonscientists that such research might best be ruled by stringent regulations — if not laws.

As a result, several years were to pass before the full power of recombinant-DNA technology got into the hands of working scientists, who by then were itching to explore previously unattainable secrets of life. Happily, the proposals to control recombinant-DNA research through legislation never got close to enactment. And when anti-DNA doomsday scenarios failed to materialize, even the modestly restrictive governmental regulations began to wither away. In retrospect, recombinant-DNA may rank as the safest revolutionary technology ever developed. To my knowledge, not one fatality, much less illness, has been caused by a genetically manipulated organism. The moral I draw from this painful episode is this: Never postpone experiments that have clearly defined future benefits for fear of dangers that can't be quantified. Though it may sound at first uncaring, we can react rationally only to real (as opposed to hypothetical) risks. Yet for several years we postponed important experiments on the genetic basis of cancer, for example, because we took much too seriously spurious arguments that the genes at the root of human cancer might themselves be dangerous to work with.

Though most forms of DNA manipulation are now effectively unregulated, one important potential goal remains blocked. Experiments aimed at learning how to insert functional genetic material into human germ cells — sperm and eggs — remain off limits to most of the world's scientists. No governmental body wants to take responsibility for initiating steps that might help redirect the course of future human evolution. These decisions reflect widespread concerns that we, as humans, may not have the wisdom to modify the most precious of all human treasures — our chromosomal "instruction books." Dare we be entrusted with improving upon the results of the several million years of Darwinian natural selection? Are human germ cells Rubicons that geneticists may never cross?

Unlike many of my peers, I'm reluctant to accept such reasoning, again using the argument that you should never put off doing something useful for fear of evil that may never arrive. The first germ-line gene manipulations are unlikely to be attempted for frivolous reasons. Nor does the state of today's science provide the knowledge that would be needed to generate "superpersons" whose far-ranging talents would make those who are genetically unmodified feel redundant and unwanted. Such creations will remain denizens of science fiction, not the real world, far into the future. When they are finally attempted, germ-line genetic manipulations will probably be done to change a death sentence into a life verdict — by creating children who are resistant to a deadly virus, for example, much the way we can already protect plants from viruses by inserting antiviral DNA segments into their genomes.

If appropriate go-ahead signals come, the first resulting gene-bettered children will in no sense threaten human civilization. They will be seen as special only by those in their immediate circles, and are likely to pass as unnoticed in later life as the now grownup "test tube baby" Louise Brown does today. If they grow up healthily gene-bettered, more such children will follow, and they and those whose lives are enriched by their exis-

tence will rejoice that science has again improved human life. If, however, the added genetic material fails to work, better procedures must be developed before more couples commit their psyches toward such inherently unsettling pathways to producing healthy children. Moving forward will not be for the faint of heart. But if the next century witnesses failure, let it be because our science is not yet up to the job, not because we don't have the courage to make less random the sometimes most unfair courses of human evolution.

Genetics and Reproductive Risk: Can Having Children Be Immoral?

LAURA M. PURDY

IS IT MORALLY PERMISSIBLE for me to have children?[1] A decision to procreate is surely one of the most significant decisions a person can make. So it would seem that it ought not to be made without some moral soul-searching.

There are many reasons why one might hesitate to bring children into this world if one is concerned about their welfare. Some are rather general, like the deteriorating environment or

the prospect of poverty. Others have a narrower focus, like continuing civil war in Ireland, or the lack of essential social support for child rearing persons in the United States. Still others may be relevant only to individuals at risk of passing harmful diseases to their offspring.

There are many causes of misery in this world, and most of them are unrelated to genetic disease. In the general scheme of things, human misery is most efficiently reduced by concentrating on noxious social and political arrangements. Nonetheless, we shouldn't ignore preventable harm just because it is confined to a relatively small corner of life. So the question arises: can it

LAURA PURDY, recently a visiting Bioethicist and Professor of Philosophy at the University of Toronto Joint Centre for Bioethics, University Health Network, Department of Philosophy, is a Professor of Philosophy at Wells College, N.Y.

From Laura Purdy, Reproducing Persons: Issues in Feminist Bioethics, *Ithaca, N.Y.: Cornell University Press, 1996. Copyright 1996 Cornell University. Used by permission of the publisher, Cornell University Press, and by Laura M. Purdy.*

be wrong to have a child because of genetic risk factors?[2]

Unsurprisingly, most of the debate about this issue has focused on prenatal screening and abortion: much useful information about a given fetus can be made available by recourse to prenatal testing. This fact has meant that moral questions about reproduction have become entwined with abortion politics, to the detriment of both. The abortion connection has made it especially difficult to think about whether it is wrong to prevent a child from coming into being since doing so might involve what many people see as wrongful killing; yet there is no necessary link between the two. Clearly, the existence of genetically compromised children can be prevented not only by aborting already existing fetuses but also by preventing conception in the first place.

Worse yet, many discussions simply assume a particular view of abortion, without any recognition of other possible positions and the difference they make in how people understand the issues. For example, those who object to aborting fetuses with genetic problems often argue that doing so would undermine our conviction that all humans are in some important sense equal.[3] However, this position rests on the assumption that conception marks the point at which humans are endowed with a right to life. So aborting fetuses with genetic problems looks morally the same as killing "imperfect" people without their consent.

This position raises two separate issues. One pertains to the legitimacy of different views on abortion. Despite the conviction of many abortion activists to the contrary, I believe that ethically respectable views can be found on different sides of the debate, including one that sees fetuses as developing humans without any serious moral claim on continued life. There is no space here to address the details, and doing so would be once again to fall into the trap of letting the abortion question swallow up all others. Fortunately, this issue need not be resolved here. However, opponents of abortion need to face the fact that many thoughtful individuals do not

see fetuses as moral persons. It follows that their reasoning process and hence the implications of their decisions are radically different from those envisioned by opponents of prenatal screening and abortion. So where the latter see genetic abortion as murdering people who just don't measure up, the former see it as a way to prevent the development of persons who are more likely to live miserable lives. This is consistent with a world view that values persons equally and holds that each deserves high quality life. Some of those who object to genetic abortion appear to be oblivious to these psychological and logical facts. It follows that the nightmare scenarios they paint for us are beside the point: many people simply do not share the assumptions that make them plausible.

How are these points relevant to my discussion? My primary concern hire is to argue that conception can sometimes be morally wrong on grounds of genetic risk, although this judgment will not apply to those who accept the moral legitimacy of abortion and are willing to employ prenatal screening and selective abortion. If my case is solid, then those who oppose abortion must be especially careful not to conceive in certain cases, as they are, of course, free to follow their conscience about abortion. Those like myself who do not see abortion as murder have more ways to prevent birth.

HUNTINGTON'S DISEASE

There is always some possibility that reproduction will result in a child with a serious disease or handicap. Genetic counselors can help individuals determine whether they are at unusual risk and, as the Human Genome Project rolls on, their knowledge will increase by quantum leaps. As this knowledge becomes available, I believe we ought to use it to determine whether possible children are at risk *before* they are conceived.

I want in this paper to defend the thesis that it is morally wrong to reproduce when we know there is a high risk of transmitting a serious disease or defect. This thesis holds that some reproductive acts are wrong, and my argument puts the burden of proof on those who disagree with it to show why its conclusions can be overridden. Hence it denies that people should be free to reproduce mindless of the consequences.[4] However, as moral argument, it should be taken as a proposal for further debate and discussion. It is not, by itself, an argument in favor of legal prohibitions of reproduction.[5]

There is a huge range of genetic diseases. Some are quickly lethal; others kill more slowly, if at all. Some are mainly physical, some mainly mental; others impair both kinds of function. Some interfere tremendously with normal functioning, others less. Some are painful, some are not. There seems to be considerable agreement that rapidly lethal diseases, especially those, like Tay-Sachs, accompanied by painful deterioration, should be prevented even at the cost of abortion. Conversely, there seems to be substantial agreement that relatively trivial problems, especially cosmetic ones, would not be legitimate grounds for abortion.[6] In short, there are cases ranging from low risk of mild disease or disability to high risk of serious disease or disability. Although it is difficult to decide where the duty to refrain from procreation becomes compelling, I believe that there are some clear cases. I have chosen to focus on Huntington's Disease to illustrate the kinds of concrete issues such decisions entail. However, the arguments presented here are also relevant to many other genetic diseases.[7]

The symptoms of Huntington's Disease usually begin between the ages of thirty and fifty. It happens this way:

> Onset is insidious. Personality changes (obstinacy, moodiness, lack of initiative) frequently antedate or accompany the involuntary choreic movements. These usually appear first in the face, neck, and arms, and are jerky, irregular, and stretching in character. Contractions of the facial muscles result in grimaces; those of the respiratory muscles, lips, and tongue lead to hesitating, explosive speech. Irregular movements of the trunk are present; the gait is shuffling and dancing. Tendon reflexes are increased. . . . Some patients display a fatuous euphoria; others are spiteful, irascible, destructive, and violent. Paranoid reactions are common. Poverty of thought and impairment of attention, memory, and judgment occur. As the disease progresses, walking becomes impossible, swallowing difficult, and dementia profound. Suicide is not uncommon.[8]

The illness lasts about fifteen years, terminating in death.

Huntington's Disease is an autosomal dominant disease, meaning that it is caused by a single defective gene located on a non-sex chromosome. It is passed from one generation to the next via affected individuals. Each child of such an affected person has a fifty percent risk of inheriting the gene and thus of eventually developing the disease, even if he or she was born before the parent's disease was evident.[9]

Until recently, Huntington's Disease was especially problematic because most affected individuals did not know whether they had the gene for the disease until well into their childbearing years. So they had to decide about childbearing before knowing whether they could transmit the disease or not. If, in time, they did not develop symptoms of the disease, then their children could know they were not at risk for the disease. If unfortunately they did develop symptoms, then each of their children could know there was a fifty percent chance that they, too, had inherited the gene. In both cases, the children faced a period of prolonged anxiety as to whether they would develop the disease. Then, in the 1980s, thanks in part to an energetic campaign by Nancy Wexler, a genetic marker was found that, in certain circumstances, could tell people with a relatively high degree of probability whether or not they had the gene for the disease.[10] Finally, in March 1993, the defective gene itself was discovered.[11] Now individuals can find out whether they carry the gene for the disease, and prenatal screening can tell us whether a given fetus has inherited it. These technological developments change the moral scene substantially.

How serious are the risks involved in Huntington's Disease? Geneticists often think a ten percent risk is high.[12] But risk assessment also depends on what is at stake: the worse the possible outcome the more undesirable an otherwise small risk seems. In medicine, as elsewhere, people may regard the same result quite differently. But for devastating diseases like Huntington's this part of the judgment should be unproblematic: no one wants a loved one to suffer in this way.[13]

There may still be considerable disagreement about the acceptability of a given risk. So it would be difficult in many circumstances to say how we should respond to a particular risk. Nevertheless, there are good grounds for a conservative approach, for it is reasonable to take special precautions to avoid very bad consequences, even if the risk is small. But the possible consequences here *are* very bad: a child who may inherit Huntington's Disease has a much greater than average chance of being subjected to severe and prolonged suffering. And it is one thing to risk one's own welfare, but quite another to do so for others and without their consent.

Is this judgment about Huntington's Disease really defensible? People appear to have quite different opinions. Optimists argue that a child born into a family afflicted with Huntington's Disease has a reasonable chance of living a satisfactory life. After all, even children born of an afflicted parent still have a fifty percent chance of escaping the disease. And even if afflicted themselves, such people will probably enjoy some thirty years of healthy life before symptoms appear. It is also possible, although not at all likely, that some might not mind the symptoms caused by the disease. Optimists can point to diseased persons who have lived fruitful lives, as well as those who seem genuinely glad to be alive. One is Rick Donohue, a sufferer from the Joseph family disease: "You know, if my mom hadn't

had me, I wouldn't be here for the life I have had. So there is a good possibility I will have children."[14] Optimists therefore conclude that it would be a shame if these persons had not lived.

Pessimists concede some of these facts, but take a less sanguine view of them. They think a fifty percent risk of serious disease like Huntington's appallingly high. They suspect that many children born into afflicted families are liable to spend their youth in dreadful anticipation and fear of the disease. They expect that the disease, if it appears, will be perceived as a tragic and painful end to a blighted life. They point out that Rick Donohue is still young, and has not experienced the full horror of his sickness. It is also well-known that some young persons have such a dilated sense of time that they can hardly envision themselves at thirty or forty, so the prospect of pain at that age is unreal to them.[15]

More empirical research on the psychology and life history of sufferers and potential sufferers is clearly needed to decide whether optimists or pessimists have a more accurate picture of the experiences of individuals at risk. But given that some will surely realize pessimists' worst fears, it seems unfair to conclude that the pleasures of those who deal best with the situation simply cancel out the suffering of those others when that suffering could be avoided altogether.

I think that these points indicate that the morality of procreation in situations like this demands further investigation. I propose to do this by looking first at the position of the possible child, then at that of the potential parent.

POSSIBLE CHILDREN AND POTENTIAL PARENTS

The first task in treating the problem from the child's point of view is to find a way of referring to possible future offspring without seeming to confer some sort of morally significant existence upon them. I will follow the convention of calling children who might be born in the future but who are not now conceived "possible" children, offspring, individuals, or persons.

Now, what claims about children or possible children are relevant to the morality of childbearing in the circumstances being considered? Of primary importance is the judgment that we ought to try to provide every child with something like a minimally satisfying life. I am not altogether sure how best to formulate this standard but I want clearly to reject the view that it is morally permissible to conceive individuals so long as we do not expect them to be so miserable that they wish they were dead.[16] I believe that this kind of moral minimalism is thoroughly unsatisfactory and that not many people would really want to live in a world where it was the prevailing standard. Its lure is that it puts few demands on us, but its price is the scant attention it pays to human well-being.

How might the judgment that we have a duty to try to provide a minimally satisfying life for our children be justified? It could, I think, be derived fairly straightforwardly from either utilitarian or contractarian theories of justice, although there is no space here for discussion of the details. The net result of such analysis would be the conclusion that neglecting this duty would create unnecessary unhappiness or unfair disadvantage for some persons.

Of course, this line of reasoning confronts us with the need to spell out what is meant by "minimally satisfying" and what a standard based on this concept would require of us. Conceptions of a minimally satisfying life vary tremendously among societies and also within them. *De Rigueur* in some circles are private music lessons and trips to Europe, while in others providing eight years of schooling is a major accomplishment. But there is no need to consider this complication at length here since we are concerned only with health as a prerequisite for a minimally satisfying life. Thus, as we draw out what such a standard might require of us, it seems reasonable to retreat to the more limited claim that parents should try to ensure something like normal health for their children. It might be thought that even this moderate claim is unsatisfactory since in some places debilitating conditions are the norm, but one could circumvent this objection by saying that parents ought to try to provide for their children health normal for that culture, even though it may be inadequate if measured by some outside standard.[17] This conservative position would still justify efforts to avoid the birth of children at risk for Huntington's Disease and other serious genetic diseases in virtually all societies.[18]

This view is reinforced by the following considerations. Given that possible children do not presently exist as actual individuals, they do not have a right to be brought into existence, and hence no one is maltreated by measures to avoid the conception of a possible person. Therefore, the conservative course that avoids the conception of those who would not be expected to enjoy a minimally satisfying life is at present the only fair course of action. The alternative is a laissez-faire approach which brings into existence the lucky, but only at the expense of the unlucky. Notice that attempting to avoid the creation of the unlucky does not necessarily lead to *fewer* people being brought into being; the question boils down to taking steps to bring those with better prospects into existence, instead of those with worse ones.

I have so far argued that if people with Huntington's Disease are unlikely to live minimally satisfying lives, then those who might pass it on should not have genetically related children. This is consonant with the principle that the greater the danger of serious problems, the stronger the duty to avoid them. But this principle is in conflict with what people think of as the right to reproduce. How might one decide which should take precedence?

Expecting people to forego having genetically related children might seem to demand too great a sacrifice of them. But before reaching that conclusion we need to ask what is really at stake. One reason for wanting children is to experience family life, including love, companionship, watching kids grow, sharing their pains and triumphs, and helping to form members of the next generation. Other reasons emphasize the validation of parents as individuals within a continuous family line, children as a source of immortality, or perhaps even the gratification of producing partial replicas of oneself. Children may also be desired in an effort to prove that one is an adult, to try to cement a marriage or to benefit parents economically.

Are there alternative ways of satisfying these desires? Adoption or new reproductive technologies can fulfill many of them without passing on known genetic defects. Replacements for sperm have been available for many years via artificial insemination by donor. More recently, egg donation, sometimes in combination with contract pregnancy,[19] has been used to provide eggs for women who prefer not to use their own. Eventually it may be possible to clone individual humans, although that now seems a long way off. All of these approaches to avoiding the use of particular genetic material are controversial and have generated much debate. I believe that tenable moral versions of each do exist.[20]

None of these methods permits people to extend both genetic lines, or realize the desire for immortality or for children who resemble both parents; nor is it clear that such alternatives will necessarily succeed in proving that one is an adult, cementing a marriage, or providing economic benefits. Yet, many people feel these desires strongly. Now, I am sympathetic to William James's dictum regarding desires: "Take any demand, however slight, which any creature, however weak, may make. Ought it not, for its own sole sake be satisfied? If not, prove why not."[21] Thus a world where more desires are satisfied is generally better than one where fewer are. However, not all desires can be legitimately satisfied since, as James suggests, there may be good reasons—such as the conflict of duty and desire—why some should be overruled.

Fortunately, further scrutiny of the situation reveals that there are good reasons why people should attempt—with appropriate social support—to talk themselves out of the desires in question or to consider novel ways of fulfilling them. Wanting to see the genetic line continued is not particularly rational when it brings a sinister legacy of illness and death. The desire for immortality cannot really be satisfied anyway, and people need to face the fact that what really matters is how they behave in their own lifetime. And finally, the desire for children who physically resemble one is understandable, but basically narcissistic, and its fulfillment cannot be guaranteed even by normal reproduction. There are other ways of proving one is an adult, and other ways of cementing marriages—and children don't necessarily do either. Children, especially prematurely ill children, may not provide the expected economic benefits anyway. Nongenetically related children may also provide benefits similar to those that would have been provided by genetically related ones, and expected economic benefit is, in many cases, a morally questionable reason for having children.

Before the advent of reliable genetic testing, the options of people in Huntington's families were cruelly limited. On the one hand, they could have children, but at the risk of eventual crippling illness and death for them. On the other, they could refrain from childbearing, sparing their possible children from significant risk of inheriting this disease, perhaps frustrating intense desires to procreate—only to discover, in some cases, that their sacrifice was unnecessary because they did not develop the disease. Or they could attempt to adopt or try new reproductive approaches.

Reliable genetic testing has opened up new possibilities. Those at risk who wish to have children can get tested. If they test positive, they know their possible children are at risk. Those who are opposed to abortion must be especially careful to avoid conception if they are to behave responsibly. Those not opposed to abortion can responsibly conceive children, but only if they are willing to test each fetus and abort those who carry the gene. If individuals at risk test negative, they are home free.

What about those who cannot face the test for themselves? They can do prenatal testing and abort fetuses who carry the defective gene. A clearly positive test also implies that the parent is affected, although negative tests do not rule out that possibility. Prenatal testing can thus bring knowledge that enables one to avoid passing the disease to others, but only, in some cases, at the cost of coming to know with certainty that one will indeed develop the disease. This situation raises with peculiar force the question of whether parental responsibility requires people to get tested.

Some people think that we should recognize a right "not to know." It seems to me that such a right could be defended only where ignorance does not put others at serious risk. So if people are prepared to forego genetically related children, they need not get tested. But if they want genetically related children then they must do whatever is necessary to ensure that affected babies are not the result. There is, after all, something inconsistent about the claim that one has a right to be shielded from the truth, even if the price is to risk inflicting on one's children the same dread disease one cannot even face in oneself.

In sum, until we can be assured that Huntington's Disease does not prevent people from living a minimally satisfying life, individuals at risk for the disease have a moral duty to try not to bring affected babies into this world. There are now enough options available so that this duty needn't frustrate their reasonable desires. Society has a corresponding duty to facilitate moral behavior on the part of individuals. Such support ranges from the narrow and concrete (like making sure that medical testing and counseling is available to all) to the more general social environment that guarantees that all pregnancies are voluntary, that pronatalism is eradicated, and that women are treated with respect regardless of the reproductive options they choose.

NOTES

1. This paper is loosely based on "Genetic Diseases: Can Having Children Be Immoral?" originally published in *Genetics Now,* ed. John L. Buckley (Washington, DC: University Press of America, 1978) and subsequently anthologized in a number of medical ethics texts. Thanks to Thomas Mappes and David DeGrazia for their helpful suggestions about updating the paper.

2. I focus on genetic considerations, although with the advent of AIDS the scope of the general question here could be expanded. There are two reasons for sticking to this relatively narrow formulation. One is that dealing with a smaller chunk of the problem may help us think more clearly, while realizing that some conclusions may nonetheless be relevant to the larger problem. The other is the peculiar capacity of some genetic problems to affect ever more individuals in the future.

3. For example, see Leon Kass, "Implications of Prenatal Diagnosis for the Human Right to Life," *Ethical Issues in Human Genetics,* eds. Bruce Hilton et al. (New York: Plenum Press, 1973).

4. This is, of course, a very broad thesis. I defend an even broader version in "Loving Future People," *Reproduction, Ethics and the Law,* ed. Joan Callahan (Bloomington, Indiana University Press, forthcoming).

5. Why would we want to resist legal enforcement of every moral conclusion? First, legal action has many costs, costs not necessarily worth paying in particular cases. Second, legal enforcement would tend to take the matter in question out of the realm of debate and treat it as settled. But in many cases, especially where mores or technology are rapidly evolving, we don't want that to happen. Third, legal enforcement would undermine individual freedom and decision-making capacity. In some cases, the ends envisioned are important enough to warrant putting up with these disadvantages, but that remains to be shown in each case.

6. Those who do not see fetuses as moral persons with a right to life may nonetheless hold that abortion is justifiable in these cases. I argue at some length elsewhere that lesser defects can cause great suffering. Once we are clear that there is nothing discriminatory about failing to conceive particular possible individuals, it makes sense, other things being equal, to avoid the prospect of such pain if we can. Naturally, other

things rarely are equal. In the first place, many problems go undiscovered until a baby is born. Secondly, there are often substantial costs associated with screening programs. Thirdly, although women should be encouraged to consider the moral dimensions of routine pregnancy, we do not want it to be so fraught with tension that it becomes a miserable experience. (See "Loving Future People.")

7. It should be noted that failing to conceive a single individual can affect many lives: in 1916, nine hundred and sixty-two cases could be traced from six seventeenth-century arrivals in America. See Gordon Rattray Taylor, *The Biological Time Bomb* (New York, 1968), p. 176.

8. *The Merck Manual* (Rahway, NJ: Merck, 1972), pp. 1363, 1346. We now know that the age of onset and severity of the disease is related to the number of abnormal replications of the glutamine code on the abnormal gene. See Andrew Revkin, "Hunting Down Huntington's," *Discover*, December 1993, p. 108.

9. Hymie Gordon, "Genetic Counseling," *JAMA*, Vol. 217, n. 9 (August 30, 1971), p. 1346.

10. See Revkin, "Hunting Down Huntington's," pp. 99–108.

11. "Gene for Huntington's Disease Discovered," *Human Genome News*, Vol. 5, n. 1 (May 1993), p. 5.

12. Charles Smith, Susan Holloway, and Alan E. H. Emery, "Individuals at Risk in Families—Genetic Disease," *Journal of Medical Genetics*, Vol. 8 (1971), p. 453.

13. To try to separate the issue of the gravity of the disease from the existence of a given individual, compare this situation with how we would assess a parent who neglected to vaccinate an existing child against a hypothetical viral version of Huntington's.

14. *The New York Times*, September 30, 1975, p. 1, col. 6. The Joseph family disease is similar to Huntington's Disease, except that symptoms start appearing in the twenties. Rick Donohue was in his early twenties at the time he made this statement.

15. I have talked to college students who believe that they will have lived fully and be ready to die at those ages. It is astonishing how one's perspective changes over time, and how ages that one once associated with senility and physical collapse come to seem the prime of human life.

16. The view I am rejecting has been forcefully articulated by Derek Parfit, *Reasons and Persons* (Oxford: Oxford University Press, 1984). For more discussion, see "Loving Future People."

17. I have some qualms about this response since I fear that some human groups are so badly off that it might still be wrong for them to procreate, even if that would mean great changes in their cultures. But this is a complicated issue that needs its own investigation.

18. Again, a troubling exception might be the isolated Venezuelan group Nancy Wexler found where, because of in-breeding, a large proportion of the population is affected by Huntington's. See Revkin, "Hunting Down Huntington's."

19. Or surrogacy, as it has been popularly known. I think that "contract pregnancy" is more accurate and more respectful of women. Eggs can be provided either by a woman who also gestates the fetus or by a third party.

20. The most powerful objections to new reproductive technologies and arrangements concern possible bad consequences for women. However, I do not think that the arguments against them on these grounds have yet shown the dangers to be as great as some believe. So although it is perhaps true that new reproductive technologies and arrangements shouldn't be used lightly, avoiding the conceptions discussed here is well worth the risk. For a series of viewpoints on this issue, including my own "Another Look at Contract Pregnancy," see Helen B. Holmes, *Issues in Reproductive Technology I: An Anthology* (New York: Garland Press, 1992).

21. *Essays in Pragmatism*, ed. A. Castell (New York, 1948), p. 73.

Worrying—and Worrying about—the Geneticization of Reproduction and Health

ABBY LIPPMAN

BIOMEDICAL RESEARCHERS are today re-defining human geography. These modern explorers are elaborating a new map of humans, a map based on genes that is likely to alter our views of the world—and our place in it—even more profoundly than did the maps generated by Columbus and other 15th and 16th century explorers. This mapmaking has already begun to alter our perceptions of self and other, of normality and abnormality, and to change our concepts of cause and prevention. This is probably more so in the area of reproduction than any other. This paper stems from work in progress in which I am examining the stories being told by today's colonizers, scientists, about their explorations and about the new world of disease, health and reproduction they are defining.

Let me note right away that I use the word "stories" not to suggest that what scientists are saying is not true; this may or may not be the case. Rather, I use it in a literary not a legal sense to capture the idea that how scientists present their observations and study results is no different from how novelists present their interpretations of the external world. Both sets of story-tellers tame, shape and interpret "raw" material to convey a message, with the construction of each reflecting their prior beliefs and the prevail-

ABBY LIPPMAN is a professor in the Department of Epidemiology & Biostatistics, McGill University.

ing social/cultural context. The stories told by scientists, therefore, are as appropriately objects of analysis as are the stories of other writers, and the stories in which I am especially interested deal with matters of health and disease.

Judging by headlines in newspapers and titles of articles in professional journals, today's stories on these issues are being told increasingly in the language of genetics. Using the metaphor of blueprints or texts, genes and DNA fragments are presented as a set of instructions to make us who and what we are, with zealots going so far as to describe human diseases as "typographical errors" (Shapiro, 1990). Through these stories, which are beginning to threaten seriously other narratives, geneticists and others are conditioning how we name, view and propose to manage a whole host of disorders and disabilities, with "genetics" increasingly identified as the way to reveal and explain health and disease, normality and abnormality (e.g. Baird, 1990). These stories are already directing how intellectual and financial resources are applied to resolve health problems but, even more critically, they are profoundly influencing our values and attitudes.

To capture this process, and to summarize the major theme of the stories, I have begun to use the term "geneticization." Very briefly, I define as geneticization the ongoing process that includes the ever-growing tendencies to name things that distinguish one person from another as genetic

Reprinted from Misconceptions: The Social Construction of Choice and the New Reproductive and Genetic Technologies, Vol. 1, Gwynne Basen, Margrit Eichler, and Abby Lippman, eds. Hull, Quebec: Voyageur Publishing, 1993. Permission granted by Abby Lippmann.

in origin, to reduce differences between individuals to their DNA codes and to define most disorders, behaviors and physiological variations as at least partly genetic in origin. It involves the use of genetic tools to look for differences between people and the application of genetic interventions and services to resolve multiple health and social problems.

Geneticization is social and political as well—maybe even more than it is—biomedical. It is also a process of colonization insofar as genetic technologies and approaches are applied to areas not necessarily genetic. Its most costly expression is the international genome program to map and sequence the 50,000–100,000 human genes . . .; its most widespread application thus far is prenatal diagnosis which comprises the multiple screening and testing procedures used to assess the physical status of the fetus or embryo during —if not before—a woman's pregnancy.

Geneticization places more and more areas of women's experiences under the territorial control of genetics, subject to genetic ideas about both the conditions for and the quality of life. While geneticization does not reverberate identically for all women, some general issues do appear to cut across racial, income, social status, ethnic and ability differences and I emphasize these common matters when I suggest it is important for us to "*worry*" about the process and the technologies of genetic screening and testing it engenders. . . .

PRENATAL TESTING

Before I consider some general sources to, and of, worry, some background about prenatal testing may be useful.

Examination of the fetus in utero probably first occurred almost 100 years ago when an x-ray picture was taken of a dead fetus. However, prenatal screening and diagnosis as we think of them now have been available "routinely" to certain groups of women, selectively to others, only since amniocentesis was first performed about twenty to twenty-five years ago.

Amniocentesis and the other technologies of prenatal screening and diagnosis currently in use provide access to fetal cells and amniotic fluid and enable the visualization of the developing fetus. Using these technologies, all recognizable chromosomal variations, many selected developmental malformations, over 150 biochemical disorders, and fetal sex can be detected before birth, with the list continuing to expand and the techniques being applied earlier and earlier in pregnancy. If prenatal diagnosis were first used for conditions generally regarded by physicians as "serious," and for which there were no effective treatments, as developers claim, it is now available for conditions with little or uncertain impact on postnatal health and functioning; for conditions that will appear, if at all, only in adulthood; and for conditions for which no treatment exists. The speed with which these new technologies have been adopted into clinical practice and the growing number of women to whom they are applied are staggering.

Amniocentesis is, to date, the most widely used procedure for obtaining fetal cells. Performed at about sixteen to twenty weeks' gestation, with studies underway to assess the safety of its earlier use, amniocentesis involves the insertion of a thin hollow needle through a woman's abdomen and into the amniotic sac to remove a small sample of fluid surrounding the developing fetus. This fluid contains cells from the fetus. Once stimulated to multiply in the laboratory, these cells can then be analyzed to determine the number of chromosomes they contain, the fetal sex, and the presence of DNA sequences associated with certain specific conditions. The growth and analysis of the fetal cells may take as long as three to four weeks so that women who decide to terminate their pregnancies following test results do not obtain an abortion until about the twentieth week, which is halfway through the pregnancy.

Chorionic villus sampling (CVS) is another way of obtaining fetal cells for diagnosis. It was said to be developed specifically to permit prenatal testing earlier in pregnancy. In CVS, a small tube (catheter) is inserted through a woman's vagina and cervix. It is then advanced under ultrasound guidance until it reaches the placenta from which a small amount of tissue (chorionic villi) is removed. Any chromosomal or DNA change can, in theory, be diagnosed with tissues obtained by CVS because the cells of the fetus and the placenta (which are formed from chorionic villi) are genetically the same.

CVS can be done as early as ten weeks after a woman's last menstrual period and, while the results of tests carried out on placental tissue could be available within hours, at least a two or three day waiting period—and more often longer—is usually required. Even so, if a woman decides to end her pregnancy following CVS, the abortion can be carried out in the first trimester. The "price" of this earlier intervention includes the somewhat less accurate test results with cells obtained from CVS than from amniocentesis, the more frequent need to repeat the diagnostic procedure following CVS, the likelihood that many women who would otherwise have a spontaneous abortion (miscarriage) must now themselves make painful decisions about continuing or terminating their pregnancies and persisting uncertainty about its total safety.

In Canada, where they are covered by public funds, the use of amniocentesis and CVS have been generally restricted to women whose age (usually 35 years, a completely arbitrary criterion) is said to put them at increased risk for having a child with Down syndrome—a group that comprises about 80–90 percent of all women currently tested—and for women known to be at risk of having a child with some specific condition that can be diagnosed via fetal cells or amniotic fluid. Neither of these two tests is done "routinely" in other groups of women.

By contrast, almost all women experience another form of prenatal testing (even if it is not so-labeled) if they have access to and receive what has become part of a standard package of prenatal care: *ultrasound examinations.* . . . During these exams, now carried out earlier and earlier in pregnancy, high frequency sound waves are projected into the uterus and the sound waves that are reflected back are resolved visually to allow one to "see" the fetus on a television-like screen (and the photograph of this image often offered to a woman as the first entry for her "baby book" is now supplemented by the sale of a videotape of the "real time" scan). As a tool for prenatal diagnosis, ultrasound can be used to identify certain malformations in fetuses known to be at risk for one of these abnormalities. It can also be used to identify fetal sex. Most subtle malformations will not be identified when ultrasound is applied on a nondiagnostic basis for pregnancy dating although more obvious changes in the body shape and size of the fetus should be detectable.

Apparently on its way to becoming another universal technology for prenatal screening in Canada, is the withdrawal of a sample of blood from a pregnant woman and its analysis for the presence of alpha-fetoprotein (AFP) and, in some jurisdictions, a limited number of other serum constituents that tend to be found in increased or decreased levels when the fetus has, respectively, a malformation of the neural tube or Down syndrome. This *MS-AFP (maternal serum AFP)* analysis, performed about 16 weeks from the first day of a woman's last menstrual period before becoming pregnant, is not diagnostic. It has rather poor predictive value and, at most, only identifies women at slightly higher than average risk of having a child with one of these conditions. Most women whose initial screening results are considered to be abnormal do not have fetuses with the conditions sought, but this is only learned after the completion of confirmatory tests (ultrasound and amniocentesis) which are recommended to all in this group to establish the diagnosis (and after these women have experienced at least a fair amount of anxiety in the interim). The application of MS-AFP screening irrespective of a woman's prior risk of having a fetus with a neural tube defect or Down syndrome in community-wide programs is acknowledged to be the first mass prenatal genetic screening (which the routine ultrasound scanning of all pregnant women is not) and is already underway in several parts of Canada.

Beyond these "established" technologies are others under development and already beginning to be marketed. A growing number of investigators have begun to report their ability to obtain and make diagnoses from *fetal cells in the mother's circulation*. With the use of increasingly sophisticated technologies, these cells, which have crossed the placental barrier and entered a woman's bloodstream, can be separated from the woman's blood cells, grown in the laboratory, subjected to procedures that amplify their genetic material, and stained with specific (fluorescent) dyes to locate the presence or absence of DNA sequences. This appears to be an "up-and-coming" approach for prenatal diagnosis, and if it does provide accurate results, it would, in principle, allow what is now a "routine" for pregnant women—having a blood sample taken—to replace a medically sophisticated and much more invasive procedure such as amniocentesis or CVS for obtaining fetal cells for prenatal diagnosis.

Another approach that may proliferate in the future is *embryo or pre-implantation diagnosis*. In this approach, which is already used in programs of technological reproduction in conjunction with IVF (and for animals as well as women . . .), a very early embryo is removed from a pregnant woman (or first created in the laboratory following *in vitro* fertilization), tested, and, if it "passes," (re)placed in the uterus to continue its development. This technology has so far only been used in Canada as a research tool for the diagnosis of certain specific genetic disorders in embryos but, should it appear not to harm the child-to-be, its further application has been endorsed by many researchers. And, given that its advocates have domesticated this problematic technique by affixing it with the acronym "BABI" (blastocyst analysis before implantation)

and then declaring it to be, potentially, a particularly welcome approach because it will circumvent abortion—only "unaffected" embryos would be (re)implanted—broader application is not an unrealistic expectation. After all, those developing prenatal testing techniques have consistently assumed, despite the absence of data on the subject, that "earlier is better." In other words, that it is "better" to know before than at or after birth that something is "wrong" with the fetus; even "better" to obtain this information earlier rather than later in pregnancy; and still "better" to know the status of the fetus before a pregnancy begins because by transferring only "good" embryos the need for abortion (of "bad" embryos??) can be averted. Unfortunately, this technology cannot be considered in any depth here, but I think it essential to worry (about) pre-implantation diagnosis. It represents a marriage between reproductive and genetic technologies and a potential offspring of this union is germline gene manipulation. For, once the fertilized egg is outside a woman's body, it is accessible to those wantig to experiment with it, and an increasingly popular area for experimentation today involves the introduction of genetic material into human cells.

WHAT'S THE WORRY

Given the collection of techniques available—and only those most likely to be used in other than rare situations have been described—there seems good reason to worry (about) geneticization, and one way to begin is to consider what these technologies mean to and for women and their childbearing.

Most generally, they raise a number of fundamental concerns related to women's health and health care simply because how, when, why, to and by whom they are applied will be conditioned by prevailing attitudes about women, their bodies and their social roles. So long as procreation, pregnancy and motherhood are (still) seen as central to being a woman in our sexist society, women will experience testing not merely as parents, but in ways peculiar to being *mothers* of children, ways that usually cut across traditional distinctions between us. And, because the world in which genetic and other reproductive technologies are developing is gendered, these technologies cannot be neutral or escape gendered use.

Thus, I worry from the start about how societal powers and privileges embedded in local screening practices shape women's plans for and experiences of maternity. Women are already, if differentially, disadvantaged, generally powerless, vulnerable to offers of services because of their diminished status, challenged by prejudicial norms surrounding motherhood and delegated responsibility for family health, and prenatal diagnosis cannot but be influenced by—and itself influence—these features of our lives. Furthermore, women have not played a major role in developing these techniques, but as children's primary caregivers, may become beholden to their use.

Beyond this, I worry because already, prenatal testing has been naturalized through stories which describe it as only a response to pregnant women at "genetic risk" who "need" some reassurance, as something women "choose" (see Lippman, 1986). But these reports, as all "stories" about prenatal testing, are not records of experiences so much as they are ways to produce meanings and so I worry about the use of these words in this context.

In North America today, where major responsibility for family health care is still allocated to women who alone are expected to do all that is recommended or available for the sake of their children, it is not surprising that a woman offered ultrasound or serum screening by an expert who implies that she really wants to have a healthy child (doesn't she?) perceives a *need* to be tested, to do all that is recommended. But can we really know if her agreement to testing in such a context is an expression of choice, an instance of conformity or a response to coercion?

Certainly, reports about prenatal testing hide the second and third possibilities (conformity and coercion) when considerations of the (macro and micro) constraints and expectations in which needs arise and choice occurs are absent from them. How and by whom has need been constructed, has choice been defined?

The interpretation of "need" is always political. Thus, feminists and others who question the prevailing interpretations and the extent of choice provided by the current practice of prenatal testing are seeking *not* to limit women's options, but to enlarge their number, insure their availability and involve women in their creation. To these critics, myself included, choice in prenatal testing requires not merely that women can themselves opt for a particular procedure but that women who reject the process are not questioned about their motives more than are women who agree immediately to testing, which is not how the women we have interviewed describe their experiences. It means that a woman can continue her pregnancy after a fetal diagnosis is made because help to support a child with a disability is guaranteed, which is not what the women we talk to perceive. And, it means that personal actions are completely severed from public agendas so that a *decrease* in "uptake" rates of testing from current levels might be seen to measure the success, not the failure, of prenatal screening, which is not how geneticists now view usage (cf Clarke, 1990).

In fact, in exploring the matter of choice in prenatal testing even further, it may be that the process in North America actually impedes or restricts free decision-making and choice. Let me explain.

In general, our reviews of medical genetics texts and of material presented to women considering the possibility of prenatal testing show that these documents convey only partial information in their highly charged stories about Down syndrome (Lippman and Brunger, 1991); about the disease-preventing capabilities of fetal diagnosis; and about the routine nature of this intervention. By aiming at entirely legitimate desires (of all women for a healthy child) and normative (if not self-serving) beliefs (that medical technology provides a way to fulfill these desires), offers of prenatal testing leave little opportunity for a woman to reflect meaningfully and develop her own knowledge of and opinions about Down syndrome or testing. Even when genetic counseling is provided prior to prenatal diagnosis (and with the huge expansion in testing programs this is becoming less and less common), the discussion is directed towards the technology, not to the range of possibilities for the pregnant woman 35 years of age or older. "Counseling," when it is provided at all, is programmed into the use of the technology rather than made available independently of this agenda. How else to explain the situation where only the women who *decline* screening are referred for genetic counseling in some jurisdictions (Green et al., 1993), where only the women who *reject* parts of the antenatal care package—if they are white and well-educated—are treated as somehow "abnormal." It would appear as if medical care providers take a Caucasian, middle-class, biomedical perspective as the norm and more easily allow African-Canadian and Asian-Canadian women to opt out, apparently assuming that *their* rejection of testing must reflect some ethnic difference from "us" to which we should be sensitive.

The minimal concern with informed choice in prenatal testing seems reflected, too, in how both the women and the counselors we have interviewed seem to regard their concerns about and reluctance towards testing as obstacles to decision-making rather than as valid expressions of the moral malaise the procedures arouse. And, it is reflected further in our observation that genetic counselors take a positive response to their question, "Have you ever heard of Down syndrome?" as sufficient evidence that a woman planning to be tested is informed about the reasons for testing. . . .

Most counseling is provided by a genetics counselor in a genetics clinics[1] (cf Scutt, 1991), and usually with enormous time pressures because of limits on what stage of pregnancy in which testing can be carried out, a situation and set of circumstances that do not foster reasoned reflection. (A not dissimilar situation exists when women who have failed to conceive as quickly as they had hoped receive counseling only in an infertility clinic; when contraceptive advice is given in a population control rather than a family planning program.)

Thus, while a woman may only exceptionally be told directly to be tested or to abort, and consequently most can give the appearance of choosing, any empowerment these women have is primarily provisional and conditional. In a society where warning labels and public advertisements constantly remind women that what they do can harm the fetus, but that if they behave responsibly, they can reduce this harm, offers of prenatal screening and testing are hardly "neutral" and even, perhaps, impossible to refuse (except for a very determined few). There are rewards and sanctions, both, implicit and explicit, that invite and encourage their use. . . .

MORE TO WORRY (ABOUT)

Prenatal testing programs express the historically-based nexus between control over reproduction and control over heredity—with the nexus located in women's bodies. Whatever may be claimed as motives, therefore, prenatal testing cannot but be eugenic. These programs are for detecting and preventing the birth of certain babies, in fact for "gatekeeping." This is most evident when the diagnosis of embryos obtained following *in vitro* fertilization and the transfer of only the "good ones" is proposed as an "advance" in prenatal testing. Even if proponents of this supposed "advance" did not generally ignore the physical risks to a woman and the documented poor success of IVF interventions in advocating it, their single-minded attention to the embryo, to what is really a quality-controlled embryo, clearly links reproductive with genetic control. . . .

But the linkage exists, too, though perhaps more subtly, in claims that routine prenatal testing is reassuring. This claim may be statistically justified, since the vast majority of fetuses will not have what is being sought, but beyond ignoring the high frequencies of false positive test results when prenatal screening is carried out in the general population of pregnant women and the anxiety these generate, it nevertheless assumes abortion when a fetus does have the condition sought; spending most of one's pregnancy awaiting the birth of a child with a detected variation does not really seem likely to allay a woman's concerns.

Related to this, and another aspect of prenatal testing to worry, and worry about, is the way stories about it restrict disability to being simply a medical problem. Much research shows that disability, most of which is not of prenatal onset, only becomes of major consequence when prevailing social, economic and political policies do not allow for a wide range of abilities and convert impairments into handicaps. Prenatal testing implicitly assumes some norm of ability, hides the social roots and political practices that create handicap and reshapes the problem of disability so that it need not be *ours* collectively to solve—what will *we* do to embrace and accommodate those among us who have or will develop disabilities?—but becomes one for an individual woman to prevent—what will *she* do to avoid having a baby who has or will develop a disability? The individual is made into an agent of the state, and this is explicit (as is the fragility of our claims of neutrality) when a 38-year-old woman gives birth to a baby with Down syndrome and we ask—even if only among ourselves, as Elizabeth Thompson has noted—why she didn't get tested.

In addition, by orienting prenatal screening specifically to the detection of particular conditions, we explicitly make a social statement about the quality or the value of a fetus and on the adult it may grow up to be based solely on its genetic/chromosomal material. Our programs say it is okay if children with certain chromosomes are not born, that being at risk to develop a particular condition is, in effect, worse than being alive (Asch, 1988). And we restate this view when we count the abortion of a fetus with some disorder as a core benefit, not a worrisome cost, in our conventional economic analyses of screening programs (cf. Modell and Kuliev, 1991).

Further, and despite our rhetoric of choice, the power to set boundaries, to make value judgments about who may or may not be born, remains disproportionately with the university researchers and for-profit laboratories developing and deploying the technologies of testing. Only the conditions for which they make tests available can be sought—with what is available determined, as in all colonialism, by prevailing social values as well as by personal goals for professional recognition or financial profit.

Medical care providers further influence attitudes to what health and abnormality mean and who should be born by what they tell parents about genetic conditions—and these tellings appear to come in what Ben Wilfond and I have called "twice-told" ways (Lippman and Wilfond, 1992). For example, the information provided to those who are considering genetic testing for Down syndrome and for cystic fibrosis differs strikingly from that provided to those who have given birth to a child with one of the conditions. In both circumstances, the overall information is correct. However, the *before* testing information is largely negative, oriented to avoiding the birth of a child with Down syndrome or cystic fibrosis by focusing on technical matters and the array of potential medical complications and physical limitations that may occur in children with the condition, while the *after* birth information tends to be more positive, oriented to caring for a child with one of these conditions by focusing on compensating aspects of the condition, highlighting the availability of medical and social resources and stressing hope for the future.

We worry about separate before and after stories and what this may signify. Granted, no single story, however balanced, can ever be neutral or value-free. But why have we chosen to tell different stories? Why not just one?

The different versions of these stories remind us that even if individual women can choose to be tested or to abort, their options have first been created by the deeds and words of others. That the birth of certain babies should be avoided would appear to be embedded inextricably in geneticists' messages no less than in the medium of testing. This should worry us enough, I suggest, that we continually question our own values and consider why aborting a fetus on the basis of its ability—its particular value[2]—is not only socially acceptable but actually encouraged. Why have we made Down syndrome, for example, a privileged reason for prenatal screening and abortion? What else shall we so privilege? If raising children with disabilities is the problem, is prenatal screening the answer? Why have we converted a problem in society—inability to accommodate disability—into a problem in the fetus?

Legitimate efforts to help a woman have a healthy baby are essential. But if healthy children really matter to us, as we say they do, does prenatal testing represent our best effort? At the collective level, the birth prevalence of low birth weight is far greater than the birth prevalence of Down syndrome or neural tube defects. Why have efforts to find every fetus with Down syndrome become so important to us that universal triple screening is entering recommended medical practice,[3] while ensuring early prenatal care for all women is still an unachieved goal? Why has preventing neural tube defects become so important that universal folate supplementation

is proposed, while sufficient income and nutrition to all (pregnant) women to decrease their probability of having a baby with growth retardation is still not guaranteed? The well-being of children is inseparable from the well-being of women, and social, political and economic neglect of women interferes more with the physical and mental development of their children than the genes they inherit. If healthy children really do matter, we must end this neglect and create the conditions in which women's agency and their choices can be fully exercised.

Thus, we should worry about prenatal testing when relying on it to insure our children's health at the collective level threatens to displace attention from society's role in creating illness. If we worry, even a bit, perhaps we will delay our initial excitement about the potential to obtain and make diagnoses from single fetal cells in maternal blood samples until the presuppositions underlying suggestions to expand prenatal screening with this approach have been uncovered, until the ways in which such screening will be of consequence to pregnant women have been explored and until the place for this screening among our overall health priorities has been debated. . . .

REFERENCES

Asch A (1988): "Reproductive Technology and Disability," in *Reproductive Laws for the 1990s,* eds. S. Cohen, N. Taub (Clifton, NJ: Humana Press), pp. 59–101.

Clarke A (1990): "Genetics, ethics and audit." *Lancet* 335: 1145–1147.

Green J, Snowdon C, Statham H (1993): "Pregnant women's attitudes to abortion and pre-natal screening." *J Reprod & Infant Psychol,* in press.

Lippman A (1986): "Access to prenatal screening services: Who decides?" *Canad J Women Law* 1: 434–445.

Lippman A, Brunger F (1991): "Constructing Down syndrome: Texts as Informants." *Santé Culture Health* VIII (1–2): 109–131.

Lippman A, Wilfond BS (1992): "'Twice-Told tales': Stories about genetic disorders." *Amer J Hum Genet* 51:936–937.

Modell B, Kuliev AM (1991): "Services for thalassemia as a model for cost-benefit analysis of genetic services." *J Inherit Metab Dis* 14:640–651.

Scutt JA (1991): "The politics of infertility 'counselling'": *Issues in Reprod and Genet Engineer* 4(3):251–256.

Shapiro, R, "The human blueprint." Lecture, Science College Public Lecture Series, Concordia Univ., Montreal, 29 November 1990.

Acknowlegment: This paper derives from previously published material, especially articles in the *American Journal of Law and Medicine, Issues in Reproductive and Genetic Engineering,* and *Social Science and Medicine* . . . Support for the research on which it is based has been provided by the Social Sciences and Humanities Research Council of Canada.

NOTES

1. This is true only for some women having amniocentesis. With general population screening using alpha-fetoprotein or other chemical markers, women give samples for testing almost always without seeing a genetic counselor beforehand. [Note: The author lives and works in Canada. Her observations may not apply to the U.S.]

2. It is interesting that we seem to be quite comfortable rejecting prenatal diagnosis for sex selection because of our values (that females are no less valued than males), and recognize this as a value judgment, but reject any suggestion that value judgments imbue other decisions about eligibility for testing.

3. It is now to be offered to all pregnant women in Ontario.

Cloning

The Science, Fiction, and Reality of Embryo Cloning

JACQUES COHEN and GILES TOMKIN

ABSTRACT. Although many scientists view cloning as a useful procedure for scientific research into early embryo development—one that cannot currently be used to produce multiple copies of humans—the popular literature has led some individuals to view it as sinister. To address the concerns of the public, various conceptions of cloning are distinguished and their basis in fact analyzed. The possible uses, benefits, and detriments of both embryo splitting and nuclear transplantation are explained. Once the nature and purposes of cloning are understood, and the distinctive ethical dilemmas created by embryo splitting and nuclear transplantation are sorted out, these procedures should be clinically implemented to assist *in vitro* fertilization treatment for those who are infertile and to further other therapeutic and investigational efforts in medicine.

MAKING IDENTICAL COPIES of molecules, cells, tissues, and even adult organisms has loosely been termed "cloning." The basic purpose of scientists in making biological copies is not generally understood. It is to avoid any variation among specimens, thereby allowing direct comparisons for scientific evaluations. Although cloning has this unambiguous rationale for investigators of biological processes, some scientific and lay persons perceive it to have unknown and sinister ends. To alleviate their fear, we wish to clarify the nature and purposes of cloning processes in general, and embryo multiplication in particular. We do so, not so much as a result of recent controversy about the prospect of human embryo cloning (Hall et al. 1993), but as a tardy response to the mistaken belief that cloning humans is currently possible. An honest discussion of the subject has probably been overdue for many years. We provide some definitions of cloning, describe the main biological processes relevant to current discussions, and consider the various uses to which cloning could be put today.[1]

JACQUES COHEN and GILES TOMKIN are at the Institute for Reproductive Medicine and Science of Saint Barnabus, West Orange, N.J.

Kennedy Institute of Ethics Journal *Vol. 4, no. 3, Sep. 1994: 194–203. Copyright 1994. Permission granted by The Johns Hopkins University Press.*

POPULAR CONCEPTIONS OF CLONING

Cloning has been defined by a number of North American reference books, works of fiction, the entertainment industry, and the scientific literature. Webster's digital dictionary explains that the word, "clone," is from the Greek *klon*, which means "twig." The term "clone" was probably first used in the botanical field to describe the process of budding. Several current uses of the term are also given, one of which is generally accepted, namely, that cloning involves creating a genetically identical individual from a single, normal, body cell. The use employed by scientists, which is less widely known, is that cloning entails asexually reproducing an identical copy of an original. Asexual reproduction is usually associated with primitive organisms such as bacteria, algae, plants, and yeast. Although it was abandoned as the only form of reproduction by such species about 500 million years ago, this method of cell division is still the only means by which the human body grows and repairs itself.

Colorful fictional depictions of human clones were developed after Aldous Huxley (1932) published his famous book on the subject, *Brave New World*. In this book, Huxley described a future society where those who continue to reproduce sexually by gestation inside the womb are designated "savages" and forced to live in special reservations; the "civilized" people are those who come to life by artificial conception and bottling as fetuses. Special laboratories provide the conditions for embryo multiplication by "budding." Birth involves "decanting" in a breeding center, and children are raised in a laboratory and conditioning center. In fact, Huxley never used the word cloning in his book.

The most controversial portrayal of cloning was given in David Rorvik's 1978 book, *In His Image: The Cloning of a Man*. Here, a millionaire called "Max" assembled a team to clone one of his body cells by inserting its genetic material into a nucleus-free egg of a donor, who then became the gestational carrier of Max's younger twin. The mixture, without acknowledgment, of facts, such as names of existing scientists, with fiction created the threatening tone of the book.[2] The book's publication coincidentally and unfairly damaged the field of assisted reproduction, which was just emerging. It has been speculated that Rorvik's book raised so much public suspicion of cloning that the American government decided in the early 1980s to halt all research on human embryos. Educated and sophisticated leaders of an advanced society were influenced by a deceptive and false tale.

The combination of *Brave New World, In His Image,* and other imaginative books, as well as science fiction fantasies in television and the cinema, generated the frightening connotations of cloning that both attract and disturb many people. These sources, which engage in a happy denial of the fact that they portray fictional and future worlds, helped to create the belief that human cloning is possible today.

If reproduction through cloning were an attractive aim, it seems unlikely that our primitive, nonhuman ancestors would have abandoned it. Modern reproductive scientists, although intrigued by the idea of creating an individual from a single body cell of an adult, have not attempted to do so because it is currently impossible.[3] Embryonic cells are initially totipotent—that is, they have the ability to develop into any kind of cell found in the body. Eventually, they lose this ability and become "differentiated" cells, such as those found in the heart or in the nervous or muscular systems. The causes of this cellular change and loss of totipotency are unknown and, therefore, cannot yet be reversed. Since cloning an individual from a single cell of an adult human being requires such reversal, it is not possible to "body-cell clone." This is the essence of the challenge that cloning presents to science. A full understanding of the process of differentiation would provide a medical magic wand, not only for cloning, but for curing or reversing malignant tumors, arterial disorders, heart disease, and ultimately the aging process.

CLONING IN THE SCIENTIFIC LITERATURE

The word "cloning" has appeared thousands of times in the scientific literature[4] and has been used in three broad areas. The first is genetic research, where scientists must make millions of identical copies of genes of molecular size in order to have sufficient material for testing ("molecular cloning"). The second is the production of cell-lines that have identical properties in order to study the biology of specific cells without bias from small dissimilarities between them ("cell cloning"). The third area where the word "cloning" has now appeared is that of embryo multiplication by nuclear transplantation, which is the process of introducing nuclei from the cells of early preimplantation embryos into unfertilized eggs from which the nuclei have been removed. Nuclear transplantation has been performed in early cattle embryos in order to produce nearly identical offspring with desirable traits.

The only exception to these categories within the scientific community occurs in the paper on blastomere separation of abnormal human embryos presented by Hall and co-workers to the annual meeting of the American Fertility Society in the fall of 1993 (Hall et al. 1993). There the word "clone" was used instead of "blastomere separation" to describe the artificial procedure of identical twinning.[5] In the hundreds of publications on "twinning"[6] or "splitting" embryos, this procedure has never previously been referred to as "cloning." It is usually called "blastomere separation" when the embryo is split at the four- or eight-cell stage and "embryo splitting" when the embryo is at the blastocyst stage, the last embryonic stage during preimplantation development. Scientists and society have never regarded natural twins as "clones." Consequently, the use of the word to refer to a procedure that could produce identical twins in an officially approved scientific context caused far more anxiety among members of the media and the public than the actual, fairly modest, procedures in the laboratory were intended to evoke. All that the investigators did was to separate the individual cells of abnormal embryos in order to investigate the potential of early human cells to grow independently of one another. The same work has been done many times in other species, dating back to 1932 (Nicholas 1932). This previous work is described as "blastomere separation" by some and "evaluation of totipotency" by others. The description of similar experiments performed in the human (Hardy 1990) does not include the term "cloning." Nevertheless, ever since the publicity given to the twinned embryos made in Washington, D.C., reference to embryo splitting as "cloning" is ineradicably becoming part of common usage throughout the world. Scientists therefore may now be forced to accept the term "cloning" to describe blastomere separation or embryo splitting as well as nuclear transplantation.

KINDS OF CLONING

Cells from early embryos called blastomeres are each able to produce a new individual. This totipotency has allowed scientists to split animal embryos into several cells through the process of blastomere separation (Figure 1). Although this technique has been used in a number of species, it has particular advantages when applied to cattle (Willadsen 1979). In the last decade, some cattle breeding companies have used this totipotent ability to increase the success rate of their embryo transfer procedures (Gray 1991). Embryo transfer involves flushing embryos from the reproductive tract of one animal and implanting them in another. The procedure is usually suc-

Blastomere separation (embryo splitting)

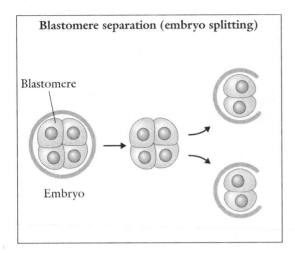

Nuclear transplantation (embryo cloning)

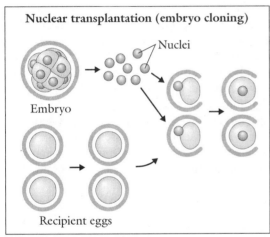

FIGURE 1

cessful, resulting in pregnancy rates of 60 percent in the recipients. Embryo splitting can increase this percentage to 100, an improvement that is both economically and biologically advantageous, since twins can be produced from select embryos. Use of this process in cattle for more than a decade has shown no disadvantages, nor defects in the offspring.

The more technically advanced form of embryo multiplication, nuclear transplantation, was developed in the early 1980s. The genetic material from recipient eggs is removed and replaced with the nucleus of a cell from an early embryo (Willadsen 1986). This procedure, like many other manipulations on single cells or embryos, is performed using micromanipulators, instruments with microscopically fine tips that are attached to a microscope. Micromanipulators enable embryologists to perform such fine procedures as inserting the sperm cell into the egg or removing the nucleus from an embryonic cell (Cohen 1992).

In theory, large numbers of identical embryos could be produced through nuclear transplantation on multiple generations of cloned embryos, each being a descendant from a single parent eight-cell-stage embryo. The limiting factor preventing this appears to be the inability of nuclei from advanced embryos (those with hundreds of cells) to be dedifferentiated and "reprogrammed" when they are placed inside an unfertilized egg, as they have lost their totipotent capability. Nuclear transplantation has been used only in the more sophisticated animal breeding stations and is successful in a small number of laboratories. Although the procedure has been associated with higher rates of congenital malformation, evidence for this is largely anecdotal. Scientists generally agree that the birth weights of calves resulting from nuclear transplantation seem to be higher than normal. Such an increase is also being reported following the application of *in vitro* fertilization (IVF) in cattle. Further development shows no apparent abnormalities in these embryo-cloned calves with higher birth weights.

POTENTIAL USES OF CLONING IN HUMANS

Reproductive specialists are interested in embryo duplication technology because the techniques that are currently used to treat infertile men and women are still largely unsuccessful. The national statistics indicate that only 15 percent of women undergoing IVF in 1991 gave birth to a child (Society for Assisted Reproductive Technology 1993).[7] Even this percentage is inflated when one considers that the chance of a live birth resulting from cases when a single embryo is transferred is less than 7 percent. Given these low rates of success, any advances are welcome, especially when the new technology already has been safely applied in a number of animal species. In our opinion, the morality of human embryo duplication by splitting should not be in doubt, much as no one doubts the morality of natural twinning or disputes the right of twins to existence. The real issue is whether the technique will improve the success rates of assisted reproductive technologies. Given that embryo duplication already works well in cattle, it is also very likely to work for human *in vitro* fertilization.

The primary human candidates to receive duplicated embryos would be patients using IVF procedures who have generated only a single embryo for transfer. These couples, however, currently constitute less than 10 percent of IVF patients; and even if patients who produced only two embryos were included, such couples still would constitute less than 20 percent of all IVF patients.[8] In practice, failures during the twinning procedure itself would reduce the percentage of recipients even further. Thus, the tangible benefits to this patient population would be limited. However, we believe that even if this method would improve the chances of pregnancy for patients with a single embryo by only 10 percent, the patients would undoubtedly consider it well worth undertaking. It should also be noted that the pregnancy complications associated with natural twinning are not a concern in embryo splitting. Such complications occur more often when twins share one placenta. Because the embryos produced by embryo splitting are completely separated and do not share a placenta, this problem would not arise from use of the technique.

Yet another benefit that might result from the use of embryo splitting is its potential to lower the costs associated with the use of advanced assisted reproductive technology. It is necessary to monitor patients' hormone levels and to examine their ovaries by ultrasound in the weeks leading up to the time of full oocyte maturation. Patients also must undergo a surgical outpatient procedure requiring anaesthesia in order to obtain a single batch of eggs. The use of embryo splitting would provide greater numbers of embryos for implantation from a single retrieval procedure and, therefore, would likely decrease the number of times that these procedures would have to be carried out. This, in turn, would decrease the costs of assisted reproduction. Furthermore, the laboratory work for *in vitro* fertilization includes careful monitoring of incubator conditions, a time-consuming task. Currently, the number of IVF procedures that can be performed by 100 health-care workers is about 1,000 per year. Any simplification of medical and laboratory procedures that could improve results would decrease the number of health care workers needed and ultimately also lower the cost per procedure.

Concern has been expressed that large numbers of identical children might result from embryo splitting. This is unlikely because the method has very limited numerical possibilities. After fertilization, embryonic cells only retain their totipotency through the next two, or at most, three cell divisions. According to current understanding, this permits a maximum number of four *viable* embryos to be obtained by splitting. While further splitting can be performed, it probably cannot result in viable embryos because the totipotent ability is lost, and the results will degenerate. At fertilization the cells commence to divide and do not go "backwards" when split into different embryos; that is, some sort of cellular count is kept of each cell division that occurs. Moreover, the ability to produce live offspring from the resulting embryos is also very limited. The live birth rate from the transfer of a single embryo is about 20 percent at the most advanced centers. Thus, even if 15 *healthy* embryos were successfully "twinned" from one embryo, which currently is not possible, and then singly transferred to 15 different wombs, the expected number of offspring would be only three.

There is also a concern that a greater proportion of congenital malformations would occur in children who result from the use of embryo splitting. Although this issue cannot be addressed fully until the procedures have been performed on a wide group of patients, the experience with cattle suggests that the concern is unfounded.

Assuming that the first trials of embryo splitting in patients with single embryos were successful, their success would be likely to affect all other *in vitro* fertilization procedures. If half of such procedures could be carried out using duplicated embryos, the standard number of oocytes needed to produce embryos would decrease dramatically. It would once again become feasible to use the natural menstrual cycle, rather than fertility drugs, to produce a sufficient number of oocytes for fertilization. With the prospect close at hand of simplifying procedures, increasing the success rates, and lessening the risks to patients, it seems almost immoral to some reproductive scientists not to allow embryo splitting trials for clinical use in human IVF laboratories.

Gynecologists and biologists are much more concerned about the use of nuclear transplantation to produce multiple embryos. Their concerns mostly involve unverified reports that many of the calves produced by nuclear transplantation have increased birth weights resulting in problems with their joints. As the calves mature, however, these problems seem to disappear, leaving the animals apparently normal. What these concerned scientists may have overlooked is that it is unusual to have a wide range in birth weights in cattle breeding, whereas birth weights have always varied widely in humans.[9] Therefore, an increase in birth weight in humans would not necessarily represent a problem. A second concern is that cattle breeders are not very successful when applying the nuclear transplantation technology. Although this is true, the

same can also be said for practitioners of human *in vitro* fertilization.

TO CLONE OR NOT TO CLONE?

Ultimately, there are many good reasons to suggest that both embryo splitting and nuclear transplantation should be implemented as soon as possible in humans at the *in vitro* fertilization centers that are currently most successful. Those scientists with demonstrated expertise in performing advanced embryology should participate. Naturally, the distinctive ethical dilemmas created by nuclear transplantation will have to be sorted out before it is used to produce embryo copies.

Although the use of embryo duplication to improve the success rates of assisted reproductive technology may have immediate clinical benefit, other potential benefits of this technique may be equally significant. The technology of removing cells from embryos and transferring nuclei between cells will expand scientists' understanding of the types of genes that determine the inheritance of characteristics and may also reveal how certain genetic diseases are activated. Other benefits seem sure to result from studying how and why embryonic cells differentiate into the specific cells of different organs. This complex process can be imitated by producing stem-cell lines from embryonic cells. The study of these stem cells is important for expanding scientists' understanding of many diseases.

We believe that irrational fears and fictional scenarios currently play a dominant role in determining ethical attitudes toward embryo splitting. The word "clone" has a negative and misleading significance for most people. Scientists and medical health-care workers, especially those who specialize in embryology and genetics, have erred by not informing the public of the real nature of cloning and its uses in assisted reproductive technology. Their own familiarity with concepts such as nuclear manipulation and genetic transfer and the great needs of the individual infertility patient has led them, all too frequently, to forget that outsiders, both lay and professional, may be disturbed by discussion of these realities. It is often easy to overlook the confusion between concepts that affects even professional practitioners in the absence of clear definitions of terms. When such confusion can occur among professionals in the field, it obviously can occur more extensively among groups without their background knowledge. It is hoped that the clarification of terms and ideas that we have presented will serve to enhance public understanding of the nature and purpose of cloning.

NOTES

1. The views contained in this article are our own and may represent a minority opinion in certain areas. Where applicable, we refer to views held by others in the field.

2. The publishers acknowledged in their foreword that they were not sure if the story were true since the persons involved wanted to remain anonymous.

3. Nuclei from adult mammalian cells, when transferred to fresh enucleated eggs from the same species cannot commence cell division and chromosome duplication and therefore do not develop. The furthest development among lower species has been accomplished in the tadpole experiments of Dr. John Gurdon (1986) from Cambridge University in the United Kingdom.

4. This estimate was derived from Mini-Medline searches and publication archives.

5. Natural identical twins are also derived from a single embryo. The process should not be confused with fraternal twinning in which multiple eggs (each genetically different) are released from the ovary and fertilized by different sperm. Fraternal twins are not genetically identical.

6. It is not certain that Hall's experiment produced identical twins. The embryonic cells that developed following separation of the abnormally fertilized egg were never tested for genetic homogeneity, which is crucial to the establishment of proof that the half-embryos were indeed identical. The abnormal embryo used in these experiments was fertilized by two sperm, which is known to cause mosaicism in animal as well as human embryos. The individual cells of a mosaic embryo are by definition all genetically different from

each other because of errors of nuclear division (Pieters 1992; Long 1993).

7. The Society for Assisted Reproductive Technology, which is part of the American Fertility Society, surveys more than 200 member programs each year.

8. This estimate was derived from analyses performed on embryos from 1200 patients using a relational database (EggCyte) at the program of Cornell University Medical Center.

9. This opinion was presented by Dr. Steen Willadsen at the workshop on embryo cloning held by the National Advisory Board on Ethics in Reproduction, Washington, D.C., 15 February 1994.

REFERENCES

Cohen, Jacques; Malter, Henry E.; Talansky, Beth E.; and Grifo, Jaime. 1992. *Micro-manipulation of Human Gametes and Embryos*. New York: Raven Press.

Gray, K. R.; Bondioli, K. R.; Betts, C. L. 1991. The Commercial Application of Embryo Splitting in Beef Cattle. *Theriogenology* 35: 37–44.

Gurdon, J. B. 1986. Nuclear Transplantation in Eggs and Oocytes. *Journal of Cell Science* 4 (supplement): 287–318.

Hall, J. L.; Engel, D.; Gindoff, P. R.; et al. 1993. Experimental Cloning of Human Polyploid Embryos Using an Artificial Zona Pellucida. The American Fertility Society conjointly with the Canadian Fertility and Andrology Society, Program Supplement, 1993 Abstracts of the Scientific Oral and Poster Sessions, Abstract o-001, S1.

Hardy, Kate; Martin, Karen L.; Leese, Henry J.; et al. 1990. Human Preimplantation Development In Vitro Is Not Adversely Affected by Biopsy at the 8-cell Stage. *Human Reproduction* 5: 708–14.

Huxley, Aldous. 1932. *Brave New World*. London: Chatto and Windus.

Long, C. R.; Pinto-Correia, C.; Duby, R. T.; et al. 1993. Chromatin and Microtubule Morphology During the First Cell Cycle in Bovine Zygotes. *Molecular Reproduction and Development* 36: 23–32.

Nicholas, J. S. 1932. Development of Transplanted Rat Eggs. *Proceedings of the Society of Experimental Biology and Medicine* 30: 1111–27.

Pieters, M. H. E. C.; Dumoulin, J. C. M.; Ignoul-Vanvuchelen, R. C. M.; et al. 1992. Triploidy after In Vitro Fertilization: Cytogenetic Analysis of Human Zygotes and Embryos. *Journal of Assisted Reproduction and Genetics* 9: 68–76.

Rorvik, David. 1978. *In His Image: The Cloning of a Man*. Philadelphia: Lippincott.

Society for Assisted Reproductive Technology, The American Fertility Society. 1993. Assisted Reproductive Technology in the United States and Canada: 1991. Results from the Society for Assisted Reproductive Technology/American Fertility Society Registry. *Fertility and Sterility* 59: 956–62.

Willadsen, Steen M. 1979. A Method of Culture of Micromanipulated Sheep Embryos and Its Use to Produce Monozygotic Twins. *Nature* 277: 298–300.
——. 1986. Nuclear Transplantation in Sheep Embryos. *Nature* 320: 63–65.

Ban Cloning? Why NBAC Is Wrong

SUSAN M. WOLF

IN ITS REPORT on cloning, NBAC [National Bioethics Advisory Commission] recommended a ban of unprecedented scope.[1] Based on commission consensus that human cloning would currently be unsafe, NBAC called for congressional prohibition throughout the public and private sectors of all somatic cell nuclear transfer with the intent of creating a child. President Clinton promptly responded by proposing legislation to enact such a ban for five years. . . .

THE REGULATORY CHALLENGE

Human cloning clearly requires regulation. Indeed, some regulation already applies. President Clinton has barred all federal funds for cloning, both research and clinical application.[2] Earlier

SUSAN M. WOLF is Professor of Law and Medicine, University of Minnesota Law School and Center for Bioethics, and Director, Joint Degree Program in Law, Health & the Life Sciences.

prohibitions on the use of federal money to create human embryos for research purposes would also impede cloning research with federal funds.[3] And federal regulations protecting human subjects would seem to block cloning in research covered by those regulations because cloning remains unsafe, at least for now.[4] This leaves two regulatory gaps that properly troubled NBAC: private sector research outside federal oversight and private clinical activity, especially infertility programs using reproductive technologies.

But by responding to these worries with a congressional ban, NBAC missed the target. Protecting human subjects in private research and regulating reproductive technologies are both long overdue. A ban on cloning just suppresses one technology, while these two systemic problems guarantee the development of other technologies in need of regulation. Some would argue that somatic cell cloning deserves to be singled out as the most threatening possibility. But that assumes a conclusion we have not had time to reach, that Dolly-style cloning raises radically more difficult problems than, for example, cloning by embryo splitting (which can also lead to a delayed twin, with cryopreservation).[5]

Instead of developing a legal response to cloning that addresses the core problems of private research and underregulated reproductive technologies, NBAC simply called for a ban of cloning itself. That skirts the central problems, while adding new ones.

THE ERROR IN A BAN

No other bioethics controversy has been addressed by a ban as broad as the one NBAC advocates and the president now proposes. Its prohibition reaches all public and private institutions, whether or not federal money is involved or FDA approval is required. Limits on the use of federal money are common, but federal prohibitions on medical and scientific work in the private sector are not.

Moreover, the ban threatens substantial damage. The president's bill prohibits "somatic cell nuclear transfer with the intent of introducing the product of that transfer into a woman's womb or in any other way creating a human being," and would impose significant fines.

. . . The policing necessary to enforce the ban will require intruding into labs and monitoring the "intent" of scientists. Research will thus be chilled. It will be chilled further by the vagueness of a prohibition that is meant to ban baby-making, but seems to reach intent to "transfer," even if a researcher knows no child will result, plus the intent to create a human being in any unspecified "other way."

Beyond the ban's breadth and potential damage, NBAC and the president have placed this weapon in the wrong hands. The ban is to be imposed by Congress itself, not a regulatory body poised to respond to developments in the technology. That turns cloning into a political football. . . .

. . . Congress may well include other technologies such as embryo splitting (which, after all, is another form of cloning and may also produce a delayed twin). Two of the three federal bills pending appear to do exactly that.[6] But embryo splitting may allow a woman undergoing in vitro fertilization to avoid repeated exposure to drugs inducing superovulation, which may reduce her risk of ovarian cancer later in life. . . .

The ban proposed thus raises serious constitutional questions. The ban's prohibition of somatic cell nuclear transfer with the wrong intent and its unavoidable chilling effect on research may infringe freedom of scientific inquiry in violation of the First Amendment.[7] And the ban as proposed by the president may well be unconstitutionally vague in its statement of the prohibited intent.[8] The ban may also represent an unconstitutional infringement on the procreative liberty of infertile couples.[9] In any case, it may exceed the limits of federal power, especially since the regulation of health and clinical practice has traditionally fallen to the states.[10]

Beyond the constitutional questions, a ban at this point is bad policy. NBAC's advocacy of this ban contradicts its call for careful study and debate in our pluralistic society. With only ninety days to report on cloning, NBAC admits more analysis is needed. Yet by calling now for a ban that is likely to sweep more broadly and last much longer than NBAC wants, the commission has in effect already yielded to those who claim cloning is wrong in all cases and for the indefinite future. This ends the important deliberation, embraces one absolutist moral perspective, and writes it into law.[11]

NBAC defends the ban as a safety measure preventing harm to potential children. But that reasoning does not justify this result. Indeed, the ban may well cause harm. A ban that inevitably chills research will prevent the development of a cloning technology that is physically safe for the children it produces. Some may protest that even physically safe cloning may threaten psychological harms. But that claim is purely speculative and can ground regulation and research, but not a ban; cloning may in fact save children from psychological difficulties involved in having an anonymous genetic parent through donor egg or sperm.

Moreover, a ban may cause harm to infertile couples, especially if it hardens into an indefinite prohibition. After all, cloning offers potential benefit in infertility cases. NBAC points to a couple each carrying a recessive gene for a serious disorder. Cloning would allow them to avoid conceiving an embryo with the disorder and facing selective abortion. In another case, a woman might carry a dominant gene for a disorder. Cloning would permit her to avoid genetic contribution from an egg donor and thus would keep the genetic parenting between the woman and her partner, something of value to many couples. Other cases would include a couple entirely lacking gametes. . . .

A federal ban on cloning thus misses the big picture. Cloning is only one of many reproductive technologies that should be safe before application, be it intracytoplasmic sperm injection, cytoplasm transfer, or beyond. The task is to devise a regulatory approach that addresses safety while permitting research and progress in a sphere of immense importance to couples. Cloning should spur us to that delicate balancing act. Simply lowering the boom on cloning does the opposite.

A BETTER MODEL

There is a better way. Certainly we need improved regulation of assisted reproduction and human subject experimentation in the private sphere.[12] But we have to combine that regulation with an advisory body providing oversight for cloning and other novel reproductive and genetic technologies.

The commission, president, and Congress should consider a model we have used before: agency regulation guided by an advisory body able to respond to improvements in the technology over time and more removed than Congress from partisan politics. Though NBAC's report compared policy options, strangely this was not among them.[13]

The Recombinant DNA Advisory Committee (RAC) is one example of such a body. RAC was formed over twenty years ago as an NIH advisory panel. When concern later erupted over human gene therapy, RAC (with its Working Group on Human Gene Therapy) showed how an advisory committee can hold the line, by refusing to consider germ-line gene therapy protocols for approval. It used not a legislative ban, but the committee's declared moratorium, continually subject to debate and reconsideration. . . .

RAC is merely one example. And it is narrower than what we need for cloning: RAC's jurisdiction has been confined to protocols requiring NIH approval. On cloning, as I have argued, we need to extend human subjects protections to private research and regulate reproductive technologies, with an advisory body for novel issues such as cloning.[14]

Certainly the details of the model can be debated. Indeed, rather than create a new advisory body, using a reinvigorated RAC, another preexisting entity, or NBAC itself (if its mission were restructured) might be considered. And some may argue we need two bodies, one for human subjects and the other for reproductive technologies. But surrendering cloning to a congressional ban, as NBAC suggests, attempts a delicate operation with far too blunt an instrument. It is slim consolation that under the president's proposal, NBAC will be continuing discussion on the sidelines.

NBAC might respond that it favored a limited ban to head off worse proposals in Congress. But a national bioethics commission should call for what is right, not merely what is expedient. Congressional bills in the panicked days after the announcement of Dolly should not drive the national bioethics agenda. . . .

REFERENCES

1. National Bioethics Advisory Commission, *Cloning Human Beings: Report and Recommendations of the National Bioethical Advisory Commission* (Rockville, Md., June 1997).

2. The White House, Office of Communications, Directive on Cloning, 4 March 1997, 1997 Westlaw 91957 (White House).

3. See "Statement by the President on NIH Recommendation Regarding Human Embryo Research," *U.S. Newswire* (2 December 1994); Omnibus Consolidated Appropriations Act, 1997, Pub. L. No. 104–208, §512, 110 Stat. 3009, 831.

4. 45 C.F.R. Part 46 (1996). These regulations cover only research that is federally funded, at institutions offering assurances that all research will be subject to the regulations, or on drugs and devices needing FDA approval.

5. NBAC's report leaves unclear the proper policy approach to embryo splitting. Chairman Shapiro's transmittal letter states, "We do not revisit . . . cloning . . . by embryo splitting." However, a report footnote ambiguously "observes that . . . any other technique to create a child genetically identical to an existing . . . individual would raise many, if not all, of the same non-safety-related ethical concerns raised by . . . somatic cell nuclear transfer" (p. iii, n. 1). One would think that "any other technique" could include embryo splitting with cryopreservation to produce a delayed genetic twin. However, the report claims that the capacity to produce a delayed genetic twin is a prospect "unique" to Dolly-style cloning, i.e., somatic cell nuclear transfer (pp. 3, 64). This leaves NBAC's approach to embryo splitting in confusion.

6. See H.B. 922, S. 368.

7. See generally Ira H. Carmen, *Cloning and the Constitution: An Inquiry into Governmental Policymaking and Genetic Experimentation* (Madison, University of Wisconsin Press, 1985); Richard Delgado and David R. Millen, "God, Galileo, and Government: Toward Constitutional Protection for Scientific Inquiry," *Washington Law Review* 53 (1978): 349–404.

8. Cf. Lifchez v. Hartigan, 735 F. Supp. 1381 (N.D. Ill.), *aff'd without opinion*, 914 F.2d 260 (7th Cir. 1990), *cert. denied sub nom.* Scholberg v. Lifchez, 498 U.S. 1069 (1991) (striking down a statute on fetal experimentation as unconstitutionally vague).

9. The shape of this argument is suggested by John A. Robertson in *Children of Choice: Freedom and the New Reproductive Technologies* (Princeton: Princeton University Press, 1994), though he questions whether cloning is so different from other forms of reproduction as to fall outside of constitutional protection for procreative liberty (pp. 169–70). On constitutional protection for reproductive technologies, see also *Lifchez*, above.

10. For the limits of federal power based on the Constitution's commerce clause, see, for example, U.S. v. Lopez, 514 U.S. 549 (1995).

11. See also Alexander Morgan Capron, "Inside the Beltway Again: A Sheep of a Different Feather," *Kennedy Institute of Ethics Journal* 7 (1997): 171–79, at 176 ("[I]t would be a mistake to say everything we believe would be wrong to do should be a wrong to do. This is particularly true of cloning.").

12. See also George J. Annas, "Regulatory Models for Human Embryo Cloning: The Free Market, Professional Guidelines, and Government Restrictions," *Kennedy Institute of Ethics Journal* 4 (1994): 235–49, 245–46.

13. NBAC did mention RAC (p. 97), but in its discussion of voluntary moratoria (and even though PAC's moratorium on germ-line gene therapy proposals has been binding on researchers seeking federal funds, not voluntary).

14. Unlike a ban on cloning, my suggested approach is likely to survive constitutional scrutiny. Research is routinely disseminated interstate with substantial commercial effects. And the terrible history of research scandals would seem to justify extending protection to subjects in private research as a matter of civil and human rights. Moreover, there is little reason to suspect infringement on researchers' freedom of inquiry from application of our current protective framework. Augmenting regulation of reproductive technologies, if carefully done to respect the constitutional need for a compelling justification to restrict access to procreative technologies, would seem defensible given extensive interstate commerce in reproductive services.

Human Cloning and the Constitution

CLARKE D. FORSYTHE

ALL CELLS IN THE HUMAN BODY start from one cell (the zygote which results from fertilization). The one-celled zygote begins to cleave, or divide, and multiply. The cells resulting from these early cleavages are called blastomeres. "Because they divide mitotically, all blastomeres contain identical chromosomes and genetic information as the original one-celled zygote." Consequently, the blastomeres are considered totipotent or "capable, on isolation, of forming a complete embryo." Eventually, this one cell, the zygote, divides into many cells, and these cells differentiate or become specialized, becoming, for example, bone, hair, or skin cells.

While there is little biological doubt that the one-celled human zygote or embryo is a separate, unique human being, in popular and legal discussions, confusion often exists between human being and person. Human being is an anthropological term that is based on biology and species, whereas "person" is a moral or philosophical term. A human being is simply a member of the species homo sapiens, and it is defined biologically, by species, not developmentally. The distinction between "human life" and "human being" is made clear by Bradley Patten and other human embryologists: "[a]lthough in a sense, an embryo preexists in the gametes from which it arises, its life as a new individual must be regarded as commencing at the moment of

CLARKE D. FORSYTHE is an attorney and president of Americans United for Life, headquartered in Chicago.

fertilization." Patten emphasizes that "[I]t is the penetration of the ovum by a sperm and the resultant mingling of the nuclear material each brings to the union that constitutes the culmination of the process of fertilization and marks the initiation of the life of a new individual."

The common law—reflected by Blackstone—was quite clear: any human creature, i.e., any offspring of human parents, is a human being and every living human being is a person. The Supreme Court departed from this longstanding tradition in its decision in Roe v. Wade. In Roe, the Court held that the human "fetus" was not a "person" and therefore not within the meaning (and protection) of the Fourteenth Amendment. Roe has now become the primary reference point for popular and academic discussion concerning the legal and moral status of unborn human beings and for the proposition that unborn human beings are not persons. Thus, much of the public debate regarding abortion and embryo experimentation including cloning) focuses, immediately and instinctively, on whether the fetus and embryo are "persons," not on whether the fetus and embryo are human beings.

As a legal matter, identifying an unborn human as a "human being" or a "person" does not determine whether states can protect the unborn through homicide law. Under the Constitution, states can protect unborn children, outside the context of abortion, without regard to the constitutional status as persons. Thus, states can protect human embryos because neither Roe

Valparaiso University Law Review, *Vol. 32, no. 2, Spring 1998. Copyright 1998, Valparaiso Law Review.*
Permission granted by Clarke D. Forsythe. Reprinted from Valparaiso University Law Review, Valparaiso,
Indiana.

nor the embryo's constitutional status limits the states in protecting human embryos outside the context of abortion.

Human cloning, and the process of developing that technology, will inevitably involve creating, manipulating, and killing individual members of the human species, i.e., human beings. It is precisely the prerogative of society to give respect to the dignity of these growing human beings and to require that other individuals give equal dignity and respect.

The compelling societal interest against human cloning cannot be protected short of a prohibition against its practice. Once cloned, the embryo's genetic identity is formed, and while subject to further possible experimentation, it cannot be altered. Once cloned, it is not possible to effectively protect the life of the extracorporeal embryo. Requiring implantation is inconceivable due to traditional legal and moral principles against battery, forced sex, or compelled medical treatment, and placing them for "adoption" would entail the use of freezing techniques that carry a high risk of death or injury. Requiring implantation would also be futile because, as soon as the embryo would be implanted, the women would have a liberty interest to abort under Roe. The only effective way to protect the human embryo is to avoid completely the perilous specter of cloning by prohibiting it altogether.

Cloning, Ethics, and Religion

LEE M. SILVER

ON SUNDAY MORNING, 23 February 1997, the world awoke to a technological advance that shook the foundations of biology and philosophy. On that day, we were introduced to Dolly, a 6-month-old lamb that had been cloned directly from a single cell taken from the breast tissue of an adult donor. Perhaps more astonished by this accomplishment than any of their neighbors were the scientists who actually worked in the field of mammalian genetics and embryology.

LEE M. SILVER is a Professor in the Department of Molecular Biology, Princeton University.

Outside the lab where the cloning had actually taken place, most of us thought it could never happen. Oh, we would say that perhaps at some point in the distant future, cloning might become feasible through the use of sophisticated biotechnologies far beyond those available to us now. But what many of us really believed, deep in our hearts, was that this was one biological feat we could never master. New life—in the special sense of a conscious being—must have its origins in a embryo formed through the merger of gametes from a mother and father. It was impossible, we thought, for a cell from an adult

Cambridge Quarterly of Healthcare Ethics, *Vol. 7, no. 2 (1998): 168–172. Copyright 1998. Reprinted with permission by Lee M. Silver and Cambridge University Press.*

mammal to become reprogrammed, to start all over again, to generate another entire animal or person in the image of the one born earlier.

How wrong we were.

Of course, it wasn't the cloning of a sheep that stirred the imaginations of hundreds of millions of people. It was the idea that humans could now be cloned as well, and many people were terrified by the prospect. Ninety percent of Americans polled within the first week after the story broke felt that human cloning should be banned.[1] And while not unanimous, the opinions of many media pundits, ethicists, and policymakers seemed to follow that of the public at large. The idea that humans might be cloned was called "morally despicable," "repugnant," "totally inappropriate," as well as "ethically wrong, socially misguided and biologically mistaken."[2]

Scientists who work directly in the field of animal genetics and embryology were dismayed by all the attention that now bore down on their research. Most unhappy of all were those associated with the biotechnology industry, which has the most to gain in the short-term from animal applications of the cloning technology.[3] Their fears were not unfounded. In the aftermath of Dolly, polls found that two out of three Americans considered the cloning of *animals* to be morally unacceptable, while 56% said they would not eat meat from cloned animals.[4]

It should not be surprising, then, that scientists tried to play down the feasibility of human cloning. First they said that it might not be possible *at all* to transfer the technology to human cells.[5] And even if human cloning is possible in theory, they said, "it would take years of trial and error before it could be applied successfully," so that "cloning in humans is unlikely any time soon."[6] And even if it becomes possible to apply the technology successfully, they said, "there is no clinical reason why you would do this."[7] And even if a person wanted to clone him- or herself or someone else, he or she wouldn't be able to find trained medical professionals who would be willing to do it.

Really? That's not what science, history, or human nature suggest to me. The cloning of Dolly broke the technological barrier. There is no reason to expect that the technology couldn't be transferred to human cells. On the contrary, there is every reason to expect that it *can* be transferred. If nuclear transplantation works in every mammalian species in which it has been seriously tried, then nuclear transplantation *will* work with human cells as well. It requires only equipment and facilities that are already standard, or easy to obtain by biomedical laboratories and freestanding in vitro fertilization clinics across the world. Although the protocol itself demands the services of highly trained and skilled personnel, there are thousands of people with such skills in dozens of countries.

The initial horror elicited by the announcement of Dolly's birth was due in large part to a misunderstanding by the lay public and the media of what biological cloning is and is not. The science critic Jeremy Rifkin exclaimed: "It's a horrendous crime to make a Xerox (copy) of someone,"[8] and the Irvine, California, rabbi Bernard King was seriously frightened when he asked, "Can the cloning create a soul? Can scientists create the soul that would make a being ethical, moral, caring, loving, all the things we attribute humanity to?"[9] The Catholic priest Father Saunders suggested that "cloning would only produce humanoids or androids—soulless replicas of human beings that could be used as slaves."[10] And *New York Times* writer Brent Staples warned us that "synthetic humans would be easy prey for humanity's worst instincts."[11]

Anyone reading this volume already knows that real human clones will simply be later-born identical twins—nothing more and nothing less. Cloned children will be full-fledged human beings, indistinguishable in biological terms from all other members of the species. But even with this understanding, many ethicists, scholars, and scientists are still vehemently opposed to the use of cloning as means of human reproduction under any circumstances whatsoever. Why do they feel this way? Why does this new reproductive technology upset them so?

First, they say, it's a question of "safety." The cloning procedure has not been proven safe and, as a result, its application toward the generation of newborn children could produce deformities and other types of birth defects. Second, they say that even if physical defects can be avoided, there is the psychological well-being of the cloned child to consider. And third, above and beyond each individual child, they are worried about the horrible effect that cloning will have on society as a whole.

What I will argue here is that people who voice any one or more of these concerns are—either consciously or subconsciously—hiding the real reason they oppose cloning. They have latched on to arguments about safety, psychology, and society because they are simply unable to come up with an ethical argument that is not based on the religious notion that by cloning human beings man will be playing God, and it is wrong to play God.

Let us take a look at the safety argument first. Throughout the 20th century, medical scientists have sought to develop new protocols and drugs for treating disease and alleviating human suffering. The safety of all these new medical protocols was initially unknown. But through experimental testing on animals first, and then volunteer human subjects, safety could be ascertained and governmental agencies—such as the Food and Drug Administration in the United States—could make a decision as to whether the new protocol or drug should be approved for use in standard medical practice.

It would be ludicrous to suggest that legislatures should pass laws banning the application of each newly imagined medical protocol before its safety has been determined. Professional ethics committees, institutional review boards, and the individual ethics of each medical practitioner are relied upon to make sure that hundreds of new experimental protocols are tested and used in an appropriate manner each year. And yet the question of unknown safety alone was the single rationale used by the National Bioethics Advisory Board (NBAC) to propose a ban on human cloning in the United States.

Opposition to cloning on the basis of safety alone is almost surely a losing proposition. Although the media have concocted fantasies of dozens of malformed monster lambs paving the way for the birth of Dolly, fantasy is all it was. Of the 277 fused cells created by Wilmut and his colleagues, only 29 developed into embryos. These 29 embryos were placed into 13 ewes, of which 1 became pregnant and gave birth to Dolly.[12] If safety is measured by the percentage of lambs born in good health, then the record, so far, is 100% for nuclear transplantation from an adult cell (albeit with a sample size of 1).

In fact, there is no scientific basis for the belief that cloned children will be any more prone to genetic problems than naturally conceived children. The commonest type of birth defect results from the presence of an abnormal number of chromosomes in the fertilized egg. This birth defect arises during gamete production and, as such, its frequency should be greatly reduced in embryos formed by cloning. The second most common class of birth defects results from the inheritance of two mutant copies of a gene from two parents who are silent carriers. With cloning, any silent mutation in a donor will be silent in the newly formed embryo and child as well. Finally, much less frequently, birth defects can be caused by new mutations; these will occur with the same frequency in embryos derived through conception or cloning. (Although some scientists have suggested that chromosome shortening in the donor cell will cause cloned children to have a shorter lifespan, there is every reason to expect that chromosome repair in the embryo will eliminate this problem.) Surprisingly, what our current scientific understanding suggests is that birth defects in cloned children could occur less frequently than birth defects in naturally conceived ones.

Once safety has been eliminated as an objection to cloning, the next concern voiced is the psychological well-being of the child. Daniel Callahan, the former director of the Hastings Center, argues that "engineering someone's entire genetic makeup would compromise his or her right to a unique identity."[13] But no such 'right' has been granted by nature—identical twins are born every day as natural clones of each other. Dr. Callahan would have to concede this fact, but he might still argue that just because twins occur naturally does not mean we should create them on purpose.

Dr. Callahan might argue that a cloned child is harmed by knowledge of her future condition. He might say that it's unfair to go through childhood knowing what you will look like as an adult, or being forced to consider future medical ailments that might befall you. But even in the absence of cloning, many children have some sense of the future possibilities encoded in the genes they got from their parents. Furthermore, genetic screening already provides people with the ability to learn about hundreds of disease predispositions. And as genetic knowledge and technology become more and more sophisticated, it will become possible for any human being to learn even more about his or her genetic future than a cloned child could learn from his or her progenitor's past.

It might also be argued that a cloned child will be harmed by having to live up to unrealistic expectations placed on her by her parents. But there is no reason to believe that her parents will be any more unreasonable than many other parents who expect their children to accomplish in their lives what they were unable to accomplish in their own. No one would argue that parents with such tendencies should be prohibited from having children.

But let's grant that among the many cloned children brought into this world, some *will* feel badly about the fact that their genetic constitution is not unique. Is this alone a strong enough reason to ban the practice of cloning? Before answering this question, ask yourself another: Is a child having knowledge of an older twin worse

off than a child born into poverty? If we ban the former, shouldn't we ban the latter? Why is it that so many politicians seem to care so much about cloning but so little about the welfare of children in general?

Finally, there are those who argue against cloning based on the perception that it will harm society at large in some way. *The New York Times* columnist William Safire expresses the opinion of many others when he says that "cloning's identicality would restrict evolution."[14] This is bad, he argues, because "the continued interplay of genes . . . is central to humankind's progress." But Mr. Safire is wrong on both practical and theoretical grounds. On practical grounds, even if human cloning became efficient, legal, and popular among those in the moneyed classes (which is itself highly unlikely), it would still only account for a fraction of a percent of all the children born onto this earth. Furthermore, each of the children born by cloning to different families would be different from each other, so where does the identicality come from?

On theoretical grounds, Safire is wrong because humankind's progress has nothing to do with unfettered evolution, which is always unpredictable and not necessarily upward bound. H. G. Wells recognized this principle in his 1895 novel *The Time Machine*, which portrays the evolution of humankind into weak and dimwitted but cuddly little creatures. And Kurt Vonnegut follows this same theme in *Galápagos*, where he suggests that our "big brains" will be the cause of our downfall, and future humans with smaller brains and powerful flippers will be the only remnants of a once great species, a million years hence.

As is so often the case with new reproductive technologies, the real reason that people condemn cloning has nothing to do with technical feasibility, child psychology, societal well-being, or the preservation of the human species. The real reason derives from religious beliefs. It is the sense that cloning leaves God out of the process of human creation, and that man is venturing into places he does not belong. Of course, the 'playing God' objection only makes sense in the context of one definition of God, as a supernatural being who plays a role in the birth of each new member of our species. And even if one holds this particular view of God, it does not necessarily follow that cloning is equivalent to playing God. Some who consider themselves to be religious have argued that if God didn't want man to clone, "he" wouldn't have made it possible.

Should public policy in a pluralist society be based on a narrow religious point of view? Most people would say no, which is why those who hold this point of view are grasping for secular reasons to support their call for an unconditional ban on the cloning of human beings. When the dust clears from the cloning debate, however, the secular reasons will almost certainly have disappeared. And then, only religious objections will remain.

NOTES

1. Data extracted from a *Time*/CNN poll taken over the 26th and 27th of February 1997 and reported in *Time* on 10 March 1997; and an ABC Nightline poll taken over the same period, with results reported in the *Chicago Tribune* on 2 March 1997.

2. Quotes from the bioethicist Arthur Caplan in *Denver Post* 1997;Feb 24; the bioethicist Thomas Murray in *New York Times* 1997;Mar 6; Congressman Vernon [Ehlers] in *New York Times* 1997;Mar 6; and evolutionary biologist Francisco Ayala in *Orange County Register* 1997;Feb 25.

3. James A. Geraghty, president of Genzyme Transgenics Corporation (a Massachusetts biotech company), testified before a Senate committee that "everyone in the biotechnology industry shares the unequivocal conviction that there is no place for the cloning of human beings in our society." *Washington Post* 1997;Mar 13.

4. Data obtained from a Yankelovich poll of 1,005 adults reported in *St. Louis Post-Dispatch* 1997;Mar 9 and a *Time*/CNN poll reported in *The New York Times* 1997;Mar 5.

5. Leonard Bell, president and chief executive of Alexion Pharmaceuticals, is quoted as saying, "There is a healthy skepticism whether you can accomplish this efficiently in another species." *New York Times* 1997;Mar 3.

6. Interpretation of the judgments of scientists, reported by Specter M, Kolata G. *New York Times* 1997;Mar 3, and by Herbert W, Sheler JL, Watson T. *U.S. News & World Report* 1997;Mar 10.

7. Quote from Ian Wilmut, the scientist who brought forth Dolly, in Friend T. *USA Today* 1997;Feb 24.

8. Quoted in Kluger J. *Time* 1997;Mar 10.

9. Quoted in McGraw C, Kelleher S. *Orange County Register* 1997;Feb 25.

10. Quoted in the on line version of the *Arlington Catholic Herald* (http://www.catholicherald.com/bissues.htm) 1997;May 16.

11. Staples B. [Editorial]. *The New York Times* 1997;Feb 28.

12. Wilmut I, Schnieke AE, McWhir J, Kind AJ, Campbell KHS. Viable offspring derived from fetal and adult mammalian cells. *Nature* 1997;385:810–13.

13. Callahan D. [op-ed]. *The New York Tmes* 1997;Feb 26.

14. Safire W. [op-ed]. *The New York Times* 1997;Feb 27.

The New Biotech World Order

LISA SOWLE CAHILL

THE GERON ETHICS ADVISORY BOARD bravely takes up the ethical big picture of genetic research: just distribution of burdens and benefits in a global market economy. Even granting that presenting new discoveries along with ethical caveats might be useful in deterring damaging public criticism, putting justice and access on the table, as Geron and its EAB have done, is valuable. It could help influence public perceptions and policy debates about new research in genetics that is fast outpacing extant moral and legislative controls.

The basic problem, however, is that just access to even one biotechnology is not something that Geron and its EAB can address or provide alone. At stake are questions of a very fundamental philosophical, cultural, and political nature that demand complex, intercultural reflection and action. To adequately address such questions clearly exceeds the expertise of the present writer. I shall, however, attempt to at least move toward greater specificity in understanding the daunting "challenge" to social ethics named by the Geron EAB. I will address three aspects of the ethics of research on biotechnologies, like stem cell research, that are driven by profits to be gained in a global context of vastly unequal access to health care and other human goods: the conceptual or philosophical definition of justice; the United States cultural context of debate about genetic justice, the market, and policy;

LISA CAHILL is the J. Donald Monan, S. J., Professor at Boston College.

and the practical political and structural conditions under which "global distribution of and access to" genetic therapies must be sought at the turn of this century.

WHAT IS JUSTICE?

Many North American bioethicists think of justice as one principle among four (justice, autonomy, beneficence, and nonmaleficence). This framework has stiffened the ethical backbone of debates about medical resources, both nationally and internationally. Many critics have observed that seemingly abstract principles need to be placed in the context of the communities that express and respect them.

The point that I want to make is somewhat different. The duties, values, or virtues indicated by the principles are interdependent rather than separate and competing, and it is possible to define justice as the category that comprehends the other three. In fact, the classical definition of justice as "giving each his or her due" implies a respect for the individual seen as part of a social whole within which benefits are to be shared and harms avoided. Thus autonomy and distributive justice should be treated together, as counterparts, and neither can be isolated from a consideration of what counts as a good for persons or society in the first place. If the right to freely choose cannot be separated from the effects of one's choice on the welfare of others, one must know what counts as a good or harm for others

The Hastings Center Report (March–April 1999): 45–48. Reprinted with permission of Lisa Sowle Cahill and The Hastings Center. Copyright 1999, The Hastings Center.

(or oneself), and one must, after all, be able to defend the proposition that free choice itself is a basic human good. Moreover, the nature of moral values, duties, and agency as interdependent and social implies that the community itself is an object of moral concern and analysis. The notion of justice as including and balancing both the good of individuals and the good of the community in which they associate can be referred to by the term "common good."

One of the conceptual and analytical difficulties we have in meeting the challenge of global justice is that we (in North America especially) tend to contrast autonomy or liberty and distributive justice as constituting different categories of obligation that are likely to be mutually incompatible. The EAB report, for instance, treats autonomy as expressing fairness and respect for persons, and holds that it is to be protected by informed consent. But although informed consent to experimentation on one's embryos is treated in relation to the intrinsic status of the embryo itself, there is little broader discussion of the way individual choice might be related to or responsible for the common good. Without this kind of discussion, it will hardly be possible to advance the consideration of global justice and access beyond a sort of impasse in which equitable access is one value and the liberty of investors another. Those with the capital will find little substantial reason to refrain from practices against which the value of liberty alone provides few concrete barriers.

As Daniel Callahan has worried, biomedical policy ethics is afraid of advancing community ideals or challenging the individualism of the rhetoric of choice and rights. In particular it has not carefully taken on the conceptions of human life, welfare, and the human future that are implicit in the biomedical research enterprise.[1] To do this is part of the challenge presented to us by the Geron EAB. Meeting this challenge will require a direct confrontation with the ways in which freedom and the market impinge on the right of all persons to participate in the common

good of an increasingly global society, as well as on the moral character of that society as such.

THE CULTURAL CONTEXT AND THE MARKET

The Geron EAB has rather tentatively implied that corporate aims and distributive justice might be on a collision course, but it has not really held up to the light the assumption that individual autonomy (of persons, groups, or corporations) is a moral priority independently of equitable access. The minimization of a link between liberty and the common good helps validate and institutionalize a free market economy, the kind upon which the business of Geron depends.

Daniel Finn has recently written that although markets are not intrinsically evil, moral markets must be subject to limits.[2] In the marketplace where buyers and sellers meet, certain kinds of activities and exchanges should be forbidden or limited. Finn refers to such restrictions as "fences" around the market. The issue is not whether market behavior should be subject to boundaries, with which even libertarians would agree, but where the fences should be erected, in consideration of both positive and negative effects. As a principle of fence construction, Finn suggests that there is a "social mortgage" on property, requiring that the basic needs of even the unpropertied be met. In this framework of the common good, liberty is not simply freedom from restraint, but the enablement of agency and communal participation, against a horizon of "communal provision" for the basic needs of all. The Geron EAB's report tacitly acknowledges this horizon and implies that in a global economic and biotechnology environment the "community" under moral consideration is in some sense global too.

Taking first a local view, one must acknowledge that the U.S. political and social environment is not particularly hospitable to ethical analyses premised on any global duty of "communal provision," or, as the EAB puts it, "global distributive justice and equitable access." Such moral ideas and ideals sit uneasily with our long-standing political traditions prizing individual civil liberties and minimizing federal or national control over access to material resources. In the assessment of Linell Cady, the political traditions of the United States follow the Enlightenment trajectory of downplaying both individual diversity and the webs of particular relationship that constitute community at the concrete and local level.[3] Instead, a public space is hypothesized that all comers enter as equal, individualized units. Moral obligation in this space becomes increasingly formal or procedural, something that can be applied identically to all persons. This ideal is reflected in the preeminent role in public bioethics of the criteria of autonomy and informed consent. It is also reflected in the difficulty we have in figuring out how to address proper limitations on freedom as exercised in market activity, especially in light of more inclusive ideals of community and shared goods. As Cady concludes, in this scenario, public life "is the individual writ large, the duplication on the macrocosmic level of its microcosmic atomism" (p. 68).

Indeed, the ideal of equitable access as expressed by the Geron EAB does not clearly envision a larger conversation about the fabric of social relations that sale of biotechnologies feeds on or promotes; nor about the dimensions of the common good that biomedical research can or should serve; nor about the sort of communal relations that exchanges of certain goods, labor, expertise, and services might reflect or produce; nor about determining criteria for deciding which possible objects of "equitable access" are deserving of communal resources. Instead, it simply asks that all individuals have equal rights to the genetic innovations that may be achieved by the research Geron funds, proposing that Geron itself and its advisors will work this out as well as possible at the ground level. The EAB report is brief, focused, and determined in large part by the parameters of previous documents and policies. Thus it may legitimately be seen as a first step in drawing to public attention some basic questions about social ethics and genetics for which Americans do not yet have a cultivated ear. But full consideration of these questions will require not only sensitive listeners but a much wider conversation.

A related point is that ethical "conversation" concludes in what can as well be called "discernment" as "judgment." Moral philosophers increasingly attend to the importance of the affective and emotional components of moral knowledge, and these are especially important in moving agents to action and establishing practices. Warren Reich describes the discernment that results in moral commitment as "a sort of prudential or practical reasoning which deals with a complex set of epistemological factors through its elements of detecting, sensing, sifting, discriminating, comparing, connecting, and deciding."[4] Within a model of broadbased and dialectical moral discernment, a variety of moral and religious stances and traditions can play a valuable role. These traditions may bring to the table a sensitivity to values in addition to autonomy, and support concern for the common good.

Themes, symbols, and ideals with a religious base—like love of neighbor, preferential option for the poor, covenant community, and stewardship—can stimulate the moral imagination and lend depth and texture to moral values and principles that may be more generally shared. James Gustafson proposes an "interactional-dialectical interpretation of a basis for ethics . . . from which persons strongly identified with a religious tradition and others can converse about medical morality."[5] The project of establishing a new consensus about social responsibility for the development, use, and consequences of biotechnology will require plumbing the resources of many traditions to arrive at a constellation of social values and priorities in which "just and equitable access" for all can be seen as a plausible common goal.

For this reason, the January 1999 ruling of the Office of General Council of the Department of Health and Human Services on federally funded stem cell research is a disappointment. Since 1995, the use of federal money for embryo research has been banned. The recent decision states that as long as stem cells are derived from embryos with private money, federal funds may be applied to research on the cells themselves. This resort to a legal technicality to avoid public discussion of the social significance and ethics of stem cell research does not advance the evolution of a wider and wiser moral perspective on biotechnology.

GLOBAL JUSTICE AND THE EMERGING WORLD ORDER

The context of international and transnational structures in which biotechnology is deployed, marketed, and barely regulated is a most important yet largely inscrutable factor in the ethical analysis. It involves the changing nature of a global "civil society" in which the market, scientific research, clinical medicine, public policy, and social control of any of them have burst the modern framework, in which global civilization is seen as a society of internally self-regulated nation states whose delegates coordinate policies at the international level. Political science literature on transnational institutions in the "new world order" can be useful in beginning to appreciate the complexity of the situation we face in meeting the Geron EAB's challenge of social justice.

The standard way of approaching regulation of scientific research and medical practice is through the federal and local governing structures of nations: for example, through legislatures, judiciaries, and professional accreditation and standards of practice. International structures come into play primarily in the form of organizations of states whose representatives make joint recommendations for law and policy at the

national level, with implementation dependent ultimately on adoption or ratification by members. But the assumption that nation states can be the primary agents of control and change in medical research or the life sciences industry is eroding. It is not responsive, for instance, to the facts that medical research is conducted across national borders, and that the purveyors and consumers of such research are internationally mobile, taking advantage of transportation and communications technologies to operate transnationally and seek out national environments that are most hospitable to their chosen enterprises.

In the view of Jeremy Rifkin, "a global life-science industry is already beginning to wield unprecedented power over the vast biological resources of the planet."[6] Many fields of research science "are being consolidated under the umbrella of giant 'life' companies in the emerging biotech marketplace" (p. 9). This time the Cassandra of modern technology rings true. His ethical concerns also converge with those of the Geron EAB, showing even more clearly why a truly intercultural approach is critical. Without broader debate and cooperative global governance, "the many special interests who have so much to gain from the speedy introduction and acceptance of their 'inventions' free themselves of any responsibility for having to ponder the merit, wisdom, or appropriateness of their 'contributions'"(p. 230).

Political scientist Jessica Mathews shows why imagination and sophistication will be as necessary as moral concern to erect the appropriate fences around the biotech marketplace. The distribution of power among states, market, and civil society has been reapportioned since the end of the Cold War. States are sharing powers with businesses, international organizations, and nongovernmental organizations. The new information technologies favor decentralized networks of power and joint action over the traditional hierarchies of government, enhancing the ability of business and research alike to operate across national boundaries and beyond the scope of national laws. More and more frequently, governments "have only the appearance of free choice when they set economic rules," since markets "are setting de facto rules enforced by their own power."[7]

For Mathews, a defining moment in the new world order was the Earth Summit in Rio de Janeiro in 1992. NGOs bridged North-South differences to mobilize public pressure and press through a treaty on greenhouse gasses that governments resisted. Mathews allows some hope for a beneficent outcome of the shifting power structure, since "a world that is more adaptable and in which power is more diffused could mean more peace, justice, and capacity to manage the burgeoning list of humankind's interconnected problems."[8] This will not happen, however, if marketplace values dominate the way power is deployed and human problems addressed. International organizations must take on larger roles, interfacing with the intersecting institutions of global "civil society" that provide and channel the conditions of daily life like security, food, shelter, and health care. Distressingly, a recent World Health Organization report that replicates the Geron EAB's position by insisting that "justice demands equitable access to genetic services," especially for those "whose needs are greatest," still envisions WHO as transmitting policy downward to member states, which then refine practices internally, in accordance with WHO principles.[9] This does little to touch the formal and informal economic institutions wherein reside the real brokers of genetic research benefits.

Exactly how biomedical marketing and consumption can be influenced toward greater equity and justice remains an unresolved question. Neither individual corporations nor nations can answer it in isolation from the other sectors of global civil society. An intercultural, international, multipronged approach has proven necessary on other issues of pressing global concern, such as the environment, ethnic conflict, human rights, and the trade in human beings. At the very least, philosophers and policy analysts in North America should pay more attention to the medical research policies of international and regional bodies like UNESCO, the United Nations Commission on Human Rights, the European Commission, and the Council of Europe. All of the above more overtly include considerations like human dignity and inviolability, the value of the embryo, and noncommodification of human life and human products in calling for limits on commercial exploitation of embryo and genetic research, than does U.S. policy. In Europe, restrictions on cloning, embryo research, and reproductive technologies apply to all relevant activities, whether privately or publicly funded.

In sum, the Geron EAB identifies the most important social justice challenge for stem cell research very accurately; it is a challenge shared with other forms of biotechnology. To meet the challenge, it will be necessary to place autonomy within an expanded concept of justice as including the common good; to give much more serious attention to appropriate limits on market behavior; and to understand medical research and therapy as occurring within "transnational" institutions of civil society that demand complex, multifocal regulation.

REFERENCES

1. Daniel Callahan, "Bioethics: Private Choice and the Common Good," *Hastings Center Report* 24, no. 3 (1994): 28–31.

2. Daniel R. Finn, "John Paul II and the Moral Ecology of Markets," *Theological Studies* 59, no. 4 (1998): 670–71.

3. Linell E. Cady, *Religion, Theology and American Public Life* (Albany, N.Y: State University of New York Press, 1993), pp. 66–68.

4. Warren Thomas Reich, with the assistance of Roberto dell'Oro, "A New Era for Bioethics: The Search for Meaning in Moral Experience," in *Religion and Medical Ethics: Looking Back, Looking Forward,* ed. Allen Verhey (Grand Rapids, Mich.: William B. Eerdmans, 1996), pp. 96–119, at III.

5. James M. Gustafson, *Intersections: Science, Theology, and Ethics* (Cleveland, Ohio: The Pilgrim Press, 1996), p. 72.

6. Jeremy Rifkin, *The Biotech Century: Harnessing the Gene and Remaking the World* (New York: Penguin Press, 1998), p. 9.

7. Jessica T. Mathews, "Power Shift," *Foreign Affairs* 76, no. (1997): 50–54; see also Anne-Marie Slaughter, "The Real New World Order," *Foreign Affairs* 76, no. 5 (1997): 183–97.

8. Mathews, "Power Shift," p. 59.

9. World Health Organization, *Proposed International Guidelines on Ethical Issues in Medical Genetics*, Report of a WHO Meeting on Ethical Issues in Medical Genetics, Geneva, 15–16 December 1997. Available at: http://www.who.int/ncd/hgn/hgnethic.htm.

Case Study Exercises

1. The age of physics has given way to the age of biochemistry, says Andrew Marr, who believes that fears of eugenics and genetic manipulation in the service of totalitarian regimes or dictators seem overblown. He contends that we may be able to cope with our increased knowledge and dexterity without disaster, arguing:

   Our strongest defence against the misuse of these discoveries is simply our democratic culture. We have learned the hard way to mistrust the state, the great misuser of science in the century just past (Chernobyl, forcible sterilisation, anthrax bombs) and we are learning to use boycotts and protests to rebuke private companies today when they push new technologies too hard and too fast. The hard questions thrown up by the genome breakthrough are not scientific ones at all. They are old-fashioned ethical and democratic ones. If you are scared by all this, then you are scared of yourself. . . . My guess is that the new genetics will bring wonderful medicines and very small shifts in the human stock, not the new eugenics or any of the nightmares based on crude and discredited thinking from a century ago. If, on the other hand, you began this piece with a spasm of furious blinking, then I am entirely wrong and the uncovering of the human genome has been a disaster. (See Andrew Marr, "Fears of a Clone: Worries about Designer Babies and Other Selective Breeding in the Wake of the Genome Project Are Overblown," *The Observer*, 2 July 2000.)

2. What are the strongest arguments for and against genetic testing of a potential husband or wife? Set out the arguments for and against making such genetic tests *mandatory* before allowing a couple to have children.

3. In an article in *The New York Times* on November 3, 1998, it was reported that medical records 30 years ago were carefully shielded. However, this is no longer the case. Dr. Abigail Zugler reported that in the summer of 1998 the federal government evidently considered assigning every citizen an electronic code to summarize his or her medical health, much as a credit report summarizes financial health—and, as she notes, presumably just as easy for interested parties to inspect. (See Abigail Zugler, "Ever Elusive, Privacy Slips from Grasp of Patients," *The New York Times*, 3 November 1998.) Set out your view on whether or not it would be wise for the government to streamline access to patient health information using an electronic code, in light of privacy considerations.

4. Should a person be able to sell his or her own genetic material? Set out the concerns regarding property rights and each person's own, unique genetic blueprint.

5. Stem-cell research holds the promise of an endless supply of new body parts. As noted by Steven H. Hall:

   Imagine, in short, a cell so protean and potent that it could theoretically generate an infinite supply of replaceable body parts—organ and skin, sinew and bone, blood and brain—to knit the tatters of disease, injury or old age. Imagine further that, with the use of controversial technologies like cloning, you might one day donate a snippet of your own skin, allowing scientists to harvest stem cells that theoretically would become a self-generated and limitless supply of transplant tissue—tissue that would make a perfect immunological match with you because, after all, it is you. These ideas have not only been imagined; patents and licensing agreements are already in place. . . . In November 1998, James Thomson of the University of Wisconsin reported the creation of human embryonic stem (or E.S.) cell line. . . . Michael Shamblott and John Gearhart, at the Johns Hopkins School of Medicine, headed a separate effort to cultivate something called "embryonic germline" (E.G.) cells, which are harvested from a tiny speck of fetal tissue from an aborted fetus and then grown in the lab. Because of the Congressional ban on federal financing for human-embryo experimentation, both teams conducted the research with financing from Geron. There are many technical hurdles to overcome. But the sheer power of the approach makes it clear that, if properly harnessed, stem cells could serve as a warehouse of spare human parts. (Steven H. Hall, "The Recycled Generation," *New York Times Magazine,* January 30, 2000.)

The research involves human embryos and is principally being done through private (corporate) money, resulting in a degree of secrecy.

Answer the following:

a. Do you think pro-life advocates are justified in their opposition to stem-cell research?

b. One concern with the privatization of the research is that public discussion of the issue has been constrained. This concern is exacerbated by abortion politics and ethical considerations raised by such research. How might we set up a public discussion (or even debate) that would allow us to examine the ethical ramifications of stem-cell research?

6. Currently there is a stampede to patent genetic information. For instance, new improved plant and animal species are being patented and this has the potential for lucrative profits for a research scientist. However, this has not proceeded without grave concerns on the part of ethicists and theologians. Set out the issues and concerns and your recommendations for how we should proceed in the matter of granting such patents.

7. Do you think we should allow animals to be genetically altered using the genetic material of another species? Discuss whether you see any ethical problems with the following case:

About 150 goats that have been bred with a spider gene are to be housed on 60 acres of a former Air Force base here [Plattsburgh, N.Y.]. Montreal-based Nexia Biotechnologies, Inc., plans for the goats to arrive Tuesday. The company said up to 1,500 genetically-altered goats may eventually live there. . . . The goats have been bred with a spider gene so their milk provides a unique protein. The company then plans to extract the protein from the milk to produce fibers—called BioSteel—for bulletproof vests, aerospace and medical supplies. Spider silk has a unique combination of strength and elasticity with an ultra-light-weight fiber. Last year, Nexia obtained the exclusive right to patents resulting from spider silk research at the University of Wyoming. The agreement included an up front payment for the university, funding for research and development expenses plus royalties on the sale of silk-based products. (See "Biotech Company to Produce 'BioSteel' Milk," *The Associated Press,* 18 June 2000.)

8. One of the consequences of learning whether one is a carrier of a genetic defect or disease is that the person may take matters into her own hands. For example, women can be tested to see if they carry the "breast cancer gene." Some women who learned that they positively were carriers of this gene elected to get mastectomies—even though they had no symptoms of breast cancer.

a. Set out the strongest case you can for a young woman getting a double mastectomy when finding out she is a carrier of the breast cancer gene.

b. Set out the strongest case against such a mastectomy.

    c. What are the societal concerns regarding giving out genetic information that people may act upon? Note the possible benefits and harms.

    d. Note the ethical issues around whether or not a physician should participate in helping seemingly healthy patients acquire genetic information so they can take steps (even extreme ones like mastectomies) to avoid underlying medical conditions that may not show up until much later.

9. In the case of *Calvert v. Johnson* (1990), Anna Johnson was a gestational surrogate for a couple (the Calverts) who provided the genetic material. The California Supreme Court ruled that Johnson had no maternal rights over the child she delivered. In short, genetics took precedence in such surrogate arrangements, and "merely" providing the service of nurturing the fetus and giving birth was relegated to a secondary role and one without any significance in establishing custodial rights to the child. State your position on whether genetics should be assigned that much significance in surrogacy (or other family) arrangements.

10. Share your thoughts on whether or not we ought to ban the cloning of human embryos. Discuss why some people find this morally repugnant, while others see it as a medical breakthrough that deserves federal support.

11. Set out the issues and concerns regarding genetic privacy. How might access to genetic information be abused (e.g., by an employer, health care provider, insurance company, and so on)? What ought we to do as a society to try to prevent possible abuses? It is anticipated that new genetic testing will make it possible to predict whether a patient will suffer a relapse of an underlying disease or enjoy complete recovery. For example, Millenium Pharmaceuticals, Inc., is said to have developed such a test for melanoma patients, based on a gene that produces melastatin. Tumors removed from the patient could be tested and, if they contain melastatin, they are most likely to be cancer free, while those with little or no melastatin could cause more serious skin cancer problems. (See Ronald Rosenberg, "Redefining Medicine with Genetic Code Mapping," *The Boston Globe,* 6 July 2000.) Do you foresee any ethical problems with such tests that have predictive value? Set out your thoughts or concerns.

12. Read the following and consider the questions below:

A new, superactive strain of mice that dash about their cages as if they are high on cocaine is yielding fresh ideas about ways to treat devastating human disorders, including drug addiction, schizophrenia and Parkinson's disease. The mice, which are at least five times as active as normal ones . . . run around for hours at a time, fail to eat enough to maintain a normal weight and sometimes drop dead from exhaustion. A Duke researcher, Dr. Marc Caron, said their frenetic state was comparable to that of a person high on cocaine or amphetamines. But in these mice, bred in the laboratory through genetic tinkering, the high is inborn rather than drug-induced . . . Circuits that would normally switch on and off are, in their case, "on" all the time. That leads to still another extraordinary trait: the mice appear completely immune to cocaine and amphetamines. (See Denise Grady, "Engineered Mice Mimic Drug Use and Mental Ills," *The New York Times,* 20 February 1996.)

    a. Are there any ethical problems with such research involving "genetic tinkering"? Share your thoughts.

    b. What sorts of benefits and risks are involved in genetic research such as in this case?

    c. Assuming we find a way to create an immunity to cocaine and amphetamines, e.g., by genetic engineering, would you recommend we consider applying this to humans?

13. British poet and waitress Donna MacLean is trying to become the first person to patent herself. Angered at the mass patenting of human genes by scientists and private companies, the woman filed an application with Great Britain's patent office. Citing the unpleasant, greedy atmosphere surrounding the mapping of the human genome, MacLean said she "wanted to see if a human being could protect their own genes in law." (See James Meek, *The Guardian* (London), 29 Feb 2000.) Whether or not you think there is any merit to her actions, the *Moore* case points out the ways in which scientists can potentially benefit financially using the genetic material of a patient or research subject. Should people be able to patent their own genetic material to prevent exploitation at the hands of others?

14. A controversial project in the eyes of indigenous groups is the Human Genome Diversity Project, which would involve collecting and storing DNA samples from hundreds of population groups. This has the potential to provide insight into human evolution and act as a springboard for medical research, according to William J. Schull, the National Research Council committee chair. However,

   Concerns have arisen about how research findings could be used against the participants. For example, health insurance might be denied to members of a group that is found to be genetically predisposed to a disease, or gene sequences could be patented for profit without any proceeds going to the group or individual donors from whom the genetic material was taken. The report recommends that the U.S. government should limit its initial funding for genetic diversity research to projects that originate in the United States, where an infrastructure of experienced investigators and well-equipped laboratories exists. (See *Public Health Reports,* Jan-Feb 1998, vol. 113, no. 1.)

   a. Native-American philosophers have expressed grave doubts about the DNA sampling of indigenous or other groups They felt there was legitimate cause for concern, whether the studies originated in the U.S. or not. Do you think it makes a significant difference in terms of the potential for abuse of individuals or groups where the studies originate?

   b. What sorts of issues arise when scientists seek to patent gene sequences for profit without compensating the individual donor(s)?

InfoTrac College Edition

1. M. Cathleen Kaveny, "Jurisprudence and Genetics"
2. Karen Wright, "Patient Medicine"
3. Joannie M. Schrof, "Remove the Mystery by Sorting the Sperm: Other Devices That Select the Sex Are Coming"
4. Anna Maria Gillis, "Finding the Right Sperm for the Job"
5. Daniel Goodkind, "On Substituting Sex Preference Strategies in East Asia: Does Prenatal Sex Selection Reduce Postnatal Discrimination?"
6. Anna Maria Gillis, "Sex Selection and Demographics: Population Biologists Use China as a Model to Theorize about Culture and Evolution"
7. David Shenk, "Biocapitalism: What Price the Genetic Revolution?"
8. Stephen G. Post, "The Judeo-Christian Case against Cloning"
9. *Public Health Reports,* "Genetic Sampling: Big Brother or Big Science?"
10. Susan Mayor, "UK Government Confirms Ban on Human Reproductive Cloning"

11. Raj S. Shiwach, "Letter to Editor of *The Lancet* on Human Cloning"
12. Thomas A. Shannon, "Ethical Issues in Genetics"
13. Susan Mayor, "UK Authorities Recommend Human Cloning for Therapeutic Research"
14. Christian Crews, "Let's Broaden Our View of Cloning"

Web Connections

For links to Genetics and Cloning Web sites, articles, cases, and more exercises go to our Genetics page at philosophy.wadsworth.com/teays.purdy/genetics

Bibliography

Chapter 1
Social Constructions of Health

Bandman, Elsie L., and Bertram Bandman. 1985. *Nursing Ethics in the Life Span.* Norwalk, CT: Appleton-Century-Crofts.

Caplan, Arthur L., H. Tristram Engelhardt, Jr., and James McCartney, eds. 1981. *Concepts of Health and Disease: Interdisciplinary Perspectives.* Reading, MA: Addison-Wesley.

Charmaz, Kathy, and Debora A. Paterniti. 1999. *Health, Illness, and Healing: Society, Social Context, and Self: An Anthology.* Los Angeles: Roxbury Publishing Co.

Ehrenreich, Barbara, and John Ehrenreich. 1970. *The American Health Empire: Power, Profits and Politics.* New York: Random House.

Emmanuel, Ezekiel. 1991. *The Ends of Human Life: Medical Ethics in a Liberal Polity.* Cambridge, MA: Harvard University Press.

Fein, Rashi. 1972. "On Achieving Access and Equity in Health Care." *Milbank Memorial Fund Quarterly,* Vol. 50, pp. 157–190.

Hardey, Michael. 1998. *The Social Context of Health.* Philadelphia: Open University Press.

Henderson, Gail E., et al. 1997. *The Social Medicine Reader.* Durham, NC: Duke University Press.

Lorber, Judith. 1997. *Gender and the Social Construction of Illness.* Thousand Oaks, CA: Sage Publications.

Marmor, Theodore R. 1993. "Health Care Reform in the United States: Patterns of Fact and Fiction in the Use of Canadian Experience." *American Review of Canadian Studies,* Vol. 23, no. 1, pp. 47–64.

Mechanic, David. 1986. *From Advocacy to Allocation: The Evolving American Health Care System.* New York: Free Press.

Morris, David B. 1998. *Illness and Culture in the Postmodern Age.* Berkeley: University of California Press.

Payer, Lynn. 1988. *Medicine and Culture: Varieties of Treatment in the United States, England, West Germany, and France.* New York: Henry Holt.

Pierce, Christine, and Donald VanDeVeer. 1988. *AIDS: Ethics and Public Policy.* Belmont, CA: Wadsworth.

Purdy, Laura M. 1996. "A Feminist View of Health," in *Feminism and Bioethics: Beyond Reproduction,* Susan M. Wolf, ed. New York: Oxford University Press.

Raffel, Marshall W., ed. 1984. *Comparative Health Systems: Descriptive Analyses of Fourteen National Health Systems.* University Park: Pennsylvania State Press.

Rodwin, Marc A. 1993. *Medicine, Money & Morals.* New York: Oxford University Press.

Singer, Peter. 1991. "How Green Is Your Grass?: A Comparative Analysis of the American and Canadian Health Care Systems." *Humane Medicine,* Vol. 7 (Winter), pp. 47–53.

Veatch, Robert M. 1989. *Cross Cultural Perspectives in Medical Ethics: Readings.* Boston: Jones and Bartlett.

Ziegenfuss, James T., Jr. 1984. *Law, Medicine and Health Care: A Bibliography.* New York: Facts on File.

Chapter 2
Rights and Obligations in Health Care

Battin, Margaret P. 1987. "Age Rationing and the Just Distribution of Health Care: Is There a Duty to Die?" *Ethics,* Vol. 97, pp. 317–340.

Binstock, Robert H., and Stephen G. Post, eds. 1991. *Too Old for Health Care? Controversies in Medicine,*

Law, Economics, and Ethics. Baltimore: Johns Hopkins University Press.

Blackstone, William T. 1976. "On Health Care as a Legal Right: Philosophical Justifications, Political Activity, and Adequate Health Care." *Georgia Law Review,* Vol. 10, pp. 391–418.

Blank, Robert. 1988. *Rationing Medicine.* New York: Columbia University Press.

Bole, Thomas J., and William B. Bondeson, eds. 1991. *Rights to Health Care.* Boston: Kluwer Academic Publishers.

Calabresi, Guido, and Philip Bobbit. 1978. *Tragic Choices: The Conflicts Society Confronts in the Allocation of Tragically Scarce Resources.* New York: W. W. Norton.

Callahan, Daniel. 1987. *Setting Limits: Medical Goals in an Aging Society.* New York: Simon & Schuster.

——. 1990. *What Kind of Life: The Limits of Medical Progress.* New York: Simon & Schuster.

Childress, James. 1984. "Ensuring Care, Respect, and Fairness for the Elderly." *Hastings Center Report,* Vol. 14 (October), pp. 27–31.

——. 1981. *Priorities in Biomedical Ethics.* Philadelphia: Westminster Press.

Churchill, Larry M. 1987. *Rationing Health Care in America: Perceptions and Principles of Justice.* Notre Dame, IN: University of Notre Dame.

Daniels, Norman. 1985. *Just Health Care.* New York: Cambridge University Press.

——. 1995. *Fair Treatment: The Lesson of AIDS for National Health Care.* New York: Oxford University Press.

——, Donald W. Light, and Arthur L. Caplan. 1996. *Benchmarks of Fairness for Health Care Reform.* New York: Oxford University Press.

Fleck, Leonard M. 1990. "Justice, HMOs, and the Invisible Rationing of Health Care Resources." *Bioethics,* Vol. 4, pp. 97–120.

Fried, Charles. 1975. "Rights and Health Care—Beyond Equity and Efficiency." *New England Journal of Medicine,* Vol. 293 (31 July), pp. 241–245.

Fuchs, Victor. 1974. *Who Shall Live? Health, Economics, and Social Choice.* New York: Basic Books.

Gordon, Suzanne, et al., eds. 1996. *Caregiving: Readings in Knowledge, Practice, Ethics, and Politics.* Philadelphia: University of Pennsylvania Press.

Green, Ronald M. 1983. "The Priority of Health Care." *Journal of Medical Philosophy,* Vol. 8, pp. 373–380.

Gutmann, Amy. 1981. "For and Against Equal Access to Health Care." *Milbank Memorial Fund Quarterly,* Vol. 59 (Fall), pp. 542–560.

Huefner, Robert R., and Margaret P. Battin, eds. 1992. *Changing to National Health Care: Ethical and Policy Issues.* Salt Lake City: University of Utah Press.

Iglehart, John K. 1992. "The American Health Care System: Managed Care." *New England Journal of Medicine,* Vol. 327 (September 3), pp. 742–747.

Jecker, Nancy S. 1991. "Age-Based Rationing and Women." *Journal of the American Medical Association,* Vol. 226, no. 21, pp. 3012–3015.

——, ed. 1991. *Aging and Ethics: Philosophical Problems in Gerontology.* Clifton, NJ: Humana Press.

Journal of Medicine and Philosophy. 1988. Special issue on the right to health care. Vol. 13.

Knowles, John H., ed. 1977. *Doing Better and Feeling Worse: Health Care in the United States.* New York: W. W. Norton.

——. "The Law and Policy of Health Care Rationing: Models and Accountability." 1992. *University of Pennsylvania Law Review,* Vol. 140, no. 5, pp. 1505–1598.

Laurence, Leslie, and Beth Weinhouse. 1994. *Outrageous Practices: How Gender Bias Threatens Women's Health.* New Brunswick, NJ: Rutgers University Press.

Menzel, Paul T. 1983. *Medical Costs, Moral Choices.* New Haven, CT: Yale University Press.

——. 1991. *Strong Medicine: The Ethical Rationing of Health Care.* New York: Oxford University Press.

Morreim, E. Haavi. 1991. *Balancing Act: The New Medical Ethics of Medicine's New Economics.* Boston: Kluwer Academic Publishers.

——, ed. 1992. "Access Without Excess." *Journal of Medicine and Philosophy,* Vol. 17, no. 1, pp. 1–6.

Orentlicher, David. 1994. "Rationing and the Americans with Disabilities Act." *Journal of the American Medical Association,* Vol. 271, no. 4, pp. 308–314.

Outka, Gene. 1974. "Social Justice and Equal Access to Health Care." *The Journal of Religious Ethics,* Vol. 2, pp. 11–32.

Pellegrino, Edmund D. 1986. "Rationing Health Care: The Ethics of Medical Gatekeeping." *Journal of Contemporary Health Law and Policy,* Vol. 2 (Spring), pp. 23–45.

President's Commission for the Study of Ethical Problems in Medicine and Biomedical and Behavioral Research. 1982. *Securing Access to Health Care: The Differences in the Availability of Health Services.*

Shelp, Earl, ed. 1981. *Justice and Health Care.* Boston: D. Reidel.

Veatch, Robert M. 1986. *The Foundations of Justice: Why the Retarded and the Rest of Us Have Claims to Equality.* New York: Oxford University Press.

Washington, D.C.: "President's Commission on Rationing Health: Social, Political and Legal Perspectives." 1992. *American Journal of Law and Medicine*, Vol. 18, nos. 1–3 (Symposium).

Weaver, Jerry L. 1976. *National Health Policy and the Underserved: Ethnic Minorities, Women, and the Elderly*. St. Louis: Mosby.

———. "The American Health Security Act: A Single-Payer Proposal." *New England Journal of Medicine*, Vol. 328 (May 20), pp. 1489–1493.

Chapter 3
Medical Experimentation: Historical Considerations

Adams, Diane, ed. 1996. *Health Issues for Women of Color*. Thousand Oaks, CA: Sage Publications.

Advisory Committee on Human Radiation Experiments. 1995. *Final Report*. Washington, D.C.: U.S. Government Printing Office.

Ahronheim, Judith C., Jonathan Moren, and Connie Zeckerman. 1994. *Ethics in Clinical Practice*. Boston: Little, Brown.

Aly, Gotz. 1994. *Cleansing the Fatherland: Nazi Medicine and Racial Hygiene*. Baltimore: Johns Hopkins University Press.

Annas, George J., and Michael A. Grodin, eds. 1992. *The Nazi Doctors and the Nuremberg Code: Human Rights in Human Experimentation*. New York: Oxford University Press.

Aziz, P. 1976. *Doctors of Death*, Vol. 2. *Joseph Mengele, the Evil Doctor*. 1976. Geneva: Ferni Publishing.

Barker-Benfield, G. J. 1976. *The Horrors of the Half-Known Life: Male Attitudes Toward Women and Sexuality in Nineteenth-Century America*. New York: Harper & Row.

Bayne-Smith, Marcia, ed. 1996. *Race, Gender, and Health*. Thousand Oaks, CA: Sage Publications.

Beecher, Henry K. 1966. "Ethics and Clinical Research." *New England Journal of Medicine*, Vol. 274, no. 24, pp. 1354–1360.

Bernadac, C. 1978. *Devil's Doctors: Medical Experiments on Human Subjects in the Concentration Camps*. Geneva: Ferni Publishing.

Bok, Sissela. 1989. *Secrets: On the Ethics of Concealment and Revelation*. New York: Vintage Books.

Brody, Baruch A. 1998. *The Ethics of Biomedical Research: An International Perspective*. New York: Oxford University Press.

Caplan, Arthur L., ed. 1992. *When Medicine Went Mad: Bioethics and the Holocaust*. Totowa, NJ: Humana Press.

Dula, Annette, and Sara Goering, eds. 1994. *"It Just Ain't Fair": The Ethics of Health Care for African Americans*. Westport, CT: Praeger.

Erwin, Edwin, Sidney Gendin, and Lowell Kleiman. 1994. *Ethical Issues in Scientific Research*. New York: Garland Publishing.

Evans, Donald. 1996. *A Decent Proposal: Ethical Review of Clinical Research*. New York: John Wiley & Sons.

Faden, Ruth, and Tom Beauchamp. 1986. *History and Theory of Informed Consent*. New York: Oxford University Press.

"Final Report of the Tuskegee Syphilis Study Legacy Committee." Vanessa Northington Gamble, chair, and John C. Fletcher, co-chair, 20 May 1996. http://www.nlm.nih.gov/pubs/cbm/hum_exp.html

Fisher, J. Walter. 1968. "Physicians and Slavery in the Antebellum Southern Medical Journal." *Journal of the History of Medicine and Allied Sciences*, Vol. 23, no. 1, pp. 36–49.

Fox, Renee C. 1998. *Experiment Perilous: Physicians and Patients Facing the Unknown*. New Brunswick, NJ: Transaction Publishers.

Genovese, Eugene. 1974. *Roll, Jordan, Roll: The World the Slaves Made*. New York: Pantheon.

Griffith, Lucille. 1962. *History of Alabama*. Northport, AL: Colonial Press.

Grodin, Michael A., and Leonard H. Glantz, eds. 1994. *Children as Research Subjects: Science, Ethics, and Law*. New York: Oxford University Press.

Harris, Seale. 1950. *Woman's Surgeon*. New York: Macmillan.

Hornblum, Allen M. 1998. *Acres of Skin: Human Experiments at Holmesburg Prison: A True Story of Abuse and Exploitation in the Name of Medical Science*. New York: Routledge.

Humphrey, David C. 1973. "Dissection and Discrimination: The Social Origins of Cadavers in America, 1760–1915." New York Academy of Medicine *Bulletin* LXIX (Sept.), pp. 819–827.

International Auschwitz Committee on Nazi Medicine. 1986. *Doctors, Victims and Medicine in Auschwitz*. New York: Ferni Publishing.

Internet resources on the Tuskegee Study: http://www.dc.peachnet.edu/%7Eshale/humanities/composition/assignments/experiment/tuskegee.html

Jones, James H. 1981. *Bad Blood: The Tuskegee Syphilis Experiment*. New York: Free Press.

Katz, Jay. 1972. *Experimentation with Human Beings: The Authority of the Investigator, Subject, Professions, and State in the Human Experimentation Process*. New York: Russell Sage Foundation.

———. 1984. *The Silent World of Doctor and Patient.* New York: Free Press.

King, J. H., Jr. 1986. *The Law of Medical Malpractice,* 2nd ed. St. Paul, MN: West Publishing.

Krugman, Saul. 1968. "Reflections on Pediatric Clinical Investigations," in *Problems of Drug Evaluation in Infants and Children,* Report of the Fifty-eighth Ross Conference on Pediatric Research, Dorado Beach, Puerto Rico, May 5–7, 1968. Columbus, OH: Ross Laboratories, pp. 41–42.

Lagnado, L. M., and S. C. Dekel. 1991. *Children of the Flames: Dr. Josef Mengele and the Untold Story of the Twins of Auschwitz.* New York: William Morrow.

Lederer, Susan E. 1995. *Subjected to Science: Human Experimentation in America before the Second World War.* Baltimore: Johns Hopkins University Press.

Levine, Lawrence W. 1977. *Black Culture and Black Consciousness.* New York: Oxford University Press.

Levine, Robert J. 1986. *Ethics and Regulation of Clinical Research.* Baltimore: Urban & Schwarzenberg.

Lifton, Robert Jay. 1986. *Nazi Doctors: Medical Killing and the Psychology of Genocide.* New York: Basic Books.

Link, Eugene P. 1969. "The Civil Rights Activities of Three Great Negro Physicians (1840–1940)." *Journal of Negro History* 521 (July): 177.

Marange, Valerie. 1991. *Doctors and Torture: Resistance or Collaboration?* London: Bellew Publishers.

McNeill, Paul M. 1993. *The Ethics and Politics of Human Experimentation.* New York: Cambridge University Press.

Mendelsohn, Robert S. 1981. *Male Practice: New Doctors Manipulate Women.* Chicago: Contemporary Books.

Mole, Robert L. 1993. *For God and Country: Operation Whitecoat: 1954–1973.* New York: Teach Services, Inc.

Muller-Hill, Benno. 1998. *Murderous Science: Elimination by Scientific Selection of Jews, Gypsies, and Others in Germany, 1933–1945.* Plainview, NY: Cold Spring Harbor Laboratory Press.

Nyiszli, M. 1986. *Auschwitz: An Eyewitness Account of Mengele's Infamous Death Camp.* New York: Seaver Books.

Perlin, Terry M. 1992. *Clinical Medical Ethics: Cases in Practice.* Boston: Little, Brown.

"Remarks by the President in Apology for Study Done in Tuskegee." Press Release, the White House, Office of the Press Secretary, 16 May 1997.

Robinson, Victor. 1946. *Victory over Pain: A History of Anesthesia.* New York: Henry Schuman.

Rothman, David J. 1991. *Strangers at the Bedside: A History of How Law and Bioethics Transformed Medical Decision Making.* New York: Basic Books.

Savitt, Todd. L. 1978. *Medicine and Slavery: The Diseases and Health Care of Blacks in Antebellum Virginia.* Chicago: Urbana.

Swanson, G. Marie, and Amy J. Ward. 1995. "Recruiting Minorities into Clinical Trials: Toward a Participant-Friendly System." *Journal of the Cancer Institute* 87: 1747–1759.

Taylor, T. 1946. "Opening Statement of the Prosecution." *Trials of War Criminals Before Nuremberg Military Tribunals Under Control Law No. 1, The Medical Case.* Washington, D.C.: U.S. Government Printing Office.

Thomas, Stephen B., and Sandra C. Quinn. 1991. "The Tuskegee Syphilis Study, 1932 to 1972: Implications for HIV Education and AIDS Risk Education Programs in the Black Community." *American Journal of Public Health,* Vol. 81, no. 11, pp. 1249–1305.

Veatch, Robert M. *The Patient as Partner: A Theory of Human-Experimentation Ethics.* Bloomington: Indiana University Press.

Ward, Robert, et al. 1958. "Infectious Hepatitis: Studies of Its Natural History and Prevention." *New England Journal of Medicine,* Vol. 258, no. 9, pp. 407–416.

Chapter 4
Contemporary Issues of Informed Consent

American Society for Reproductive Medicine. 1998. *Guidelines for Gamete and Embryo Donation.* Birmingham, AL: American Society for Reproductive Medicine.

Annas, G., and S. Elias. 1989. "The Politics of Transplantation of Human Fetal Tissue." *New England Journal of Medicine,* Vol. 320, no. 16, pp. 1079–1082.

Bauer, Arthur R. 1994. *Legal and Ethical Aspects of Fetal Tissue Transplantation.* Austin, TX: R. G. Landes Co.

Beauchamp, Tom L. 1997. "Opposing Views on Animal Experimentation: Do Animals Have Rights?" *Ethics Behavior,* Vol. 7, no. 2, pp. 113–121.

———, and L. Walter, eds. 1989. *Contemporary Issues in Bioethics,* 3rd ed. Belmont, CA: Wadsworth.

Boss, Judith A., and Alyssa V. Boss. 1994. "Paradigm Shifts, Scientific Revolutions and the Moral Justification of Experimentation on Nonhuman Animals." *Between Species,* Vol. 10, no. 3–4, pp. 119–130.

Brassard, Ed. 1996. *Body for Sale: An Inside Look at Medical Research, Drug Testing, and Organ Transplants and How You Can Profit from Them.* Boulder, CO: Paladin Press.

Brody, Baruch A. 1998. *The Ethics of Biomedical Research: An International Perspective.* New York: Oxford University Press.

Buchanan, A., and D. Brock. 1989. *Deciding for Others: The Ethics of Surrogate Decisionmaking.* New York: Cambridge University Press.

Burk, Judith, Seymour L. Zelezn, and Edward O. Terino. 1985. "More than Skin Deep." *Plastic and Reconstructive Surgery,* Vol. 76, no. 2, pp. 271–275.

Byar, D. P., D. A. Schoenfeld, S. B. Green, et al. 1990. "Design Considerations for AIDS Trials." *New England Journal of Medicine,* Vol. 323, no. 19, pp. 1343–1348.

Campbell, Courtney S. 1992. "Body, Self, and the Property Paradigm." *Hastings Center Report,* Vol. 22, no. 5, pp. 34–42.

Canterbury v. Spence, 464 F.2d 772 (D.C. Cir.), cert. denied, 409 U.S. 1064 (1972).

Caplan, Arthur L. 1994. *If I Were a Rich Man, Could I Buy a Pancreas? And Other Essays on the Ethics of Health Care.* Bloomington: Indiana University Press.

Catlin, Don H., and Thomas H. Murray. 1996. "Performance-Enhancing Drugs, Fair Competition, and Olympic Sport." *Journal of the American Medical Association,* Vol. 276, no. 3, pp. 231–237.

Clune, Alan C. 1996. "Biomedical Testing on Nonhuman Animals: An Attempt at a 'Rapprochement' between 'Utilitarianism' and Theories of Inherent Value." *Monist,* Vol. 79, no. 2, pp. 230–235.

Cobbs v. Grant, 8 Cal. 3d 229 104 Cal. Rptr. 505, 502 P.2d 1 (1972).

Cole, Norman M. 1988. "Informed Consent: Considerations in Aesthetic and Reconstructive Surgery of the Breast." *Plastic and Reconstructive Breast Surgery,* Vol. 15, no. 4, pp. 541–548.

D'Antonio, Michael. 1993. *Atomic Harvest: Hanford and the Lethal Toll of America's Nuclear Arsenal.* New York: Crown Publishing.

Donnelley, Strachan, Charles R. McCarthy, and Rivers Singleton, Jr. 1994. "The Brave New World of Animal Biotechnology." *Hastings Center Report,* Vol. 24, no. 1, Supp., pp. 1–31.

Dorney, Maureen S. 1990. "*Moore v. the Regents of the University of California:* Balancing the Need for Biotechnology Innovation Against the Right of Informed Consent." *High Technology Law Journal,* Vol. 5, no. 2, pp. 333–370.

Eichstaedt, Peter H. 1990. *If You Poison Us: Uranium and Native Americans.* Santa Fe, NM: Red Crane Books.

Erwin, Edwin, Sidney Gendin, and Lowell Kleiman. 1994. *Ethical Issues in Scientific Research.* New York: Garland Publishing.

Faden, Ruth, and Tom Beauchamp. 1986. *History and Theory of Informed Consent.* New York: Oxford University Press.

Fox, Renee C., and Judith P. Swazey. 1992. *Spare Parts: Organ Replacement in American Society.* New York: Oxford University Press.

Fradkin, Phillip L. 1989. *Fallout: An American Nuclear Tragedy.* Tucson: University of Arizona Press.

Freedman, Benjamin. 1975. "A Moral Theory of Informed Consent." *Hastings Center Report,* Vol. 5 (August), pp. 32–39.

Gold, E. Richard. 1996. *Body Parts: Property Rights and the Ownership of Human Biological Materials.* Washington, D.C.: Georgetown University Press.

Hacker, Barton C. 1987. *The Dragon's Tail: Radiation Safety in the Manhattan Project, 1942–1946.* Berkeley: University of California Press.

Hershberg, James. 1993. *Harvard to Hiroshima and the Making of the Nuclear Age.* New York: Alfred Knopf.

Hillebrecht, John M. 1989. "Regulating the Clinical Uses of Fetal Tissue: A Proposal for Legislation." *The Journal of Legal Medicine,* Vol. 10, no. 2, pp. 269–322.

Hilts, Philip J. 1992. "Strange History of Silicone Held Many Warning Signs." *The New York Times,* 18 January, p. A8.

Hyman, David. 1990. "Aesthetics and Ethics: The Implications of Cosmetic Surgery." *Perspectives in Biology and Medicine,* Vol. 33, no. 2, p. 193.

John Moore v. Regents of the University of California, 202 Cal.App.3d 1230.

Johnson, Charles W., and Charles O. Jackson. 1981. *City Behind a Fence: Oak Ridge, Tennessee, 1942–1946.* Knoxville: University of Tennessee Press.

Jorgensen, O. L., and Jens L. Christiansen. 1993. "Growth Hormone Therapy—Brave New Senescence: GH in Adults." *Lancet,* Vol. 341, no. 8855, pp. 1247–1248.

Josefson, Deborah. 1998. "Concern Raised About Performance Enhancing Drugs in the US." *British Medical Journal,* Vol. 317, no. 7160, p. 702.

Kahn, Jeffrey P., Anna C. Mastroianni, and Jeremy Sugarman. 1998. *Beyond Consent: Seeking Justice in Research.* New York: Oxford University Press.

Kathren, Ronald L., Jerry B. Gough, and Gary T. Benefiel, eds. 1984. *The Plutonium Story: The Journals of Professor Glenn T. Seaborg, 1939–1946.* Columbus, OH: Battelle Press.

Kerns, Thomas A. 1997. *Ethical Issues in HIV Vaccine Trials.* New York: St. Martin's Press.

———. 1993. "Animal Models in Biomedical Research: Some Epistemological Worries." *Public Affairs Quarterly,* Vol. 7, no. 2, pp. 113–130.

Lindee, Susan. 1994. *Suffering Made Real: American Science and the Survivors of Hiroshima.* Chicago: University of Chicago Press.

Lombardo, Paul. A. 1981. "Consent and Donations from the Dead." *Hastings Center Report,* Vol. 11, no. 6, pp. 9–11.

MacDonald, June Fessenden. 1992. *Ethics and Patenting of Transgenic Organisms.* Ithaca, NY: National Agricultural Biotechnology Council.

McNeill, Paul M. 1993. *The Ethics and Politics of Human Experimentation.* New York: Cambridge University Press.

Magel, C. R. 1981. *A Bibliography on Animal Rights and Related Matters.* Washington, D.C.: University Press of America.

Mastroianni, Anna C., Ruth R. Faden, and Daniel D. Federman. 1994. *Women and Health Research: Ethical and Legal Issues of Including Women in Clinical Studies.* Washington, D.C.: National Academy Press.

Munzer, Stephen R. 1994. " An Uneasy Case Against Property Rights in Body Parts." *Social Philosophy and Policy,* Vol. 11, no. 2, pp. 259–286.

Natanson v. Kline, 186 Kan. 393, 350 P.2d 1093, the opinion on denial of motion for rehearing, 187 Kan. 186 354 P.2d 670 (1960).

Ozar, David T. 1985. "The Case Against Thawing Unused Frozen Embryos." *Hastings Center Report,* Vol. 15, no. 4, pp. 7–12.

Palmer, Louis J. 1999. *Organ Transplants from Executed Prisoners: An Argument for the Creation of Death Sentence Organ Removal Statutes.* Jefferson, NC: McFarland.

Petchesky, Rosalind Pollack. 1987. "Foetal Images: The Power of Visual Culture in the Politics of Reproduction." In Michelle Stanworth, ed., *Reproductive Technologies: Gender, Motherhood and Medicine.* Minneapolis: University of Minnesota Press.

Potts, John T. 1997. *Non-Heart-Beating Organ Transplantation: Medical and Ethical Issues in Procurement.* Washington, D.C.: National Academy Press.

Preece, Rod, and Lorna Chamberlain. 1995. *Animal Welfare and Human Values.* Waterloo, Ontario: Wilfrid Laurier University Press.

Prottas, Jeffrey. 1994. *The Most Useful Gift: Altruism and the Public Policy of Organ Transplants.* San Francisco: Jossey-Bass.

Public Responsibility in Medicine and Research. 1989. *People as Products: The Ethical, Legal and Social Issues in Reproductive Technologies and Other Procedures Involving the Commercialization of Body Parts and Tissues.* Boston: Public Responsibility in Medicine and Research.

Radin, Margaret J. 1982. "Property and Personhood." *Stanford Law Review,* Vol. 34 (May), pp. 957–1015.

Roberts, James David. 1988. "The Intentional Creation of Fetal Tissue for Transplants: The Womb as a Fetus Farm?" *The John Marshall Law Review,* Vol. 21, no. 4, pp. 853–880.

Rosenberg, Howard L. 1980. *Atomic Soldiers: American Victims of Nuclear Experiments.* Boston: Beacon Press.

Schloendorff v. Society of New York Hospital, 211 N.Y. 125, 105 N.E. 92, 95 (1914).

Shanks, Niall, and Hugh LaFollette. 1996. *Brute Science: Dilemmas of Animal Experimentation.* New York: Routledge.

Smyth, Henry DeWolf. 1989. *Atomic Energy for Military Purposes: The Official Report on the Development of the Atomic Bomb under the Auspices of the United States Government: 1940–1945.* Stanford, CA: Stanford University Press.

Sordillo, Peter P., and Kenneth F. Schaffner. 1981. "The Last Patient in a Drug Trial." *Hastings Center Report,* Vol. 11, no. 6, pp. 21–23.

Sperlinger, D., ed. 1991. *Animals in Research: New Perspectives in Animal Experimentation.* New York: John Wiley & Sons.

Stannard, J. Newell. 1988. *Radioactivity and Health: A History.* Oak Ridge, TN: Office of Scientific and Technical Information.

Starr, Paul. 1982. *The Transformation of American Medicine.* New York: Basic Books.

Udall, Stewart L. 1994. *The Myths of August: A Personal Exploration of Our Tragic Cold War Affair with the Atom.* New York: Pantheon Books.

Underkuffler, Laura S. 1990. "On Property." *Yale Law Journal,* Vol. 100 (Oct.), pp. 127–148.

U.S. Congress, Office of Technology Assessment. 1987. *New Developments in Biotechnology: Ownership of Human Tissues and Cells—Special Report.* Washington, D.C.: U.S. Congress, Office of Technology Assessment.

Vawter, Dorothy E. 1990. *The Use of Human Fetal Tissue: Scientific, Ethical, and Policy Concerns.* Minneapolis, MN: Center for Biomedical Ethics, University of Minnesota.

Weisgall, Jonathan. 1994. *Operation Crossroads.* Annapolis, MD: Naval Institute Press.

Weiss, R. 1991. "Breast Implant Fears Put Focus on Biomaterials." *Science,* Vol. 252, no. 5010, pp. 1059–1060.

White, Gladys. 1993. "Human Growth Hormone: The Dilemma of Expanded Use in Children." *Kennedy Institute of Ethics Journal,* Vol. 3, no. 4, p. 401.

Chapter 5
Death and Dying

Ackerman, Felicia. 1997. "Goldilocks and Mrs. Ilych: A Critical Look at the 'Philosophy of Hospice,'" *Cambridge Quarterly of Healthcare Ethics,* Vol. 6, no. 3, pp. 314–324.

Amundsen, D. W. 1978. "The Physician's Obligation to Prolong Life: A Medical Duty Without Classical Roots." *Hastings Center Report,* Vol. 8, pp. 23–30.

Annas, George J. 1994. "Death by Prescription: The Oregon Initiative." *New England Journal of Medicine,* Vol. 331, no. 18, pp. 1240–1243.

———. 1995. "How We Lie." *Hastings Center Report,* Vol. 25, no. 6, pp. S12–S14.

Anonymous. 1988. "It's Over, Debbie." *Journal of the American Medical Association,* Vol. 259, no. 14, pp. 2094–2098.

Bailey, Don V. 1990. *The Challenge of Euthanasia: An Annotated Bibliography on Euthanasia and Related Subjects.* Lanham, MD: University Press of America.

Baird, Robert M., and Stuart E. Rosenbaum, eds. 1989. *Euthanasia: The Moral Issues.* Buffalo, NY: Prometheus Books.

Bartholome, William G. 1997. "Still Here/Above Ground." *Bioethics Forum,* Vol. 13, no. 1, pp. 31–37.

Battin, Margaret Pabst. 1995. *Ethical Issues in Suicide.* Englewood Cliffs, NJ: Prentice-Hall.

———, Rosamund Rhodes, and Anita Silvers. 1998. *Physician-Assisted Suicide: Expanding the Debate.* New York: Routledge.

Beauchamp, Tom L., ed. 1996. *Intending Death: The Ethics of Assisted Suicide and Euthanasia.* Upper Saddle River, NJ: Prentice-Hall.

Berger, Arthur S., and Joyce Berger, eds. 1990. *To Die or Not to Die? Cross-Disciplinary, Cultural and Legal Perspectives on the Right to Choose Death.* New York: Praeger.

Bouvia v. Superior Court, 255 Cal. Rptr. 297, 306 (1986).

Brock, Dan W. 1992. "Voluntary Active Euthanasia." *Hastings Center Report,* Vol. 22, no. 2, pp. 10–22.

Brody, Baruch A., ed. 1989. *Suicide and Euthanasia: Historical and Contemporary Themes.* Boston: Kluwer Academic Publishers.

Brophy v. New England Sinai Hospital, Inc., 497 N.E. 2d 626 (Mass. 1986).

Callahan, Daniel. 1989. "Mercy, Murder, & Morality: Perspectives on Euthanasia. Can We Return Death to Disease?" Special Supplement. *Hastings Center Report,* Vol. 19, no. 1, suppl., pp. 4–6.

———. 1990. *What Kind of Life: The Limits of Medical Progress.* New York: Simon & Schuster.

Cantor, Norman L., and George C. Thomas III. 1996. "Pain Relief, Acceleration of Death, and Criminal Law." *Kennedy Institute of Ethics Journal,* Vol. 6, no. 2, pp. 107–128.

Cassell, E. 1982. "The Nature of Suffering and the Goals of Medicine." *New England Journal of Medicine,* Vol. 306, no. 11, pp. 639–645.

Compassion in Dying v. Washington, 79 Fed 790 (9th Circ. 1996).

Cruzan v. Harmon, 760 S.W. 2d 408 (Mo. 1988), *aff'd sub. nom. Cruzan v. Director,* 497 U.S. 261 (1990).

Devettere, Raymond J. 1990. "Neocortical Death and Human Death." *Law, Medicine & Health Care,* Vol. 18, no. 1–2, pp. 96–104.

Diekstra, R. F. 1993. "Assisted Suicide and Euthanasia: Experience from the Netherlands." *Annals of Medicine,* Vol. 25, no. 1, pp. 5–9.

Dworkin, Gerald. 1998. *Euthanasia and Physician-Assisted Suicide.* Cambridge: Cambridge University Press.

Emanuel, Linda L. 1998. *Regulating How We Die: The Ethical, Medical, and Legal Issues Surrounding Physician-Assisted Suicide.* Cambridge, MA: Harvard University Press.

Engelhardt, H. Tristram, Jr. 1989. "Fashioning an Ethic for Life and Death in a Post-Modern Society." *Hastings Center Report,* Special Supplement (Jan–Feb), pp. 7–9.

Fenigsen, R. 1989. "A Case Against Dutch Euthanasia." *Hastings Center Report,* Vol. 19, no. 1, pp. 522–530.

Grossman, D. 1995. "On Killing: The Psychological Cost of Learning to Kill." Boston: Little, Brown.

Hendin, Herbert. 1997. *Seduced by Death: Doctors, Patients, and the Dutch Cure.* New York: W. W. Norton.

Humphry, Derek, and Ann Wickett. 1986. *The Right to Die: Understanding Euthanasia.* New York: Harper & Row.

Ikuta, Sandra Segal. 1989. "Dying at the Right Time: A Critical Legal Theory Approach to Timing-of-Death Issues." *Issues in Law and Medicine,* Vol. 5, no. 1, pp. 3–66.

Kamisar, Y. 1995. "Against Assisted Suicide, Even in a Very Limited Form." *University of Detroit Mercy Law Review,* Vol. 72, pp. 735–769.

Kevorkian, Jack. 1991. *Prescription: Medicine: The Goodness of Planned Death.* Buffalo, NY: Prometheus Books.

Kuhse, Helga. 1987. *The Sanctity-of-Life Doctrine in Medicine: A Critique.* Oxford: Clarendon Press.

Leone, Daniel A. 1999. *The Ethics of Euthanasia.* San Diego, CA: Greenhaven Press.

Lo, B. 1995. "Improving Health Care Near the End of Life: Why Is It so Hard?" *Journal of the American Medical Association,* Vol. 274, no. 20, pp. 1634–1636.

McGee, Ellen. 1997. "Hospice Narratives of Good Dying." *Bioethics Forum,* Vol. 13, no. 3, pp. 36–42.

Miles, Steven H., and Allison August. 1990. "Courts, Gender and the Right to Die." *Law, Medicine and Health Care,* Vol. 18, no. 1–2, pp. 85–95.

Murray, Tom, and Arthur Caplan, eds. 1985. *Which Babies Shall Live?* Clifton, NJ: Humana.

O'Brien, L.A., et al. 1995. "Nursing Home Residents' Preference of Life-Sustaining Treatments." *Journal of the American Medical Association,* Vol. 274, no. 22, pp. 1775–1779.

Paust, Jordan J. 1995. "The Human Right to Die with Dignity: A Policy-Oriented Essay." *Human Rights Quarterly,* Vol. 17, no. 3, pp. 463–487.

Quill v. Vacco, 80 E3d 716 (2d Circ. 1996).

Quill, Timothy. 1991. "Death and Dignity." *New England Journal of Medicine,* Vol. 324, no. 10, pp. 691–694.

———. 1996. *A Midwife Through the Dying Process.* Baltimore, MD: Johns Hopkins Press.

Rachels, James. 1986. *The End of Life: Euthanasia and Morality.* New York: Oxford University Press.

Rahman, Fazlur. 1989. *Health and Medicine in the Islamic Tradition: Change and Identity.* New York: Crossroad.

re Quinlan, 70 NJ 10, 355 A. 2d 647 (1976).

Royal Dutch Medical Association. 1995. *Euthanasia in the Netherlands,* 4th ed. Utrecht: Royal Dutch Medical Association.

Scherer, Jennifer M. 1999. *Euthanasia and the Right to Die: A Comparative View.* Lanham, MD: Rowman and Littlefield.

Singer, Peter A., and Mark Siegler. 1990. "Euthanasia—A Critique." *New England Journal of Medicine,* Vol. 322, no. 26, pp. 1881–1883.

Smith, George P., II. 1989. "All's Well That Ends Well: Toward a Policy of Assisted Rational Suicide or Merely Enlightened Self-Determination?" *U.C. Davis Law Review,* Vol. 22 (Winter), pp. 275–419.

Thomasma, David C. 1998. *Asking to Die: Inside the Dutch Debate about Euthanasia.* Dordrecht, Netherlands: Kluwer Academic Publishers.

Tolle, S. W. 1996. "Legalizing Assisted Suicide: Views of Physicians in Oregon." *New England Journal of Medicine,* Vol. 334, no. 5, pp. 310–315.

U.S. Catholic Bishops. 1994. "Ethical and Religious Directives for Catholic Health Care Services." *Origins,* Vol. 24 (December 15), p. 458.

Wainey, Deborah A. 1989. "Active Voluntary Euthanasia: The Ultimate Act of Care for the Dying." *Cleveland State Law Review,* Vol. 37, pp. 645–682.

Wennberg, Robert N. 1989. *Terminal Choices: Euthanasia, Suicide, and the Right to Die.* Grand Rapids, MI: Eerdmans.

Chapter 6
Abortion and Reproductive Freedom

Annas, George. 1982. "Forced Cesareans: The Most Unkindest Cut of All." *Hastings Center Report,* Vol. 12, no. 3, pp. 16–17.

Arras, John D. 1990. "AIDS and Reproductive Decisions: Having Children in Fear and Trembling." *Milbank Memorial Fund Quarterly,* Vol. 68, no. 3, pp. 353–382.

Baehr, Nina. 1990. *Abortion Without Apology: A Radical History for the 1990's.* Boston: South End Press.

Bell, Susan. 1984. "Birth Control," in *Our Bodies, Ourselves.* Boston Women's Health Book Collective, ed. New York: Simon & Schuster, pp. 220–262.

Bondeson, William B., H. Tristram Engelhardt, Jr., Stuart Spicker, and Daniel Winship, eds. 1983. *Abortion and the Status of the Fetus.* Boston: Kluwer Academic Publishers.

Callahan, Daniel. 1970. *Abortion: Law, Choice and Morality.* New York: Macmillan.

Callahan, Joan C., and James W. Knight. 1989. *Preventing Birth.* Salt Lake City: University of Utah Press.

Corea, Gena. 1985. *The Hidden Malpractice.* Updated ed. New York: Harper & Row.

Daniels, Cynthia R. 1993. *At Women's Expense: State Power and the Politics of Fetal Rights.* Cambridge, MA: Harvard University Press.

Dixon, Nicholas. 1997. "The Morality of Anti-Abortion Civil Disobedience." *Public Affairs Quarterly,* Vol. 11, no. 1, pp. 21–38.

Djerassi, Carl. 1981. *The Politics of Contraception.* 2nd ed. San Francisco: W.H. Freeman.

Doerr, Edd, and James W. Prescott, eds. 1989. *Abortion Rights and Fetal Personhood.* Long Beach, CA: Centerline Press.

Dworkin, Ronald. 1993. *Life's Dominion: An Argument about Abortion, Euthanasia, and Individual Freedom.* New York: Alfred Knopf.

Eisenstadt v. Baird, 405 U.S. 438, 453 (1972).

Feinman, Clarice, ed. 1992. *The Criminalization of a Woman's Body.* Binghamton, NY: Harrington Park Press.

Fried, Marlene Gerber. 1990. *From Abortion to Reproductive Freedom: Transforming a Worldwide Movement.* Boston: South End Press.

Gallagher, Janet. 1987. "Prenatal Invasions and Interventions: What's Wrong with Fetal Rights." *Harvard Women's Law Journal,* Vol. 10 (Spring), pp. 9–58.

Garfield, Jay L., and Patricia Hennessey, eds. 1984. *Abortion: Moral and Legal Perspectives.* Amherst: University of Massachusetts Press.

Ginsburg, Faye D. 1989. *Contested Lives: The Abortion Debate in an American Community.* Berkeley: University of California Press.

Gordon, Linda. 1990. *Woman's Body, Woman's Right: A Social History of Birth Control in America,* rev. ed. New York: Penguin Books.

Grisez, Germain. 1970. *Abortion: The Myths, the Realities, and the Arguments.* New York: Corpus Books.

Griswold v. Connecticut, 381 U.S. 479 (1965).

Harris v. McCrae, 448 U.S. 297 (1980).

Harrison, Beverly Wildung. 1983. *Our Right to Choose: Toward a New Ethic of Abortion.* Boston: Beacon Press.

Hartmann, Betsy. 1987. *Reproductive Rights and Wrongs: The Global Politics of Population Control and Contraceptive Choice.* New York: Harper & Row.

Holmes, Helen Bequaert. 1992. *Issues in Reproductive Technology I: An Anthology.* New York: Garland Publishing.

Jaggar, Alison. 1997. "Regendering the U.S. Abortion Debate." *Journal of Social Philosophy,* Vol. 28, no. 1, pp. 127–140.

Kolder, Veronika E., Janet Gallaher, and Michael T. Parsons. 1987. "Court-Ordered Obstetrical Interventions." *New England Journal of Medicine,* Vol. 316, no. 19, pp. 1192–1196.

Luker, Kristin. 1984. *Abortion and the Politics of Motherhood.* Berkeley: University of California Press.

McDonnell, Kathleen. 1984. *Not an Easy Choice: A Feminist Re-examines Abortion.* Boston: South End Press.

Mintzes, Barbara, and Anita Hardon. 1992. *A Question of Control: Women's Perspectives on the Development and Use of Contraceptive Technologies.* Amsterdam, Netherlands: Women's Health Action Foundation.

Moskowitz, Ellen H., and Bruce Jennings, eds. 1996. *The Ethics of Long-Term Contraception: Guidelines for Public Policy.* Washington, D.C.: Georgetown University Press.

Murphy, Timothy F. 1995. "Abortion and the Ethics of Genetic Sexual Orientation Research." *Cambridge Quarterly of Healthcare Ethics,* Vol. 4, no. 3, pp. 340–350.

Newman, L. F., ed. 1985. *Women's Medicine: A Cross-Cultural Study of Indigenous Fertility Regulation.* New Brunswick, NJ: Rutgers University Press.

Petchesky, Rosalind Pollack. 1985. *Abortion and Woman's Choice: The State, Sexuality, and Reproductive Freedom.* Boston: Northeastern University Press.

Planned Parenthood v. Danforth, 428 U.S. 52 (1976).

Rhoden, Nancy K. 1986. "The Judge in the Delivery Room: The Emergence of Court-Ordered Cesareans." *California Law Review,* Vol. 74, no. 6, pp. 1951–2030.

Schott, Lee A. 1988. "The Pamela Rae Stewart Case and Fetal Harm: Prosecution or Prevention?" *Harvard Women's Law Journal,* Vol. 11 (Spring), pp. 227–245.

Seaman, Barbara, and Gideon Seaman. 1978. *Women and the Crisis in Sex Hormones.* New York: Bantam Books.

Shannon, Thomas. 1997. "Fetal Status: Sources and Implications." *Journal of Medicine and Philosophy,* Vol. 22, no. 5, pp. 415–422.

Shaw, Margery. 1984. "Conditional Prospective Rights of the Fetus." *The Journal of Legal Medicine,* Vol. 5, no. 1, pp. 63–116.

Smith, Katharine V., and Jan Russell. 1997. "Ethical Issues Experienced by HIV-Infected African-American Women." *Nursing Ethics,* Vol. 4, no. 5, pp. 394–402.

State of New York v. Schweiker, 557 F. Supp. 354 (S.D.N.Y. 1983).

Steinbock, Bonnie. 1992. *Life Before Birth: The Moral and Legal Status of Embryos.* New York: Oxford University Press.

Sumner, L. W. 1983. *Abortion and Moral Theory.* Princeton, NJ: Princeton University Press.

Tong, Rosemarie. 1997. *Feminist Approaches to Bioethics.* Boulder, CO: Westview Press.

Tooley, Michael. 1983. *Abortion and Infanticide.* Oxford: Oxford University Press.

Tribe, Laurence H. 1990. *Abortion: The Clash of Absolutes.* New York: W. W. Norton.

Wardle, Lynn D. 1980. *The Abortion Privacy Doctrine: A Compendium and Critique of Federal Court Abortion Cases.* Buffalo, NY: William S. Hein.

Wolf, Susan M., ed. 1996. *Feminism & Bioethics.* New York: Oxford University Press.

Yanoshik, Kim, and Judy Norsigian. 1989. "Contraception, Control, and Choice: International Perspectives," in K. S. Ratcliff, ed., *Healing Technology: Feminist Perspectives*. Ann Arbor, MI: University of Michigan Press.

Chapter 7
Reproductive Technology and Surrogacy

Alpern, Kenneth D., ed. 1992. *The Ethics of Reproductive Technology*. New York: Oxford University Press.

Andrews, Lori. 1989. *Between Strangers: Surrogate Mothers, Expectant Fathers & Brave New Babies*. New York: Harper & Row.

Arditti, Rita, Renate Duelli Klein, and Shelley Minden, eds. 1984. *Test-Tube Women*. London: Pandora.

Assisted Reproductive Technologies: Analysis and Recommendations for Public Policy. 1998. New York: The Task Force.

Bartels, Dianne M., Reinhard Priester, Dorothy E. Vawter, and Arthur L. Caplan, eds. 1990. *Beyond Baby M: Ethical Issues in New Reproductive Technologies*. Clifton, NJ: Humana Press.

Baruch, Elaine Hoffman, Amadeo F. D'Adamo, Jr., and Joni Seager, eds. 1988. *Embryos, Ethics, and Women's Rights*. Binghamton, NY: Harrington Park Press.

Bayles, Michael D. 1984. *Reproductive Ethics*. Englewood Cliffs, NJ: Prentice Hall.

Berkowitz, Jonathan M., and Jack W. Snyder. 1998. "Racism and Sexism in Medically Assisted Conception." *Bioethics*, Vol. 12, no. 1, pp. 25–44.

Callahan, Joan C., ed. 1995. *Reproduction, Ethics, and the Law*. Bloomington: Indiana University Press.

Chadwick, Ruth, ed. 1987. *Ethics, Reproduction, and Genetic Control*. New York: Croom Helm.

Chesler, Phyllis. 1988. *Sacred Bond: The Legacy of Baby M*. New York: Times Books.

Cohen, Cynthia, ed. *New Ways of Making Babies: The Case of Egg Donation*. Bloomington: Indiana University Press.

Cohen, Sherill, and Nadine Taub, eds. 1989. *Reproductive Laws for the 1990s*. Clifton, NJ: Humana Press.

Corea, Gena. 1985. *The Mother Machine*. New York: Harper & Row.

Dickens, Bernard. 1997. "Interfaces of Assisted Reproduction Ethics and Law," in F. Shenfield and C. Sureau, eds., *Ethical Dilemmas in Assisted Reproduction*. New York: Pantheon.

Fiandaca, Sherylynn. 1998. "In Vitro Fertilization and Embryos: The Need for International Guidelines." *Albany Law Journal of Science & Technology*, Vol. 8, p. 337.

Field, Martha. A. 1990. *Surrogate Motherhood*. Expanded Edition. Cambridge, MA: Harvard University Press.

Freedman, Warren. 1991. *Legal Issues in Biotechnology and Human Reproduction: Artificial Conception and Modern Genetics*. Westport, CT.: Quorum Books.

Gostin, Larry, ed. 1988. *Surrogate Motherhood*. Bloomington, IN: Indiana University Press.

Holmes, Helen B. 1988. "In Vitro Fertilization: Reflections on the State of the Art." *Birth*, Vol. 15, no. 3, pp. 134–145.

———, ed. 1992. *Issues in Reproductive Technology I: An Anthology*. New York: Garland Publishing.

Holmes, Helen B., Betty B. Hoskins, and Michael Gross, eds. 1980. *Birth Control and Controlling Birth*. Clifton, NJ: Humana Press.

———. 1981. *The Custom-Made Child?* Clifton, NJ: Humana Press.

Holmes, Helen B., and Laura M. Purdy, eds. 1992. *Feminist Perspectives in Medical Ethics*. Bloomington, IN: Indiana University Press.

Hull, Richard, ed. 1990. *Ethical Issues in the New Reproductive Technologies*. Belmont, CA: Wadsworth.

King, Leslie, and Madonna Harrington-Meyer. 1997. "The Politics of Reproductive Benefits: U.S. Insurance Coverage of Contraceptive and Infertility Treatments." *Gender and Society*, Vol. 11, no. 1, pp. 8–30.

Lauritzen, Paul. 1993. *Pursuing Parenthood: Ethical Issues in Assisted Reproduction*. Bloomington, IN: Indiana University Press.

Leach, Gerald. 1972. *The Biocrats*. Middlesex, England: Penguin.

Lorber, Judith. 1992. "Choice, Gift, or Patriarchal Bargain? Women's Consent to in Vitro Fertilization," in *Feminist Perspectives in Medical Ethics*, Helen B. Holmes and Laura M. Purdy, eds. Bloomington, IN: Indiana University Press.

Lublin, Nancy. 1998. *Pandora's Box: Feminism Confronts Reproductive Technology*. Lanham, MD: Rowman and Littlefield.

Mahowald, Mary. 1993. *Women and Children in Health Care*. New York: Oxford University Press.

Meyer, Cheryl L. 1997. *The Wandering Uterus: Politics and the Reproductive Rights of Women*. New York: New York University Press.

Nelson, James Lindemann. 1998. "The Meaning of the Act: Reflections on the Expressive Force of Reproductive Decision Making and Policies." *Kennedy Institute of Ethics Journal*, Vol. 8, no. 2, pp. 165–182.

Overall, Christine. 1987. *Ethics and Human Reproduction*. Boston: Allen & Unwin.

———. 1993. *Human Reproduction: Principles, Practices, Policies.* Toronto: Oxford University Press.

Packard, Vance. 1977. *The People Shapers.* Boston: Little, Brown.

Peterson, Kerry, ed. 1997. *Intersections: Women on Law, Medicine and Technology.* Brookfield, VT: Ashgate.

Pollitt, Katha. 1990. "When Is a Mother Not a Mother?" *The Nation* (December 31), pp. 840–846.

Purdy, Laura M. 1996. *Reproducing Persons.* Ithaca, NY: Cornell University Press.

Roberts, Dorothy. 1997. *Killing the Black Body: Race, Reproduction, and the Meaning of Liberty.* New York: Pantheon.

Robertson, John. 1994. *Children of Choice.* Princeton, NJ: Princeton University Press.

Rothman, Barbara Katz. 1989. *Recreating Motherhood.* New York: W. W. Norton.

Sandelowski, Margarete. 1991. "Compelled to Try: The Never-Enough Quality of Conceptive Technology." *Medical Anthropology Quarterly,* New Series, Vol. 5, no. 1, pp. 29–47.

Shannon, Thomas A. 1988. *Surrogate Motherhood: The Ethics of Using Human Beings.* New York: Crossroads.

Sherwin, Susan. 1992. *No Longer Patient.* Philadelphia: Temple University Press.

Shildrick, Margrit. 1997. *Leaky Bodies and Boundaries: Feminism, Postmodernism and (Bio)Ethics.* New York: Routledge.

Singer, Peter, and Deane Wells. 1985. *Making Babies.* New York: Scribners.

Singer, Peter, and Helga Kuhse. 1998. "Choosing the Sex, Race, and Sexual Orientation of Our Children." *Bioethics,* Vol. 12, no. 1, pp. iii–v.

Silver, Lee. 1997. *Remaking Eden: Cloning and Beyond in a Brave New World.* New York: Avon Books.

Spallone, Patricia. 1989. *Beyond Conception.* Granby, MA: Bergin & Garvey.

———, and Deborah Lynn Steinberg, eds. 1987. *Made to Order: The Myth of Reproduction and Genetic Progress.* Oxford: Pergamon.

Stanworth, Michelle, ed. 1987. *Reproductive Technologies.* Minneapolis: University of Minnesota Press.

Walters, LeRoy. 1991. "Ethical Issues in Human Gene Therapy." *Journal of Clinical Ethics,* Vol. 2 (Winter), pp. 267–274.

Warnock, Mary. 1984. *Report of the Committee of Inquiry into Human Fertilisation and Embryology.* London: Her Majesty's Stationery Office.

Warren, Mary Anne. 1988. "IVF and Women's Interests: An Analysis of Feminist Concerns." *Bioethics,* Vol. 2 (January), pp. 37–57.

Chapter 8
Genetics

Agius, Emmanuel, and Salvino Busuttil, eds. *1998. Germ-Line Intervention and Our Responsibilities Toward Future Generations.* Boston: Kluwer Academic Publishers.

Anderson, W. French. 1989. "Human Gene Therapy: Why Draw a Line?" *Journal of Medicine and Philosophy,* Vol. 14, no. 6, pp. 681–693.

Andrews, Lori B. 1998. "Mom, Dad, Clone: Implications for Reproductive Privacy." *Cambridge Quarterly of Healthcare Ethics,* Vol. 7, no. 2, pp. 176–186.

Annas, George, and Sherman Elias. 1992. *Gene Mapping: Using Law and Ethics as Guides.* New York: Oxford University Press.

Annas, George J. 1998. "Commentaries: Human Cloning: A Choice or an Echo?" *University Of Dayton Law Review,* Vol. 23, no. 2, pp. 247–275.

Asch, Adrienne. 1988. "Reproductive Technology and Disability," in *Reproductive Laws for the 1990s,* Sherrill Cohen and Nadine Taub, eds. Clifton, NJ: Humana Press.

———. 1989. "Can Aborting 'Imperfect' Children Be Immoral?" in *Ethical Issues in Modern Medicine,* John Arras and Nancy Rhoden, eds. Mountain View, CA: Mayfield Publishing.

Babu, M. N. 1998. "Human Cloning: An Ethically Negative Feat in Genetic Engineering." *Philosophy and Social Action,* Vol. 24, no. 2, pp. 46–55.

Bosk, Charles L. 1992. *All God's Mistakes: Genetic Counseling in a Pediatric Hospital.* Chicago: University of Chicago Press.

Broyde, Michael. 1998. "Cloning People: A Jewish Law Analysis of the Issues." *Connecticut Law Review,* Vol. 30 (Winter), pp. 503–535.

Cahill, Lisa Sowle, Albert Moraczewski, and Gilbert Meilaender. 1998. "Religion-Based Perspectives on Cloning of Humans." *Ethics and Medicine,* Vol. 14, no. 1, pp. 8–25.

Callahan, Daniel. 1998. " Cloning: Then and Now." *Cambridge Quarterly of Healthcare Ethics,* Vol. 7, no. 2, pp. 141–144.

Callahan, Sidney. 1979. "An Ethical Analysis of Responsible Parenthood," in *Genetic Counseling: Facts, Values, and Norms,* Alexander M. Capron, Marc Lappe, and Robert F. Murray, eds. New York: Alan R. Liss.

Capron, Alexander Morgan. 1997. "Inside the Beltway Again: A Sheep of a Different Feather." *Kennedy Institute of Ethics Journal,* Vol. 7, no. 1, pp. 171–179.

Carmen, Ira H. 1985. *Cloning and the Constitution: An Inquiry into Governmental Policymaking and Genetic*

Experimentation. Madison, WI: University of Wisconsin Press.

Chadwick, Ruth. 1982. "Cloning." *Philosophy,* Vol. 57 (April), pp. 201–210.

———, ed. 1987. *Ethics, Reproduction and Genetic Control.* London: Croom Helm.

Cohen, Cynthia. 1996. "'Give Me Children or I Shall Die!' New Reproductive Technologies and Harm to Children." *Hastings Center Report,* Vol. 26, no. 2, pp. 19–27.

Council for Responsible Genetics, Human Genetics Committee. 1993. "Position Paper on Human Germ Line Manipulation." *Human Gene Therapy,* Vol. 4, no. 1, pp. 35–37.

Council on Ethical and Judicial Affairs, American Medical Association. 1991. "Use of Genetic Testing by Employers." *Journal of the American Medical Association,* Vol. 266 (Oct. 2), pp. 1827–1830.

Feinberg, Joel. 1986. "Wrongful Life and the Counterfactual Element in Harming." *Social Philosophy and Policy,* Vol. 4, pp. 145–178.

Fitzgerald, Kevin T. 1998. "Human Cloning: Analysis and Evaluation." *Cambridge Quarterly of Healthcare Ethics,* Vol. 7, no. 2, pp. 218–222.

Glannon, Walter. 1998. "The Ethics of Human Cloning." *Public Affairs Quarterly,* Vol. 12, no. 3, pp. 287–305.

Glover, Jonathan. 1984. *What Sort of People Should There Be?* Harmondsworth, England: Penguin.

Harris, John. 1998. "Cloning and Human Dignity." *Cambridge Quarterly of Healthcare Ethics,* Vol. 7, no. 2, pp. 163–167.

Hauerwas, Stanley. 1986. "Suffering the Retarded: Should We Prevent Retardation?" in *Suffering Presence: Theological Reflections on Medicine, the Mentally Handicapped, and the Church,* Stanley Hauerwas, ed. Notre Dame, IN: University of Notre Dame Press.

Heyd, David. 1992. *Genethics.* Berkeley: University of California Press.

Holm, Soren. 1998. "A Life in the Shadow: One Reason Why We Should Not Clone Humans." *Cambridge Quarterly of Healthcare Ethics,* Vol. 7, no. 2, pp. 160–162.

Howard, Ted, and Jeremy Rifkin. 1977. *Who Should Play God? The Artificial Creation of Life and What It Means for the Future of the Human Race.* New York: Dell Publishing Co.

Humber, James M. 1998. *Human Cloning.* Totowa, NJ: Humana Press.

Hyde, Margaret O., and Lawrence E. Hyde. 1984. *Cloning and the New Genetics.* Hillside, NJ: Enslow Publishers.

Kass, Leon. 1985. *Toward a More Natural Science: Biology and Human Affairs.* New York: Free Press.

Katz, Katheryn D. 1997. "The Clonal Child: Procreative Liberty and Asexual Reproduction." *Albany Law Journal of Science & Technology,* Vol. 8.

Kerr, Susan M. 1997. "Mammalian Cloning: Implications for Science and Society." *Science and Engineering Ethics,* Vol. 3, no. 4, pp. 491–498.

Macklin, Ruth. 1995. "Cloning without Prior Approval: A Response to Recent Disclosures of Noncompliance." *Kennedy Institute of Ethics Journal,* Vol. 5, no. 1, pp. 57–60.

Maha, F. Munayyer. 1997. "Genetic Testing and Germ-Line Manipulation: Constructing a New Language for International Human Rights." *American University Journal of International Law & Policy,* Vol. 12, p. 687.

Millen, David R. 1978. "God, Galileo, and Government: Toward Constitutional Protection for Scientific Inquiry." *Washington Law Review,* Vol. 53, pp. 349–404.

Mitchell, C. Ben. 1998. "A Protestant Perspective on Cloning." *Ethics and Medicine,* Vol. 14, no. 1, pp. 26–30.

Moen, Elizabeth. 1991. "Sex Selective Abortion: Prospects in China and India." *Issues in Reproductive Genetic Engineering,* Vol. 4, no. 3, pp. 231–249.

National Bioethics Advisory Commission. 1997. *Cloning Human Beings: Report and Recommendations of the National Bioethics Advisory Commission.* Rockville, MD: National Bioethics Advisory Commission.

Nelkin, Dorothy, and Susan Lindee. 1998. "Cloning in the Popular Imagination." *Cambridge Quarterly of Healthcare Ethics,* Vol. 7, no. 2, pp. 145–149.

Nussbaum, Martha, and Cass Sunstein, eds. 1998. *Clones and Clones.* New York: Oxford University Press.

O'Neill, Onora, and William Ruddick, eds. 1979. *Having Children.* New York: Oxford University Press.

Parfit, Derek. 1984. *Reasons and Persons.* Oxford, England: Clarendon Press.

Pence, Gregory. 1998. *Flesh of My Flesh: The Ethics of Cloning Humans: A Reader.* Lanham, MD: Rowman and Littlefield.

Purdy, Laura M. 1996. *Reproducing Persons.* Ithaca, NY: Cornell University Press.

Roberts, Melinda A. 1996. "Human Cloning: A Case of No Harm Done?" *Journal of Medicine and Philosophy,* Vol. 21, no. 5, pp. 537–554.

Rorvik, David M. 1978. *In His Image: The Cloning of a Man.* Philadelphia, PA: Lippincott.

Schroten, Egbert. 1998. "Ethical Aspects of Genetic Modification of Animals: Opinion of the Group of Advisers on the Ethical Implications of Biotechnology of the European Commission." *Cambridge Quarterly of Healthcare Ethics,* Vol. 7, no. 2, pp. 194–198.

Silva-Ruiz, Pedro F. 1998. "The Protection of Persons in Medical Research and Cloning of Human Beings." *American Journal of Comparative Law,* Vol. 46, p. 151.

Steinbock, Bonnie, and Ron McClamrock. 1994. "When Is Birth Unfair to the Child?" *Hastings Center Report,* Vol. 24, no. 6, pp. 16–22.

Stepanuk, Natalie Anne. 1998. "Genetic Information and Third Party Access to Information: New Jersey's Pioneering Legislation as a Model for Federal Privacy Protection of Genetic Information." *Catholic University Law Review,* Vol. 47, no. 3, pp. 1105–1144.

Stock, Gregory, and John H. Campbell. 1999. *Engineering the Human Germline: An Exploration of the Science and Ethics of Altering the Genes We Pass to Our Children.* New York: Oxford University Press.

Strong, Carson. 1998. "Cloning and Infertility." *Cambridge Quarterly of Healthcare Ethics,* Vol. 7, no. 3, pp. 279–293.

The White House, Office of Communications, Directive on Cloning, 4 March 1997. Westlaw 91957 (White House).

Warren, Mary Anne. 1985. *Gendercide.* Totowa, NJ: Rowman and Allanheld.

Wilson, James Q. 1998. *The Ethics of Human Cloning.* Washington, D.C.: AEI Press.

Wu, Lawrence. 1998. "Family Planning Through Human Cloning: Is There a Fundamental Right?" *Columbia Law Review,* Vol. 98, no. 6, pp. 1461–1515.